FUNCTION AND STRUCTURE OF THE IMMUNE SYSTEM

ADVANCES IN EXPERIMENTAL MEDICINE AND BIOLOGY

Recent Volumes in this Series

FUNCTION AND STRUCTURE OF THE IMMUNE SYSTEM

Edited by

Wolfgang Müller-Ruchholtz
and
Hans Konrad Müller-Hermelink

University of Kiel
Kiel, Germany

PLENUM PRESS • NEW YORK AND LONDON

Library of Congress Cataloging in Publication Data

International Conference on Lymphatic Tissue and Germinal Centers in Immune
Reactions, 6th, Damp/Kiel, 1978.
Function and structure of the immune system.
(Advances in experimental medicine and biology; v. 114)
"Proceedings."
Includes index.
1. Immunology – Congresses. 2. Immunocompetent cells – Congresses. 3. Can-
cer – Immunological aspects – Congresses. I. Müller-Ruchholtz, Wolfgang.
II. Müller-Hermelink, Hans Konrad. III. Title. IV. Series. [DNLM: 1. Immunity,
Cellular – Congresses. 2. Lymphocytes – Immunology – Congresses. W1 AD559
v. 114 / QW568 I59 1978f]
QR180.3.I53 1978   616.07′9   79-4272

Proceedings of the Sixth International Conference on Lymphatic Tissues and
Germinal Centers in Immune Reactions held in Damp/Kiel, Germany, June
11-16, 1978

© 1979 Plenum Press, New York
Softcover reprint of the hardcover 1st edition 1979
A Division of Plenum Publishing Corporation
227 West 17th Street, New York, N.Y. 10011

ISBN 978-1-4615-9103-0   e-ISBN 978-1-4615-9101-6 (eBook)
DOI 10.1007/ 978-1-4615-9101-6

Preface

This volume represents the Proceedings of the VI. International Conference on Lymphatic Tissues and Germinal Centers in Immune Reactions. The Meeting took place in Damp, a small resort with great facilities on the shores of the Baltic Sea near Kiel on June 11 - 16, 1978. Both, the Genius loci and the God of Weathers were charming enough to stimulate the many participants from all continents and also to facilitate the establishment and/or maintenance of close contacts outside the sessions.

The organizers of this Conference have tried to remind the scientific community of the necessity to (re-) consider sufficiently the role of morphological studies for a thorough understanding of immune reactions. Furthermore, they have been anxious to emphasize a closer connection between analytical work and biological relevance of the phenomena observed. Thus, three main trends were formulated: (1) connections and correlations between function and structure, (2) in-vivo relevance of in-vitro models and (3) clinical relevance of experimental models.

The programme, induced by these outlines and reflected by the contents of this volume, covers a remarkably broad field of interests and activities. It is set in order under nine session chapters. Each of them may allow the reader to answer for himself the question how far the above trends have been recognized, especially when considering the variety of new methodological approaches reported.

Although the usefulness of publishing proceedings such as these has sometimes been challenged, it is believed that the present volume provides a variety of stimuli for future experimental and clinical work on the function and structure of the immune system. Considering that scientific progress depends on both the generation of falsifiable hypotheses and the dissemination and experimental analysis of these, it is hoped that these proceedings will make a worthwhile contribution to these objectives.

W. Müller-Ruchholtz

H.K. Müller-Hermelink

Contents

SESSION A 2

IMMUNOLOGICAL FUNCTION OF CELL SURFACE STRUCTURES

Chairpersons: J.J. Marchalonis and R.M.E. Parkhouse

SESSION A 3

IMMUNOLOGICAL TOLERANCE (SUPPRESSION/DELETION)

Chairpersons: J.R. Batchelor and W. Müller-Ruchholtz

SESSION A 4

IN VIVO RELEVANCE OF NON-LYMPHOID CELLS IN THE IMMUNE REACTION

Chairpersons: H. Dvorak and H. Fischer

SESSION A 5

SOLUBLE MEDIATORS OF IMMUNITY

Chairpersons: J. David and A. de Weck

SESSION B 1

FUNCTIONAL AND MORPHOLOGICAL ASPECTS OF MALIGNANT LYMPHOMAS

Chairpersons: M. Seligmann and K. Lennert

SESSION B 2

IMMUNOPATHOLOGY OF PARASITIC DISEASES

Chairpersons: A.C. Allison and V. Houba

SESSION C

IMMUNOLOGICAL REACTIONS AND IMMUNOTHERAPY OF MALIGNANT DISEASES

Chairpersons: Eva Klein and M.D. Hanna, Jr.

SESSION D

IMMUNOPROPHYLAXIS AND THERAPY OF INFECTIOUS DISEASES

Chairperson: G.J.V. Nossal

CLOSING SESSION

CONCLUSIONS AND OUTLOOK

INTRODUCTORY REMARKS

Karl Lennert

Speaker of Special Research Area 111, University of Kiel;
Institute of Pathology, University of Kiel, Kiel,
W. Germany

The germinal center conference is being held this year near the
place where the germinal centers were originally detected and the
term "germinal center" was born. The person responsible for this
was Walther Flemming, Professor of Anatomy at the University of Kiel,
and the time was nearly a hundred years ago (1884 and 1885).

The germinal center conferences have been of a special nature
from the very beginning - they are not just meetings at which immunologists present highly sophisticated experimental data. These
conferences provide an opportunity for morphologists to sit at the
same table with immunologists. Morphology and function - two aspects
of one phenomenon - are the pillars of this construction, which offers
us a vital chance, viz.: that of applying or translating experimental
data to human pathology. Together, they help to check the danger of
immunology becoming an esoteric branch of science that is not related
enough to man.

At first glance, morphology appears to provide only a rough
framework for the functional data we obtain from good experiments.
It actually offers much more than that, however, if we take advantage
of all technical possibilities. This does not mean using thick,
hematoxylin-eosin-stained sections of material that has been poorly
embedded in paraffin. It means applying the best methods available,
not only in experiments, but also in the morphological investigation
of the corresponding cells and tissues. We need proper embedding,
in certain instances even in plastic, special stainings of sections
and imprints, and histochemical and cytochemical analyses. In
addition, we need electron microscopical investigations, but not
without previous careful histological examination. A combination of

histological stainings with new methods, such as the immunoperoxidase technique, may be of great help in correlating histological findings with functional data.

If we pursue morphologiy as I have just indicated, in other words, by paying as much attention to the methods as one does to in vitro techniques, it will not only be easier to find correlates of experimental data, but it will also be possible to contribute some suggestions and corrections to experimental research. There would then be a give-and-take between the two sides.

At present, morphology is widely underestimated. This has many reasons. One of the main reasons is that researchers who are highly competent in the experimental/functional field are not always as proficient in morphology. According to Egon Brunswik, there are two scientific talents: a rational and a ratiomorphic one. Experimental work is chiefly based on a rational approach - curves have to be analyzed, numbers and percentages have to be interpreted. The ratio-morphic approach, on the other hand, means interpreting given pictures. This requires good eyes and the corresponding aptitude. Not very many people are born with these prerequisites.

Many people believe that everyone's eyes are the same. That is not true, however, which may be readily understood if we think of our ears. Everyone knows that there are differences in the ability to distinguish between different tones. Some people are not musical at all; many can sing quite well; others can play the violin in a string quartet; and only a very few have absolute pitch. The same is true of our eyes - there are many different degrees of seeing ability.

Conferences like this one are of particular importance, because some of us have been born with good eyes and some of us can present the convincing curves and numbers obtained from functional studies. So, if each of us makes his or her own special contribution, the result will be more than just the sum of the facts - there will be a multiplicative effect and our understanding will be deepened.

Organizers of such a conference have several obligations, but also a number of privileges and opportunities. A special privilege is to give a talk that is not under the control of the program committee and in which one can throw out some personal ideas or ask stupid questions. In German, one would say that I have been given "Narrenfreiheit" - I am free to play the fool. I am going to take bold advantage of this opportunity and present some findings in human lymph node reactions that I do not understand and that have not, to my knowledge, been observed or studied enough in animals. I would like to ask you experimenters to think about the interpretation of these findings.

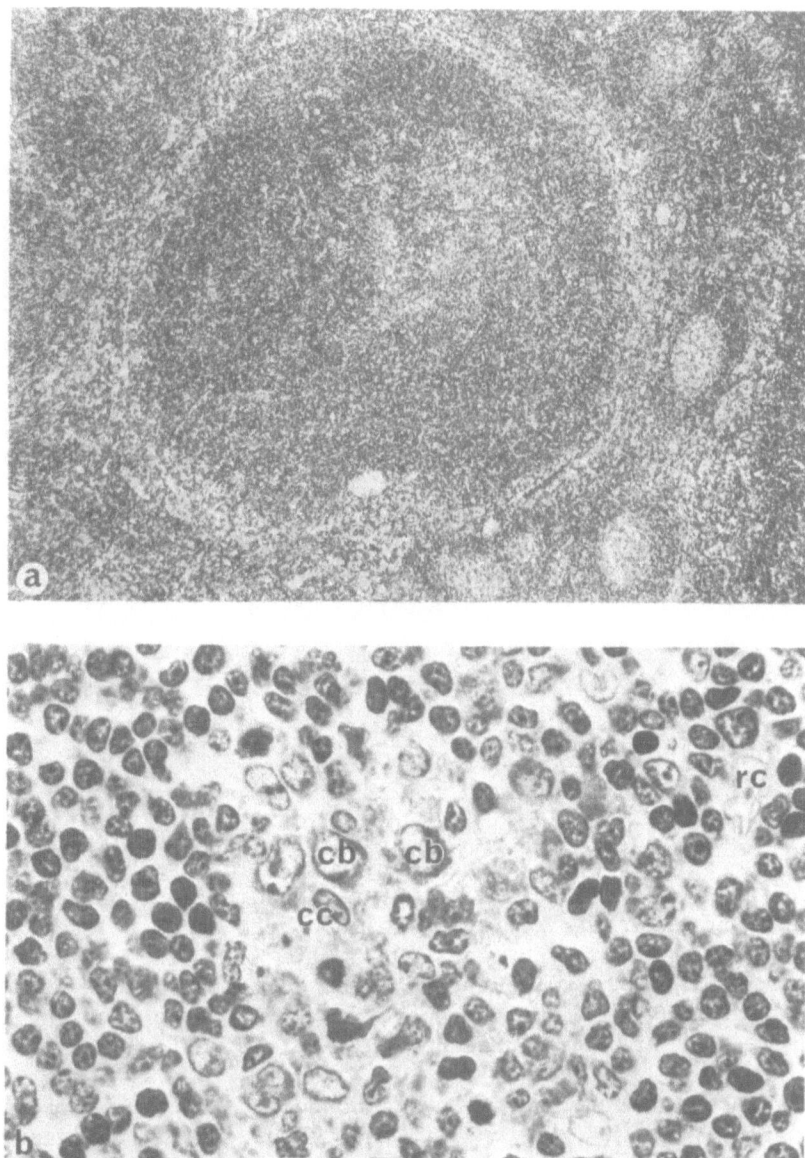

FIG. 1: (a) Large progressively transformed germinal center in the
middle. Small typical germinal centers at lower right. Gomori,
X 35. (b) Detail of a progressively transformed germinal center
with Giemsa staining. Some centroblasts (cb) and centrocytes (cc).
One dendritic reticulum cell (rc). X 880.

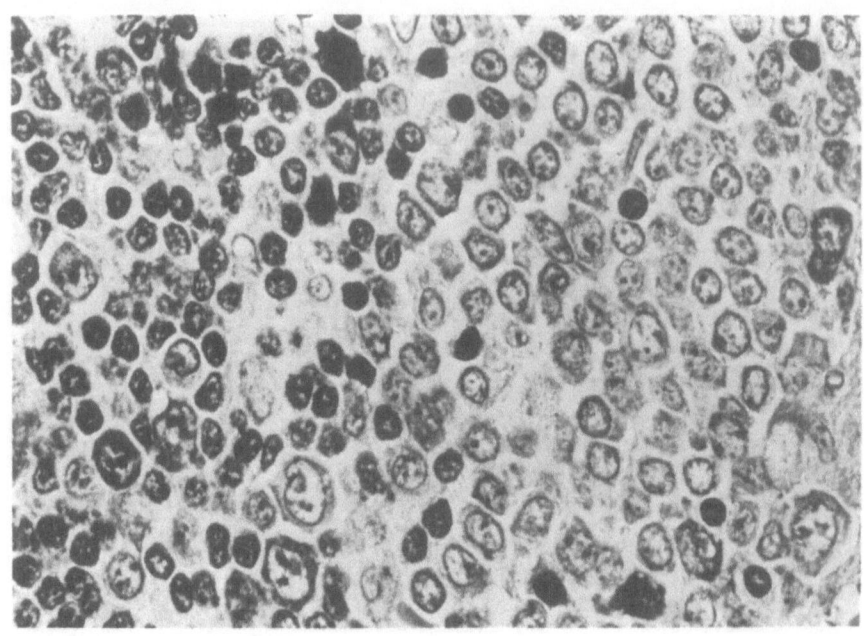

FIG. 2: Nest of "T-associated plasma cells" on the right. On the
left, numerous lymphocytes and some immunoblasts. Giemsa, X 880.

     The first phenomenom is a lymph node structure that we call
"progressively transformed germinal center" (Fig.1). This is a large
nodule-like structure, which consists chiefly of lymphocytes, but
also contains some remnants of germinal centers (centroblasts, centrocytes) and dendritic reticulum cells. Such nodules are found in
a number of cases of lymph node hyperplasia (6). The question I
would like to ask you is: Have you ever encountered such nodules in
animal experiments? Might they have something to do with the observations made by William Ehrich during the last year of his life?

     The second phenomenon is the focal accumulation of lymphoid cells
found exclusively in T-regions, in the thymus, and in malignant
lymphomas derived from the T-cell series (2,3). The cells are somewhat larger than lymphocytes and have a more abundant, moderately
basophilic (pyroninophilic) cytoplasm (Fig.2). On electron microscopy,
they reveal a moderate amount of rough endoplasmic reticulum. We
therefore proposed the term "T-associated plasma cell" (4,7),intending
it as more of a provocation than a final name. Apparently, however,
these cells do not secrete immunoglobulin; at least we have not been
able to demonstrate immunoglobulin in such cells in sections by means
of the immunoperoxidase technique. - Have you ever seen such cells in
animal experiments? Do you have any idea what they might secrete?
Might they be T-helper cells?

The third phenomenon is observed in the sinuses of human lymph nodes - dense collections of cells (Fig.3) that are clearly distinguishable from sinus histiocytes. The cells have smaller nuclei than sinus histiocytes and sparse cytoplasm that stains gray-blue with Giemsa. Their cytoplasm does not contain nonspecific esterase or acid phosphatase activity. At first, we called these cells "immature sinus histiocytes" (2); but electron microscopical investigations with Mori (5) later showed that they are not histiocytes but rather a special variety of lymphocytes. - How should we interpret these cells? They are probably special functional forms of lymphocytes. Do they belong to the B-cell or the T-cell series? What is their function in the sinuses? Do you know of corresponding cells in animals from your experiments?

The fourth phenomenon is the epithelioid cell reaction. At this point, I should first give a definition, because many morphologists do not use the term "epithelioid cell" and just call these cells "histiocytes" or "macrophages". We think those names are not precise enough. In our opinion, the epithelioid cell "was" a histiocyte or macrophage that no longer has a full capacity to phagocytose, but is instead highly capable of secreting. This functional difference between epithelioid cells and histiocytes or macrophages corresponds to differences in their light microscopical, cytochemical, and ultrastructural features. The cytoplasm of epithelioid cells is oxyphilic and often contains a large PAS-positive Golgi body. In contrast to the strongly nonspecific esterase- and acid phosphatase-positive macrophages, epithelioid cells are only weakly positive. On electron microscopy, one does not find phagolysosomes; but there are many vesicles containing substances of variable electron density. In addition, there are strands of rough endoplasmic reticulum and one large, or even multiple Golgi bodies, which is a characteristic marker of secretory activity. The surface of epithelioid cells displays long thin processes.

Just as we do not call plasma cells "lymphocytes", although they are in fact transformed lymphocytes, we should no longer call the cells I have just described "macrophages". If we keep this definition of epithelioid cells in mind and look for them in pathological conditions in man, we shall find that there are many diseases and reactions in which epithelioid cells are of essential importance.

In humans one has to distinguish two varieties of epithelioid cell reactions (2). The first is a focal variant - the cells occur in small clusters. Toxoplasmosis is the most common disease of this type. The second is a granulomatous variant that is typical of tuberculosis and sarcoidosis.

In order to understand the epithelioid cell reaction in tuberculosis it may be helpful to study special conditions in which epithelioid cell formation is insufficient or even lacking. Examples of

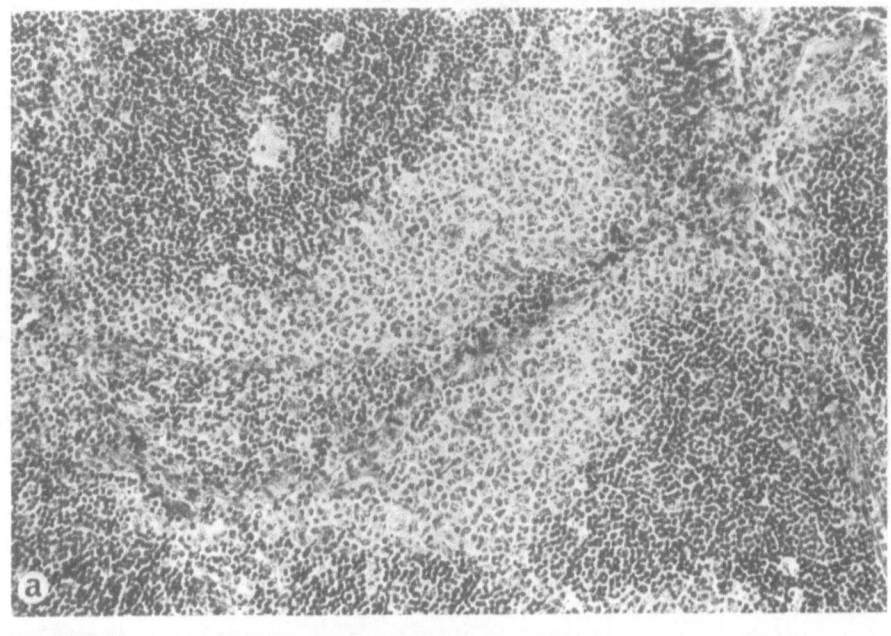

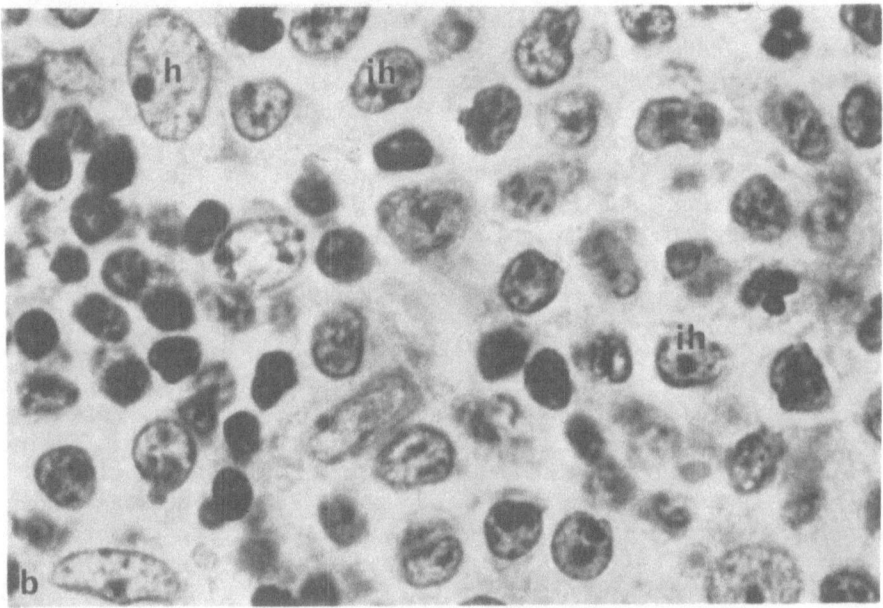

FIG. 3a and b: "Immature sinus histiocytosis". (a) Two light
areas representing "immature histiocytosis" of intermediary sinuses.
Giemsa, X 140. (b) High magnification. "Immature histiocytes"
(ih). Large true histiocytic cell (h). Azure-eosin, X 1250.

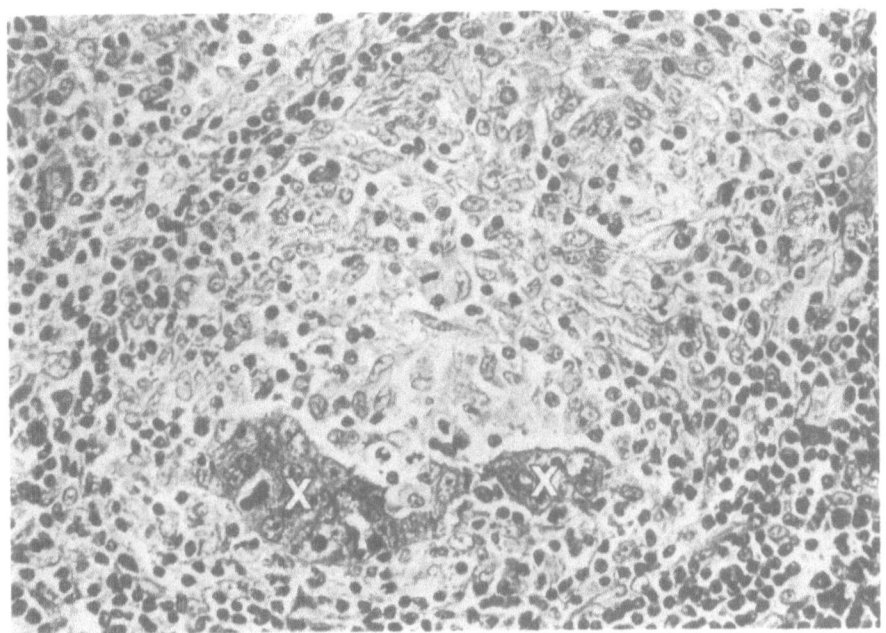

FIG. 4: Epithelioid cell granuloma containing a group of tumor cells (x). Lymph node metastasis of lymphoepithelial carcinoma ("nasopharyngeal carcinoma"). Giemsa, X 350.

such conditions are sepsis tuberculosa acutissima Landouzy and BCG histiocytosis. In BCG histiocytosis, immense numbers of macrophages with a myriad of mycobacteria are found instead of epithelioid cells. The macrophages contain large amounts of nonspecific esterase and acid phosphatase. The reason for the absence of epithelioid cell formation is not clear; there is probably a defect in the number or function of T-lymphocytes.

The questions that arise here are: What is the function of T-lymphocytes in epithelioid cell reactions? Why do we find either focal or granulomatous, small or large accumulations of epithelioid cells?

Epithelioid cell reactions are of particular interest in malignant tumors. In one type of tumor they occur almost as a rule and may therefore even be considered to be a diagnostic criterion. I am speaking of seminoma, which nearly always shows a granulomatous epithelioid cell reaction in the stroma of the tumor.

Another tumor, namely, lymphoepithelial carcinoma (Schmincke's tumor), shows an especially frequent occurrence of tuberculoid lesions

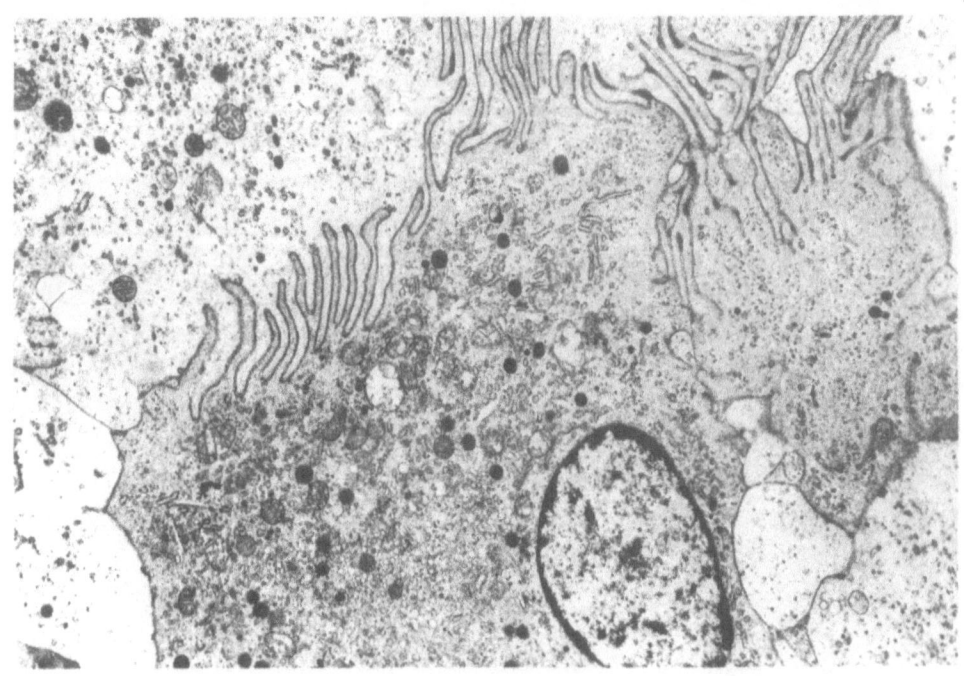

FIG. 5:   Epithelioid cell in lymph node of BCG-treated guinea pig
with malignant hepatoma two weeks after BCG treatment.   Specimen
kindly provided by Dr. M.G. Hanna, Jr., Frederick, Maryland, U.S.A.
Photographed by Dr. E. Kaiserling, Kiel.   X 11,400.

in regional lymph nodes, sometimes even with caseation necrosis. The
epithelioid cell granulomas (Fig.4) in this tumor often contain
residual living tumor cells, some even in mitosis, which are probably
destroyed by the epithelioid cell reaction.

The very interesting experiments of Hanna and his group (1,8)
might give us an answer to the question about the significance of
epithelioid cell reactions in malignant tumors. Hanna et al. studied
the influence of BCG injections into malignant tumors and found a
marked so-called histiocytic reaction in the regional lymph nodes.
Hanna was kind enough to send us a series of these lymph nodes for
investigation with our techniques. The studies have not yet been
completed, but I can present some findings that might be interesting
in this context. In Giemsa-stained sections the histiocyte-like
cells are oxyphilic; in cytochemical preparations they are slightly
positive for nonspecific esterase and acid phosphatase. On electron
microscopy (Fig.5) these cells correspond to the preepithelioid cells
and epithelioid cells we described in human lymph nodes (5).

In man, epithelioid cells occur in malignant tumors with a
relatively good prognosis. The experiments of Hanna et al. also
showed that epithelioid cells are a favorable prognostic sign. All
the data I have presented here underline the importance of attaining
a better understanding of the functional basis of the biologically
significant epithelioid cell reaction.

To conclude - I have asked you a number of questions. Perhaps
this conference will already answer all, or some of them. If not,
we may look forward to the VII International Conference on Lymphatic
Tissues and Germinal Centers in Immune Reactions. Above all, however,
I hope that I have generated a slight stimulus and that the experimenters among you will be encouraged to think more about the phenomena
in human immunopathology. That would certainly be of advantage for
the understanding of human diseases.

REFERENCES

1.   Hanna, M.G., Jr., Zbar, B., Rapp, H.J. J. nat. Cancer Inst. 48
      (1972) 1441.
2.   Lennert, K. in: Handbuch der Speziellen pathologischen Anatomie
      und Histologie, I/3A. Uehlinger, E., ed. Berlin-Göttingen-
      Heidelberg: Springer (1961).
3.   Lennert, K. in collaboration with Stein, H., Mohri, N.,
      Kaiserling, E., Müller-Hermelink, H.K. Malignant Lymphomas
      Other than Hodgkin's Disease. New York-Heidelberg-Berlin:
      Springer (1978).
4.   Lennert, K., Kaiserling, E., Müller-Hermelink, H.K. Letter to
      the Editor, Lancet I, pp. 1031-1032 (1975).
5.   Mori,Y., Lennert, K. Electron Microscopic Atlas of Lymph Node
      Cytology and Pathology. Berlin-Heidelberg-New York: Springer
      (1969).
6.   Müller-Hermelink, H.K., Lennert, K. in: Lennert, K. Malignant
      Lymphomas Other than Hodgkin's Disease, pp. 1-71. New York-
      Heidelberg-Berlin: Springer (1978).
7.   Müller-Hermelink, H.K., Kaiserling, E., Lennert, K. Virchows
      Arch. B 14 (1973) 47.
8.   Snodgrass, M.J., Hanna, M.G., Jr. Cancer Res. 33 (1973) 701.

SESSION   A 1

LYMPHOID CELL DIFFERENTIATION AND TRAFFIC

CHAIRPERSONS:

Maria A.B. de Sousa

J.L. Gowans

INTRODUCTION - ON THE 20TH ANNIVERSARY OF A SCIENTIFIC DISCOVERY

Maria de Sousa

Laboratory of Cell Ecology, Sloan-Kettering Institute

for Cancer Research, New York, N.Y. 10021, U.S.A.

I have suggested to the organizers of the conference that the title of this introduction could be adopted as the subtitle of the session. I shall lead you into my reasons for this request by quoting a short passage taken from the recent Steinbeck's translation into modern English of Sir Thomas Mallory's Winchester manuscripts on "The Acts of King Arthur and his noble nights" (1):

> "You cannot know a venture from its beginning"
> Merlin said, "Greatness is born little."

Greatness in the venture of the recirculation of lymphocytes was born so little that, at first it was not recognized.

Indeed, the first experiments indicating that lymphocytes traveled from the blood to the thoracic duct lymph in the rat published twenty years ago (2,4) met with criticism. It was feared that lymphocytes behaved abnormally in animals infused with heparin and stressed by confinement in restraining cages (5). It was said that the evidence for a blood-to-lymph circulation of lymphocytes was indirect, and that no individual lymphocyte had been followed in detail along its supposed route from blood to lymph. Gowans, between his first papers in the late fifties and the paper published with Knight in 1964, on "The route or recirculation of lymphocytes" not only silenced the noise of criticism with impeccable experimental data, but opened a door into a vast new room in this big house of science.

Twenty years later we have for the first time the combined bonus of having the words lymphocyte traffic in the title of a session of this Conference and Gowans co-chairing it.

I am using the privilege of being the chairperson of this session to dedicate it to my co-chairman.

Each of the papers to follow will thus be presented in the spirit of a birthday present to celebrate the anniversary of a discovery. I think we are by far too concerned with the making of our own discoveries, to take the time to celebrate and acknowledge the discoveries of others. But if science is to continue as a civilized, and civilizing activity of the type those of my generation learned in England, in one way or another, with John Humphrey, competition, of the type that may make nations successful economically, cannot be the only ground rule. Contributions made in the spirit of giving and sharing seem to be just as needed as those made in the spirit of taking.

As we were reminded by the inaugural presentation on W. Flemming's behalf, the possibility that lymphocytes circulated continuously between blood and lymph was first discussed in 1885 (6). I would like to remind you, however, of the conclusions based on experimental data that transformed the lymph node into a true 20th century structure (4):

"The route taken by lymphocytes in passing from the blood into the lymph is not known. Sjovall (7) argued from circumstantial evidence that lymphocytes were normally formed at a low rate in the lymph nodes and that in order to maintain the output of lymphocytes from the lymph ducts, they must recirculate from the blood to the lymph. He proposed that lymphocytes entered the tissue spaces and returned to the blood via the peripheral lymphatics. A slow recirculation of this kind probably does take place through most of the tissues of the body, but it is not large enough to account for more than a fraction of the thoracic duct output. Thus, Yoffey and Drinker (8) found only a few lymphocytes in the peripheral lymph from the hind limbs of dogs and cats and Baker (9) noted small numbers in the peripheral lymphatics of the cat intestine. Since large numbers of lymphocytes were added to lymph as it passed through a lymph node and new lymphocytes are formed at a low rate in the nodes, it is possible that the main channel of recirculation is through the lymph nodes."

Thus, the prevailing XIX century notion that the lymph nodes were exclusive sites of lymphopoiesis started to be questioned.

The same paper (4) concludes with the following comment about large and small lymphocytes, "however, it has never been demonstrated

that the larger lymphocytes are the precursors of the small and it
is possible that the life histories of the two groups are quite
distinct".

In the last twenty years we have learned that the distinction
between large and small lymphocytes is mostly a morphological one
but the concept that distinct groups of lymphocyte have distinct life
histories is well and alive and the papers in the first half of this
session will attest to that (10-17). In species where alloantisera
are not available for the characterization of lymphocyte sets,
techniques are being developed for the separation by velocity sedimentation of purified cell subpopulations with distinct functional
characteristics (18,19).

Largely under the influence of Gowans' early ideas on the
function of lymphocyte circulation considerable progress has been
made in understanding the role of the circulation of lymphocytes in
the development and propagation of the immune response (20).

Research in the field of lymphocyte circulation, however, is
moving on to understanding basic mechanisms of control of circulation
in the absence of obvious antigenic motivation (21-25). There is
also a growing interest in the question of distribution of lymphocytes
in man. In the paper by Dwyer, Wade and Thakur (26) we will find
details of labeling and tracing of guinea pig lymphocytes with In[111],
a radioisotope with a short half life, low toxicity and rapid incorporation into cells which is already being sucessfully utilized for
lymphocyte tracing studies in man.

From our own work with cell surface markers on the distribution
of lymphocytes in the peripheral blood and spleen of patients with
Hodgkin's disease (27-29) we have postulated that lymphocyte migration
may be influenced by the interaction of lymphocytes with iron and iron
binding proteins (30,31). I was therefore very interested to see that
later on in the meeting Jankovic, Popeskovic and Isakovic will be
presenting work on cation induced immunosuppression.

The possibility that lymphocytes and other cells of the immune
system can recognize, utilize, and compete for metal cations indis-
pensible for bacterial growth (32) and cell division (33) is worth
exploring because at the end of the exploration we may find a very
simple basis for immune surveillance and for some of the discrepancies
that have surrounded it. In connection with this point of recognition
of metal ions by lymphocytes, it is perhaps worth remembering that
some routine materials we are all using in our laboratories such as
concalavilin A and viruses owe much of their activities to the metal
in their structure (34,35).

The idea that lymphocytes may play basic physiological roles involving the recognition of metals and synthesis of matalloproteins is just starting to emerge from recent work in my laboratory (31,36). We may have to wait another twenty years to prove it. Before that, I will conclude by returning to King Arthur's feast:

> "Do not dishonour your feast by ignoring what
> comes to it.   Such is the law of quest."

Such is the law, I hope, that will prevail in this Conference.

REFERENCES

1.   Steinbeck, J.   The Acts of King Arthur and his Noble Knights. p. 101. Ballantine Books. (1976).
2.   Gowans, J.L.   Brit. J. Exp. Pathol. 43 (1957) 424.
3.   Gowans, J.L.   Brit. Med. Mull. 15 (1959a) 50.
4.   Gowans, J.L.   J. Physiol. 146 (1959b) 54.
5.   Gowans, J.L., Knight, E.J.   Proc. Roy. Soc. B. 159 (1964) 257.
6.   Brockendahl, A., Drews, R., Mobius, O., Paulsen, E., Schendel, J., Flemming, W. (1885) Reprinted 1978. This vol.
7.   Sjövall, H.   Acta. Path. Microbiol. Scand. Suppl. 27 (1936).
8.   Yoffey, J.M., Drinker, C.K.   Anat. Rec. 73 (1939) 417.
9.   Baker, R.D.   Anat. Rec. 55 (1933) 207.
10. Von Gaudecker, B., Muller-Hermelink (1975) This vol.
11. Scollay, R., Kochen, M., Weissman, I.   (1978) This vol.
12. Boyd, R.L., Ward, H.A. (1978) This vol.
13. Schauenstein, K., Wick, G., Pfeilschifter (1978) This vol.
14. Smithyman, A.M., Carr, K., Forman, D., White, R.G. (1978) This vol.
15. Gastkemper, N.A., Wubbena, A.S., Nienwenhuis, P. (1978) This vol.
16. de Sousa, M., Freitas, A., Huber, B., Cantor, H., Boyse, E.A. This vol.
17. Reske-Kunz, A.B., Scheid, M.P., de Sousa, M., Boyse, E.A. (1978) This vol.
18. Cooper, E.L., MacDonald, H.R., Soront, B. (1978).
19. Leene, W., Pohell, P.J.M. (1978).
20. Ford, W.L. Progress in Allergy 19 (1978) 1.
21. Butcher, E., Scollay, R., Weissman, I.   (1978) This vol.
22. Anderson, A.O., Anderson, N.I., White, J.I. (1978) This vol.
23. Smith, M.E., Ford, W.L. (1978) This vol.
24. Curtis, A.S.G., Davies, M., Wilkinson, P.C. (1978) This vol.
25. Sainte-Marie, G. (1978) This vol.
26. Dwyer, J.M., Wade, M., Taker, M.   (1978) This vol.
27. de Sousa, M., Yang, M., Lopez, C., Corrales, E., Tan, C., Hansen, J.A., Dupont, B., Good, R.A. Clin. Exp. Immunol. 27 (1977) 143.

28. de Sousa, M., Tan, C.T.C., Siegal, F.P., Filippa, D., Tan, R., Good, R.A. Ped. Res. (1978).
29. Tan, C.T.C., de Sousa, M., Tan, R., Hansen, J.A., Good, R.A. Cancer Res. 38 (1978) 886.
30. de Sousa, M., Smithyman, A.M., Tan, C.T.C. Am. J. Pathol. 90 (1978) 497.
31. de Sousa, M. in Symp. Soc. Exp. Biol. on 'Cell-Cell Recognition' 32 (1978) 393. Ed. A.S.G. Curtis, Cambridge University Press.
32. Neilands, J.B. in: Microbial iron metabolism (Neilands, J.B. ed.) pp. 3-34 (1974) Academic Press.
33. Fernandez- Pol, J.A. Feb Letters 88 (1978) 345.
34. Becker, J.W., Reeke, G.N., Cunningham, B.A., Edelman, G.M. Nature 259 (1976) 406.
35. Racker, E., Krimsky, I. J. Exp. Med. 85 (1947) 715.
36. de Sousa, M., Nishiya, K. Cell. Immunol. 38 (1978) 203.

ONTOGENETIC DIFFERENTIATION OF EPITHELIAL AND NON-EPITHELIAL CELLS

IN THE HUMAN THYMUS

B. von Gaudecker and H.K. Müller-Hermelink[1]

Institute of Anatomy and [1]Institute of Pathology,

University of Kiel, Kiel, W. Germany

Most electron microscopical and functional reports dealing with the ontogenesis of the thymus in laboratory animals and man (1,2) consider almost only the differentiation of its typical "lymphoid" organization. The aim of the present study was to determine whether the main epithelial and mesenchymal structures develop before, or at the same time as the first lymphoid cells are seen in the thymus, i.e. whether the differentiation of a characteristic microecology may be regarded as a necessary prerequisite for lymphoid colonization.

Thymuses from 50 human fetuses were investigated by light and electron microscopy. The ages of the fetuses was calculated from the crown-heal length and ranged from the 8th to 28th week of gestation. Fetuses were obtained from abortions and hysterectomies.

The thymus anlage of the 8th gestational week (g.w.) contains almost exclusively immature epithelial cells (Fig.1a) being arranged at the periphery as a regular row of prismatic cells and in the central area having a random distribution. On electron microscopy, the cytoplasmic processes of the central cells are closely interwoven with each other. The cells are connected by short desmosomes and single bundles of tonofilaments can be seen. Microvilli and sometimes solitary cilia project into widened intercellular spaces. Even at this stage, myoid cells have been found.

In fetuses of about the 9th g.w., basophilic round cells are distributed evenly throughout the thymus anlage among the epithelial cells. In the central part of the thymus, the epithelial cells are more spindleshaped. The first Hassall's corpuscles may be found in this region.

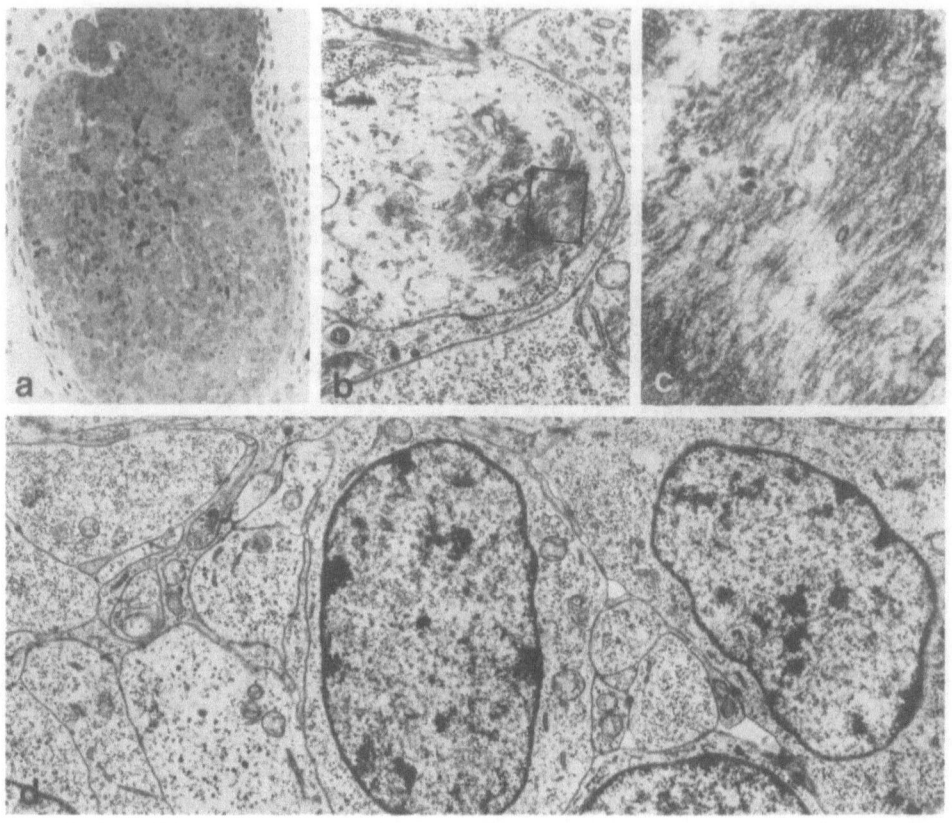

FIG. 1:   Thymus of the 8th g.w.:   a) Semithin section from one lobe
of the thymus anlage (75 x).   b) Myoid cell (12,000 x).   c) Area
with myofilaments, marked in b) (60,000 x).   d) Central epithelial
cells (8,000 x)

     During the next weeks of gestation, the periphery of the thymus
becomes indented by mesenchymal septae. At the 12th g.w., small
lymphocytes are more abundant in the centrum of the organ than at
the periphery, which mainly contains cells with weakly stained large
nuclei. Mitoses are distributed over the whole section. In the
presumptive medulla, one recognizes a region that is composed mainly
of spindle-shaped epithelial cells. Medullary epithelial cells in
the centrum of the organ are also frequently spindle-shaped. Their
cytoplasm contains abundant tonofilaments. In this area

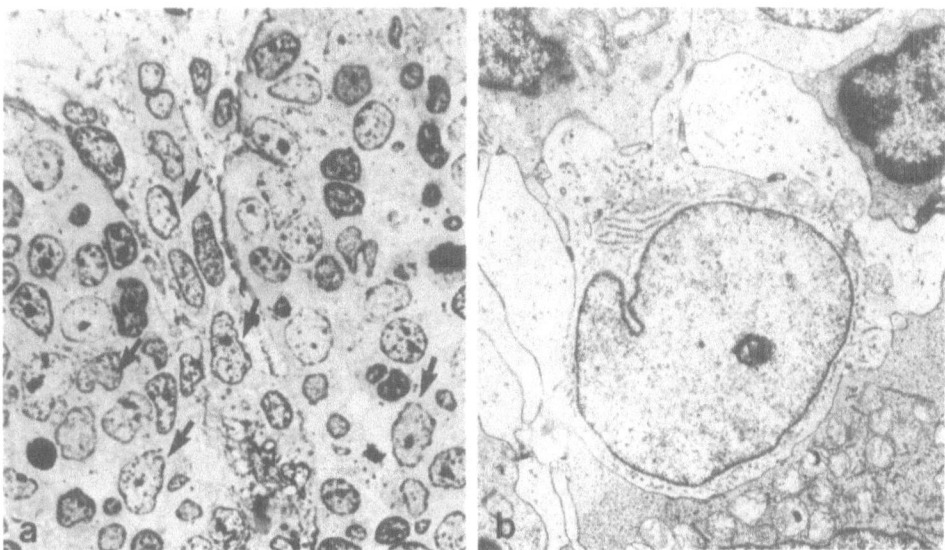

FIG. 2: Thymus of the 12th g.w.: a) Silver impregnation of a semithin section from a mesenchymal septum. Large cells with irregularly shaped nuclei (arrows) are located both in the septum and in the medullary region (1120 x). b) Interdigitating reticulum cell (7800 x).

tubular formations with epithelial cells containing microvilli can be seen. Epithelial cells at the periphery of the thymus anlage have relatively blunt cytoplasmic protrusions. Their nuclei have finely dispersed chromatin and the cytoplasm is electron-lucent. Together with large lymphoblasts, these cells cause the lightly stained aspect of the peripheral regions of the thymus anlage. As seen after silver impregnation of the surrounding basal laminae (Fig.2a), the mesenchymal septae do not reach very far into the thymus anlage. Sometimes they seem to be "open" at the end facing the epithelial part of the thymus. Large electron-transparent cells (Fig.2a, arrows) with irregularly shaped nuclei are found both in the mesenchymal septae and in the presumptive medullary regions of the thymus anlage. These cells have some mitochondria and a few profiles of rough and smooth endoplasmic reticulum, the cytoplasm frequently contains small dark granules assembled in the Golgi field. Irregular interdigitating cytoplasmic projections begin to extend between the other cell types. These ultrastructural features resemble those of interdigitating reticulum cells of peripheral lymphatic tissue.

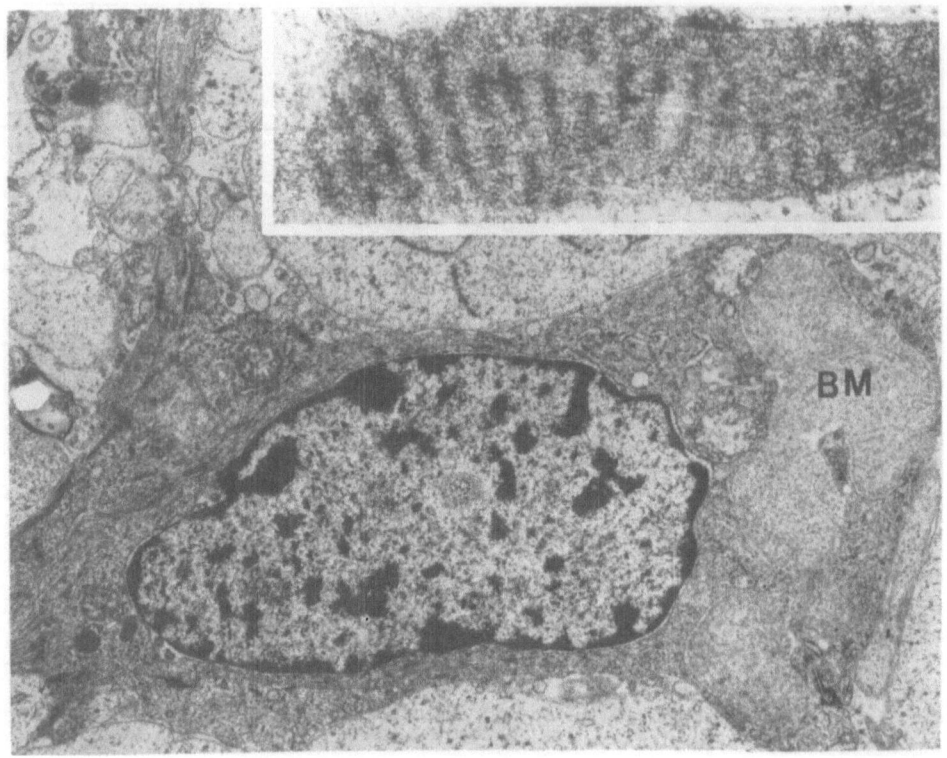

FIG. 3:   Thymus of the 14th g.w.:   Medullary epithelial cells
enclosing basement membrane material (BM) (12,000 x).
Inset: Basement membrane material with a periodicity of about
80 nm (30,000 x).

During the next two weeks, the typical cortical and medullary
differentiation becomes obvious. The mesenchymal septae have reached
the cortico-medullary junction, where they branch and widen. They
contain blood vessels and various hemopoietic cell types. Cellular
diapedeses may also be seen: Mesenchymal precursor cells with a
large, electron-lucent, irregularly shaped nucleus enter the epithelial
region of the thymus, and lymphocytes are leaving the thymus anlage
and wandering towards the mesenchymal septum. The direction of these
moving cells is indicated by their so-called hand-mirror shape: the
cytoplasm is going ahead, and the nucleus is being drawn behind.
Characteristic differences between cortical and medullary epithelial
cells may be seen at the 15th g.w.   The medullary epithelial cells
have long slender processes and their cytoplasm is relatively darkly
stained (Fig.3). They are associated with basement membranes, which

are composed of fine filamentous material sometimes showing the
periodicity of about 80 nm (Fig.3, inset). In contrast, cortical
epithelial cells have a translucent cytoplasm with only a few
tonofilaments and rare desmosomes. Inside the cortical constituent
no association between epithelial cells and basement membranes is
seen.

At the 15th to 18th g.w., the cytologic differentiation of the
thymus constituents is complete. Numerous well differentiated
interdigitating reticulum cells can be found in the thymic medulla.
Their ultrastructure has been described elsewhere (3,4). Some of
them have a more darkly stained cytoplasm owing to numerous free
ribosomes. The permeation of the thymic medulla by non-epithelial
reticular cells occurs concurrently with the formation of morphologically different cortical and medullary epithelial cells.

In fetuses at the 18th g.w., lymphoid cells of cortex and
medulla show the same differences as in the postnatal thymus (4).
Even at this stage, "open" mesenchymal septae with diapedeses at
the cortico-medullary junction are found; these are not seen in
the postnatal thymus.

CONCLUSIONS

These findings indicate that the cortex and medulla contain
different epithelial cells. In addition, the thymic medulla shows
cells with the same morphology as the interdigitating reticulum
cells of peripheral lymphatic tissue. Both the differentiation of
epithelial cells and the invasion of mesenchymal cells into the
thymic medulla occur before and concurrently with the lymphoid
colonization and are complete before the typical "lymphoid-defined"
structure of the thymus is formed. The different microecologies of
the thymic cortex and medulla provide a structural basis for
explaining the occurrence of different types of "homing" cells.

REFERENCES

1.   Haar, J.L. Anat. Rec. 179 (1974) 463.
2.   Hoshimo, T., Takeda, M., Abe, K., Ito, T. Anat. Rec. 164
      (1969) 47.
3.   Kaiserling, E., Stein, H., Müller-Hermelink, H.K. Cell. Tiss.
      Res. 155 (1974) 47.
4.   von Gaudecker, B., Cell. Tiss. Res. 186 (1978) 507.

ANTIGENIC CHANGES ASSOCIATED WITH CHICKEN B LYMPHOCYTE DEVELOPMENT

R.L. Boyd[1] and H.A. Ward

Department of Pathology and Immunology, Monash Medical School, Melbourne, Australia

[1]Present Address: Department of General and Experimental Pathology, University of Innsbruck, Austria

INTRODUCTION

Analysis of changes in specific antigenic determinants during ontogeny constitutes one of the most practical methods for investigating lymphocyte differentiation pathways. Such studies have been very successful in mice, using alloantisera specific for T cells (reviews 1,2), but those of B cells have been largely restricted to alteration in immunoglobulin subclasses (3). We have approached this problem by identifying heteroantigens specific for B or T lymphocyte subpopulations using the chicken as a model (4) because of the clear lymphoid tissue dichotomy. These determinants were the chicken B lymphocyte-specific antigen (CBLA), chicken mature B lymphocyte-specific antigen (CMBLA), chicken foetal-associated antigen (CFAA), chicken T lymphocyte-specific antigen (CTLA) and chicken thymus-specific antigen (CTOA). From the analysis of the adult cellular representation and tissue localization of these determinants and immunoglobulin (Ig) and IgG (4), there appeared to be a progression of cells bearing immature to mature markers, each subclass being associated with different elements of the microenvironment. This was particularly evident for B cells within the bursa: CBLA-positive cells were present in both the cortex and medulla but those with CFAA were only in cortex, in association with a specific reticulin fibre framework (5) while Ig-, IgG- and CMBLA-bearing cells were restricted to the medulla which has a supporting framework of reticular epithelial cells. This problem of B cell differentiation has been examined further by an

ontogenic study of the B lymphocyte markers in cell suspensions and
tissue sections.

MATERIALS AND METHODS

Lymphoid Tissues

Bursa, thymus, spleen, bone marrow, blood and gut-associated
lymphoid tissue (GALT) were obtained from 12, 15 or 18 day embryonic-
or 1 day- or 3 week old Australorp/White Leghorn F_1 hybrids (Musgrove
Chicks, Victoria, Australia). Cell suspensions in Hanks' balanced
salt solution (HBSS, pH 7.6) or cryostat tissue sections were
prepared as previously described (4). In experiments requiring
yolk sac, the "area-vasculosa" was rinsed free of yolk by 4 washings
in cold HBSS at 4°C and teased out. The resultant cell suspension
was washed a fruther three times with cold HBBS, by centrifuging at
170 g_{av} for 5 min each time to remove remaining yolk granules.

Immunohistology

Rabbit antisera to CBLA, CMBLA, CFAA, Ig and IgG, and the
fluorescein-labelled goat anti-rabbit globulin were prepared as
described previously (4). Standard membrane and section immunofluorescence tests were performed according to Nairn (6). Parallel
control preparations were treated with phosphate-buffered saline
(pH 7.2), HBSS or preimmune rabbit antisera. Specimens were
examined by narrow band blue or darkground ultraviolet fluorescence
microscopy (6). Each result is the mean from at least 3 experiments
in which tissues from 6-12 embryos or 3 post-hatch chickens were
pooled.

RESULTS

Bursa

The ontogenic development of the B cell antigens in the bursa
is summarized in Tab. 1. A relatively high percentage of CFAA-
positive cells were present in the 12-day embryo and at this and
subsequent embryonic ages were localized in the mesenchyme of the
tunica propria (developing cortex) in the vicinity of epithelial
medullary follicles. The latter were negative throughout. The
CFAA-bearing cells declined in later foetal stages but rose markedly
again at hatching, at which time fluorescence of the cortical mantle
of lymphocytes was clearly visible, similar to that observed in the
adult bursa (4).

TAB. 1:   Ontogenic development of B lymphocyte antigens in the
bursa (percentage positive cells by immunofluorescence).

Antigen	Embryonic Age (Days)			1 day old	6 weeks old
	12	15	18		
CFAA	12	9	2	31	41
CBLA	19	39	63	81	95
Ig	1	8	22	83	80
IgG	-	1	1	18	58
CMBLA	-	1	1	23	60

CBLA-positive cells increased steadily with age from approximately 1% in 12-day embryos to nearly the adult value at hatching,
with an associated increase in membrane concentration of this
antigen. Initially they were localized in the tunica propria,
similar to that observed for CFAA, but by day 15 many were associated
with the larger developing follicles, the extent of which increased
by day 18. In one day old bursas, the larger follicles with a well
defined cortex gave a similar fluorescence to that in the adult (4)
having positive cells in both the cortex and medulla.

Anti-Ig stained cells were first observed in the 12-day
embryonic bursa but only in very low numbers. From day 15 there
was a rapid increase in these cells particularly around hatching;
on tissue sections they were localized only in the medullary
follicules. IgG- and CMBLA- positive cells first appeared in significant levels at hatching. As for Ig, they were restricted to
the medulla of the follicles.

Bone Marrow

CFAA-bearing cells were found in high numbers in the bone
marrow throughout development, there being 41% by day 15 of incubation and 51% at hatching (Tab. 2) Since this antigen appears to
be associated with immature cells (4), this finding may reflect the
precursor source of this organ. A low, but consistent percentage
of CBLA-positive cells was present during embryogenesis, this
markedly rising to the adult value in day old chicks. Ig-, IgG-
and CMBLA- bearing cells, however, were virtually absent in the
embryonic bone marrow and were found only after hatching.

TAB. 2:   Ontogenic development of B lymphocyte antigens in the bone
marrow (percentage positive cells by immunofluorescence)

Antigen	Embryonic Age (Days)			1 day old	6 weeks old
	12	15	18		
CFAA	18	41	32	51	60
CBLA	5	3	2	16	13
Ig	–	–	–	10	15
IgG	–	–	–	3	8
CMBLA	–	–	–	1	6

Spleen

In the developing spleen (Tab. 3) there was a gradual decrease
in the percentage of anti-CFAA stained cells, while CBLA-positive
cells were found in only very low numbers - those in day 12
embryos being large, basophilic, granular cells with no lymphocytic
characteristics. Again, after hatching there was a marked increase
in CBLA- and Ig-positive cells and the first appearance of IgG- and
CMBLA-bearing cells. On tissue sections, however, despite this
increase in B lymphocytes in one day old chicks, the B-dependent
periellipsoidal sheaths and germinal centres were not yet organized;
these were fully established by 3 weeks of age.

Other Lymphoid Tissues

The development of cells bearing B lymphocyte markers in the
blood closely paralleled that in the spleen, but the GALT was the
last to develop, no B cells being observed in this tissue even by
hatching. The characteristic primary follicles and germinal centres
found in the adult (4) were again fully evident in 3 week old
chickens. The thymus was virtually negative throughout, although
older birds (10-12 weeks) showed 5-6% cells positive for CBLA and
Ig.   Of the non-lymphoid tissues, CBLA-positive cells were found
in 6-day yolk sac preparations, well prior to bursa formation, and
also 12-day foetal liver. Neither of these were studied in greater
detail.

DISCUSSION

This ontogenic study illustrates further the developmental
relationship between chicken B lymphocyte subpopulations expressing

TAB. 3:   Ontogenic development of B lymphocyte antigens in the
spleen (percentage positive cells by immunofluorescence)

| Antigen | Embryonic Age (Days) | | | 1 day old | 6 weeks old |
	12	15	18		
CFAA	13	9	2	1	-
CBLA	7	1	3	9	29
Ig	-	-	4	10	34
IgG	-	-	-	4	14
CMBLA	-	-	-	4	14

different membrane antigens. The temporal appearance of CBLA and
Ig determinants in the bursa agrees well with that found by others
(7,8,9,10) and the localization within this organ of the additional
antigens investigated here, provides information on the differing
interactions of these subclasses with specific elements of the
microenvironment. As a result, a scheme for B cell differentiation
in the chickens can be proposed (Tab. 4).

Precursors, at least some of which may express CFAA since cells
bearing this antigen have been shown to differentiate into B lymphocytes in vitro (unpublished observations), enter the bursa in the
tunica propria or cortical region. Here, possibly as a result of
interaction with a specific reticulin component (5), they are
induced to express CBLA. These CFAA, CBLA- positive, Ig-negative
cells are found only in the bursa cortex. On subsequent differentiation they appear to migrate into the medulla where, in close
association with a framework of reticular epithelial cells, they
acquire surface Ig, probably IgM, and lose the immature foetal
antigen.

These cells are the last stage reached during embryogenesis,
but are also found in the adult peripheral lymphoid tissue e.g.
bone marrow and spleen. The final step, prior to differentiation
into antibody-secreting plasma cells, would be the induction of
memory cells after antigen stimulation, probably beginning soon
after hatching. Associated with this is a transient increase in
CBLA concentration as indicated by germinal centre staining on the
adult (4), and the appearance of IgG and the mature marker, CMBLA.

Thus, a characteristic feature of chicken B lymphocyte differentiation appears to be the alteration in membrane antigenicity of
these cells, each subpopulation localizing in distinct regions
within the lymphoid tissues. It remains to be determined what the
exact regulatory mechanisms are, but, within the bursa, reticular
epithelial cells and/or associated products appear to be of prime

TAB. 4:   Summary of antigenic changes associated with B lymphocyte development

Antigen	Stem Cells	Foetal Bursa Cortex	Bursa Medulla, Peripheral	1 day old adult Bursa Medulla, Peripheral
CFAA	? +	+	–	–
CBLA	–	++	++	++
Ig	–	–	+	+
IgG	–	–	–	+
CMBLA	–	–	–	+

importance. It is also still not known why B cells actually migrate from the bursa and localize within specific areas. The striking influence of hatching on both the maturation of lymphocytes within the bursa and their seeding to the peripheral lymphoid tissues suggests a role of antigen stimulation but this requires further clarification. An alternative explanation could be that maturation of the non-lymphocyte elements within the secondary tissues is a prerequisite for establishment of the B-independent areas.

REFERENCES

1.   Schlesinger, M.,Prog. Allergy 16 (1972) 214.
2.   Greaves, M.F., Owen, J.J.T., Raff, M.C., T and B Lymphocytes: Origins, Properties and Roles in Immune Responses. American Elsevier Publishing Company, New York (1973).
3.   Lawton, A.R., Kincade, P.W., Cooper, M.D., Fed. Proc. 34 (1975) 33.
4.   Boyd, R.L., Ward, H.A., Immunol. 34 (1978) 9.
5.   Boyd, R.L., Ward, H.A., Muller, H.K., Int. Arch. Allergy 50 (1976) 129.
6.   Nairn, R.C., Fluorescent Protein Tracing, 4th edn. Churchill Livingstone, Edinburgh (1976).
7.   Kincade, P.W., Cooper, M.D., J. Immunol. 106 (1971) 1421.
8.   Albini, B., Wick, G., Int. Arch. Allergy 44 (1973) 804.
9.   Hudson, L., Roitt, I.M., Europ. J. Immunol. 3 (1973) 63.
10. Albini, B., Wick, G., Int. Arch. Allergy 48 (1975) 513.

ACKNOWLEDGEMENTS

We are indebted to Mr. P.H. Atkin and Mrs. J.C. Mackowiak for preparation of fluorescein conjugates. This work was supported by a grant from the Australian Research Grant Committee.

EVIDENCE FOR SURFACE ANTIGEN(S) SPECIFIC FOR A SUBPOPULATION OF PERIPHERAL B AND T LYMPHOCYTES IN THE CHICKEN

K. Schauenstein, R. Pfeilschifter and G. Wick

Institute for General and Experimental Pathology

University of Innsbruck, Austria

INTRODUCTION

Previous work in this laboratory was dedicated to the serological classification of chicken lymphoid cells by means of specific heteroantisera. The original purpose of those attempts was to make use of such antibodies for the elucidation of the pathogenetic mechanisms in certain autoimmune phenomena, viz. the spontaneously occurring autoimmune thyroiditis in chickens of the Obese strain (1). Taking advantage of the clearcut anatomical separation of the bursa and thymus system in the chicken, antisera against bursa (ABS) and thymus cells (ATS) had been raised in turkeys, which - after proper absorptions - were shown to be strictly specific for the respective cell type (2). These reagents turned out to be perfectly suited for both the in vitro delineation of B and T cells in various lymphoid organs and the peripheral blood of chickens (3), as well as for the specific in vivo suppression of B and T cell functions most probably due to the ability of avian sera to fix chicken complement (4). In addition, these antisera have been successfully used for the analysis of the expression of antigenic surface determinants during the ontogeny of the lymphoid system (5). In continuation of these studies the present paper deals with serologically detectable differences in the expression of surface antigens during the maturation of central bursa and thymus cells to B and T lymphocytes in the peripheral blood and the peripheral lymphoid organs. The results of these experiments speak for pronounced quantitative differences for B and T markers as detected by ABS and ATS on central and peripheral lymphoid cells respectively and, furthermore, rabbit antisera prepared against peripheral splenic lymphocytes were shown to react with surface determinants on about 30% peripheral lymphocytes, which are absent from bursa and thymus cells.

TAB. 1

Absorption with spleen cells v/v cells/serum	MeIF titres of			
	ABS on		ATS on	
	BURSA	SPLEEN	THYMUS	SPLEEN
0	256	128	256	128
1/8	256	128	128	64
1/4	128	64	128	64
1/2	128	64	128	64
1/1	128	64	32	0
2/1	64	64	16	0
4/1	32	32	16	0
6/1	32	8	0	0
8/1	32	0	0	0

EXPERIMENTAL APPROACH

Antisera

Specific ABS and ATS prepared as described earlier (2) were subjected to differential absorptions with twofold increasing amounts (1/8 - 8/1, v/v, cells/serum) of peripheral lymphocytes from spleens of adult normal White Leghorn (NWL) chickens according to a method described by Raff and Wortis (6).

Rabbit antisera were raised against peripheral lymphocytes (ASS) by three weekly intracutaneous injections of cells from one half spleen of an adult NWL chicken after nylon wool passage. The cells were incorporated in complete Freund's adjuvant (1/1, v/v). The animals were bled prior to each injection and were exsanguinated 10 days after the last immunization. The resulting antisera were pre-absorbed with glutaraldehyde crosslinked chicken serum (80 mg/ml), with chicken erythrocytes (1/5, v/v) and then absorbed consecutively in an analogous manner with bursa and thymus cells (1/8 - 4/1, v/v, cells/serum).

Immunofluorescence Tests

Indirect membrane fluorescence tests (MeIF) were performed with differentially absorbed ABS, ATS and ASS on living bursa, thymus and spleen cells from 3-4 week old NWL chicken donors. The tests were done

TAB. 2

Absorption with bursa + thymus v/v cells/serum	MeIF titres of ASS on		
	SPLEEN	BURSA	THYMUS
0	512	512	512
1/8	512	512	512
1/4	512	256	128
1/2	512	32	32
1/1	256	0	0
2/1	128	0	0
4/1	128	0	0

using a semi-automated procedure described earlier (7). The following conjugates were used: (1) A FITC labelled chicken anti-turkey Ig γ-globulin, prepared in this laboratory, with 16 standard precipitating units and a molar fluorescein/protein (F/P) ratio of 6.9; (2) A commercial FITC tagged goat anti-rabbit Ig γ-globulin (Code no. F.2190, Dakopatts, Copenhagen, Denmark; 8 precipitating units, F/P ratio 2.6); (3) For double staining experiments a TRITC goat anti-rabbit Ig γ-globulin (Code no. 7077, Cappel Labs. Inc., Downington, Pa., USA; 32 precipitating units and a ratio of optical densities 280/550 nm of 4.13).

RESULTS AND DISCUSSION

Table 1 summarizes the reactivities in MeIF of ABS and ATS with central and peripheral lymphocytes. It is evident that both sera could be rendered specific for the respective central cell type against which they had been raised by exhaustive absorption with splenic lymphocytes. ATS does no longer react with spleen cells at an absorption ratio of 1/1 while still reacting with thymocytes after absorption with spleen cells at a ratio of 4/1. With ABS an analogous effect was observed only after absorption with much higher amounts of spleen cells (6/1 and 8/1). This is most likely due to the small percentage of B cells (20-30%) in the spleen as compared to that of T cells (60-70%) (3).

Although the requirements of a classical "exhaustive absorption" are met in these experiments, which would indicate qualitative differences of the antigens detected by the unabsorbed and absorbed sera, further endeavour is needed to definitely prove this assumption.

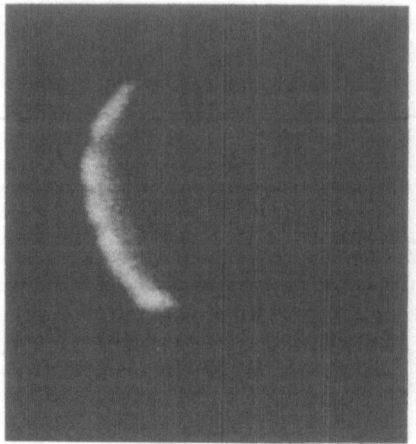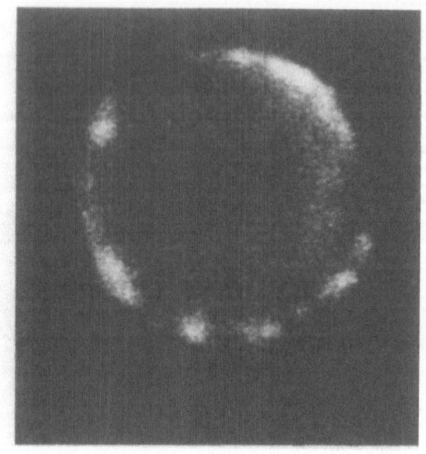

FIG. 1:   A splenic T lymphocyte stained with ATS at capping
conditions (37°C) (A) and with ASS (B) in presence of 0.02 M NaN₃
to prevent capping. Note the independent distribution of both
surface antigens.

    The results for one of the rabbit ASS are given in Table 2.
Exhaustive absorption with bursa and thymus cells made this serum
specific for splenic lymphocytes. Enumeration of fluorescent cells
revealed a proportion of 30-40% of spleen cells to carry this
(these) surface determinant(s) detected by the absorbed ASS.

    Two further ASS reacted in essentially the same manner.
Furthermore, this antigenicity was detected to be present also on a
similar proportion of lymphocytes in the peripheral blood (27.4+8%)
and was verified by a second approach, i.e. complement dependent
cytotoxicity as determined by ⁵¹Cr release assays (not shown).

    In order to investigate possible relationships between the
expression of B and T markers and the peripheral lymphocyte specific
antigen(s), MeIF double staining and cocapping experiments were
performed on spleen cells with turkey ABS and ATS detected by a
fluorescein conjugate, and with rabbit ASS detected by a rhodamine
labelled anti-rabbit Ig antibody. The results of these experiments
speak for an entirely independent representation of the two kinds
of surface determinants as the peripheral lymphocyte antigen(s) was/
were detected on both B and T cells and no significant cocapping
could be obtained with either ABS or ATS (Fig.1).

    Separate enumeration of ABS and ATS positive cells double
stained with ASS revealed almost all (92.5+2%) of peripheral B

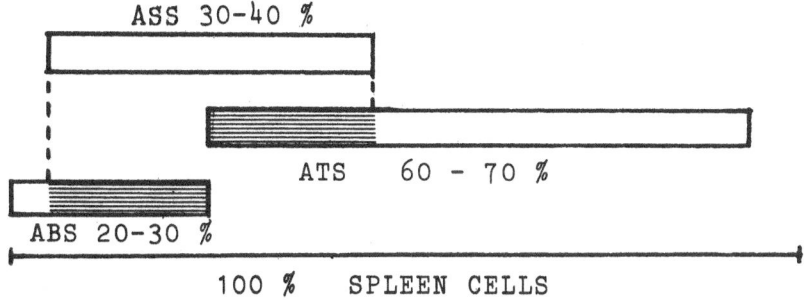

FIG. 2:   Schematical representation of quantitative staining of
spleen cells with ABS, ATS and ASS.

lymphocytes to carry the periphery specific antigen(s), whereas only
a minor percentage (48.0+14%) of T cells appeared to react with ASS.
Accordingly, the distribution of this subpopulation within the B and
T compartment could be imagined as schematically depicted in Fig.2.

Experiments are presently in progress to find correlations
between the expression of this new membrane determinant and certain
immunological functions of peripheral lymphocytes in vitro and in
vivo.

REFERENCES

1.   Wick, G., Sundick, R., Albini, B., Clin. Immunol. Immunopathol.
     3 (1974) 272.
2.   Wick, G., Albini, B., Milgrom, F., Clin. Exp. Immunol. 15 (1973)
     237.
3.   Albini, B., Wick, G., J. Immunol. 112 (1974) 444.
4.   Wick, G., Albini, B., Johnson, W., Immunology 28 (1975) 305.
5.   Albini, B., Wick, G., Int. Arch. Allergy 48 (1975) 513.
6.   Raff, M.C., Wortis, H.H., Immunology 18 (1970) 931.
7.   Schauenstein, K., Wick, G., Kink, H., J. Immunol. Meth. 10 (1976)
     143.

SEPARATION OF GERMINAL CENTRES FROM CHICKEN SPLEEN

[1]A.M. Smithyman, [2]K. Carr, D. Forman and [3]R.G. White

[1]Sloan-Kettering Institute, 1275 York Avenue, New York

[2]Department of Anatomy and [3]Department of Bacteriology
and Immunology, Glasgow University, Glasgow, Scotland

INTRODUCTION

The role of germinal centres in immune reactions has intrigued
immunologists for almost a hundred years, since Flemming's classical
monograph of 1885 (1), and has been a central theme throughout this
Conference series. Such interest derives from the implication of
these structures in the following aspects of the immune response:

1. Expansion of population of immunocompetent cells (2,3)
2. Generation of B-memory cells (4)
3. Induction of immunological tolerance (5)
4. Long-term retention of antigen (6,7)
5. Multiple antigen retention (8)
6. Antibody production (7)
7. Feedback control of antibody production (9,10)
8. Homing of Bursa-derived cells (11)
9. T-B cell interaction (12)
10. Antigen-B cell interaction (13)

As demonstrated in the present meeting many of the old problems
still remain. For example, the nature and role of the antigen-bearing
dendritic cells, and of the rapidly dividing lymphoid cells within
germinal centres are as yet unresolved.

A major limitation on past investigation of germinal centre
function has been the lack of a suitable in vitro study system, in
which the germinal centre could be studied as a separate entity. By
taking advantage of the fact that chicken lymphoid tissue germinal
centres are more clearly delineated from the surrounding tissues

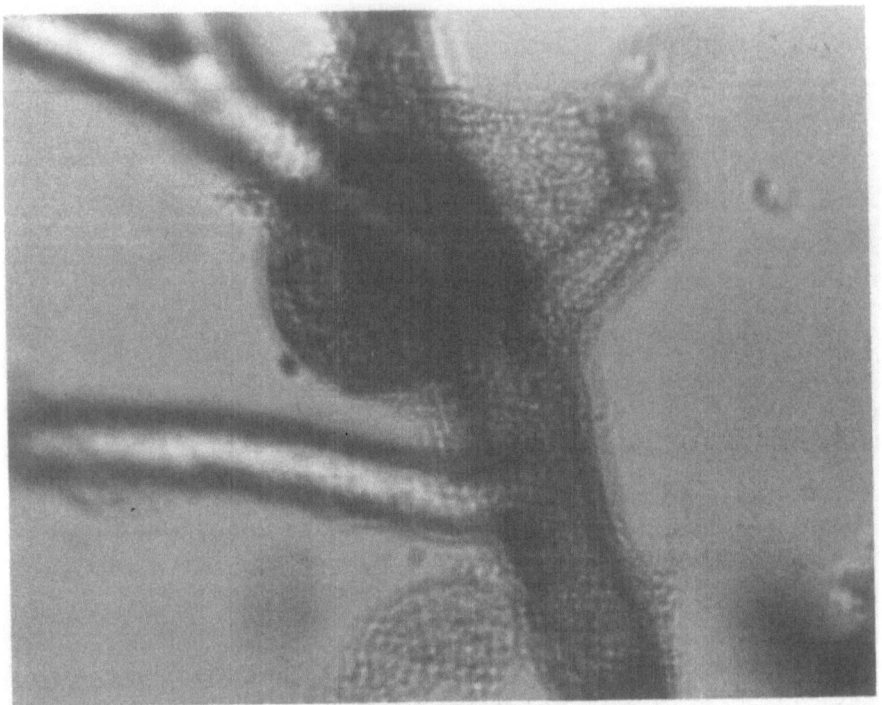

FIG. 1:   Germinal centre sitting at the fork of a penicillary and central arteriole during the final isolation procedure.   x 350.

than in other species, we have devised a simple and rapid method for the separation and isolation of these structures from the chicken spleen.

MATERIALS AND METHODS

Animals and immunisation schedule: Six week old White Leghorn chickens of both sexes were used.   Some birds were immunised 5 days prior to kill with an intravenous injection of 10 mgms of human serum albumin (HSA) (Behringwerke, Marburg, W. Germany) in 1 ml of saline.

Isolation procedure: Details of the isolation procedure have been published elsewhere (14).   Briefly, each bird was killed by an intravenous overdose of sodium pentabarbitone (Nembutal, Abbot Laboratories, U.S.A.), the spleen removed, and placed in a petri dish containing 5 ml of ice-cold Eagle's medium.   The splenic capsule

was gently peeled away from the spleen mass and the pulp tissue
gradually teased out into the surrounding medium, as in the preparation of a spleen cell suspension. This cell suspension is
decanted and the teasing out procedure repeated with fresh medium
until the arterial tree can be seen (with the naked eye) as a pale-
white, branched structure, devoid of attached pulp tissue. This
final preparation was examined under the 4 x or 10 x objectives of
an ordinary light microscope (with the light diaphragm almost closed).
The germinal centres are easily visible at the forks made by the
penicillary with the central arterioles, as large spheres, closely
attached to the vessel walls (Fig.1).

Scanning Electron Microscopy: Fragments of the above preparation were fixed in either 10% formol saline or 2% glutaraldehyde
in phosphate-buffered saline (pH 7.2), critical point dried, and
splutter coated using a gold/pallidium target. Mounted specimens
were viewed in a Phillips Scanning Electron Microscope.

RESULTS AND DISCUSSION

The isolated centres were studied by both light and scanning
electron microscopy. They appeared as distinctive, spherical units,
between 150-300 μm in diameter, encased in a smooth connective tissue
capsule which apparently arises from the adventitia of adjacent
arteriolar vessels (Figs. 2 and 3). The centres were invariably
found at the same sites, at the junctions of the penicillary and
central arterioles, a position which is easily confirmed in histological sections. Prior immunisation resulted in an overall increase
in the number of germinal centres separated. In suspension the
centres proved to be rather robust, elastic structures, strongly
attached to the vascular tree, though it was possible with practise
to cut off individual centres.

The main value of the present method lies in the investigation
of germinal centre function and the following suggestions are put
forward:

1.   Culture of individual isolated centres and investigation of the
effect on the contained cells of various additions to the culture
medium, such as antigens, T-cells, and lymphokines.

2.   Isolation of a pure population of germinal centre lymphoid cells
for lymphocyte traffic and transfer of memory studies.

These ideas are not entirely new. Fagreus (15) and Thorbecke
and her colleagues (16) have used dissected mammalian splenic white
pulp for similar studies, but the separation technique presented
here may offer greater flexibility. In the final lecture at the
last Germinal Centre Conference (17), Humphrey, in discussing germinal

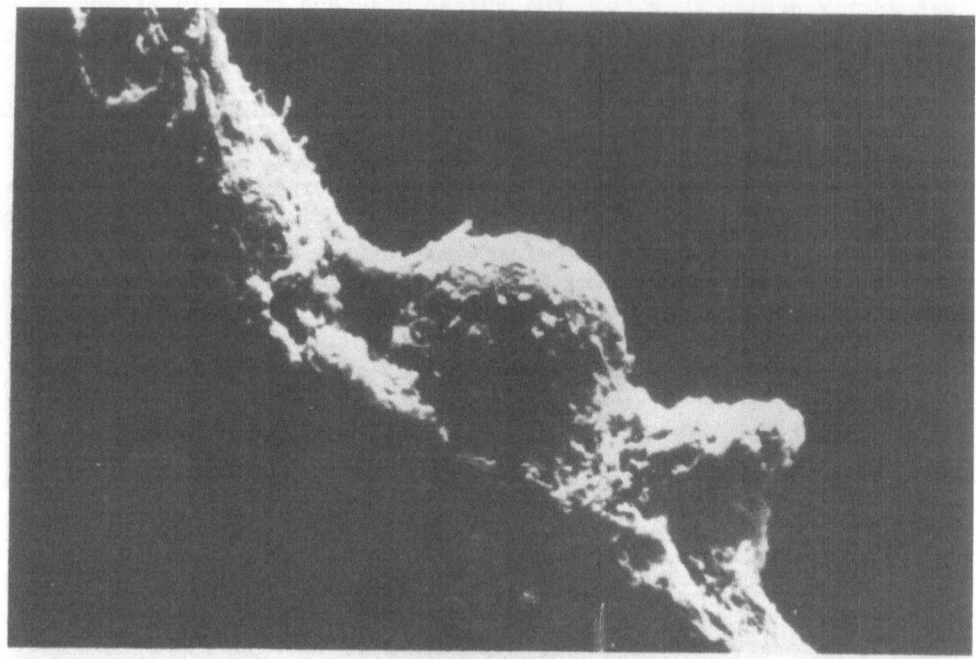

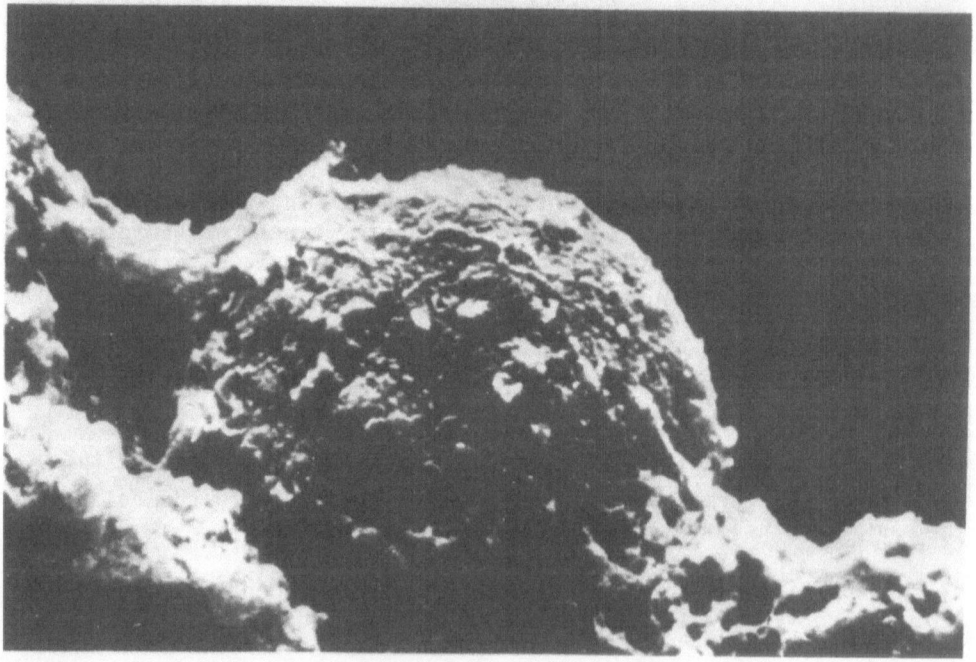

<u>FIGS. 2 and 3</u>:   Scanning electron micrographs of an isolated ger-
minal centre from chicken spleen.   x 400 and 100 (Reduced 20%
for purposes of reproduction.).

centres, suggested that "we shall need to understand much more about the ecology of lymphocytes in the micro-environment of lymphoid tissues before the mystery is finally revealed". The study of isolated germinal centres in vitro may prove valuable in this respect.

REFERENCES

1. Flemming, W. Archiv. f. Mikros. Anat. Entwicklung. 24 (1885) 50.
2. White, R.G., In: Mechanisms of Antibody Formation. M. Holub, L. Jaraskova (Eds.).Prague. Czechoslovak Acad. p.25 (1960).
3. Good, R.A., Cain, W.A., Perey, D.Y., Dunt, P.B., Menwissen, H.J., Rodey, G.E., Cooper, M.D., In: Lymphatic Tissue and Germinal Centers in Immune Responses. L. Fiore- Donati and M.G. Hanna, Jr. (Eds.). Plenum Press, New York, p. 33 (1969).
4. Thorbecke, G., Lerman, S.P., In: The Reticuloendothelial System in Health and Disease: Functions and Characteristics. S.M. Reichard, M.R., Escobar, H. Friedman (Eds.). Plenum Press, New York, p. 83 (1976).
5. Ada, G.L., Parish, C.R., Proc. Nat. Acad. Sci. 61 (1968) 556.
6. Ada, G.L., Williams, J.M., Immunology 10 (1966) 417.
7. White, R.G., French, V.I., Stark, J.M., J. Med. Microbiol. 3 (1) (1970) 65.
8. Henderson, D.C., Smithyman, A.M., J. Immunol. Methods 6 (1974) 115.
9. Sinclair, N.R.St.C., Chan, P.L., In: Morphological and Functional Aspects of Immunity. K. Lindahl-Kiessling, G. Alm, M.G. Hanna, Jr. (Eds.). Plenum Press, New York, p. 609 (1971).
10. White, R.G., In: Immunopotentiation. Ciba Foundation Symp. 18. ASP, Amsterdam. p.47 (1973).
11. Durkin, H.G., Theis, G.A., Thorbecke, G.J., See reference 9,p.119.
12. Gutman, G.A., Weissman, I.L., See reference 9, p.
13. Smithyman, A.M., J. Immunol. Methods. 12 (1977) 217.
14. Smithyman, A.M., J. Dev. Comp. Immunology 1 (1977) 263.
15. Fagreus, A., Acta Med. Scand. (suppl.) 204 (1930).
16. Thorbecke, G.J., Keuning, F.J., J. Infect. Dis. 98 (1956) 157.
17. Humphrey, J.H., Adv. Exp. Med. Biol. 66 (1976) 711.

GERMINAL CENTRES AND THE B-CELL SYSTEM: A SEARCH FOR THE GERMINAL

CENTRE PRECURSOR CELL IN THE RAT

Nicolette A. Gastkemper, Auk S. Wubbena and Paul
Nieuwenhuis
The Department of Histology, State University of
Groningen, Groningen, The Netherlands

INTRODUCTION

Previous work (1) suggested that Germinal Centres (GC) play a
role in B-cell differentiation (Fig.1). On the afferent side GC
are supposedly dependent upon an influx of bone marrow (BM) derived
cells: Germinal Centre Precursor Cells (GCPC). On the other hand,
lymphocytes produced by a GC are defined as Germinal Centre Derived
Cells (GCDC). Earlier experiments have shown that these cells can
perform as Antibody Forming Cell Precursors (AFCP) (1), as well as
memory cells (2). Thus, GCDC form at least part of the pool of
mature B-cells. Next to this pathway of B-cell differentiation,
mature B-cells may also originate without the intermediate stage
of a GC, as e.g. is clearly shown in germfree (GF) animals (3).

While focussing on the GC, our eventual interest is to elucidate
the role of these lymphocytic structures in the whole of the B-cell
differentiation.

The objective of the work described in this paper is to
characterize the GCPC. As a likely source for GCPC we used BM of a
highly inbred rat strain; Thoracic Duct Lymphocytes (TDL) were used
as an alternative source of B-cells.

MATERIALS AND METHODS

Rats: 8-16 weeks old rats of a highly inbred AO strain.

Experimental System: In short, various types of lymphocyte

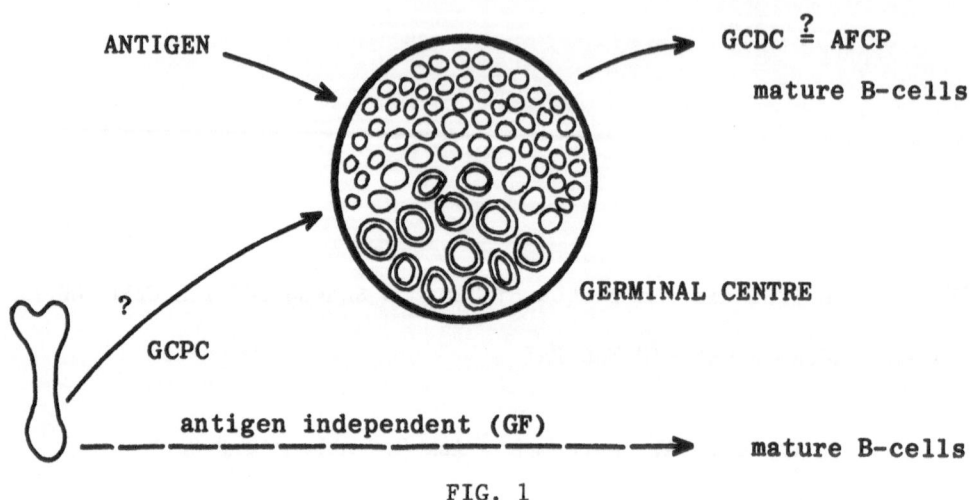

ANTIGEN

GCDC $\overset{?}{=}$ AFCP

mature B-cells

GERMINAL CENTRE

?

GCPC

antigen independent (GF)

mature B-cells

FIG. 1

cell suspensions were tested for their capacity to form GC, using a cell transfer system: cells were i.v. injected into lethally (900 rads) irradiated rats, 24 hours after irradiation, and challenged with SRBC (10^9).   Spleen samples were taken 7 or 14 days later and studied histologically for the presence of Germinal Centres.   Controls received no antigen.

Cell Suspensions:

T-cell depleted BM (BM^{T-}):   adult thymectomized rats were cannulated and drained for 7 days.   By this procedure T-cell depleted bone marrow cell suspension (BM^{T-}) can be obtained (4).

TDL: thoracic duct lymphocytes;   first overnight collection following cannulation (about 40% s-Ig$^+$).

T-TDL: sublethally (400 rads) irradiated rats with an indwelling thoracic duct cannula were given TDL (2×10^9) i.v..   TDL collected from these rats over the first 18 hours after TDL transfer, were found to be enriched for T-cells (about 5% s-Ig$^+$).

B-TDL: thymectomized, lethally (900 rads) irradiated, BM^{T-} reconstituted rats (B-rats), were cannulated 6-8 weeks after reconstitution.   The first overnight collection contained over 95% s-Ig$^+$ cells.

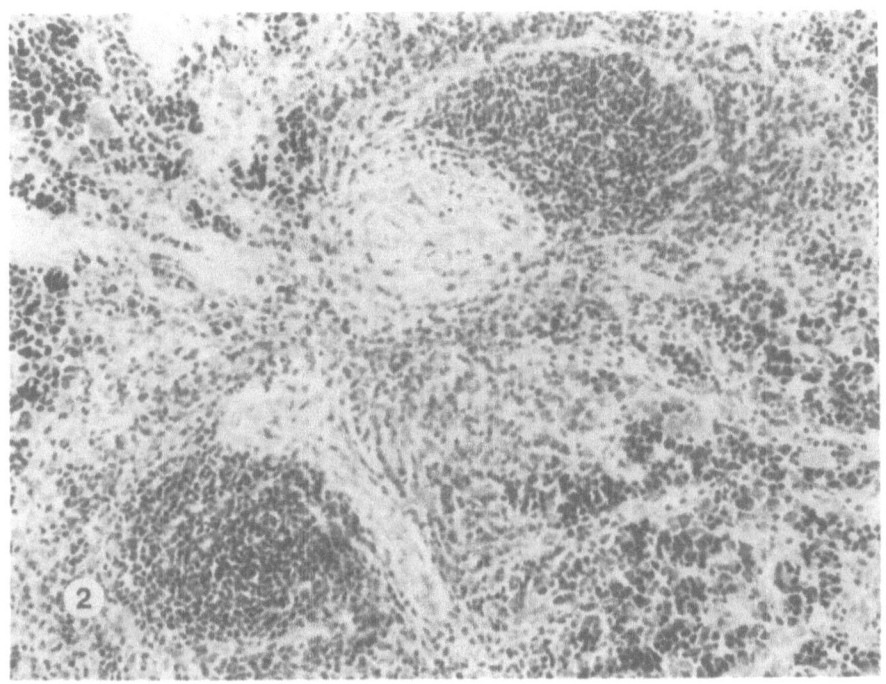

FIG. 2:   Spleen of a lethally irradiated (900 rads) rat, 14 days
after reconstitution with BM^{T-} ($5x10^7$) and challenge with SRBC
(10^9).   x 500.

RESULTS

Reconstitution experiments using BM and TDL

Our first attempt was to see whether BM cells could give rise
to GC development. 2 weeks after syngeneic BM ($5x10^7$) reconstitution
and antigenic stimulation (SRBC 10^9) newly formed primary follicles
were present in the spleen (Fig.2) Much to our surprise no GC
activity was observed. By this time, the periarteriolar lymphocyte
sheath (T-cell area) was still depleted.

In a second series of experiments we used TDL, a population
known to contain mature B-cells. Again the results were against
our expectations: now, already 7 days after cell transfer and
antigenic stimulation, active GC were present (Fig.3).

Without antigenic challenge upon TDL transfer, both B- and T-
cell areas were repopulated, however, without signs of GC activity,
once more indicating the antigen dependency of GC formation.

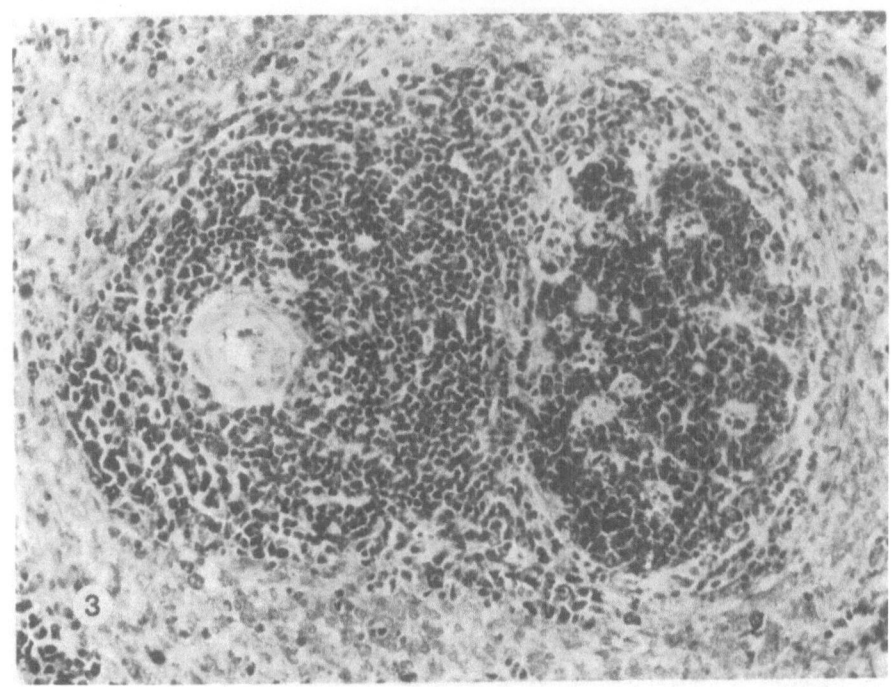

FIG. 3:   Spleen of a lethally irradiated (900 rads) rat 7 days
after reconstitution with TDL (10^8) and challenge with SRBC (10^9).
x 500.

So far, these experiments have shown that BM^{T-} reconstitution
did not restore the capacity for GC formation, i.e. over the short
period observed (14 days), and TDL apparently contain GCPC.

Reconstitution experiments using T-TDL and B-TDL

To further characterize the GCPC as present in TDL, animals
were reconstituted with T-TDL and/or B-TDL in our standard assay
system. Upon reconstitution with T-TDL, no B-cell structures were
recognizable 7 days later (Fig.4a). Only T-dependent areas were
populated. Identical results were obtained 7 days after transfer
of a thymus cell suspension. GCPC, therefore, are not considered
to be T-cells.

Upon reconstitution with B-TDL, the white pulp was found to
contain primary follicles, however, without any GC activity (Fig.4b);
T-dependent areas are empty.

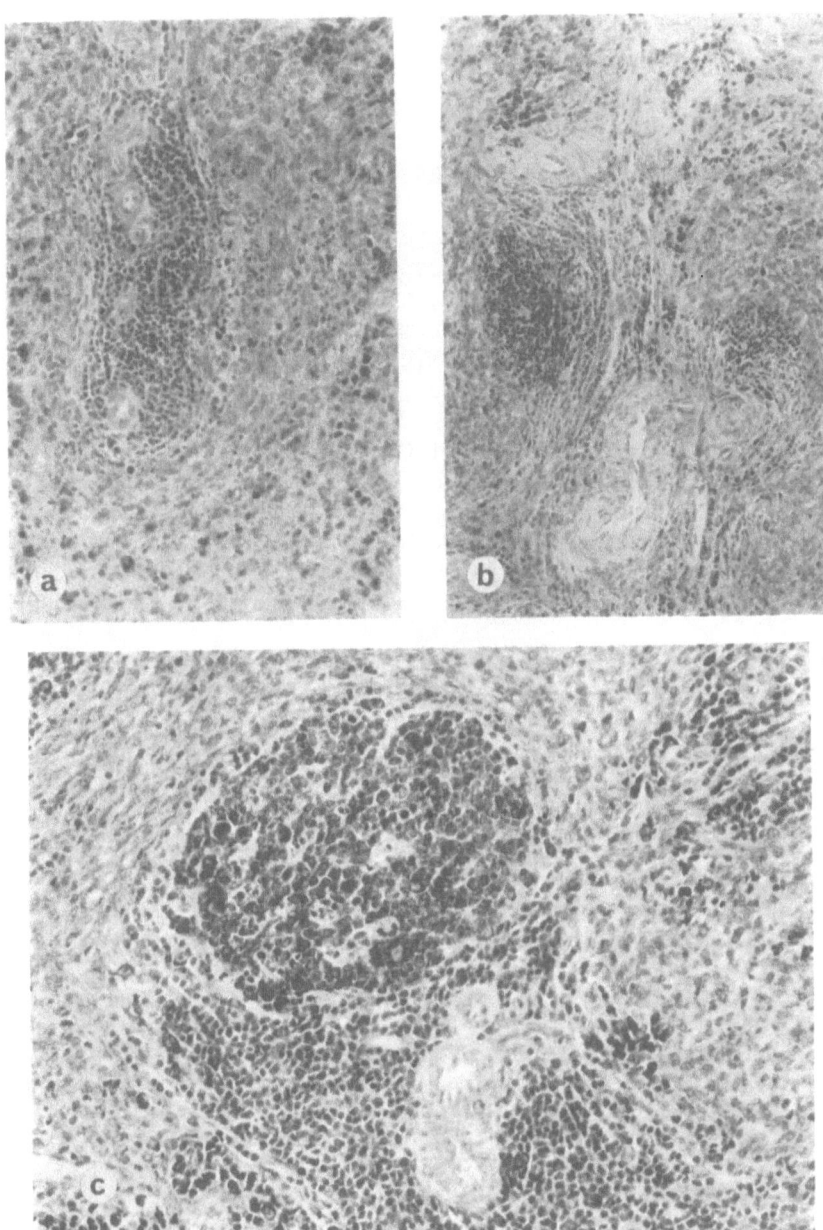

FIG. 4:   Spleens of lethally irradiated (900 rads) rats, 7 days
after challenge with SRBC (10^9) and reconstitution with :

a: T-TDL ($3x10^7$).   x 360.
b: B-TDL ($1x10^8$).   x 300.
c: T-TDL ($3x10^7$) and B-TDL ($1x10^8$).   x 500.

Upon transfer of a combination of T-TDL and B-TDL, and antigenic stimulation, well developed GC reactions were seen (Fig.4c), as after normal TDL transfer (Fig.3).

DISCUSSION

The above data clearly indicate that next to antigen both B-TDL and T-TDL are necessary for GC formation. Although formal proof is lacking, we feel that GCPC as present in TDL are not T-cells but contained within the B-cell compartment. This interpretation is supported by experiments in nude mice, where reconstitution with T-cells also led to the restoration of GC forming capacity.

Our observation of absence of GC formation shortly after BM reconstitution (up to 14 days) also can be explained by a lack of (helper?) T-cells, as B-cell regeneration well preceeds T-cell regeneration. With longer intervals, in non-thymectomized lethally irradiated animals, BM cell transfer eventually leads to restored GC forming capacity, indicating an ultimate BM origin for GCPC.

Presently, we hope to answer the following questions:

(i)   are GCPC as present in TDL s-Ig$^+$?

(ii) are $GCPC_{BM}=GCPC_{TDL}$?

Answering these questions might shed some more light on the possible significance of GC in the whole of B-cell differentiation. Recent reviews (5-8) do not take into account a possible contribution of GC to the establishment of a complete B-cell compartment. Only few (7,8) suggest antigen dependence for some stage in B-cell differentiation.

Characterisation of GCPC as part of the B-cell system and comparing its characteristics with other B lymphocytes might help to fill in the gap.

SUMMARY

At least three conditions were found to be essential for GC activity to develop:

1.   a GCPC: presumably BM derived; possibly a B-cell; present in TDL.

2.   presence of antigen,

3.   presence of T-cells.

REFERENCES

1. Nieuwenhuis, P., Keuning, F.J., Immunol. 26 (1974) 509.
2. Thorbecke, G.J., et al., Progress in Immunol. II vol. 3 (1974) 25.
3. Gordon H.A., Wostmann, B.S., Anat. Rec. 137 (1960) 65.
4. Howard, J.C., Scott, D.W., Immunol. 27 (1974) 903.
5. Parkhouse, R.M.E., Cooper, M.D., Immunol. Rev. 37 (1977) 105.
6. Vitetta, E.S., Uhr, J.W., Immunol. Rev. 37 (1977) 50.
7. Strober, S. Progress in Immunol. III (1977) 183.
8. Nossal, G.J.V., et al., Immunol. Rev. 37 (1977) 187.

MIGRATORY PATTERNS OF THE Ly SUBSETS OF T LYMPHOCYTES IN THE MOUSE

M. de Sousa, A. Freitas, [1]B. Huber, [1]H. Cantor and
E.A. Boyse

Sloan-Kettering Institute for Cancer Research, 1275 York
Avenue, New York, N.Y. 10021, U.S.A.

[1]Farber Cancer Center, Harvard Medical School

INTRODUCTION

In the preceeding paper by Gastkemper, Wubbena and Nieuwenhaus the requirement for adequate T cell 'help' in germinal center formation in the rat was illustrated (1). In the present short communication we describe briefly the results of a study of the tissues of B mice selectively reconstituted with Lyt-1 (helper) or Lyt-23 (suppressor) cell sets and demonstrate that germinal center formation appears to be related to selective reconstitution with Lyt-1, helper cells. In addition, we examine the distribution of radiolabeled Lyt-1 on Lyt-23 cells in intact syngeneic recipients.

MATERIALS AND METHODS

Preparation of selected T cell suspensions: C57 BL/6 (B6) mice were used for selection of T cell sets have been published elsewhere (2,3).

Radiolabeling of cells in vitro and autoradiographic analysis. Suspensions of Lyt-1 cells and Lyt-23 cells were labeled in vitro with ^{3}H adenosine for autoradiography according to Shand and de Sousa (4), and injected intravenously into syngeneic B6 mice (2 x 10^6 labeled cells per recipient). Sections of spleen, mesenteric lymph node, inguinal lymph nodes, lungs and Peyer's patches from B 6 mice killed 24 hrs after the i.v. injection of ^{3}H-adenosine-labeled cells were prepared for autoradiography by the technique routinely used in this laboratory (4). Labeled cell counts in the spleen and lymph

nodes were made under a Leitz Ortholux microscope, using the X40
objective, and an eyepiece equipped with a grid covering an area of
1 sq cm divided in four 0.5 x 0.5 cm squares. The numbers of labeled
cells were counted in at least eight 2.5 x 2.5 mm squares (range 4-48
squares) over randomly-selected sites within the major splenic and
lymph node regions (see below).

    Histological analysis.   Coded tissue samples of spleen and
lymph nodes from groups of 6B mice, prepared and selectively reconstituted with unselected T cells or Lyt cell sets according to Huber
et al (2), were screened particularly for the following features:
number and size of germinal centers, regional lymphoid or plasmacell repopulation, and erythropoiesis (in the spleen). The four
major splenic regions considered were: (a) red pulp; (b) marginal
zone, at the interface of the red and white pulp, surrounding the
white pulp or Malpighian bodies; (c) the outer region of the
Malpighian body, which consists mostly of B cells and where germinal
centers develop; and (d) the region which immediately surrounds the
central arteriole and is the thymus-dependent area (TDA) normally
occupied by recirculating T lymphocytes. In lymph nodes, the
corresponding four major areas are: (a) the medulla consisting of
sinuses and cords, occupied mostly by maturing B cells, plasma cells
and macrophages; (b) the deep cortical region or cortico-medullary
junction located at the interface of the cortical and medullary
regions, probably corresponding to the marginal zone in the spleen,
(c) the outer cortical area of primary nodules which consist mostly
of B cells, where germinal centers develop, corresponding to the
outer region of the Malpighian body in the spleen.

                                 RESULTS

    Autoradiography.   No statistically significant differences
were observed between the distributions of ^{3}H-adenosine labeled
unselected T or Lyt-1 cells. Both in the spleen and lymph nodes
the highest numbers of T and Lyt-1 cells were formed in the thymus-
dependent areas. Labeled Lyt-23 cells, however, did not show a
clearcut ecotaxis pattern to thymus-dependent areas but were found
in similar numbers in the outer Malpighian follicle (B cell) area
and in lymph node primary nodules. In a few animals labeled Lyt-23
cells were seen in close association with recipient polymorph
aggregates in the gut lamina propria and in the medullary cords of
lymph nodes.

    Histology.   The following histological results relate to a
period of 16-20 weeks after T cell reconstitution. After this period
of time, differences were apparent between the four major groups
examined, namely, B mice, B mice reconstituted with T cells, B mice
reconstituted with Lyt-1 or Lyt-23 cells.

B mice: The spleen and lymph node sections from B mice were
easily identified by the characteristic depletion of lymphocytes in
the TDA of spleen and lymph nodes, and the absence of germinal
centers in the B cell areas. The red pulp of the spleen showed
prominent areas of erythropoiesis and myelopoiesis.

B mice reconstituted with unselected or selected T cell sets.
The highest numbers of germinal centers were found in the spleen and
peripheral lymph nodes of B mice reconstituted with Lyt-1 cells.
Although germinal centers were also present in the tissues of B mice
reconstituted with T cells their numbers were lower than in the
spleen and lymph nodes of B Lyt-1 mice. Differences were also
observed between the ratio of red pulp and white pulp areas in the
spleens from the three groups of reconstituted B mice. The highest
proportion of splenic red pulp occupied by erythropoietic tissue was
found in the spleens of the B mice reconstituted with unselected T
cells.

DISCUSSION

The two major classes of lymphocytes, T cells and B cells, have
the capacity to ecotax, i.e., to migrate and arrange themselves in
specific environments of the peripheral lymphoid tissues (5). It has
been suggested that lymphocyte ecotaxis is a property acquired during
differentiation and related to the acquisition of specific surface
phenotypes (5).

The present results confirm that T cells known to be prepro-
grammed to perform selected T immune functions and to express different Lyt surface phenotypes (6-8) do have distinct destinations in
the spleen and lymph nodes. The autoradiographs were only examined
at 24 hours after intravenous injection and it is necessary to
examine tissues of recipients killed at later times to determine
whether the finding of Lyt-23 cells in B cell areas represents their
final ecotaxis pattern or a slower rate of migration through the
white pulp. On the other hand, the finding of fewer and smaller
germinal centers in the tissues of B mice selectively reconstituted
with Lyt-23 or in mice with pathological inbalances of T cell sets
(9) indicates that Lyt-23 cells may interact directly with cells in
B cell areas.

The finding of considerably higher amounts of erythropoietic
tissue in the spleen of B mice reconstituted with T cells than in B
mice or B mice reconstituted with Lyt-1 or Lyt-23 cells is also of
interest in the light of the recent evidence indicating that T cells
participate not only in immunological co-operation but in the
regulation of erythropoiesis (10).

REFERENCES

1. Gastkemper, N.A., Wubbena, A.S., Niewenhuis, P. Adv. Exp. Biol. Med. (1978) Present volume.
2. Huber, B., Cantor, H., Shen, F.W., Boyse, E.A. J. Exp. Med. 144 (1976) 1188.
3. Shen, F.W., Boyse, E.A., Cantor, H. Immunogenetics 2 (1975) 591.
4. Shand, J.A., de Sousa, M. J. Immunol. Methods 6 (1974) 141.
5. de Sousa, M. Contemp. Topics Immunobiol. 2 (1973) 119.
6. Boyse, E.A., Cantor, H. in: The Molecular Basis of Cell-Cell Interactions: Proc. of the First Int. Conference, La Jolla, Calif., p. 249 (1978).
7. Cantor, H., Boyse, E.A. J. Exp. Med. 141 (1975) 1376.
8. Cantor, H., Boyse, E.A. Contemp. Topics Immunol. 7 (1977) 47.
9. Reske-Kunz, A.B., Scheid, M.P., de Sousa, M., Boyse, E.A. Adv. Exp. Biol. Med. (1978) Present volume.
10. Nathan, D.G., Hess, L., Hillman, D.G., Clarke, B., Beard, J., Merler, E., Housman, B.E. J. Exp. Med 142 (1978) 324.

ACKNOWLEDGEMENTS

The present work was done with support from the following NIH grants: CA 08748, CA 10267 and RR 05534.

CORRELATION OF IMMUNOGENETIC AND HISTOLOGICAL CHANGES IN IMMUNO-DEFICIENT MUTANT hr/hr MICE

Angelika B. Reske-Kunz, Margrit P. Scheid, Maria de Sousa and Edward A. Boyse

Memorial Sloan-Kettering Cancer Center, 1275 York Avenue, New York, N.Y. 10021, USA

INTRODUCTION

At least the majority of peripheral T lymphocytes of the mouse can be classified serologically into three sets of cells that express different Lyt surface phenotypes, denoted Lyt-1, Lyt-23 and Lyt-123 (1). Each of these three sets is programmed for different immune functions (2). In brief, cells of the Lyt-1 set have helper-amplifier effects, whereas the functions of the Lyt-23 set are concerned with cell-mediated cytotoxicity and with suppression; the present view of the Lyt-123 set is that it constitutes an inter-mediary pool from which the two other T-cell sets are derived; other possible functions of this set are less well defined.

Considering that the peripheral T-cell population comprises cell sets with different genetic programs, in which distinctive surface phenotypes and functions are manifest, it seems highly probable that there are hereditary immunological disorders in which one particular T-cell set is affected selectively, or in which the natural balance between the three cell sets is disturbed, as a result of mutation.

This was the reason why we undertook a study of the represent-ation of the Lyt sets in mice of the HRS/J strain which carry the mutation hairless (hr). In the homozygous state, this mutation causes complete loss of hair in the first few weeks of life. More-over, these mice undergo a premature decline in immunocompetence (3), and it has been proposed that this may be responsible for the higher incidence of leukemia in mutant homozygotes as compared with heterozygous hr/+ littermates (5).

MATERIALS AND METHODS

Mice.   HRS/J breeders were obtained from the Jackson
Laboratory, Bar Harbor, Maine. All matings were female haired
(hr/+) and male hairless (hr/hr) mice, resulting in 50% mutant
progeny.

Antisera.   For details of preparation and use of antisera to
Lyt-1.2 and Lyt-3.2 see Shen et al (6).

Antibody-complement-dependent cytotoxicity assay.   50 µl spleen
cells at 5 x 10^6/ml (Tris-ammonium chloride-treated, ^{51}Cr-labeled for
30 minutes with 250 µCi per 30 x 10^6 cells in Medium 199 containing
2% heat-inactivated fetal calf serum) were incubated with 50 µl antiserum (pre-determined dilution in phosphate buffered saline (PBS);
or as control with normal mouse serum (NMS)) for 30 minutes on ice,
washed once, brought up in 0.1 ml freshly thawed rabbit serum (pre-
determined dilution in PBS) and incubated for an additional 30
minutes at 37°C. The rabbit serum (source of complement) was
selected for low natural cytotoxicity against mouse cells and for
high complement activity. Percent lysis was calculated by the
formula:

$$\frac{cpm \ (antisera) \ - \ cpm \ (NMS)}{cpm \ (freeze\text{-}thaw) \ - \ cpm \ (NMS)} \ x \ 100$$

Calculation of the Lyt subsets (1).   The proportion of cells
displaying one or more Lyt antigens were estimated from the lytic
effects of anti-Lyt-1 and anti-Lyt-3 antisera used either alone or
in combination.

Histology.   Spleen sections were stained with methyl green
pyronine (4). Coded specimens were examined especially for number
and size of germinal centers.

RESULTS AND DISCUSSION

Enumeration of the Lyt subsets

The following data on Lyt set distribution represent comparisons
of age-matched and sex-matched hairless homozygotes with heterozygous
littermates not exhibiting hair loss. We shall focus on the Lyt-1
and Lyt-123 sets, because the representation of Lyt-23 cells in the
HRS strain, as in other strains of mice, is too small for accurate
estimation by present conventional serological methods.

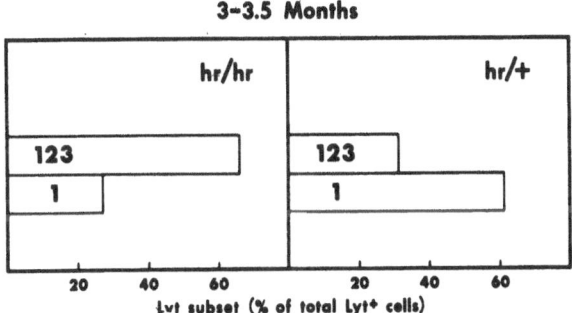

FIG. 1:   Proportional representation of Lyt subsets in spleens of hr/hr compared with hr/+ mice at 3-3.5 months of age.   (Other data show no striking differences between hr/hr and hr/+ numbers of Thy-1[+] T cells or of B cells present in spleens.)

Up to the age of about 2 1/2 months the relative proportions of Lyt-1 and Lyt-123 sets are similar in both genotypes.

Around the age of 3-3 1/2 months, however, there is a dramatic difference between the two genotypes. Fig.1 shows the Lyt set composition in spleens of hr/hr homozygotes (left-hand panel) and of hr/+ littermates (right-hand panel). These data are calculated as percentage of the total Lyt[+] population present in spleen. In hr/hr homozygotes there is a highly significant comparative increase in Lyt-123 cells, and an equally substantial comparative decrease in Lyt-1 cells. These changes in the proportions of Lyt-1 and Lyt-123 cells are not accompanied by any marked change in the proportion of Thy-1[+] T-cells or of B-cells.

In older mice, selected for absence of obvious leukemic changes, the subset composition is again similar in the two genotypes. Our tentative interpretation is that the mutation hr is not fully recessive and that the shift in proportional representation of Lyt subsets occurs also in hr/+ heterozotes, but at a later age.

Histology

In other studies lack of Lyt-1 cells has been associated histo-logically with scarcity and small size of germinal centers in spleen (M. de Sousa et al, this volume, and manuscript in preparation).

The results of similar histological studies of HRS mice may be summarized as follows:

Up to around two months of age the number and size of germinal centers is similar in spleen of hr/hr and hr/+ origin. In hr/hr mice, however, abnormal aggregates of lymphoid cells begin to develop in red pulp sinuses and around the marginal zone. The nature of the aggregates is not yet clear.

From about 3 months of age onward, the decline of Lyt-1 cells in hr/hr mice is paralleled by scarcity of germinal centers. The lymphoid cell aggregates are now more prominent. Further histo-logical findings suggest that the ability to form germinal centers is similarly diminished in heterozygotes at a later age.

Thus a direct relationship may exist between the aberration in representation of T-cell sets and changes in splenic morphology. We are now studying the question of whether the Lyt subset disturbance we have described accords with alterations in functional capacities as revealed by tests of immune function in vitro.

REFERENCES

1.   Cantor, H., Boyse, E.A., J. Exp. Med., 141 (1975) 1376.
2.   Cantor, H., Boyse, E.A., Cold Spring Harbor Symp. Quant. Biol. XLI (1976) 23.
3.   Heiniger, H.J., Meier, H., Kaliss, N., Cherry, M., Chen, H.W., Stoner, R.D., Cancer Research 34 (1974) 201.
4.   Lillie, R.D., Fullmer, H.M., Histopathologic Technic and Practical Histochemistry. McGraw Hill Book Co., New York (1976).
5.   Meier, H., Myers, D.D., Huebner, R.J., Proc. Nat. Acad. Sci. USA 63 (1969) 759.
6.   Shen, F-W., Boyse, E.A., Cantor, H., Immunogenetics 2 (1976) 591.

ACKNOWLEDGEMENTS

We acknowledge the technical assistance of Ms. P. Good in the preparation of the histological material.

This work was supported in part by grants AI-00270, CA-08748, CA-22241, and HD-08415 from the National Institutes of Health. EAB is American Cancer Society Research Professor of Cell Surface Immunogenetics.

MORPHOLOGY OF THE EXTRAFOLLICULAR ZONE AND PSEUDO-FOLLICLES OF THE RAT LYMPH NODE, AND THEIR ROLE IN LYMPHOCYTE TRAFFIC

G. Sainte-Marie and F.-S. Peng

Université de Montréal, Département d'Anatomie,

C.P. 6128, Montréal, Québec, Canada

In a previous 3-dimensional study of the histology of the rat node (1,2), we reported that the small lymphocyte population of the cortex is mainly distributed into two morphologycally distinguishable components which we named : the extrafollicular zone and the pseudo-follicles. These lymphocytes are distinguished, on the other hand, into B and T cells which are said to be concentrated, respectively, in a B and T zone (paracortex) whose outlinings remain to be precised. An aim of further works was to complete the morphological study of the pseudo-follicles. Another objective was to attempt clarifying the topographical relation existing between the B and T zones, and the actual morphological structures which are the extrafollicular zone and the pseudo-follicles. A third goal was to determine the respective role of the latter two morphological components in the lymphocyte traffic within nodes.

Three types of investigations were carried out : a 3-dimensional study of the morphology of pseudo-follicles (in preparation) ; secondly, experiments dealing with the in vivo RNA labelling of the lymphocyte population of both components (in preparation) ; and, thirdly, experiments involving the transfer of labelled lymphoid cells (3-6).

It was found that each pseudo-follicle is centered on the opening of an afferent lymphatic vessel (Fig.1) and, that pseudo-follicles vary in number from one to several per node. The 3-dimensional study further revealed that postcapillary venules are concentrated at the periphery of these structures while they are regularly distributed in the extrafollicular zone.

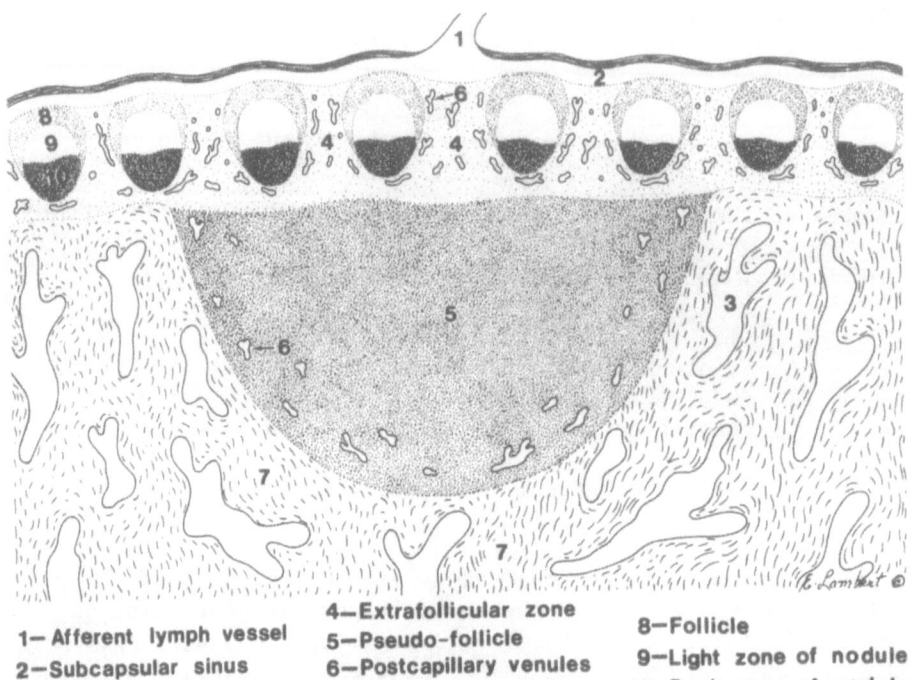

1— Afferent lymph vessel	4—Extrafollicular zone	8—Follicle
2—Subcapsular sinus	5—Pseudo-follicle	9—Light zone of nodule
3—Medullary sinus	6—Postcapillary venules	10—Dark zone of nodule
	7—Medullary cords	

FIG. 1:   Schematic illustration of the architecture of the rat node.

While the usual procedure for in vivo RNA labelling fails to label tissue lymphocytes, we succeeded in doing so by combining an injection of a large dose of tritiated uridine or cytidine (10 - 20 μC/gbw) with long radioautographic exposure times (150 - 250 days). Then, unlike those of the extrafollicular zone, the lymphocytes of the pseudo-follicles are strongly labelled (Figs.2,3). Hence, the results revealed that the overall lymphocyte population of the two morphologically distinguishable components behave differently with respect to the rate of incorporation of these RNA precursors. If the current concept that lymphocytes strongly labelled with uridine are T cells is correct, the results would demonstrate that pseudo-follicles are T zones whereas the extrafollicular zone and the follicles around nodules are B zones. The alternative explanation is that the strong labelling reveals not so much the origin of the cells in the pseudo-follicles than their greater metabolic activity. Interestingly, the lymphocyte population of the thymus of the same animals was much less labelled than that of pseudo-follicles.

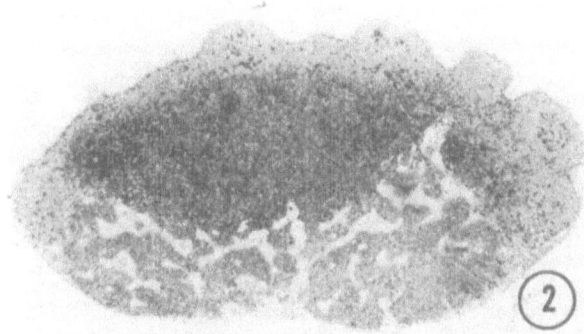

FIG. 2:   Rat node. Unlike the extrafollicular zone, the pseudo-follicle is strongly labelled with uridine-³H (unstained radio-autograph).

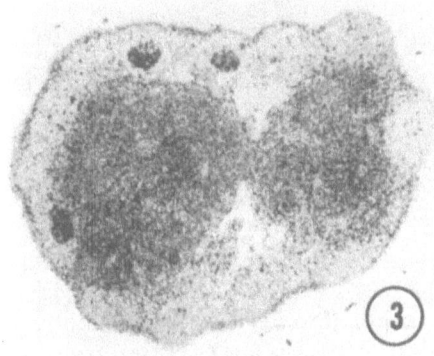

FIG. 3:   Same but, due to cutting incidence, the two pseudo-follicles do not show a typical semi-spheric shape. Note that nodules (arrow) are also strongly labelled.

Particularly less labelled were the thymic medullary lymphocytes which, as to be seen later, do migrate into pseudo-follicles.

    Observations on the traffic, into nodes, of transferred labelled lymphoid cells revealed a further physiological difference between the extrafollicular zone and the pseudo-follicles. During the first hours after transfusion of labelled medullary small lymphocytes, such cells became scattered in the extrafollicular zone and the pseudo-follicles (Fig.4). Then, labelled cells were seen in the subcapsular sinus as well as in the wall of the postcapillary

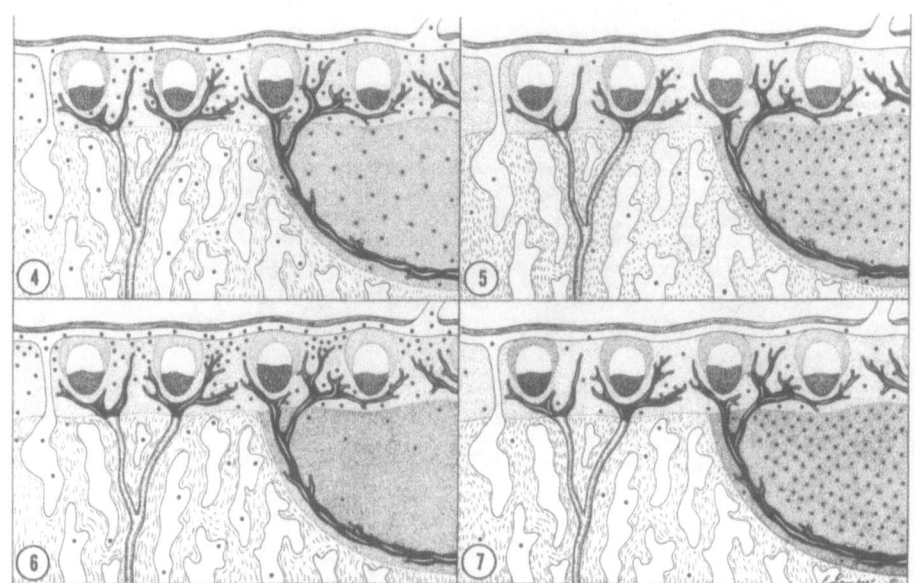

FIGS. 4 and 5:   Distribution in nodes of labelled medullary small
thymocytes (black dots), respectively, 3 and 24 hr after transfusion.

FIGS. 6 and 7:   Same, but in draining nodes after local injection.

venules which indicated that they had entered the nodes by both ways.
At 24 hours, however, labelled cells were few in the extrafollicular
zone while many were concentrated in the centers of the pseudo-
follicles (Fig.5). The latter observation resembled that of others
(7). In a second experiment, similar cells were transferred but in
the mediastinum. Five minutes later, labelled cells were present in
the subcapsular sinus of draining nodes; and, at 15 minutes, some
were present in the underlining peripheral layer of the extrafollicular zone. At 3 hours, labelled cells were scattered in the extrafollicular zone and some had entered the pseudo-follicles (Fig.6).
At 24 hours, as was the case in preceeding experiment, the labelled
cells had become rare in the extrafollicular zone but a large number
was concentrated in the center of pseudo-follicles (Fig.7). The
observations thus revealed that cells can migrate within a few hours
from the subcapsular sinus through the thickness of the extrafollicular zone ; and, that transferred cells entering a node via its
subcapsular sinus can be accumulated in its pseudo-follicles 24 hours
later. The results further showed that part of the incoming cells

leaves a node from 30 minutes to a few hours later, while part remains in the pseudo-follicles. The latter cells could represent the fraction of circulating lymphocytes that have become involved in an immunological process occurring in a node. Hence, in both above experiments, the extrafollicular zone appeared as a zone of rapid migration of lymphocytes whereas the pseudo-follicles appeared as a zone of retention of part of the circulating lymphocytes. The particular behavior of the pseudo-follicles was also observed in an experiment in which labelled cells from the thymic cortex as well as medulla were injected in the mediastinum. The findings were similar to those of preceeding experiment except that, at 24 hours, labelled cells were rare in the pseudo-follicles while abundant in medullary cords. Here, the pseudo-follicles had been penetrated by few of the transferred cells. Probably only the small minority of lymphocytes from the thymic medulla had done so for, being mature, they could participate in an immunological process.

In conclusion, the results demonstrated that, on the whole, the extrafollicular zone and the pseudo-follicles are two morphologically distinguishable components with a lymphocyte population having a somewhat different physiological behavior. However, while we sofar considered a pseudo-follicle as a homogeneous structural unit, some results now suggest to us that one should possibly distinguish the periphery from the center of the structure. Indeed, the periphery differs morphologically from the center by its abundance of post-capillary venules in which it resembles the extrafollicular zone. Moreover, experiments on transfer of labelled lymphocytes revealed that such cells accumulate only in their centers. Again, the periphery of pseudo-follicles resembles the extrafollicular zone as it also appears as a zone of rapid lymphocyte migration. Both facts can indicate that the periphery of a pseudo-follicle could be considered as an extension of the extrafollicular zone surrounding a differently behaving component restricted to the central portion of a pseudo-follicle.

REFERENCES

1. Sainte-Marie et al. Structures of the lymph node and their possible function during the immune response. Rev. Can. Biol. 27 (1968) 191.
2. Sainte-Marie et al. Structures of the lymph node and their possible function during the immune response. In "Regulation of haematopoiesis". Edit. by A.S. Gordon Appleton-Century-Crofts, N.Y. 2 (1970) 1339.
3. Sainte-Marie et al. A study of the mode of lymphocyte recirculation in the dog. Ann. Immunol. (Inst. Pasteur) 126C (1975) 481.

4.   Sainte-Marie et al.   Migration of intramediastinally injected
     thymocytes in draining nodes.   Ann. Immunol. (Inst. Pasteur)
     126C (1975) 501.
5.   Sainte-Marie et al.   Migration into pseudo-follicles of draining
     lymph nodes of medullary small thymocytes injected in the medi-
     astinal cavity.   Rev. Can. Biol. 34 (1975) 205.
6.   Sainte-Marie et al.   Migration into pseudo-follicles of lymph
     nodes of transfused medullary small thymocytes.   J. Ret. End.
     Soc. 20 (1976) 51.
7.   Gowans, J.L., Knight, E.J., The route of re-circulation of
     lymphocytes in the rat.   Proc. roy. Soc. B, 159 (1964) 257.

LYMPHOCYTE-HIGH ENDOTHELIAL VENULE INTERACTIONS:

EXAMINATION OF SPECIES SPECIFICITY

Eugene Butcher, Roland Scollay, and Irving Weissman

Department of Pathology, Stanford Medical School

Stanford, California 94305

INTRODUCTION

Lymphocytes enter lymph nodes from the blood by adhering to and migrating through the specialized endothelium of post-capillary high endothelial venules (HEV). Recently, two in vitro assays of this lymphocyte-HEV interaction have been developed, one utilizing arterial perfusion of labeled lymphocytes through an isolated mesenteric lymph node chain (1), and the other measuring adherence of lymphocytes to HEV in glutaraldehyde fixed frozen sections of rat lymph nodes (2). The availability of these in vitro techniques makes it possible to examine many aspects of lymphocyte/high endothelial cell recognition and interaction. In the present study we have combined these techniques (modified for use in mice) with in vivo homing assays to investigate the evolutionary conservation of lymphocyte-HEV adherence mechanisms. We have compared the ability of lymphocytes from several species to interact with mouse HEV. In principle, these studies will provide the background for more detailed investigations of the molecular basis of this cell-cell interaction.

MATERIALS AND METHODS

Six to eight week old Balb/c x C57BL/Jackson Fl mice, 5-8 week old Lewis rats, 6-10 week old White Leghorn or New Hampshire Red chickens, and 6 week old or one year old New Zealand White rabbits were used in the present experiments. Human spleen was obtained from laparotomy specimens from young (15 and 24 year old) patients with Hodgkin's disease, in which there was no macroscopic abdominal involvement.

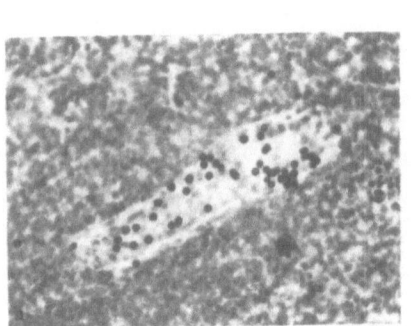 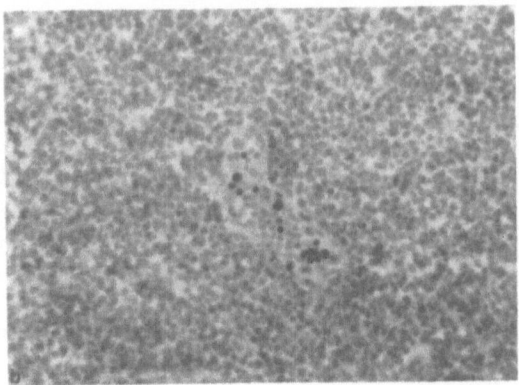

FIG. 1:   Lymphocytes adhering to HEV in frozen sections of mouse
mesenteric node after in vitro incubation at 7°C.   a) mouse mesenteric node cells, and b) chicken spleen cells.

In vivo experiments: Donor lymphocytes were labeled with
^{3}H-uridine and/or ^{3}H-leucine and 0.8-1.0 x 10^8 viable cells were
injected i.v. into mice. At various time points, organs were
removed, fixed, and sectioned for autoradiography. Developed
autoradiographs were stained with hematoxylin and eosin. Mesenteric
node sections from 15 minute and 4 hour time points were randomly
scanned with a 40x objective. In order to quantitate initial HEV
adherence and subsequent transmural migration by sample cells, the
number of cells in HEV, in the number of cells in the paracortical
parenchyma, and the percent paracortex in each field were determined.

Frozen section technique: 100 microliters of a sample cell
suspension (2-2.5 x 10^7 cells/ml in BSS containing 1% BSA) were
incubated at 7°C for 30-45 minutes on freshly cut unfixed 10 micron
thick frozen sections of mouse mesenteric node in wax pencil circles
approximately 1.2 cm in diameter. The medium was removed and the
adherent cells were fixed to the section with 1% glutaraldehyde in
cold PBS for at least 10 minutes. After fixation, nonadherent cells
were gently rinsed off the section, which could then be stained with
Giemsa or thionine for light microscopy (Fig.1). To allow quantitative comparisons, an internal standard population of fluorescent
mouse lymphocytes (labeled by incubation with 60 micro g/ml fluorescein   isothiocyanate (FITC) for 15 minutes at 37°C, or 5-50 micro
g/ml rhodamine isothiocyanate (RITC) for 15 minutes at room temper-

ature) was mixed with each sample population prior to in vitro incubation on frozen sections. A positive control sample of mesenteric
node lymphocytes (MNL), and a negative control sample of erythrocytes
or formalin fixed lymphocytes were included in each experiment. After
incubation and fixation, solitary fluorescent standard cells or unlabeled sample cells adherent over HEV were counted by fluorescence
and dark field microscopy. Data from at least 5 separate mesenteric
node sections were pooled for each sample. The data were expressed
as the specific adherence ratio (SAR):

$$SAR = \frac{\text{sample cells on HEV/standard cells on HEV}}{\text{sample cells in suspension/standard cells in suspension}}$$

In order to simplify comparisons between experiments, a specific adherence index (SAI) was calculated for each sample population
relating the adherence ability of the sample to that of the positive
control (MNL).

$$SAI = \frac{\text{SAR (sample cells) - SAR (negative control cells)}}{\text{SAR (MNL) - SAR (negative control cells)}}$$

The standard deviation of each ratio was calculated by the
delta method. In another study we have extensively characterized
this frozen section assay and have demonstrated its reproducibility
(Butcher and Weissman, in preparation).

Perfusion system: A trocar was inserted into the left
ventricle of an anesthetized mouse, and the right atrium was incised
to allow efflux of the perfusate (3). The trocar was attached to
an i.v. infusion apparatus allowing control of perfusion at 2-3
ml/minute and 37°C, and a mixture of 10^8 ^{3}H-leucine labeled sample
cells, 10^8 RITC labeled standard cells, and 10^8 formalin fixed FITC
labeled thymocytes (as an internal negative control) were perfused
in 15 ml medium 199 containing 1% BSA. The mesenteric node was
removed and 6 micron frozen sections were cut, fixed, and processed
for autoradiography. Sections were developed after exposure proportional to the observed cpm/10^6 cells of each sample, and solitary
standard (RITC labeled) and sample (radiolabeled) cells in HEV of
several sections were counted.

RESULTS AND DISCUSSION

Species specificity of lymphocyte-HEV interactions as studied by in
vivo homing experiments

In vivo homing studies were carried out to determine if xenogeneic lymphocytes were capable of recognizing, adhering to, and
migrating through mouse HEV. After i.v. injection both syngeneic
and xenogeneic lymphocytes were seen in mouse mesenteric node HEV.

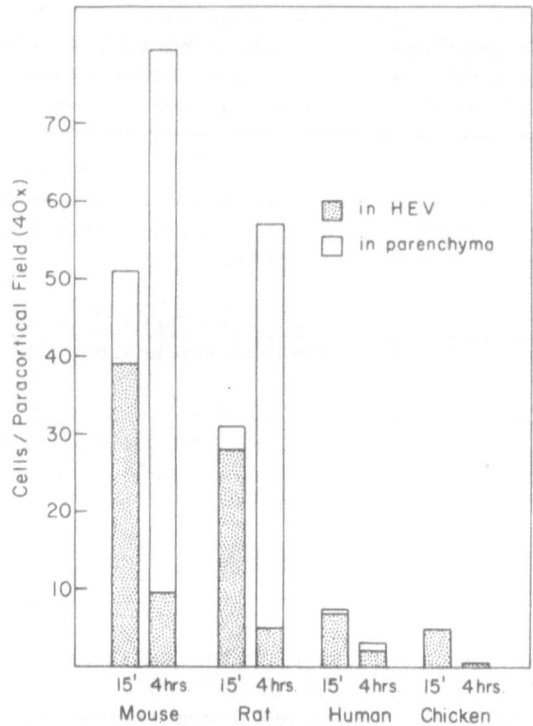

FIG. 2:   Localization of radio-labelled syngeneic and xenogeneic lymphocytes in mouse mesenteric lymph node paracortex 15 minutes and 4 hours after i.v. injection.

The number of cells localizing in HEV 15 minutes after injection was inversely related to the evolutionary distance between the lymphocyte donor and the mouse host (Fig.2).   These results may reflect the relative ability of cells to recognize and adhere to mouse HEV, but could also be due to variable sequestration or destruction of lymphocytes in the liver, lung or spleen.   This point will be clarified by the in vitro studies described below.

There were also differences in the ability of the lymphocyte populations to cross the venule wall into the paracortex.   In this respect, mouse and rat lymphocytes behaved similarly: large numbers were seen in HEV at 15 minutes, but by 4 hours the majority of lymphocytes in the section were in the lymph node parenchyma.   On the other hand, human and chicken lymphocytes demonstrated a relative inability to migrate through the HEV wall.   At 4 hours, the ratio of cells in the paracortex to cells in HEV was 7 for mouse lympho- cytes, 10 for rat lymphocytes, and 0.5 for human lymphocytes (Fig.2). In over 30 microscope fields of mesenteric node taken 4 hours after injecting mice with chicken cells, only 4 labeled cells were seen

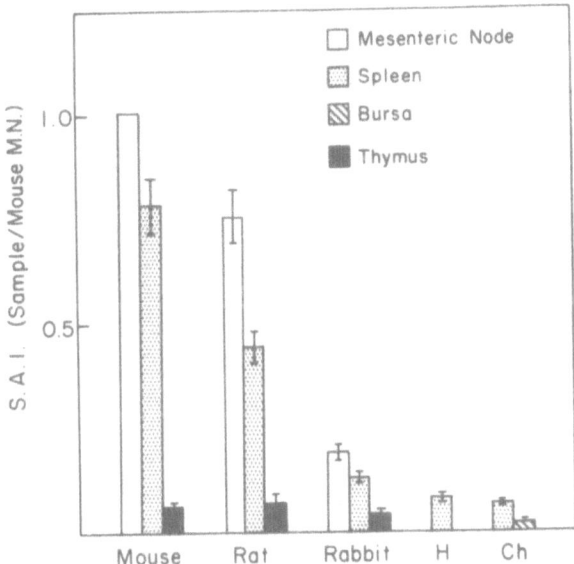

FIG. 3: Comparison of HEV adherence of syngeneic and xenogeneic lymphocytes in the <u>in vitro</u> frozen section assay. Except for the thymuses, the bursa,and the human spleen, the bar for each sample represents pooled data from 2 to 3 replicate determinations.

which appeared to be outside HEV. Seven cells per field would have been expected if the cells which had initially adhered had behaved like mouse lymphocytes. Thus the ability of xenogeneic lymphocytes to enter the lymph node was not proportional to their initial HEV adherence.

Three possible explanations are suggested for this seeming disparity between initial HEV adherence and subsequent transmural migration.

1. It is possible that lymphocyte entry into lymph nodes involves at least two independent events: a) adherence to HEVs; b) transmural migration into the lymph node parenchyma. The adherence property could have been conserved to a greater degree during evolution than the property of specific transmural migration.

2. Interaction with the host immune system may have immobilized the lymphocytes or destroyed them soon after adherence (e.g. with "natural" antibodies).

3. Rapid release of HEV-adherent human or chicken lymphocytes could have prevented transmural migration. The total number of human or chicken cells per field decreased between 15 minutes and

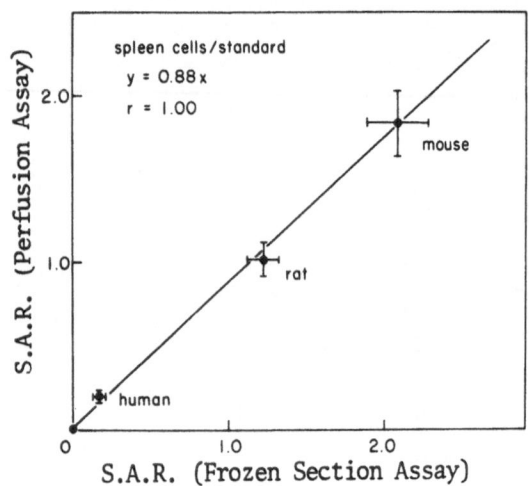

FIG. 4:   Comparison of the frozen section and vascular perfusion
assays of HEV adherence: the relative HEV adherence of mouse, rat,
and human spleen cells was nearly identical at 7°C on a frozen
section and at 37°C during single pass vascular perfusion.   The
results of two separate perfusions were pooled for each sample.

4 hours (in contrast to a marked increase in total rat and mouse
lymphocytes), suggesting that lymphocyte-HEV adherence may be
reversible and adherent cells may return to the blood.   (However,
we could not exclude the possibility that the observed decrease in
human and chicken lymphocytes was due to cell death).

Species specificity of lymphocyte-HEV interactions as studied by in vitro frozen section technique

    In order to quantitate the effect of evolutionary divergence,
we compared the ability of spleen and, where available, lymph node
cells from mouse, rat, rabbit, human,and chicken to adhere to mouse
HEV using the in vitro frozen section technique.   Immature (thymic
and bursal) lymphocytes were included in the study for comparison
with the mature spleen and lymph node populations (Fig.3).   Comparing
the data for spleen cells, SAI decreases as the evolutionary separation increases (in the order presented in the figure).   Thus in
vitro quantitation confirmed the in vivo results described above.
The data also demonstrated in all cases examined that adherence
remained a property more highly expressed by lymphocytes from
secondary (lymph node and spleen) than from primary (thymus, bursa)

lymphoid organs, suggesting that we were indeed measuring a specific functional property of mature (presumably recirculating) lymphocytes.

Comparison of frozen section and perfusion assays

In order to determine, as nearly as possible, the in vivo relevance of the quantitative results obtained in the frozen section assay, we compared the ability of mouse, rat, and human spleen cells to adhere to mouse HEV in both the frozen section technique and the single pass systemic vascular perfusion system. The results are shown in Fig. 4. The two systems give statistically indistinguishable results, suggesting that the in vitro system is an adequate model for investigation of in vivo lymphocyte-HEV adherence mechanisms.

CONCLUSION

We have demonstrated that the ability of xenogeneic lymphocytes to adhere to and to migrate through mouse HEV decreases with evolutionary separation (in the order mouse, rat, rabbit, human, and chicken). It is remarkable that chickens, which are separated from mice by over 500 million years of evolution and which lack well organized lymph nodes of the mammalian type, nonetheless have lymphocytes capable of recognizing and adhering to mouse HEV.

Complex cell-cell recognition and interaction phenomena of several types are known to cross species barriers - e.g. tissue specific reaggregation of dissociated xenogeneic embryonic cells (4), and long term xenograft acceptance by nude mice (5). However, precise quantitation of these interactions among cells of widely divergent species has not been performed. The interaction of lymphocytes with the endothelial cells of postcapillary venules is an example of a complex cell/cell recognition phenomenon which lends itself to quantitative in vitro study. It is hoped that further study will provide insight into the molecular basis of this interaction, as well as an understanding of the rate and the mechanism of co-evolution of these very different cell types.

REFERENCES

1. Sedgley, M., Ford, W.L., Cell Tissue Kinet. 9 (1976) 231.
2. Stamper, H.B., Woodruff, J.J., J. Exp. Med. 144 (1976) 828.
3. Van Ewijk, W., Verzijden, W.H.M., Van der Kwast, Th.H., Luijex-Meijer, S.W.M., Cell Tiss. Res. 149 (1974) 43.
4. Moscona, A.A., Proc. Natl. Acad. Sci. U.S. 43 (1957) 184.
5. Rygaard, J., Thymus and Self, John Wiley and Sons, London (1973).

ACKNOWLEDGEMENTS

    E.B. is a Post-Doctoral Fellow in Experimental Pathology.
R.S. is a Leukemia Society of America Special Fellow. It is a
pleasure to acknowledge the excellent secretarial assistance of
M. Beers and D. Chestnut.

BASIC MECHANISMS OF LYMPHOCYTE RECIRCULATION IN LEWIS RATS

Arthur O. Anderson, N.D. Anderson and J.D. White

USAMRIID, Fort Detrick, Maryland 21701, and the
John Hopkins Hospital, Baltimore, Maryland 21205, USA

INTRODUCTION

Recirculating lymphocytes emigrate from the blood into lymph nodes by selectively crossing the walls of high endothelial venules (HEV) (1). This process depends upon the ability of lymphocytes to attach to endothelium via membrane receptors (2,3) and on the capacity of the lymphocytes to propel themselves across HEV. We studied the role of microfilaments and microtubules (4-10) in attachment and migration of recirculating lymphocytes by using the cytoskeletal probes cytochalasin-A (CA) and colchicine (Col). The results indicate that both CA and Col inhibit entry of lymphocytes into lymph nodes. However, CA interferes with locomotion more than it affects recognition, and Col blocks recognition without significantly affecting locomotion.

MATERIALS AND METHODS

The adherent cell index for rat lymphocytes was determined in isolated perfused mesenteric lymph nodes prepared for scanning (SEM) and transmission (TEM) electron microscopy by previously described techniques (2). Thoracic duct lymphocytes (TDL) were collected from Bollman fistulae (1) for 2 days, after which the rats were euthanized. TDL were washed and resuspended in media to equal 1×10^8 cells/ml. ^{3}H-Uridine (spec. activity, 21 Ci/mmol) was added to a final concentration of 10 uCi/ml and the culture was incubated at 37° for 1 hour. The cells were washed and resuspended, 4×10^8 labeled lymphocytes were injected IV. Labeled and unlabeled TDL were used fresh or after incubation in media containing:

73

a)   cytochalasin-A (0.2 - 10.0 µg/ml),

b)   colchicine (10^{-8} - 10^{-2} M),

c)   lumicolchicine (10^{-4} M) prepared by the method of Wilson and
      Friedkin (7), or

d)   TDL incubated at 50° for 20 minutes.

Each suspension was assessed for viability by trypan blue dye
exclusion, spontaneous locomotion during 10-minute incubation at
37°, and examined by SEM and TEM. All lymphoid tissues, liver and
lungs were excised at timed intervals, weighed and disrupted in a
tissue homogenizer. Aliquots were counted in a Beckman LS-233
scintillation counter. Lymph nodes for autoradiography were fixed,
embedded in methacrylate and sectioned at 1.0-µm thickness. Sections
were dipped in Kodak NTB-2 liquid emulsion and exposed for 8 - 12
weeks at 4°. After developing and fixing, the slides were stained
and the distribution of labeled lymphocytes was tabulated per 10
high-powered fields.

                                RESULTS

     Characterization of TDL used in these studies.   Untreated TDL,
which were 98.6% viable by trypan blue dye exclusion, exhibited
15.6 $\pm$ 3.2 % (mean $\pm$ SD) spontaneous locomotion during 10 minutes
of viewing by phase microscopy at 37°. Locomotion began when a
lymphocyte placed its hyaline pseudopod onto the surface. This
initiated a wave of cytoplasmic contraction which flowed from front
to rear as the cell advanced. Each cell rounded up after every 3 - 9
minute cycle of movement. SEM of moving lymphocytes confirmed the
presence of this avillous constriction ring (Fig. 1a). Stationary
TDL were rounded and had numerous microvilli on their surfaces
(Fig. 1b). In TEM studies, microvilli and cortical cytoplasm
excluded ribosomes and other organelles, but did not appear to
contain obvious microfilaments or microtubules. However, approximately 12 segments of 25-nm microtubules were seen within a 1.0-µm
radius from the centrioles in cells where the centrioles could be
located.

     Cytochalasin-A (0.2 - 8.0 µg/ml) treated lymphocytes showed
markedly reduced spontaneous locomotion. Some TDL exhibited asymmetric and distorted locomotion. Blebs were extruded and retracted
along lateral surfaces of moving lymphocytes. Doses of CA above
4.0 µg/ml completely immobilized TDL without affecting viability
(Tab. 1). The effects of CA on locomotion were not reversed by
washing and re-incubation in fresh media. SEM showed loss of
microvilli and zeiotic blebbing (Fig. 1c). Doses above 2.0 µg/ml

TABLE 1:   In Vitro Effects of Cytochalasin-A on Lymphocytes

Dose µg/ml	Phase microscopy of living cells		% loss of MV	Ultrastructure % with blebs	Aggregated microfilaments
	% viable	% motile			
0	98.6	15..6	0	0	0
0.2	95.8	6.1	17.1	8.3	0
2.0	96.4	3.7	51.7	33.2	+
4.0	96.7	0.3	77.3	65.0	++
6.0	97.2	0	80.5	61.2	++++
8.0	94.8	0	89.7	65.1	++++

TABLE 2:   In Vitro Effects of Colchicine on Lymphocytes

Dose M	Phase microscopy of living cells		Ultrastructure % SEM changes	Microtubule No.
	% viable	% motile		
0	98.0	15.6	0	12.0
10^{-8}	95.3	14.9	0	9.9
10^{-6}	98.2	15.7	0	6.7
10^{-4}	94.6	14.7	0	1.3
10^{-2}	64.3	0	15	0.5

TABLE 3:   Rheological Determination of Adherent Luminal Lymphocytes

	Perfusion conditions	ACI ± SE
A.	Normal rat nodes (no cells added) Flushed with dextran/saline (DS)	0.235 ± 0.03
B.	Normal rat nodes (+ transfused TDL)	
	Flushed with DS 30 minutes after CA-TDL, IV	0.535 ± 0.09
	Flushed with DS 30 minutes after Col-TDL, IV	0.150 ± 0.01
C.	Nodes from rats given 1 µg/g Col, IP (no cells added) Flushed with DS	0 ± 0

Adherent cell index (ACI) = $\dfrac{\text{No. adherent lymphocytes}}{\text{No. endothelial cells}}$

revealed partial separation of the microfilament mat from the
plasmalemma, and formation of dense aggregates of 5 - 7 nm microfilaments by TEM.   Fasces were usually seen crossing bases of
zeiotic blebs (Fig. 1d).

Colchicine (10^{-8} - 10^{-2} M) treated lymphocytes did not show
significant reduction of spontaneous locomotion until the dose
reached toxic levels (Tab. 2).   Hyaline pseudopods were extended
but did not "stick" to the substratum, and lymphocytes with pseudopods did not appear to translocate.   There were few gross changes
in the surface appearance of colchicinized TDL by SEM.   TEM studies
revealed progressive reduction in the mean number of pericentriolar
microtubules with increasing doses of colchicine.   Lumicolchicine-
treated TDL were indistinguishable from normal TDL in every respect.

Lymphocyte attachment.   Approximately 80% of the lymphocytes
found in the lumens of HEV retained their connections with the
endothelial surfaces after all nonadherent blood elements were
flushed away by 10% dextran/0.9% saline (DS) perfusion (Fig. 1e).
The adherent cell index (Tab. 3) was 0.235 $\pm$ 0.03 in light microscopic and SEM preparations of perfusion-flushed lymph nodes.
Normal rats which had received transfusion of CA-treated TDL 30
minutes prior to DS perfusion had significantly more adherent
luminal lymphocytes than control nodes.   Some of these adherent
lymphocytes were smooth surfaced and resembled the in vitro preparations of CA-treated TDL shown previously (Fig. 1f).   In rats
transfused with colchicine-treated TDL, the ACI was not different
from normal DS-perfused HEV.   In contrast, no adherent lymphocytes
were found on the luminal surfaces of lymph node HEV from rats which
were injected IP with colchicine 1 hour previously (Fig. 1g).   TEM
examination of this endothelium revealed absence of cytoplasmic
microtubules and there were fasces of 10-nm filaments coursing
through the cytoplasm.

Lymphocyte traffic studies.   Immediately after transfusion of
4 x 10^8 untreated ^{3}H-labeled TDL, there was a rapid accumulation of
label in the lung, liver and spleen, reflecting the blood flow to
these organs (Fig.2).   Traffic to the spleen was indicated by an
initial period of high splenic labeling which then tapered off.   In
contrast, there was progressive "selective" accumulation of lymphocytes in lymph nodes which peaked 18 hours postinfusion.   TDL
treated with 4.0 µg/ml CA failed to accumulate in lymph nodes in
appreciable numbers, and splenic uptake was also reduced.   Liver
uptake of CA-treated lymphocytes was not different from normal
which attested to the viability of CA-treated TDL.   Heat-killed
lymphocytes were sequestered in the liver by Kupfer cells at the
expense of all other tissues.   Lymphocytes treated with 10^{-4} M
colchicine showed depressed accumulation in lymph nodes, which was
significantly reduced until 8 hours after infusion.   When untreated

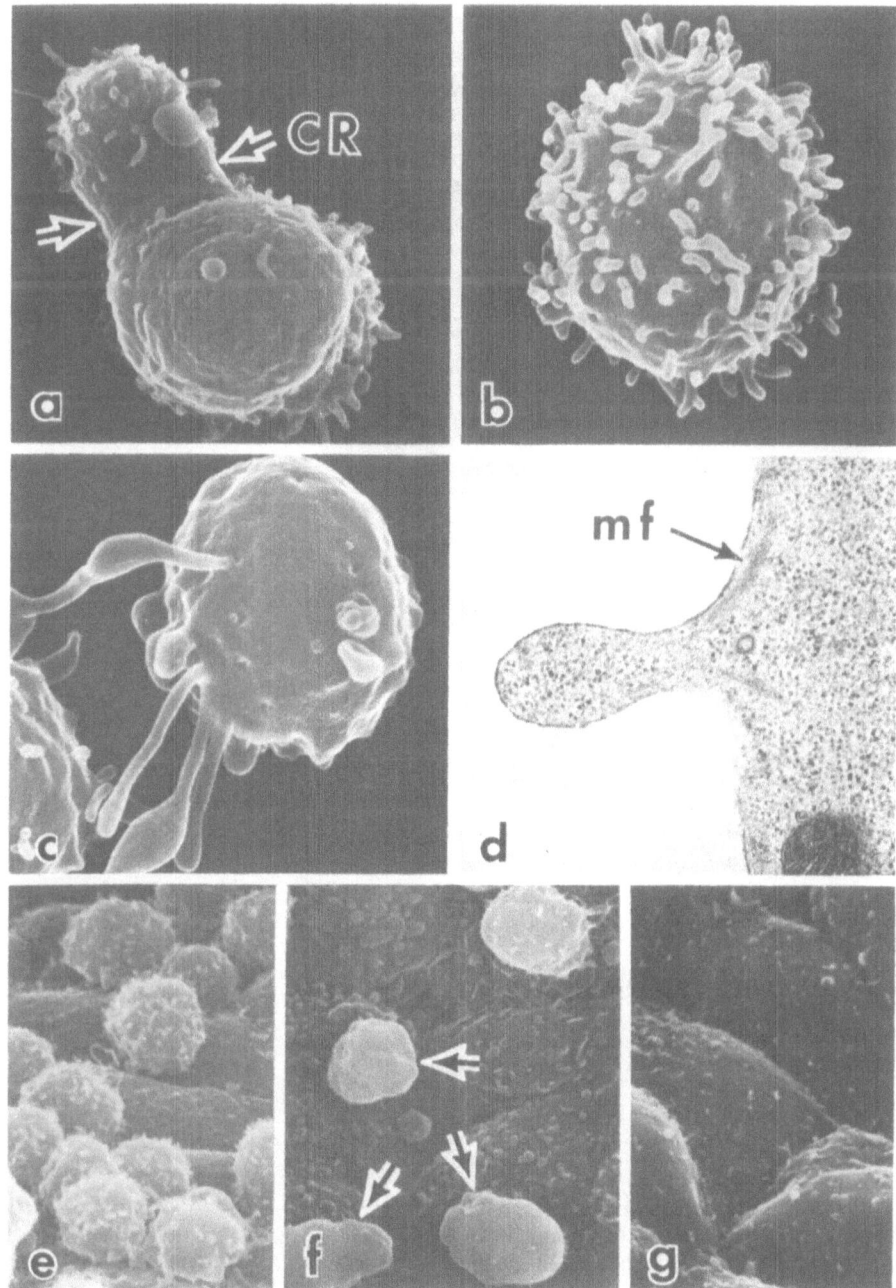

FIG. 1: SEM of untreated migrating (CR, contraction ring) (a) and sessile (b) TDL. SEM/TEM of CA TDL, showing blebs and microfilament aggregates (mf) (c and d). SEM of HEV lumina showing untreated (e), CA-treated (f) TDL (arrows). HEV from Col-treated rat (g).

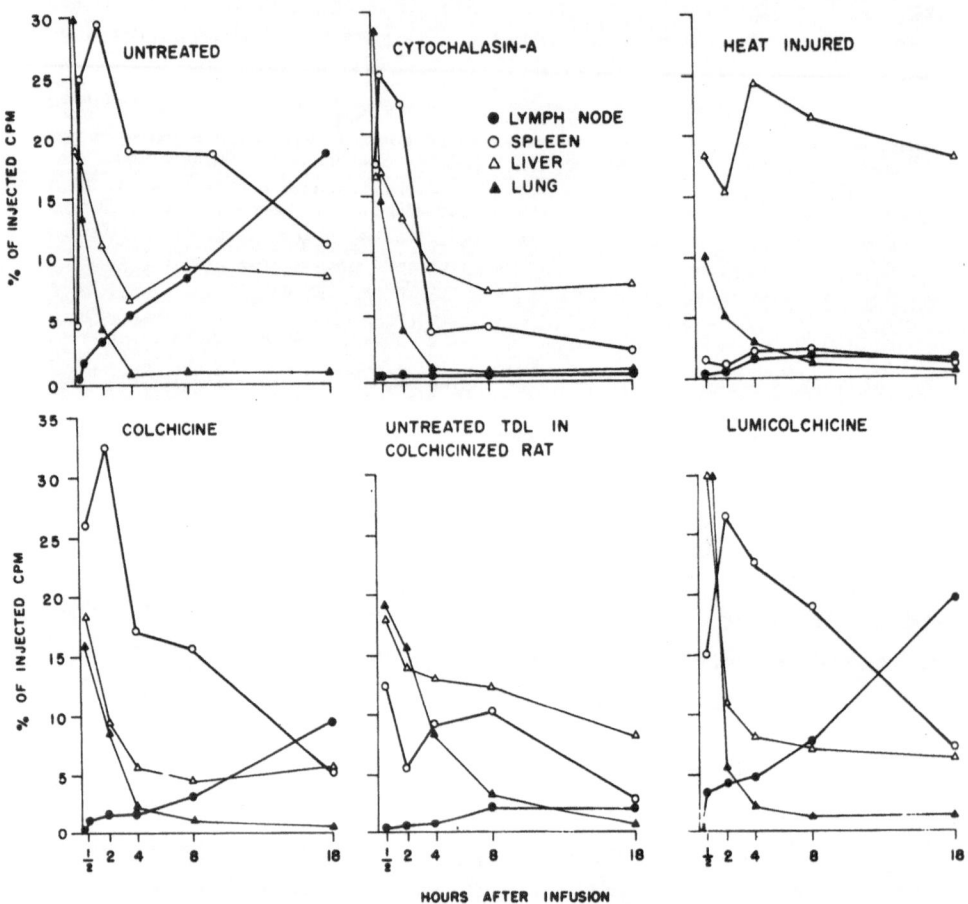

FIG. 2:   Tissue radioactivity after IV infusion of TDL treated as shown.

TDL were infused into rats given IP colchicine at 1.0 µg/g body weight, both lymph node and splenic uptake was depressed. In contrast, 10^{-4} M lumicolchicine-treated TDL migrated normally when infused into untreated rats.

Autoradiography.   Autoradiography of lymphocyte entry into lymph nodes after IV infusion was quantitated. The data for untreated, CA-treated and Col-treated TDL are shown in Tab. 4. Untreated TDL were rapidly cleared from the vascular lumen by 30

TAB. 4:   Intranodal distribution of labeled lymphocytes after IV
infusion (effects of cytochalasin A and colchicine)

| Time | Mean no. labeled lymphocytes/10 HPF | | | | | | | | |
| min. | HEV lumen | | | HEV wall | | | Node cortex | | |
	TDL	CA	Col	TDA	CA	Col	TDL	CA	Col
3	10.1	27.6	1.8	15.8	7.6	0.3	1.0	0.5	0
30	1.8	27.1	3.6	27.8	36.1	4.1	28.8	19.3	1.4
60	0.4	18.3	4.2	12.1	21.5	6.4	150.8	15.6	11.7
240	2.2	14.5	0.8	12.0	19.1	0.9	302.8	57.8	10.0

minutes postinfusion. Migrating labeled cells were a constant proportion of interendothelial lymphocytes, and accumulated in the
surrounding parenchyma in a nearly linear fashion. Lymphocytes
treated with 4.0 µg/ml cytochalasin-A persisted in significant
numbers along luminal surfaces of HEV. Increases in interendothelial
cells were also seen, and a small percentage of the CA-treated TDL
gained access to the lymph node cortex. Lymphocytes treated with
10^{-4} M colchicine showed reduced luminal accumulation at 3 minutes
postinfusion, but failed to accumulate appreciably in the node
parenchyma during the 4-hour study.

TEM of lymph nodes. In normal lymph nodes, some lymphocytes were
seen which appeared to be in the process of migrating through the HEV
at the time of fixation. These cells were structurally polarized
and some had cytoplasmic constrictions with thickened microfilament
mats indenting the nucleus on both sides (Fig. 3a). In lymph nodes
from rats which received CA-treated TDL 30 minutes earlier, rare
migrating lymphocytes were seen which had alterations consistent
with CA effects. These cells were elongated, distorted and exhibited
asymmetric distribution of microfilament bundles at sites of contact
with the endothelium (Fig. 3b). In addition, smooth surfaced luminal
lymphocytes in these nodes appeared to make contact only where
aggregated microfilaments retained their connections with the
membrane. No grossly abnormal lymphocytes were seen in TEM of
lymph nodes from rats transfused with colchicinized TDL.

DISCUSSION

Long-lived lymphocytes recirculate continuously between the
blood and lymph by entering lymphatic tissues through high endothelial venules (2,8). This phenomenon has received considerable
attention (9) following Gowan's original demonstration (1).

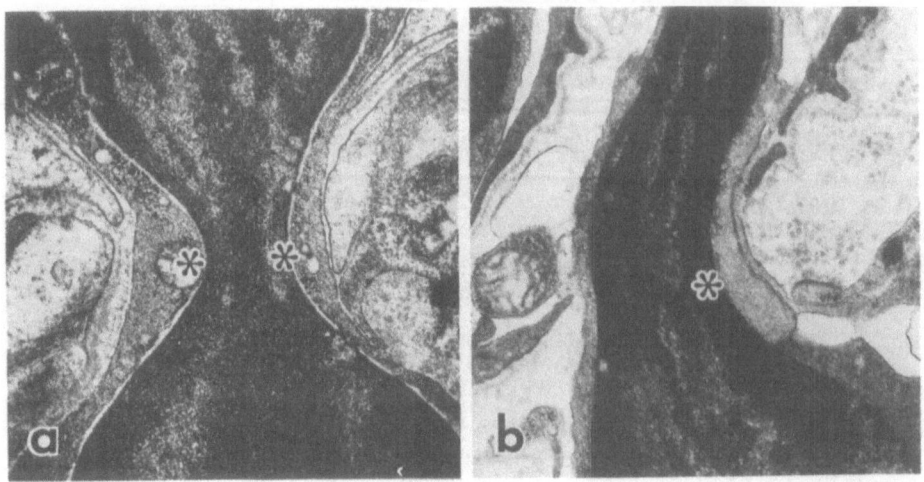

FIG. 3:   Appearance of microfilament bundles (*) at contraction
ring of untreated (a) and CA-treated (b) migrating lymphocytes.

However, relatively little is known about the molecular events
associated with attachment and locomotion of lymphocytes in vivo.

   In the present studies we have attempted to dissect the role
of microfilaments and microtubules in lymphocyte recirculation
using cytochalasin-A and colchicine. CA was used in these studies
because it has been reported to cause prolonged disruption of
microfilament function without altering hexose and nucleoside
membrane transport (10). Its relative irreversibility and reduced
metabolic effects made it useful for in vivo studies. Cytochalasins
are thought to interfere with actin or myosin interactions with an
integral membrane protein, possibly ∝-actinin; actin-binding protein
or tropomyosin (10). Colchicine has well-documented effects on
microtubule polymerization (6) and recent studies have shown that
Col also affects the distribution of 10-nm filaments which apparently
anchor to microtubules (10).

   Cytochalasin-A clearly blocks lymphocyte locomotion without
completely preventing lymphocyte homing. Despite the absence of
microvilli, some of these lymphocytes retain the capacity to recognize and attach to HEV surfaces via segments of membrane which have
intact networks of underlying microfilaments. CA-treated lymphocytes
were not seen adhering via the membranes of zeiotic blebs. These
bulbous structures are thought to result from herniation of endoplasm
at sites where broken microfilament connections expose unsupported
membrane. It is not known if adhesive receptors are present in

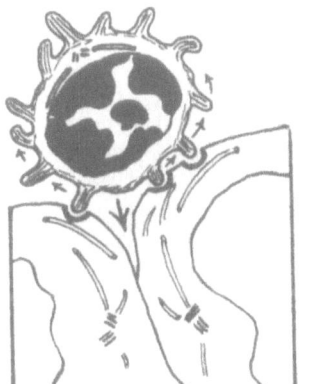 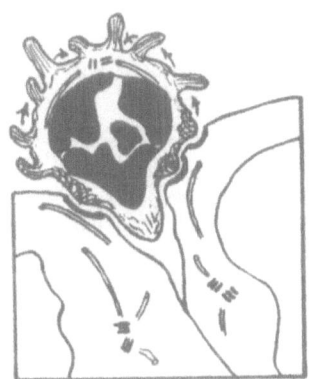 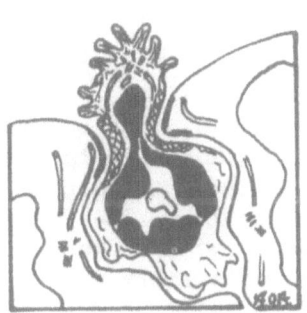

FIG. 4:   Hypothetical mechanism of lymphocyte attachment and emigration _in vivo_.

zeiotic membranes; however, recent studies suggest that a major surface glycoprotein (fibronectin) is released into the media by treatment with cytochalasin (11). These observations indicate that the attachment receptor molecules, which are also trypsin- and EDTA-sensitive (2,3), may be linked to cytoplasmic actin- myosin filaments.

Colchicine has differential effects on attachment and locomotion, depending on the method of administration. IP injection of Col prior to transfusion with normal TDL blocks homing to spleen and lymph nodes, while Col-treated TDL showed normal motility _in vitro_ but reduced homing into lymph nodes after IV infusion. This is in contradiction to _in vitro_ studies by Woodruff et al. who suggested that homing receptors on lymphocytes were not affected by colchicine when treated cells were incubated on fixed frozen sections of HEV at 7° (3). We have ruled out any direct effects of colchicine binding to membranes through use of lumicolchicine, which has all the pharmacological characteristics of Col except the ability to alter microtubules. The reported role of microtubules in anchoring or stabilizing membrane receptors may help explain this effect of Col on homing. Microtubules apparently prevent ligand-induced receptor redistribution on lymphocytes and other cells; colchicine treatment releases these receptors from direct or indirect micro- tubule restraint, and capping occurs (6). If adhesive receptors on lymphocytes were released from localization on microvilli, this might lessen the likelihood of circulating lymphocytes adhering to HEV surfaces. Reciprocally, if complementary receptors on endothe- lial cells were free to diffuse in the membrane, lymphocytes might not "see" the correct receptor density or have a stabilized series

of membrane receptors against which the force of locomotion may be
applied.

We propose a model of lymphocyte emigration using concepts of
transmembrane cytoskeletal control of receptor movement (4-11)
(Fig. 4). Normal lymphocytes attach to pits on HEV surfaces via
receptors located on microvilli (2,12). Contact or some other
stimulus, such as chemotactic gradient emanating from between
endothelial cells (13) may signal locomotion. A wave of cytoskeletal contraction moves lymphocyte surface receptors toward the
centriole. The force of receptor movement gains leverage against
the resistance of microtubule and/or 10-nm filament stabilized
complementary sites on lateral endothelial surfaces. This scheme
is consistent with descriptions of lymphocyte locomotion in vitro
(14); descriptions of the distorted asymmetric motion of CA-treated
lymphocytes fit the contraction-wave concept, since deformation
occurs toward residual connections of microfilaments with the
membrane.

SUMMARY

Lymphocyte locomotion in vivo depends upon an intact network of
subplasmalemmal contractile microfilaments which are linked through
the membrane to surface receptors, and the distribution and stabili-
zation of recognition receptors may be controlled by microtubules
and/or 10-nm filaments in the cytoplasm. The differential effects
of cytochalasin-A and colchicine on lymphocyte homing and locomotion
have proven useful in dissecting the subcellular events underlying
the process of lymphocyte recirculation.

REFERENCES

1.   Gowans, J.L., J. Physiol., 146 (1959) 54.
2.   Anderson, A.O., Anderson, N.D., Immunol. 31 (1976) 731.
3.   Woodruff, J.J., Katz, I.M., Lucas, L.E., Stamper, H.B., Jr.,
     J. Immunol., 119 (1977) 1603.
4.   Singer, S.J., Annu. Rev. Biochem. 43 (1974) 805.
5.   Nicholson, G.L., Biochem. Biophys. Acta. 457 (1976) 57.
6.   Edelman, G.M., Yahara, I., Wang, J.L., Proc. Natl. Acad. Sci.
     USA 70 (1973) 1442.
7.   Wilson, L., Friedkin, M. Biochemistry 5 (1966) 2463.
8.   Gowans, J.L., Int. Rev. Exp. Pathol. 5 (1966) 1.
9.   Sprent, J., In:B and T Cells in Immune Recognition, p59 (1977)
     (Loor, F.,Roelants, G.E., eds), John Wiley & Sons, London.

10. Goldman, R., Pollard, T., Rosenbaum, J. (eds) (1976). Cell Motility, Cold Spring Harbor Conferences on Cell Proliferation, Vol 3A. Cold Spring Laboratory, Cold Spring Harbor, N.Y.
11. Kurkinen, M., Wartiovaara, J., Vaheri, A., Exp. Cell Res., 111 (1978) 127.
12. Van Ewijk, W., Brons, N.H.C., Rozing, J., Cell Immunol., 19 (1975) 245.
13. Anderson, A.O., Anderson, N.D., Amer. J. Pathol., 80 (1975) 387.
14. Lewis, W.H., Bull. Johns Hopkins Hosp., 49 (1931) 29.

THE EFFECT OF CYTOSKELETAL INHIBITORS ON THE MIGRATION OF LYMPHO-CYTES ACROSS VASCULAR ENDOTHELIUM

M.E. Smith and W.L. Ford

Department of Pathology, University Medical School

Manchester, England

Recirculating lymphocytes leave the blood in large numbers by crossing the high walled endothelium of post-capillary venules in the cortex of lymph-nodes and the endothelium of small vessels in the marginal zone of the spleen. The nature of the interaction between lymphocytes and specialized vascular endothelium can be investigated either by exposing the lymphocates in vitro to various agents in an attempt to alter the cell surface in some defined way or alternatively by attempting to alter the endothelial surface either by perfusion of an isolated lymph node or by treatment of a whole animal prior to the injection of lymphocytes. We have previously described the consequences for the migratory properties of lymphocytes of treatment in vitro with sodium azide (1), trypsin (2), papain and dextran sulphate (1). In agreement with the results of others (3) all these agents were found to inhibit the early localization of lymphocytes in lymph nodes. In each case the treated cells recovered their migratory properties in vivo so that by 24 hours after injection their organ distribution resembled that of untreated cells. Dextran sulphate inhibited migration into lymph nodes more effectively when injected into recipients than when applied to lymphocytes in vitro.

The starting point of the present study was that the inhibition of lymph node localization following treatment with sodium azide suggested that metabolic activity by the lymphocyte is required in order to cross high endothelial venules (HEVs) in lymph nodes. This prompts the question of whether the microtubules and microfilaments of lymphocytes are active in their selective adhesion to HEVs and their translation across the vessel wall. Conceivably cytoskeletal activity by specialized endothelial cells may be important. The

TAB. 1:   Cytochalasin B $20\mu g\ ml^{-1}$ in vitro

Time, hours after injection	Lymph nodes	Spleen	Blood	Lung	Liver	Small gut (~pp)
0.5	0.82 (.78–.84)	1.05 (1.02–1.08)	1.05 (1.02–1.08)	0.92 (.91–.94)	1.04 (.94–1.12)	0.97 (.89–1.01)
2.5	0.83 (.75–.88)	1.00 (.98–1.01)	1.21 (1.19–1.25)	1.00 (.96–1.03)	1.05 (.99–1.12)	1.08 (1.02–1.12)
24	1.04 (1.03–1.07)	0.96 (.95–.98)	1.07 (1.00–1.14)	1.03 (1.00–1.05)	1.05 (.95–1.20)	1.02 (1.00–1.05)

Ratio of   radioactivity associated with treated lymphocytes
           radioactivity associated with untreated lymphocytes

Geometric mean and range (n = 6)

TAB. 2: Colchicine 10^{-4}M in vitro

Time, hours after injection	Lymph nodes	Spleen	Blood	Lung	Liver	Small gut (-pp)
0.5	0.69 (.63-.73)	0.91 (.87-.93)	0.85 (.82-.89)	1.47 (1.37-1.54)	0.92 (.90-.93)	0.54 (.45-.61)
2.5	0.72 (.68-.75)	0.98 (.96-1.02)	0.94 (.80-1.10)	2.22 (2.00-2.40)	1.08 (.98-1.14)	0.64 (.59-.67)
24	0.88 (.84-.90)	1.10 (1.06-1.12)	0.91 (.86-.92)	0.97 (.93-.99)	1.04 (.97-1.15)	0.77 (.75-.81)

Ratio of $\dfrac{\text{radioactivity associated with treated lymphocytes}}{\text{radioactivity associated with untreated lymphocytes}}$

Geometric mean and range (n = 6)

TAB. 3:   Cytochalasin + Colchicine in vitro

Time, hours after injection	Lymph nodes	Spleen	Blood	Lung	Liver	Small gut (-pp)
0.5	0.41 (.33–.52)	0.85 (.82–.87)	0.81 (.74–.88)	1.96 (1.94–1.99)	0.94 (.85–1.05)	0.78 (.59–1.02)
2.5	0.47 (.37–.59)	0.99 (.91–1.03)	1.33 (1.01–1.76)	3.27 (3.17–3.38)	1.15	0.67
24	0.88 (.85–.92)	0.94 (.87–1.01)	0.90 (.85–.95)	0.84 (.80–.89)	1.02	0.63 (.51–.78)

Ratio of radioactivity associated with treated lymphocytes
radioactivity associated with untreated lymphocytes

Geometric mean and range (n = 6)

TAB. 4: Colcemid in vivo 1h before cells

Time, hours after cell injection	Lymph nodes	Spleen	Blood	Lung	Liver	Small gut (-pp)
0.5	0.21	0.45	1.12	1.78	1.16	0.71
2.5	0.29	0.80	1.26	1.42	1.43	0.64
24	1.00	0.92	0.93	1.09	1.19	0.75

$$\frac{\text{Ratio of radioactivity recovered from treated animals}}{\text{radioactivity recovered from control animals}}$$

results of treating lymphocytes in vitro with colchicine and cytochalasin B and the effect of treating recipients with Colcemid are
reported.

Lymphocytes were centrifuged from thoracic duct lymph obtained
by cannulation of inbred rats. They were labelled in vitro with
^{3}H-uridine or ^{14}C-uridine (4) before incubation with colchicine or
cytochalasin B. After washing they were combined with alternatively
labelled control lymphocytes and injected i.v. into syngeneic
recipients which were killed at 0.5, 2.5 and 24 hours after injection.
By scintillation counting the localization of treated and control
cells could be compared to the radioactivity associated with each
population injected. A simultaneous experiment with isotope reversal
was performed (5). In tables 1-3 a ratio of less than 1.0 signifies
a deficit of treated cells in the tissue compared to the distribution
of control cells.

The exposure of lymphocytes to cytochalasin B at 20µg ml^{-1} for
1h at 37°C produced a marginal but consistent impairment in their
ability to enter lymph nodes (Tab.1). Both at 0.5h and 2.5h after
injection there was a 20% deficit of the treated cells in lymph-nodes
in the face of a slight excess in the blood.

By contrast treatment of lymphocytes for 1h with 10^{-4}M colchicine
(Tab.2) resulted in a deficit of the treated cells in the blood early
after injection. This appeared to be a consequence of higher numbers
in the lungs probably because of prolonged retention there. There
was again a slight deficit in the lymph node localization of treated
cells but this may have been partly or wholly because of the deficit
in the blood.

Combined treatment with cytochalasin B and colchicine affected
lymphocyte migration as shown in Table 3. The size of the early
deficit of treated cells in lymph nodes suggests not synergy but
rather a simple additive effect of the two reagents as would be
expected from the distinct mechanisms of inhibition we have suggested.
The excess of treated cells in the lung was striking although it
represented only 3.6% of the injected activity at 2.5h.

Recipients were injected intraperitoneally with Colcemid (4mg
Kg^{-1}) one hour before the i.v. injection of ^{51}Cr labelled syngeneic
lymphocytes and their distribution was compared to that in untreated
recipients (Tab.4). The early localization in lymph nodes was deeply
depressed in the face of a moderate surplus in the blood, the lungs
and the liver. Localization in the spleen was less markedly depressed
and preliminary experiments have shown that the relative blood flow
to the spleen (but not to lymph nodes) was reduced to about half after
Colcemid treatment. Since colchicine treatment in vitro of lymphocytes had a barely significant effect on their lymph node localization,

it appeared probable that an action of Colcemid on HEVs in lymph nodes impeded the entry of lymphocytes.

By studying the adherence of lymphocytes to HEVs in frozen sections of lymph nodes Woodruff and her colleagues observed that treatment of lymphocytes with either sodium azide or cytochalasin B inhibited the interaction whereas colchicine was entirely without effect (6). Our results suggest that these three agents have similar consequences for the capacity of lymphocytes to interact with HEVs in vivo, with some reservations stemming from the smallness of the inhibition produced by cytochalasin B. As a whole these results indicate that the microfilament system of lymphocytes is required to be active to enable their selective migration across HEVs. The microtubule system of lymphocytes does not apparently play a necessary part in this process. However, the microtubules of specialized endothelial cells may have a role in facilitating the high volume traffic of lymphocytes across HEVs in lymph nodes.

REFERENCES

1. Ford, W.L., Smith, M.E., Andrews, P. in: Cell-cell Recognition. Ed. A.S.G. Curtis. Cambridge University Press, p. 359 (1978).
2. Ford, W.L., Sedgley, M., Sparshott, S.M., Smith, M.E. Cell Tiss. Kinetics 9 (1976) 351.
3. Freitas, A.A., de Sousa, M.A.B. Cell. Immunol. 31 (1977) 62 and Cell. Immunol. 22 (1976) 345.
4. Ford, W.L. Chapter 23 in Handbook of Experimental Immunology. Ed. D.M. Weir. Blackwell. (1978).
5. Atkins, R.C., Ford, W.L. J. Exp. Med. 141 (1975) 664.
6. Woodruff, J.J., Katz, I.M., Lucas, L.E., Stamper, H.B. J. Immunol. 119 (1977) 1603.

NEW EVIDENCE ON CONTROL MECHANISMS IN LYMPHOCYTE TRAFFIC

A.S.G. Curtis, M. Davies and P.C. Wilkinson

Departments of Cell Biology and of Bacteriology &
Immunology, Glasgow University,
Glasgow G12 800, U. K.

Interaction modulation factors from murine lymphocytes were
first described by Curtis & De Sousa (1973, 1975). These factors
are low molecular weight glycoproteins secreted by lymphocytes in
short term culture and which can be detected in body fluids and
adsorbed to certain cell types, Curtis (1978). In earlier work it
was shown that these substances specifically diminish the adhesion
of lymphocytes of the opposite type. Thus the T interaction modulation factor from thymocytes or T cells decreases the adhesion of
B lymphocytes, not only to each other but also to other types of
cell surface. Conversely the B interaction modulation factor
diminishes the adhesion of thymocytes and of peripheral T cells.
It was suggested by Curtis & De Sousa (1975) that these substances
might play a role in the control of lymphocyte circulation and a
certain amount of evidence supporting this interpretation was
described by Curtis (1978).

This paper describes fuller evidence which shows that the T
interaction modulation factor can play an important role in lymphocyte circulation and positioning in vivo, and reveals more about the
manner in which this factor interacts with cells and with the
relationship between this type of system for controlling cell-cell
recognition and histocompatibility systems.

T interaction modulation factor, hereafter called T IMF, was
prepared from short term (1 hour) cultures of highly viable lymphocytes derived from the thymus by techniques described by Curtis &
De Sousa (1975). In recent preparations an activity of 30,000 units
per microgram of protein has been obtained.

TAB. 1:   The Effect of Intravenously Injected Thymocyte IMF

Time (hours)	Treat- ment	Blood Leucocyte (x 10^{-6})/ml	% Ig Positive Lymphocytes Peripheral Blood	Spleen
2	Saline	2.92±0.71	34.9	55.2
2	TIMF	4.06±1.00 $p = 0.009$	64.25	34.7
24	Saline	3.7 ±1.13	36.8	53.7
24	TIMF	3.34±0.7 $p =$ Non-significant	46.9	38.4

Effects on lymphocyte circulation in vivo

Three different types of experiment were carried out.   In the first T IMF was injected in isotonic saline by tail vein.   Samples of blood were obtained from freshly killed animals at various intervals thereafter and the total count of white cells, and the proportion of Ig positive cells was measured.   The proportion of Ig positive and T cells in spleens was also measured.   Results are shown in Tab.1.

In essence these results show that injection of T factor produces an extensive leucocytosis in the blood which is partly composed of an increased number of B cells while T cells remain at a normal level.   Effects on leucocytes are less long-lasting than on the changes in the B:T proportion.   The effects in the spleen are apparently complementary to those in the blood which suggests that the spleen is probably the source of the cells.   Histological changes occur in the spleen which suggest that the B dependent areas may be extensively cleared of cells.   The results are those that would be expected if the effect of T IMF in vivo is to reduce the adhesion of B cells and of leucocytes while leaving T cells unaffected.

In the second type of experiment T factor was injected together with ^{51}Cr labelled LN lymphocytes or spleen B cells.   Organs were sampled for radioactivity at various intervals after injection of the cells by tail vein.   Results are shown in Tab.2.

This table shows that injection of factor together with cells changes the localisation of the lymphocytes.   Effects are partic- ularly noticeable on spleen and lymph node localisation.   The effects

TAB. 2:   The Effect of Intravenously Injected Thymocyte IMF on the Localisation of ^{51}Chromium Labelled Lymph Node Cells

| Time (hours) | Treatment | % of labelled cells in | | | |
		Spleen	Liver	Peripheral Lymph Nodes	Total Recovery
1	Control	28.5	13.05	3.1	68.0
1	Thymocyte IMF 122 7000 units	32.0	16.0	1.97*	73.3
4	Control	31.05	11.78	5.18	61.7
4	Thymocyte IMF 122 7000 units	36.08**	14.27**	4.29**	67.7
24	Control	17.98	10.36	8.62	57.2
24	Thymocyte IMF 122 7000 units	19.28	10.30	8.51	57.5

p values of significance of difference   * < 0.05
                                        ** < 0.01
                                        *** < 0.001

S. deviations $< 2.6\%$

on B cell trapping can be easily explained if it is presumed that the T IMF makes these cells less adhesive. The increase in localisation of lymph node cells, presumably of the T proportion of these populations, can be explained if the T IMF reduces the host's own population of B cells in various lymphoid organs so that there are now fewer B cells to depress the adhesiveness of approaching T cells.

However, these experiments are open to the objection that it is not clear whether the injected factor alone or the modified cells have the main effect. So in the third type of experiment we pretreated ^{51}Cr labelled cells with T IMF and removed excess T IMF before injection. Results are shown in Tab. 3.

Tab. 3 shows that the effects noted in the second experiment persist and may even be accentuated so that it must be concluded that a main effect must be determined by the nature of the surface of the injected cell and not necessarily by modification of existing host lymphoid cells. Recently we have shown that the T IMF has

TAB. 3:   The Effects of Intravenous Thymocyte IMF and the Pretreatment of Cells with Thymocyte IMF on the Localisation of
^{51}Chromium Labelled Lymph Node Lymphocytes

Time (hours)	Treatment	% of labelled cells in			
		Spleen	Liver	Lymph Nodes	
				Peripheral	Mesenteric
4	Control	28.53	11.32	5.30	3.76
4	Thymocyte IMF 126 21000 units	28.83	14.17***	2.83***	2.61***
4	Thymocyte IMF 126 + one wash	31.94	13.01**	3.13**	2.31

p values of significance of difference ** < 0.01   Total
                                       *** < 0.001   recovery
S. deviations   < 4.4%   approx. 60%

chemokinetic effects on B cells: this introduces new possibilities
on the possible modes of action of these factors and also serves to
link chemokinesis and chemotaxis to the adhesive states of the cells
involved.

The histocompatibility relationships of T IMF

We found by chance that T IMF from one mouse strain will
diminish the adhesiveness of thymocytes and T cells from other
strains of mice unless the strains are matched at H-2D. See Tab.4.

Antibodies against a given T IMF will bring about complement
induced lysis of target cells if these are producers of T IMF and
of the same H-2D nature as the T IMF used to raise antibody. See
Tab.5.

Both these experiments suggest that H-2D is involved in the
action of the T IMF. The simplest interpretation is that the T IMF
is an H-2D product. The first experiment shows that T IMF will
diminish the adhesion of thymocytes, provided that they are not
matched at H-2D, the second experiment shows the antibodies will
only complement lyse cells if they are of the same H-2D type as
the cells that were the source of the IMF used to immunise rabbits.

TAB. 4:   H-2 Relationship of IMFs; Allogeneic Effects of IMFs
on Adhesion of Thymus Cells

Target cell strain type	IMF origin	Adhesion	H-2 mismatch	Congenic
B10.A,A	B10.A,A	13.8	None	–
	B10.A(2R)	0.0	D only	Yes
	B10.A(4R)	2.1	All except K & IA	Yes
	A/WySn	4.8	None	No
B10.A(2R)	B10.A(2R)	27.4	None	–
	B10.A,A	0.0	D only	Yes
	B10.A(4R)	13.9	IB, IJ, IE, IC, S & G	Yes
B10.A(4R)	B10.A(4R)	11.8	None	–
	B10.A(2R)	14.9	IB, IJ, IE, IC, S & G	Yes
	B10.A,A	0.0	All except K & IA	Yes
B10.G	B10.G	10.7	None	–
	B10.AKM	11.0	All except D	Yes
	AQR	0.0	All except K	No
A/WySn	A/WySn	9.4	None	–
	AQR	8.7	K	Yes
	B10.AKM	0.03	IC, S, G & D	No
	B10.A(5R)	9.0	K, IA & IB	No

Adhesion measured as collision efficiency percentages. Measurements
made with IMF yields of c. 1×10^5 cells on 1×10^6 cells. Haplotype compositions compared at K, IA, IB, IJ, IE, IC, S, G & D.

Since there is now good evidence that T IMF can be prepared as a
single molecular species we appear to have a substance which only
diminishes adhesion if the target cell is:

a)   of the same tissue type but different histocompatibility type, or

b)   is from the same or a syngeneic animal but of different tissue
      type or

c)   differs in both respects.

It is tempting to conclude that the similarity of effect seen in
a) and b) implies that T and B and other cell types in a single

TAB. 5:   Immune Cytolysis of Thymocytes by Anti-T IMF Antibodies

Antibody against	Target cell strain	Cytolysis (%)	H-2 mismatch
CBA/ca	CBA/ca	94.0	None
	B10.AKM	0.0	D
	B10.A(4R)	0.0	All except K & IA
	B10.A(2R)	1.8	IC, S, G & D
	AQR	21.0	K, IE, IC, S, G & D
BALB/c	BALC/c	94.2	None
	C57 BL10/ScSn	2.0	All
	B10.A(5R)	96.8	K, IA, IB
	B10.S(7R)	87.0	All except D

Cytolysis expressed as maximum cytolysis with a range of antibody concentrations less background cytolysis. Background cytolysis in no case exceeded 12% of the total number of cells. Antibodies raised in rabbits.

animal differ in the display of the set histocompatibility antigens belonging to that genotype and that this difference determines adhesive differences. This also suggests that the prime role of the histocompatibility system may lie in controlling tissue inter-actions. It is also of interest to note that there are some similarities between T IMF and the low molecular weight soluble Ia antigens isolated by Parish (1976).

CONCLUSIONS

These results go a long way to proving the original proposals put forward by Curtis & De Sousa (1975) about the probable actions of IMFs. The results also establish that there is good reason to think that these glycoproteins may be the natural control system used in lymphocyte positioning in addition, since they are found in body fluids and in abnormal concentrations in certain diseases (Curtis, in press).

These results also serve to point out that lymphocyte recir-culation does not only involve trapping at the endothelium but also may involve questions of release from the lymphoid organs and sorting-out within them.

Finally it is of considerable relevance that these substances are linked to the histocompatibility system; because :

A. of the known involvement of the H-2 system, etc., in other T:B interactions. Now we may wonder to what extent some of these involvements may be based on the adhesive effects of soluble products or on histocompatibility antigens as receptors in cell adhesion

B. it raises the question of differences in histocompatibility antigen expression in different cell types within one organism, and thus;

C. the possibility that the prime function of the histocompatibility system is on tissue positioning in the organism.

REFERENCES

1. Curtis, A.S.G., Symp. Soc. Exp. Biol. 32 (1978) 51.
2. Curtis, A.S.G., De Sousa, M.A.B., Nature New Biology 244 (1973) 45.
3. Curtis, A.S.G., De Sousa, M.A.B., Cellular Immunol. 19 (1975) 282.
4. Parish, C.R. et al, Immunogenetics 3 (1976) 455.

ACKNOWLEDGEMENTS

This work was supported by the Wellcome Trust Grant 5533.

SEPARATION OF EARTHWORM COELOMOCYTES BY VELOCITY SEDIMENTATION

E.L. Cooper, H.R. MacDonald and B. Sordat

Unit of Human Cancer Immunology, Lausanne Branch,
Ludwig Institute for Cancer Research and Swiss
Institute for Experimental Cancer Research,
1066 Epalinges s/Lausanne, Switzerland

INTRODUCTION

Earthworm leukocytes (coelomocytes) are heterogeneous morphologically (1,2) and participate in diverse functions including
graft rejection (3), phagocytosis (1), formation of rosettes with
SRBC (4), and mitogen responsiveness (5,6). Specific cells
mediating these responses are controversial, thus we have developed
a procedure for separating coelomocytes by velocity sedimentation
at unit gravity. This separation technique, widely applicable in
mammalian systems,selects cells primarily on the basis of size (7,
8). By this isolation procedure, we have enriched for at least two
distinct coelomocytic types, basophils and granulocytes which
participate in graft rejection (3). After enriching for distinct
coelomocytes, we now have a method for subjecting them to various
immunobiological tests.

MATERIALS AND METHODS

Coelomocytes were isolated by submerging unanesthetized worms
in a buffered medium free of Ca^{++} and MG^{++} that was modified to
prevent clumping (9). It contained NaCl, 6.5 g; Hepes, 10 mM;
EGTA, 5 mM; trypsin, 0.05%; K_2HPO_4, 10 mM; KH_2PO_4, 10 mM; pH,
7.2. After worms shed coelomocytes through integumentary pores at
room temperature (22°C), the coelomocytes were decanted into fresh
medium through cheese cloth to remove debris. For separation by
velocity sedimentation at unit gravity, approximately 10×10^6
coelomocytes were suspended in 30 ml of medium supplemented with 5%
(v/v) fetal calf serum and then applied to a buffered step gradient

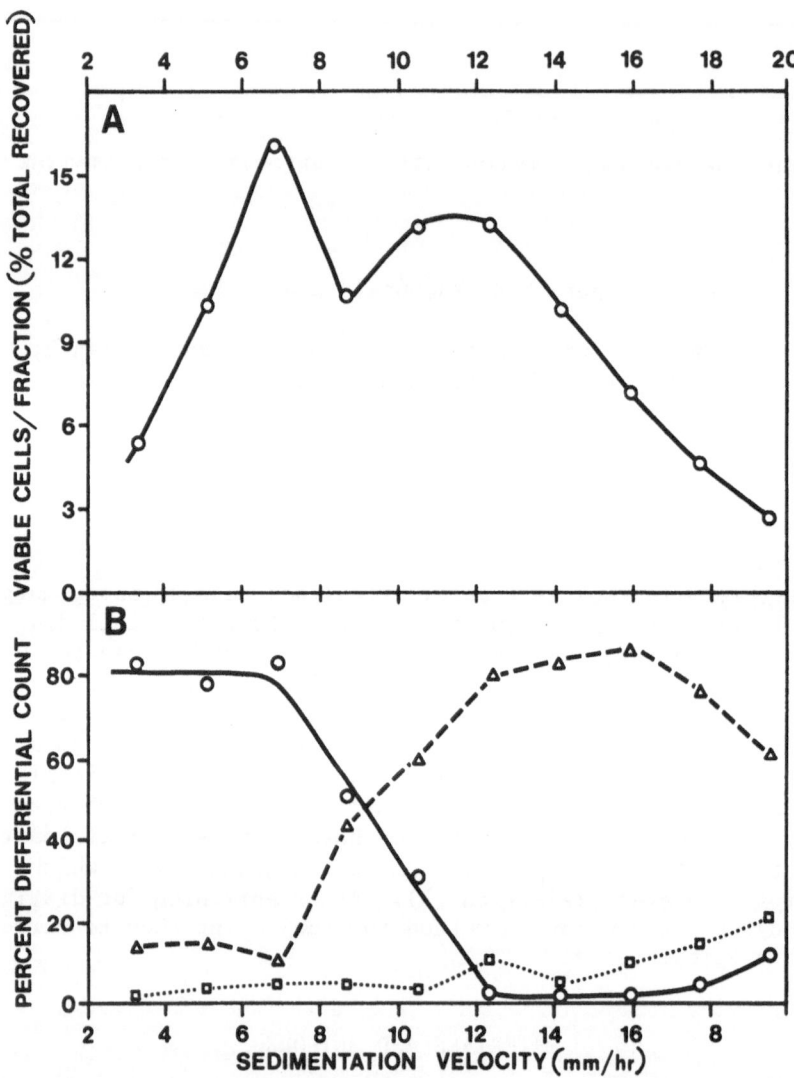

FIG. 1:   Velocity sedimentation analysis of earthworm coelomocytes.
Viable (dye-excluding) cells arbitrarily normalized (A).   Cells (2 -
5 x 10⁴) were differentially counted (B).   Basophils o-o;   Granulocytes △ - △ ;   Neutrophils ▫..▫ .   Unseparated control preparations
contained 50% basophils, 29% granulocytes and 9.4% neutrophils.

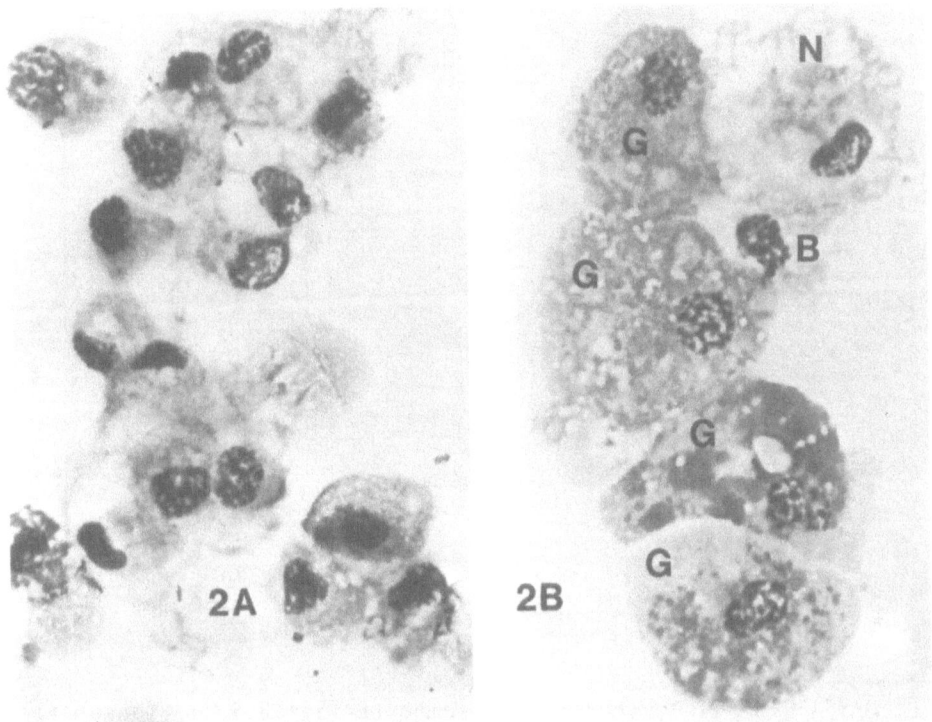

FIG. 2A: Basophils showing vacuoles and filamentous pseudopodia.
1800 X;   sedimentation velocity 6.9 mm/hr.

FIG. 2B: Four granulocytes (G), one basophil (B) and one neutrophil
(N). Note pseudopodial extensions which appear as clear ectoplasm.
1800 X;   sedimentation velocity 15.9 mm/hr. Enrichment for basophils
and granulocytes was approximately 80%.

consisting of 7 - 30% calf serum in the medium in a siliconized glass
chamber of 11 cm diameter. After 1.5 - 2 hours sedimentation at 4°C,
the cone volume was discarded and 30 ml fractions were collected and
concentrated to 1 ml by centrifugation. Individual fractions were
then cytocentrifuged, stained with May-Grunwald-Giemsa and differentially counted.

RESULTS

Coelomocytes were heterogeneous in sedimentation velocities
(Fig.1A). Viable cells were recoverd in a range of 2 - 20 mm/hour
and were broadly distributed into two major peaks, one at approxi-

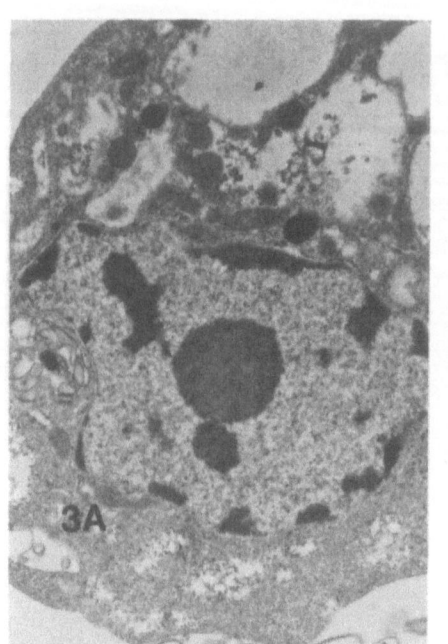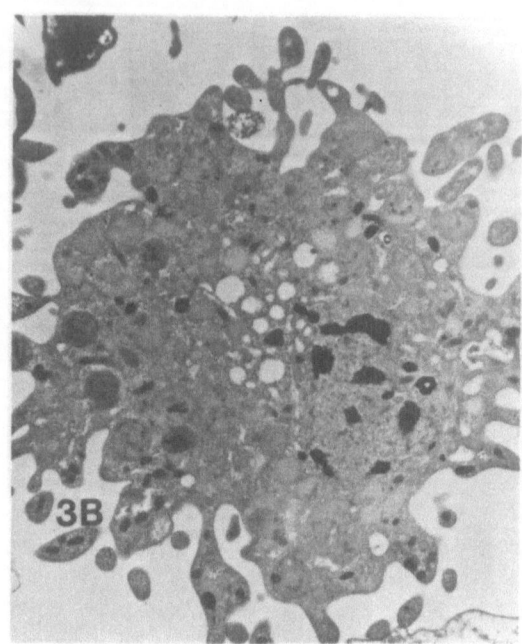

FIG. 3A: Type II lymphocytic coelomocyte (5 - 8.5 μm) (basophil)
resembles the smaller Type I.   Note the nucleolus in the centrally
located nucleus, rough endoplasmic reticulum, mitochondria.   13,500
X;   sedimentation velocity 12.3 mm/hr.

FIG. 3B: Type II granulocytes (7 - 9 μm) are stellate, showing
elaborate pseudopodial extentions, granules and empty vacuoles.
6,000 X;   sedimentation velocity 12.3 mm/hr.

mately 6 - 7 mm/hour and the second at 10 - 13 mm/hour. We recovered
approximately 40% of total cells after separation. Basophils comprised the first peak, whereas the second consisted almost exclusively of granulocytes and neutrophils. Significant enrichment (2 -
3 fold) was observed and highly purified populations obtained in
certain fractions (Fig.1B). For example, basophils were enriched
almost two-fold in slowly sedimenting fractions and both granulocytes
and neutrophils were enriched 3-fold in rapidly sedimenting fractions.
In absolute terms, the purity of basophils and of granulocytes was
greater than 80% in the most enriched fractions. These cells showed
the typical structure as observed in previous light microscopic
preparations (Figs.2A,B). Acidophils constituted 6.6% of the unseparated population and were mainly found in rapidly sedimenting
fractions (data not shown). Chlorogogen and transitional cells in
the unseparated fractions were present in low frequency as has been
found previously. However, upon separation

we observed no significant enrichment. We confirmed the ultrastructural appearance of cell types using the following terminology:
Types I and II lymphocytic coelomocytes correspond to basophils in
light microscopy ranging in size from about 4 - 9 µm with numerous
membrane limited vacuoles, smooth and rough endoplasmic reticulum,
Golgi vesicles and pseudopodial formations (Fig.3A). Granulocytes
and neutrophils were variable and granulocytes ranged from 9 - 15
µm. The cytoplasm contained dark granules, endoplasmic reticulum
Golgi.

DISCUSSION AND SUMMARY

We confirmed the existence of five major categories of earthworm coelomocytes (1), and developed a physical method for separating them by sedimentation velocity at unit gravity. Subfractions
are significantly enriched for at least two coelomocytic types,
basophils and granulocytes, showing two major peaks. The distribution in gross velocity sedimentation implies the presence of at
lease two coelomocytic types, a distribution similar to that of
leukocytes in mammalian bone marrow and peripheral blood. This
procedure should now allow significantly newer approaches to the
immunobiological properties of invertebrate immunocytes.

REFERENCES

1.   Stein, E., Avtalion, R.R., Cooper, E.L., J. Morphol.153 (1977)
      467.
2.   Linthicum, D.S., Stein, E.A., Marks, D.H., Cooper, E.L., Cell
      Tiss. Res., 185 (1977) 315.
3.   Linthicum, D.S., Stein, E.A., Marks, D.H., Cooper, E.L., Eu.
      J. Immunol., 7 (1977) 871.
4.   Cooper, E.L., Symposium on non-specific factors influencing
      host resistance. Braun, W., Ungar, J., (eds) Bern (1973).
5.   Rcoh, Ph., Valembois, P., DuPasquier, L., Adv. Exp. Med. Biol.
      64 (1975) 45.
6.   Toupin, J., Lamoureux, G., Phylogeny of thymus and bone
      marrow-bursa cells. Wright, R.K., Cooper, E.L., (eds) Elsevier/
      North Holland Biomedical Press Amsterdam (1976).
7.   Miller, R.G., Phillips, R.A., J. Cell. Physiol. 73 (1969) 191.
8.   MacDonald, H.R., Miller, R.G., Biophys 10 (1970) 834.
9.   Roch, P., Valembois, P., Dev. Comp. Immunol. 2 (1978) 51.

ACKNOWLEDGEMENTS

Supported in part by NIH Grant HD 0933-04 and a Brown Hazen Grant to ELC, recipient of an Eleanor Roosevelt Fellowship from UICC, on leave from Department of Anatomy, School of Medicine, University of California, Los Angeles, 90024. We thank Dr. J. Mauel, Institut de Biochimie, Université de Lausanne, for purchasing the earthworms.

TWO SUBPOPULATIONS OF CORTISONE-RESISTANT LYMPHOID CELLS IN THE RABBIT THYMUS

W. Leene, P.J.M. Roholl, K.A. Hoeben and T.M. Hogenes

Lab. of Histology, University of Amsterdam

Amsterdam, The Netherlands

INTRODUCTION

The final product of lymphoid cell differentiation in the thymus along common or separate (1) maturation pathways is the small lymphocyte. A minor, cortisone-resistant (CR), part of small thymic lymphocytes contributes to the generation of immuno-competent peripheral T cells, a high, cortisone-sensitive (CS), proportion of incompetent small cells appears to die within the thymus (2,3). Candidate (precursor) cells for the functionally various classes of T cells are to be found within the category of CR small thymic lymphocytes, which, in the present study, was analysed with physical and morphological methods. Evidence for a possible separation and identification of two subpopulations of CR small thymic lymphocytes will be presented.

MATERIALS AND METHODS

Female rabbits (Chinchilla Strain) 6-8 weeks of age were used throughout. Corticosteroid treatment was achieved by daily i.v. injections of dexamethasone (Organon-Oss, Holland) 5 mg/kg body weight. Thymus cell suspensions were prepared and separated according to density as described earlier (4). Thymus tissue fragments and pellets of cell suspensions were fixed with glutaralde-hyde and tannic acid (5), dehydrated and embedded in Epon 812. Thin sections were stained with bismuth subnitrate (6) or with uranyl acetate and lead citrate.

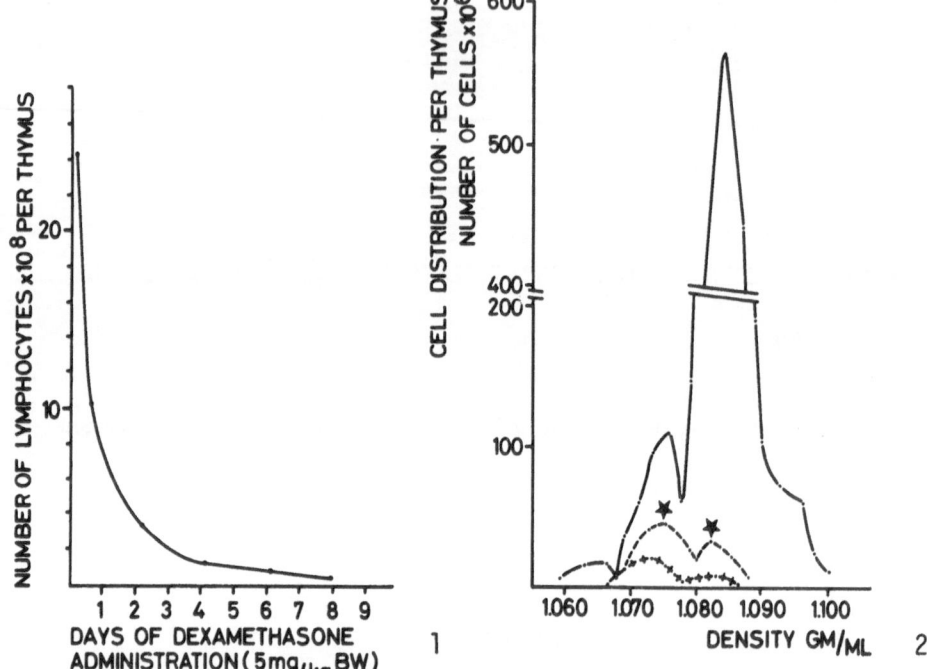

FIG. 1:   Effect of prolonged dexamethasone treatment upon number
of lymphocytes per thymus.

FIG. 2:   Density distribution of rabbit thymocytes after 0 (———),
48 (----) and 96 hr (++++) dexamethasone treatment.

RESULTS

To investigate cytological details and anatomical localization
of CR lymphoid cells in the rabbit thymus, cells were killed in the
thymus by treating the animals with the synthetic corticosteroid
dexamethasone. Fig.1 shows the effect of daily injections of the
drug upon the total number of lymphoid cells isolated from the
rabbit thymus; after 2 d dexamethasone administration the total
number of lymphoid cells present in both thymus lobes is approx.
10% of the original number. It should be noted that the further
decrease of the cell number upon prolonged treatment cannot be
explained to be the result of a continued degradation of lymphoid
cells in situ as visible signs of cell death in cortex and medulla
were observed exclusively during the first 36 hr of dexamethasone
treatment (vide infra).

Using a linear Ficoll-Metrizoate gradient (4) we were able to
separate rabbit thymus lymphoid cells into three distinct classes

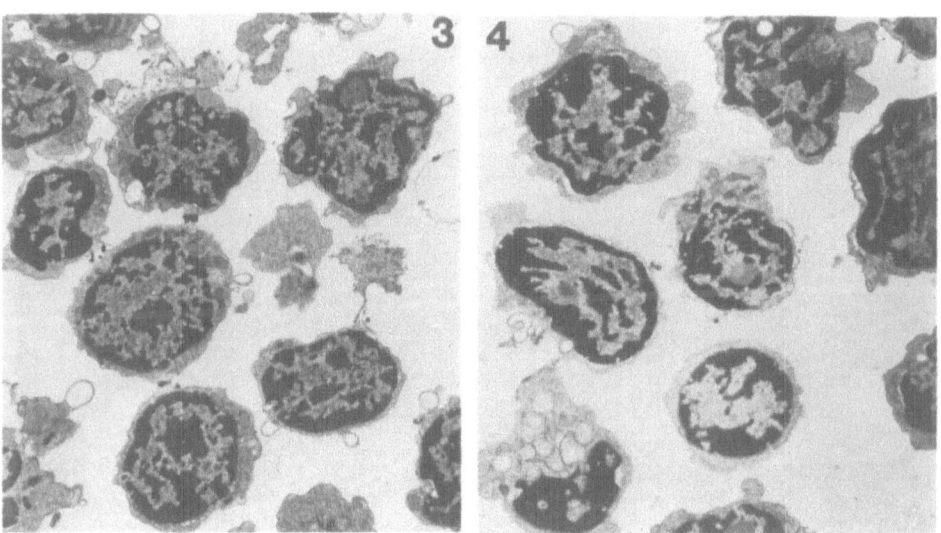

FIG. 3:   CR lymphocytes from medium density fraction (Fig.2
asterisk at the left).

FIG. 4:   CR lymphocytes from high density fraction (Fig.2 asterisk
at the right).

(Fig.2, continuous line) of high (peak at 1.084 g/ml), medium
(1.074- 1.077 g/ml) and low (1.064 - 1.067 g/ml) density. From
the density profiles of the thymus cells after 2 d dexamethasone
administration (Fig.2 ----) and that of the control (———) it can
be calculated that the high density class consists of approx.
4.5% CR cells and the medium density class of approx. 35% CR cells.
EM-investigation of the peak fractions of high and medium density
CR cells (Fig.2, asterisks) revealed interesting differences in
nuclear morphology, especially when the bismuth subnitrate staining
was used: nuclei of lymphoid cells of high density were characterized
by a marginally located compact mass of heterochromatin (Fig.4),
nuclei of lymphoid cells of medium density by a more disperse heterochromatin distribution (Fig.3).

     The anatomical localization of CR lymphoid cells in the thymus
was studied by comparing the cellular composition of cortex and
medulla of dexamethasone treated (16-24-36-48 hr) and control animals.
In controls and 48 hr treated animals no signs of cell damage could
be detected, but an extensive depletion of lymphoid cells in the
cortex and a moderate depletion in the medulla was observed after 48
hr dexamethasone treatment.

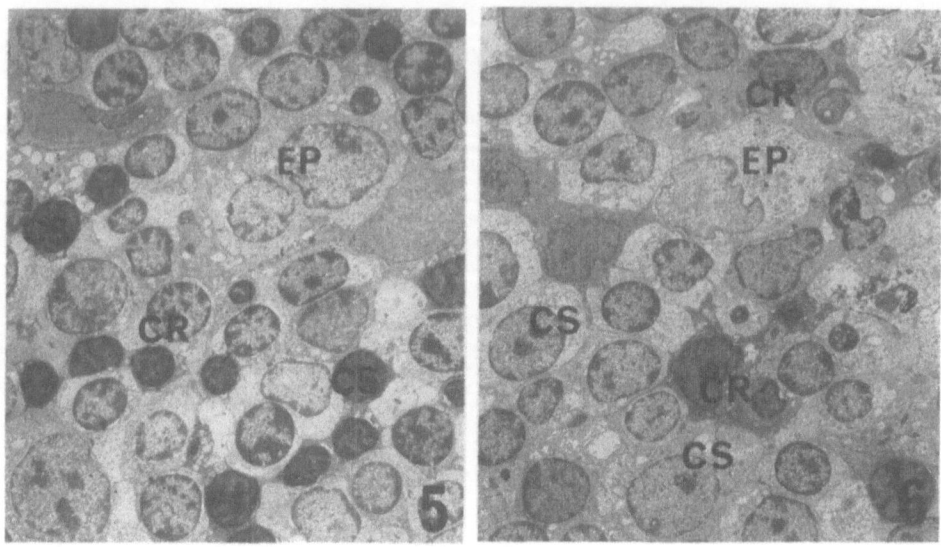

FIG. 5:   Control thymus cortex.   FIG. 6:   Control thymus medulla.

        During the first 36 hr of dexamethasone administration,
however, cells (to be indicated as CS cells) in various stages of
degradation were present in cortex as well as in medulla;   CS cells
in the cortex being invariably of the smallest type of lymphocyte
present in this region, showing pycnosis and karyorrhexis (Fig.7,
CS, compare with Fig.5, CS),   in contrast with CS cells in the
medulla belonging to the large and medium sized type of lymphocyte
and showing signs of cytoplasmic swelling and karyolysis (Fig.8 and
6, CS).   Comparing the nuclear morphology of the undamaged cells
(to be indicated as CR cells) present during the first 36 hr of
dexamethasone treatment (Fig. 7 and 8) with the nuclear structure
of the cells of the peak fractions of high and medium density (Fig.
4 and 3), it is obvious that the CR medullary cells are of the
medium and the CR cortical cells are of the high density type.   It
is concluded therefore that within the rabbit thymus two subpopulations of CR lymphocytes are present, a minor one located in the
cortex (cells with compact heterochromatin patterns) apparently
corresponding to the high density class of CR cells, and a major
one located in the medulla (cells with disperse heterochromatin
patterns) apparently corresponding to the medium density class of
CR cells.

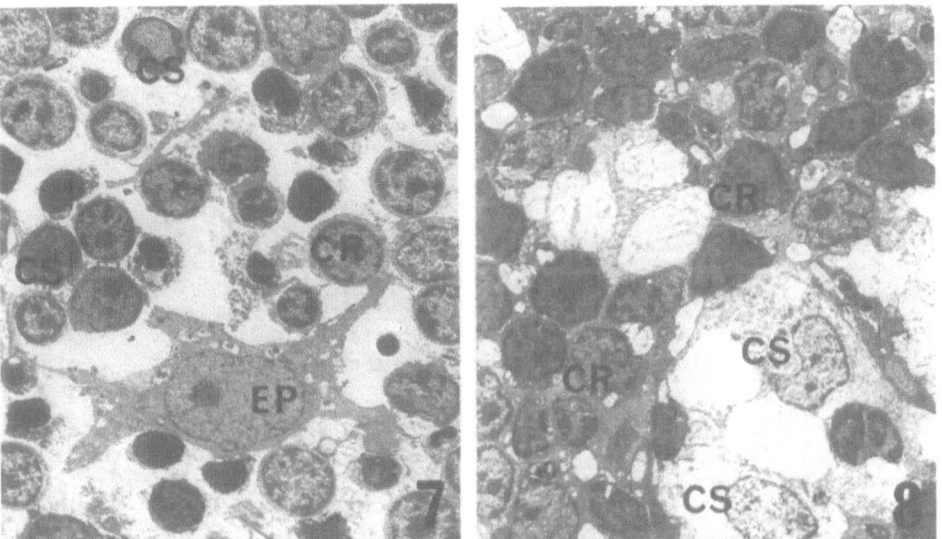

FIG. 7:   Degradation of small cortical cells (CS) after 24 hr
dexamethasone, compare with Fig.5 (CS).

FIG. 8:   Degradation of large and medium medullary cells (CS) after
24 hr dexamethasone, compare with Fig.6 (CS).   CR = CR cell,   EP
= epithelial cell.

DISCUSSION

Small thymic lymphocytes are generally subdivided into two subpopulations, CS cortical and CR medullary cells (2,3). The present
results provide evidence for the existence of a third subpopulation
of small thymocytes, a minor pool of CR cortical cells. The
functional significance of this subpopulation is questionable: it
may be speculated that the CR cortical cells are precursors of the
CR medullary cells, although the cell types appeared to be morphologically different; on the other hand, it should be considered that
the CR cortical lymphocytes may correspond to the spleen-seeking,
non-recirculating cells of relatively high density and the CR
medullary cells to the lymphnode seeking, recirculating cells of
relatively low density (7). Morphological criteria to distinguish
small cortical from small medullary thymocytes were presented earlier
by Abe and Ito (8) and were based mainly on cytoplasmic details;
our criteria are based on the patterns of heterochromatin distribution
of the nuclei of small thymocytes visualized with a tannic acid
fixation. Studies on the relation between the two categories of

morphological criteria are in progress. Moreover, functional parameters and surface antigens (8) of the two CR subpopulations will
be investigated to evaluate their stage of maturation and possible
role in the generation of peripheral lymphocytes.

REFERENCES

1.   Shortman, K., Progr. in Immunol. III, p.197 Austr. Ac. Sci.
      (1977).
2.   Field, E.J., J. Anat. 90 (1956) 428
3.   Blomgren, H., et al., Exp. Cell Res. 57 (1969) 185.
4.   Leene, W., et al., Ann. Immunol. (Inst. Pasteur) 127 C (1976)
      911.
5.   Futaesaku, Y., et al., Proc. Int. Congr. Histo-Cytochem. 4
      (1972) 155.
6.   Ainsworth, S.K., et al., J. Histochem. Cytochem 20 (1972) 995.
7.   Schlezinger, M., et al., Europ. J. Immunol. 3 (1973) 335.
8.   Abe, K., Ito, T., Z. Zellforsch. 110 (1970) 321.
9.   Roholl, P., et al., In: Dev. Immunobiol. p. 163, Elsevier Asd.
      (1977).

DEVELOPMENT OF AN ISOTOPE DILUTION ASSAY TO DETERMINE THE T-CELL MASS IN GUINEA PIGS

[1]J.M. Dwyer, M. Wade and M. Thakur

Departments of Medicine and Nuclear Medicine,
Yale University School of Medicine, New Haven,
Connecticut, U.S.A. 06510

[1]Investigator for the Howard Hughes Medical Institute

Evidence is accumulating which suggests that T-lymphocytes, both in humans and animals, have a remarkably long lifespan (1-4). Large numbers of T-lymphocytes with unstable chromosome forms have been observed in patients ten years after receiving radiotherapy (5) and some abnormal T-cells persisted 25 years after atomic bomb radiation in survivors from Hiroshima and Nagasaki (6). Thus a number of workers have suggested that the maximum lifespan of the small lymphocyte may well approach that of the animal and that after maturity T-cell clones may well be irreplaceable (2). In humans the serum level of the thymic hormone thymosin is stable until the age of 15 but then it declines steadily (7,8). The levels observed at 30 years are below those found to be effective in laboratory assays of thymosin activity (9).

Drainage of human thoracic duct lymph has been found in many studies to cause significant long-lasting immunological impairment (10,11). It seems that the loss of as few as 50×10^9 T-cells can result in long-lasting immunosuppression and there is now considerable evidence to suggest that in the adult the thymus cannot replace these lost cells.

To place T-cell loss from such causes as irradiation, blood donations, etc., in their correct perspective, knowledge of the total T-cell mass in humans will be necessary. Reported here are initial attempts to develop an isotope dilution assay in guinea pigs that will eventually be suitable for the study of T-cell movement and loss in humans.

Purified T-cells have been labelled with the isotope Indium^{III} as Indium Oxine. Indium ^{III} is cyclotron produced and is commercially available in a form free of carrier substances. The half-life of the isotope is 2.8 days. It emits gamma rays of optimum energies for detection with scanning gamma cameras (12,13). Indium oxine is soaked up through cell membranes nonspecifically because of its lipophilic nature (14). The label stays in lymphocytes tenaciously and does not impair the cells normal migration through lymphoid tissues (15).

Every known form of Indium^{III} has a very high affinity for the plasma protein transferrin and quite strong affinity for other proteins such as albumin. In order to label lymphocytes efficiently, the cells must be separated from other cells and suspended in protein-free medium. Indium^{III} does not leak significantly from live cells and isotope that does escape is rapidly bound to transferrin and other proteins and is not reusable by previously unlabelled cells.

Experiments with this isotope were designed to:

1.   find the optimal conditions for labelling purified guinea pig T-cells with Indium^{III};

2.   to determine the effects of the incorporated isotope on the function of the labelled cells;

3.   to examine the in vivo distribution and equilibration of the labelled cells to determine if a reproducible dilution assay was feasible.

Lymphnodes were surgically removed from outbred Harley guinea pigs two weeks after a footpad injection of Freund's adjuvant. T-cell purification was obtained by centrifuging cells rosetted with papaine-treated rabbit red blood cells through Ficoll Hypaque with subsequent lysis of the red cells. The T-cells so obtained were held with 0.5 μci of Indium^{III} per 10^6 cells for 30 minutes in a protein free media. 60% uptake of isotope was achieved in 15 minutes. Dilution studies with non-labelled cells revealed that Indium^{III} was distributed evenly among the labelled cells. Spontaneous leakage in vitro was only 5% of label in 24 hours. Thus if these conditions could be repeated in vivo the dilution of the isotope amongst T-cells could be used to calculate the T-cell pool into which the labelled cells had been distributed.

To determine the effects of the isotope on both the membrane characteristics and the function of labelled T-cells, lymphocytes were examined before and after labelling for their ability to

TAB. 1:   Relative Radioactivity/Gram of Various Tissues

| | Groups of Animals Studied | | | |
	T1	T2	T3	T4
% viable, mature T-cells among injected cells	nt	58	60	82
# animals	4	2	2	4
TISSUES				
liver	31	5.4	3.6	.4
spleen	36	5.4	9	1.2
lymphnodes	1.0	1.0	1.0	1.0
kidney		4.0	3.5	.2
lung	8	.6	1.2	.1
thymus	.2	.3	.2	.02
blood	.6	.08	.07	<.01
foot or muscle	.9	<.01	.1	<.01

rosette rabbit red blood cells, and to respond to the mitogen phytohemagglutinin.   No abnormalities were noted.

Fifteen experiments were performed in which guinea pigs received 10×10^6 Indium^{III} labelled autologous T-cells intravenously. Equilibration occurred after 24 hours and lymphnode, spleen and liver labelling could be visualized by gamma scanning.   No significant free isotope was present in the serum of animals examined 1-5 days after the injection of labelled cells.   As can be seen from Tab.1, in some experiments a significant amount of the Indium was recovered from the liver but histological examination of the tissue and Ficoll Hypaque sedimentation of homogenized liver did not reveal lymphocyte accumulation so that almost certainly these counts represented uptake by the reticuloendothelial system of damaged cells.   Allowing labelled cells to recover for 24 hours in tissue culture from the trauma associated with their purification and labelling considerably improved the distribution of the lymphocytes among lymphoid tissue.   Only 3% of the administered Indium^{III} was associated with T-cells in blood while the thymus did not contain any labelled cells.   Careful recovery of as much lymphoid tissue as possible for direct counts of the number of T-cells present never gave values in excess of 1×10^9 cells.   As this is a very small number of T-cells it is obvious that direct counting is extremely inefficient.

After mathematical adjustment to exclude the Indium^{III} counts that had accumulated in the liver repeated studies of the isotope dilution in the spleen, lymphnode and blood consistently suggested a total T-cell mass of 10-15 x 10^9 T-cells in the guinea pig. In Tab.1 the relative amount of radioactivity/gram of various tissues studied is detailed. The number of counts obtained from the lymphnodes of the animals has been equated to 1.0 and all the other figures given are compared to this standard. In the four experiments reported (T1-T4) note that improved technique associated with improved viability among T-cells injected in the animals resulted in better distribution of the isotope among lymphoid tissues and less uptake by the liver.

Indium labelled lymphocytes are already being injected into humans suffering from various forms of lymphoid malignancy and preliminary evidence would suggest that there may be even less damage to human lymphocytes and less uptake by the reticuloendothelial system than in the animals studied here. We are confident the approach reported here can be used to examine similar questions in humans.

REFERENCES

1. Ford, W.L., Lymphocyte migration and immune response. Progress in Allergy 19 (1975) 1.
2. Otteson, L.W., The age of human white cells in peripheral blood. Acta.Physiol. Scand. 32 (1954) 75.
3. Elves, M.W., The Lymphocytes. 2nd ed. Chicago (1972) Yearbook Medical Publishers Inc.
4. Caffrey, R.W., Rieke, W.O., Everett, N.B., Radioautographic studies of small lymphocytes in the thoracic duct of the rat. Acta. Haemat. 28 (1962) 145.
5. Buckton, K.E. et al., Lymphocyte survival in men treated with x-rays for ankylosing spondylitis. Nature 214 (1967) 470.
6. Awa, A.A. et al., Chromosome aberration frequency in cultured blood cells in relation to radiation dose of A-bomb survivors. Lancet ii (1971) 903.
7. Bach, J.F., Thymic hormone - from myth to facts. (editorial) Clin. Immunol. Immunopathol. 50 (1976) iii.
8. Schulof, R.S., Goldstein, A.L., Thymosin and the Endocrine Thymus. Adv. Int. Med. 22 (1977) 121.
9. Bach, J.F., et al., Isolation, biochemical characteristics, and biological activity of a circulating thymic hormone in the mouse and in the human. Ann. N.Y. Acad. Sci. 274 (1976) 186.

10. Sarles, H.E., et al., Depletion of lymphocytes for the
     protection of renal allografts. Arch. Int. Med. 125 (1970) 443.
11. Sarles, H.E., et al., Suppression of cellular immunity by lymph
     duct drainage in man. Clin. Res. 16 (1968) 323.
12. Goodwin, D.A., et al., Preparation, physiology and dosimetry of
     ^{III}In-labelled radiopharmaceuticals for cisternography. Radiol-
     ogy. 198 (1973) 91.
13. MacDonald, N.S., et al., Methods for compact cyclotron pro-
     duction of indium-III for medical use. Int. J. Appl. Radiat.
     Isot. 26 (1975) 631.
14. Albert, A., et al., The influence of chemical constitution of
     anti-bacterial activity Part VII. The site of action of 8-
     hydroxy-quinoline (oxine). Brit. J. Exp. Path. 35 (1954) 75.
15. Rannie, G., et al., Radiolabels for lymphocyte migration
     studies. Clin. Exp. Immunol. (in press).

ACKNOWLEDGEMENTS

This work was supported in part by NIH Grant AI 11785.

LYMPHOCYTE PRODUCTION AND ORGAN DISTRIBUTION OF NEWLY FORMED LYMPHOCYTES AFTER SELECTIVE ^{3}H-DEOXYCYTIDINE LABELLING OF MESENTERIC LYMPH NODES

R. Pabst[1] and F. Trepel[2]

[1]Division of Functional and Applied Anatomy, Medical School of Hannover, D 3000 Hannover 61, Postfach 610180

[2]Division of Clinical Morphology, University of Ulm, D 7900 Ulm/D, West Germany

Systemic labelling procedures with DNA precursors showed lymphocytopoiesis in normal lymph nodes. For quantitative aspects of lymphocyte production in lymph nodes, the rate of exit from the lymph nodes and entry of newly formed lymphocytes from other organs must be known. For rat lymphatic tissue, a preferential labelling of lymphocytes with a rapid turnover rate by tritiated deoxycytidine ([3]HdCy) application was demonstrated (1). In the present study mesenteric lymph nodes of young pigs were selectively labelled with 125 μCi (specific activity 20 Ci/mM) of [3]HdCy. The organ distribution of radioactively labelled lymphocytes one or two days later indicated the migration pattern of newly formed lymph node lymphocytes, and by summing up all labelled lymphocytes the total amount of lymphocytopoiesis could be estimated. In normal young pigs (about 23 kg body weight) mesenteric lymph nodes were labelled by about 50 minute injections of [3]HdCy into the parenchyma. Two pigs were killed 24 and two 48 hours after labelling by bleeding to death. The relative number of newly formed lymphocytes was determined autoradiographically on imprints or histologic sections of the following organs: labelled mesenteric lymph nodes, unlabelled mesenteric, cervical and inguinal lymph nodes, spleen, thymus, bone marrow, tonsil, jejunum, ileum, colon, liver, lung and serial samples of peripheral blood. The technical details of the operation, autoradiography and evaluation were comparable to those used in a previous study on splenic lymphocytopoiesis (5). The labelling indices determined on histological sections were corrected according to the method of Modak et al. (3). The absolute number of emigrated newly formed lymphocytes was calculated on the basis of a previous

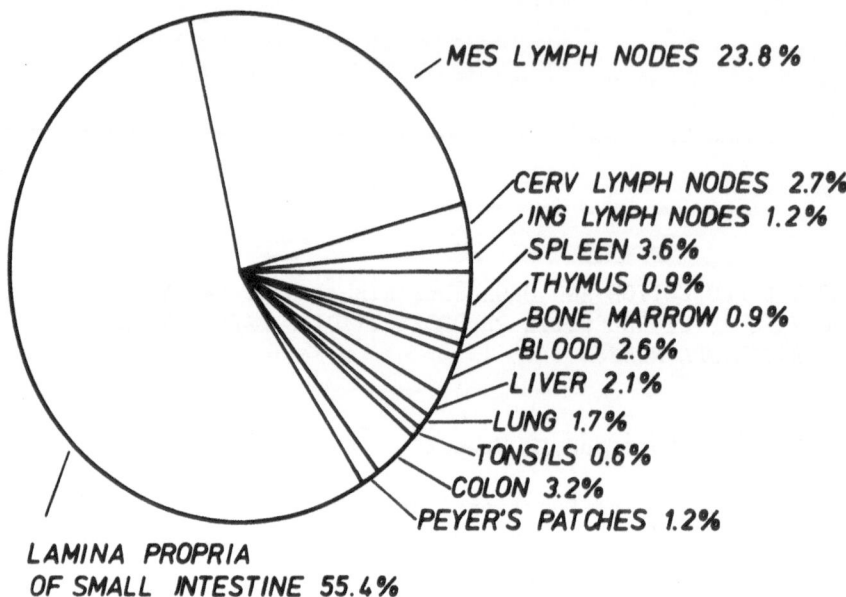

FIG. 1:   Organ distribution (%) of labelled lymphocytes found 24
h after local labelling of mesenteric lymph nodes (initially
labelled mesenteric nodes excluded). (Mes cerv and ing lymph nodes
are mesenteric, cervical and inguinal lymph nodes).

calculation of the total number of lymphocytes in these organs in
similar young pigs (4).

    As evidence for the selectivity of the labelling procedures the
following findings were made : absence of labelling in epithelial
cells of the intestinal mucosa, in lymphoid blast and plasma cells
of the spleen and in cells of the erythroid and granulocytic series
in the bone marrow. The injection of [3]HdCy into the lymph node
parenchyma resulted in no obvious destruction or hemorrhage into the
lymph nodes.

    Lymphoid cells of germinal centers were preferentially labelled
but labelled cells could also be found in other areas of the lymph
nodes. The preference of [3]HdCy seemed not to be as marked as in
rats (1). No obvious differences could be seen after 24 or 48 hours
in the distribution of labelled cells in injected mesenteric lymph
nodes or in the organ distribution of emigrated, newly formed cells.
From 3 hours after labelling labelled lymphocytes were found in the
peripheral blood and remained at a rather constant level from about
6 hours onwards. The relative and absolute number of lymphocytes

TAB. 1: Relative and absolute number of labelled lymphoid cells found 24 or 48 hours after selectively labelling of mesenteric lymph nodes(GALT = Gut-associated-lymphoid-tissue). Each column represents the data of one pig.

ORGAN	24 HOURS AFTER LABELLING LABELLING INDEX (%)		LABELLED CELLS x 10⁶		48 HOURS AFTER LABELLING LABELLING INDEX (%)		LABELLED CELLS x 10⁶	
LYMPH NODES								
mesenteric "labelled"	3.6	4.0	990	1020	2.8	2.2	962	934
mesenteric "unlabelled"	0.32	0.25	176	138	0.12	0.15	64	83
cervical	0.09	0.07	21	15	0.07	0.10	20	29
inguinal	0.09	0.06	10	7	0.07	0.11	8	12
SPLEEN	0.09	0.06	28	19	0.08	0.04	25	14
THYMUS	0.004	0.004	6	6	0.004	0	6	0
BONE MARROW	0.07	0	12	0	0	0	0	0
BLOOD	0.23	0.1	24	10	0.12	0.13	12	13
GALT								
PEYER'S PATCHES	0.07	0.14	5	10	0.06	0.11	4	8
LAMINA PROPRIA OF SMALL INTESTINE	–	–	250	480	–	–	305	236
COLON	–	–	29	13	–	–	8	7
TONSILS	–	–	3	5	–	–	5	6
LUNG	–	–	17	5	–	–	5	9
LIVER	–	–	8	20	–	–	20	9
TOTAL			1579	1748			1452	1360

TAB. 2:   Regional distribution of labelled lymphocytes (%)   (PALS = Periarteriolar lymphatic sheath).

| | | | Time after labelling | | |
		24 hours		48 hours	
SPLEEN	PALS	57%	52%	43%	49%
	CORONA	10%	12%	11%	10%
	MARGINAL ZONE	22%	22%	32%	23%
	FOLLICLES	0%	11%	4%	3%
	RED PULP	11%	3%	9%	12%
CERVICAL LYMPH NODES	PARACORTICAL	78%	76%	74%	76%
	CORONA	19%	14%	8%	14%
	FOLLICLES	0%	3%	2%	1%
	OTHERS	3%	7%	16%	9%
MESENTERIC LYMPH NODES	PARACORTICAL	79%	60%	60%	69%
	CORONA	18%	29%	20%	16%
	FOLLICLES	0%	0%	6%	5%
	OTHERS	3%	11%	13%	10%
TONSILS	PARAFOLLICULAR	65%	75%	57%	52%
	CORONA	27%	9%	17%	23%
	FOLLICLES	0%	6%	4%	3%
	SUBEPITHELIAL	8%	9%	23%	23%
PEYER'S PATCHES	PARAFOLLICULAR	69%	59%	59%	64%
	CORONA	10%	20%	20%	15%
	FOLLICLES	0%	4%	12%	11%
	DOME	20%	17%	7%	5%

(The left-hand bracket spanning CERVICAL, MESENTERIC and TONSILS/PEYER'S groups is labelled **UNLABELLED**.)

produced by mesenteric lymph nodes are given in Tab.1.   The labelling index for the injected lymph nodes was determined on imprints of 27 different tissue samples.   For an estimation of the lymphocyte production of all mesenteric lymph nodes the data actually found had to be corrected, because not all nodes were injected and due to the intraparenchymal injection technique not all areas of these nodes could be reached by the label sufficiently.   The mean of the labelling indexes of the six tissue samples with the highest indexes was assumed to be representative for optimally labelled areas.   Thus, the total number of labelled lymphocytes found had to be corrected with these two factors which resulted in 6.2×10^9 and 4.5×10^9 lymphocytes for 24 and 48 hours respectively or 11% and 8.5% of all lymphocytes in mesenteric lymph nodes. About 40% of all newly formed lymphocytes have already left the mesenteric lymph nodes 24 hours after labelling in comparison to about 17% of newly formed splenic lymphocytes (5).

The relative organ distribution of the newly formed lymphocytes one day after labelling is shown (in Fig.1). A preferential homing to the small intestine (55%) and to the primarily unlabelled mesenteric lymph nodes (24%) is obvious. This preference supports previous findings of labelling blasts from the mesenteric lymph in vitro, which migrated predominantly back to the gut, which led to the hypothesis to classify lymphocytes into somatic and gut lympho-cytes (2). On histological slides at least 100 labelled lymphocytes were scored per organ, to which area the newly formed cells homed. In the thymus 98% of the labelled lymphocytes were found in the medulla, most of them near to the corticomedullary junction. In all organs studied: spleen, cervical unlabelled mesenteric lymph node, tonsils and Peyer's patches, the newly formed cells were predominantly found in "T" cell regions (Tab.2).

Only few studies are known in which a selective labelling of lymph nodes with DNA precursors was performed (such as 6), but a calculation of the total production and organ distribution was not attempted. Even when not taking account of cell death during the time studied and reutilization, one can conclude that in normal young pigs the rate of lymphocytopoiesis is high in mesenteric lymph nodes, a considerable number of the newly produced lymphocytes leave the organ within 24 hours, show a preferential homing to the gut associated lymphoid tissue and a preference to "T" cell regions of lymphoid organs.

REFERENCES

1. Amano, M., Everett, N.B., Cell Tissue Kinet. 9 (1976) 167.
2. Hall, J.G., Hopkins, J., Orlans, E., Biochem. Soc. Trans. 5 (1977) 1581.
3. Modak, S.P., Lever, W.E., Therwath, A.M., Uppuluri, V.R.R., Exp. Cell Res. 76 (1973) 73.
4. Pabst, R., Trepel, F., Blut 31 (1975) 77.
5. Pabst, R., Munz, D., Trepel, F., Cell Immunol. 33 (1977) 33.
6. Werdelin, O., Acta path. microbiol. scand. Sect. A., Suppl. 232 (1972).

ACKNOWLEDGEMENTS

This study was supported by the Deutsche Forschungsgemeinschaft (Pa 240/1).

GERMINAL CENTERS AND THE B-CELL SYSTEM: B CELL DIFFERENTIATION IN RABBIT APPENDIX GERMINAL CENTERS

Davine Opstelten, Dieuwertje van der Heijden, Rita Stikker and Paul Nieuwenhuis

Department of Histology, State University of Groningen, Groningen, The Netherlands

INTRODUCTION

Recently a choice of B cell differentiation models has become available (1,2,3). In general, peripheral mature (a.o. surface immunoglobulin- and complement receptor-bearing) B cells are thought to derive from relatively undifferentiated though committed (containing cytoplasmic IgM, no surface markers) pre-B cells as present in the bone marrow (4,5). Usually this process is considered to be antigen independent and to occur also in germfree animals (6). Antigen dependent B cell differentation is mainly restricted to terminal differentiation of mature B cells (antibody forming cell precursors, AFCP's) into actually antibody forming cells (AFC's or plasmacells). In some instances, however, (7,8) it is suggested that antigen may also be instrumental in the earlier stages of B cell maturation, and there are some indications that spleen B cells from germfree animals cannot do all the tricks that B cells from conventionally reared animals can, i.e. respond to LPS stimulation by polyclonal antibody formation (9). It should be noted that due to a lack of antigenic stimulation germfree animals are also germinal center free (10).

Previous work (11,12) suggested that at least in the rabbit part of the primary IgM AFCP-pool may derive from germinal centers (GC's) a.o. as present in the appendix. Whether GC processing of these cells involves maturation of immature bone marrow derived cells to AFCP or simply amplification was not established at that time (see also: 13). On the other hand, there is a wealth of information relating GC to memory cell production (14). Thus, some data are available as to the characteristics of the cell(s) produced in GC (GC-Derived Cells, GCDC's). Also quite a lot is known about the

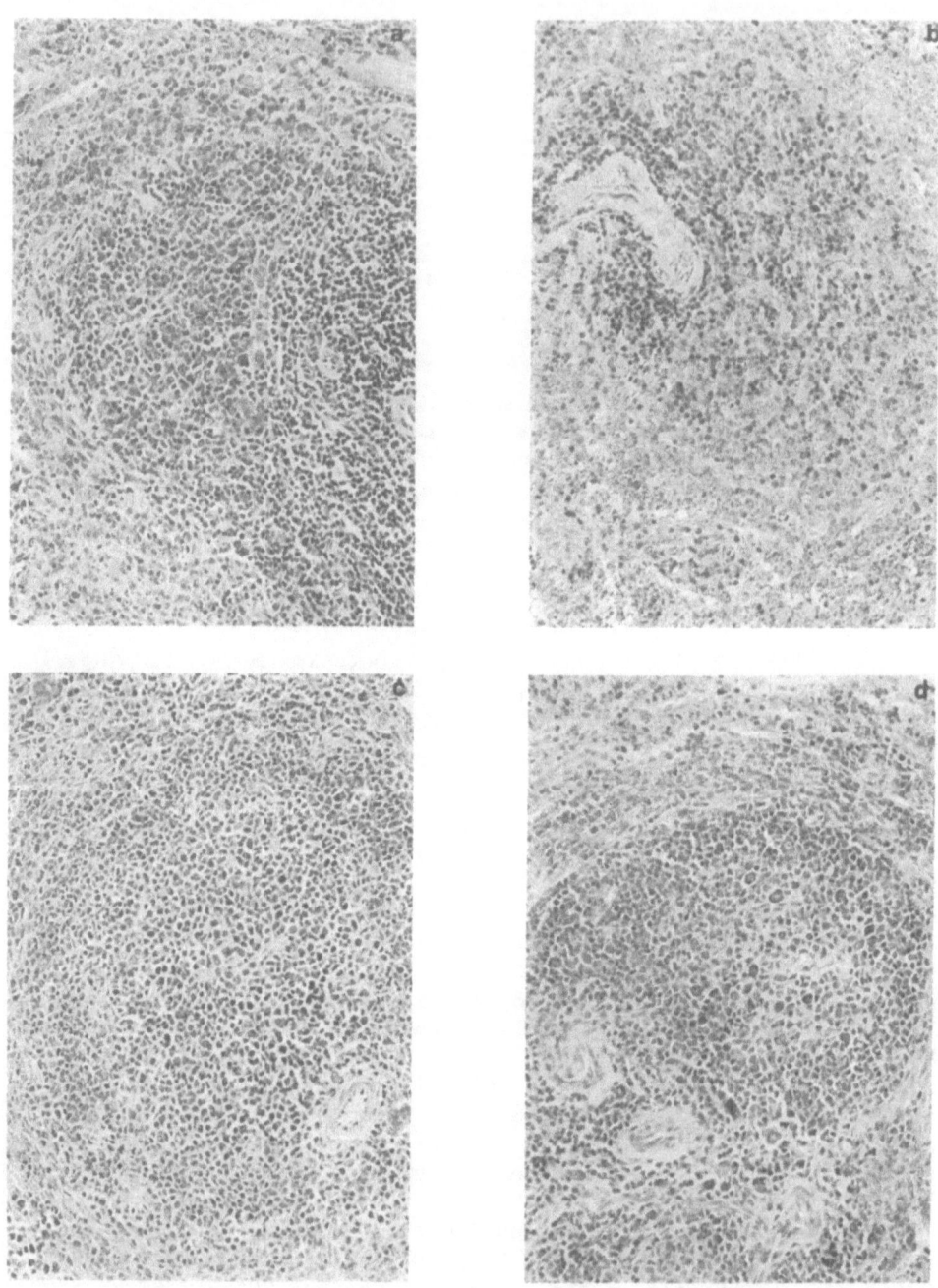

FIG. 1:   Regeneration of follicular structure in the rabbit spleen
7 days after 450 rads whole body X-irradiation. a) Ax X AGCC. b)
As X.   c) Ax X AGCC injected i.v. with Salmonella flagellar antigen
1 day after X-irradiation.   d) As X likewise antigen-stimulated (x 240).
(Reduced 20% for purposes of reproduction.).

prerequisites for germinal center formation a.o. antigenic stimulation, factors involved in antigen trapping and T cells (14).

Little is known, however, about the cell(s), from which GC
originate (GC-Precursor Cells, GCPC). In mammals, available evidence
indicates GCPC to be ultimately bone marrow derived, but further
characteristics are completely lacking. Our present aim is twofold:
1) to characterize the GCPC and, by comparing its characteristics
with those of GCDC, to gain more insight in the events taking place
inside a GC (proliferation, maturation?) and 2) to investigate how
this antigen dependent phase of B cell production as occuring in GC
fits in the overall scheme of B cell differentiation from stem cell
to mature B cell.

EXPERIMENTAL DESIGN

To answer these questions, a source of GCPC is needed. In this
paper we focus on the GC compartment of follicles in the rabbit
appendix, where GCPC's as such might still be present. Using the
stripping technique as devised by Ozer and Waksman (13), the GC
compartment could be isolated. Following 450 rads whole body X-
irradiation, the appendix GC cell suspension (AGCC) was reinjected
into the donor animal (code: Ax X AGCC; control: Ax X). Spleen
histology following reconstitution, with or without antigenic
stimulation, was studied as well as functional consequences as to
primary antibody forming capacity and memory cell production. For
comparison, rabbits X-irradiated with the appendix shielded (code:
As X; control: X) were studied. In this model, cells from the
appendix migrate to other peripheral lymphoid tissues under more or
less physiological conditions. Previous results (11) indicate that
(the majority of) these appendix-leaving cells are actually derived
from appendix GC and thus might constitute a reference population
of GCDC.

RESULTS AND DISCUSSION

Post-irradiation regeneration of follicular structures in the
spleen. Upon injection of AGCC, at first primary follicles, and
from 7 days onwards also rapidly expanding GC were seen in the spleen,
even without exogenous antigen administration (Fig.1a,c). Heat
killing of AGCC totally abolished GC formation. In non-reconstituted
appendectomized control animals, deficient regeneration of follicular
structure in the spleen was observed. In rabbits X-irradiated with
the appendix shielded, enhanced regeneration of follicular structure
was observed in the spleen (Fig.1b) as compared to whole body X-
irradiated controls (not shown). Antigenic stimulation was necessary

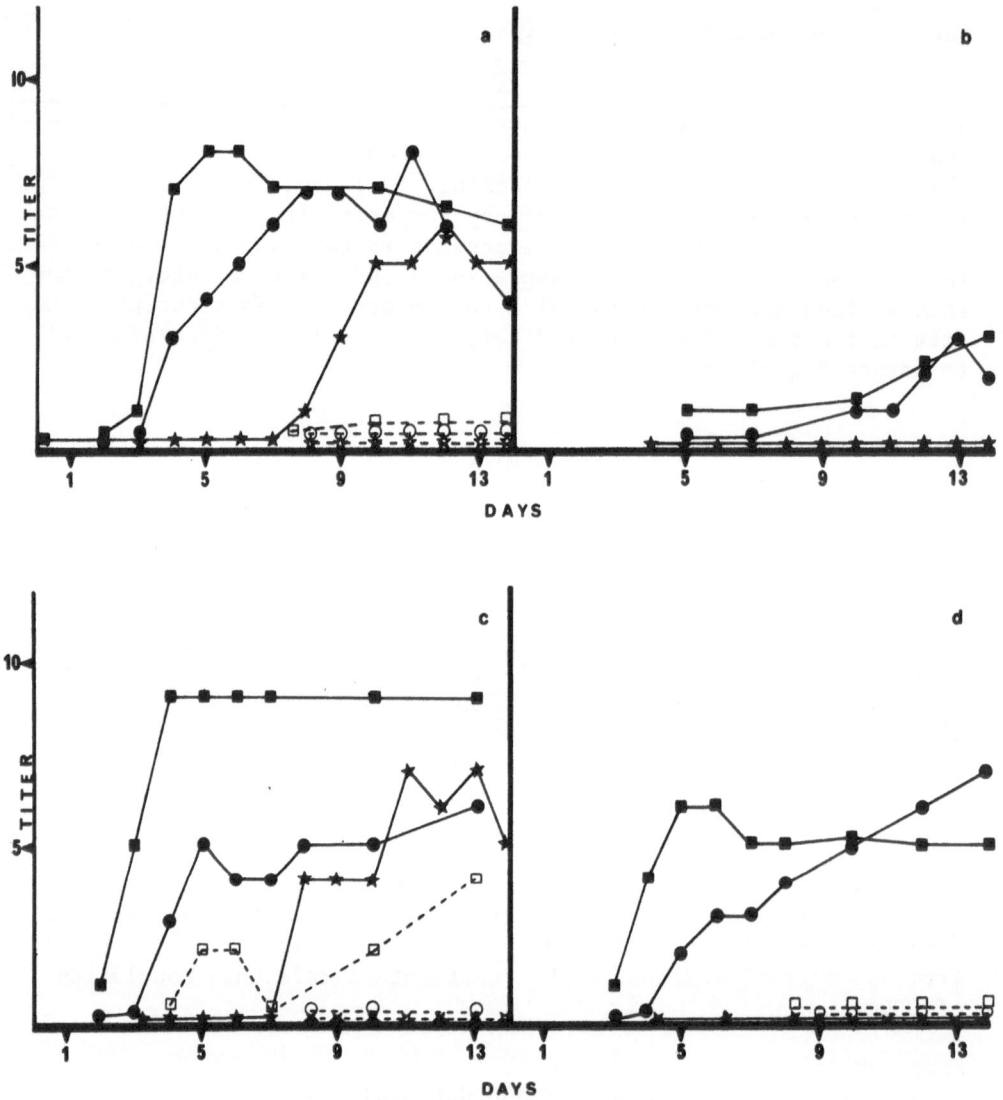

FIG. 2: Regeneration of primary responsiveness in 450 rads X-irradiated rabbits. a) Ax X AGCC. b) Ax X (control). c) As X. d) X
(control). Salmonella flagellar antigen was given i.v. 1 day (★), 7
days (●) or 14 days (■) after irradiation. In the following two weeks
serum-H-agglutinin titers (total——and 2-mercapto-ethanol resistant
---) were determined. Titers were expressed as $\log_2$ of the reciprocal
of the highest dilution showing visible agglutination. Results within
each group of animals (at least five individuals) are presented as
median titers. Day 0: day of antigen administration.

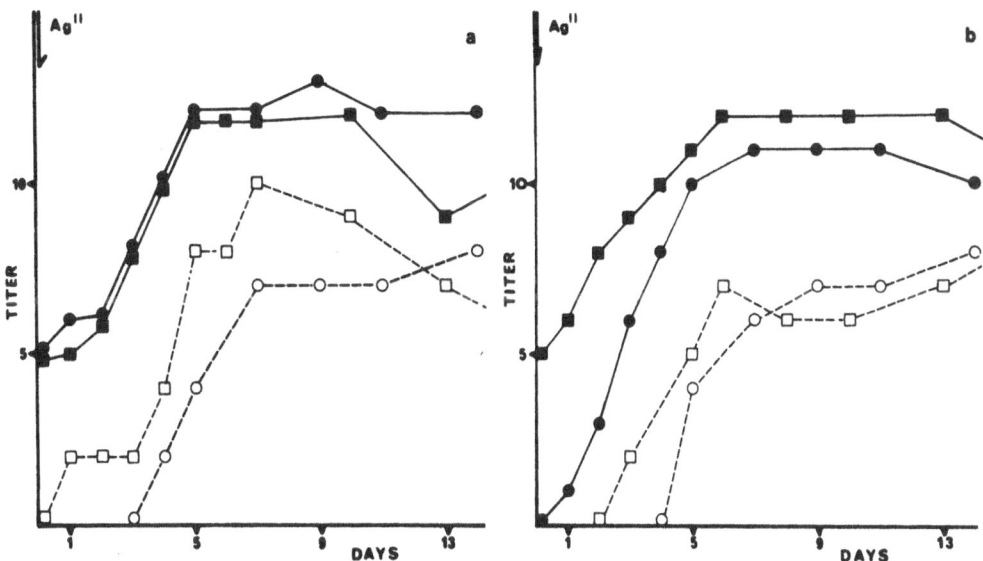

FIG. 3: Regeneration of secondary responsiveness in X-irradiated rabbits. Rabbits were primed with Salmonella flagellar antigen i.v. 1 day after irradiation and challenged 10 (●) or 14 (■) days later. Titers are expressed as described in legends to Fig.2. a) Ax X AGCC. b) As X.

to induce GC formation (Fig.1d). Apparently, both AGCC and appendix-(GC?)-derived cells, when appropriately stimulated, are capable of GC-formation.

Post irradiation regeneration of immune responsiveness. In both groups (Ax X AGCC and As X) primary immune responsiveness was restricted to IgM antibody synthesis, which was low and of late onset (day 7) when tested 1 day after irradiation, but near normal when tested 14 days after irradiation (Fig.2). In all instances, responsiveness was well above controls. These data indicate that in As X-rabbits the shielded appendix with its highly active GC's is responsible for a continuous production (and delivery) of IgM-precursors, a process which after injection of AGCC is mimicked by the rapidly expanding GC as observed in the spleen of reconstituted rabbits. Upon priming (day 1) and subsequent challenge (day 10 or 14), both groups showed an excellent secondary response (both IgM and IgG) (Fig.3), presumably due to B memory cell production deriving from specifically induced GC in the spleen.

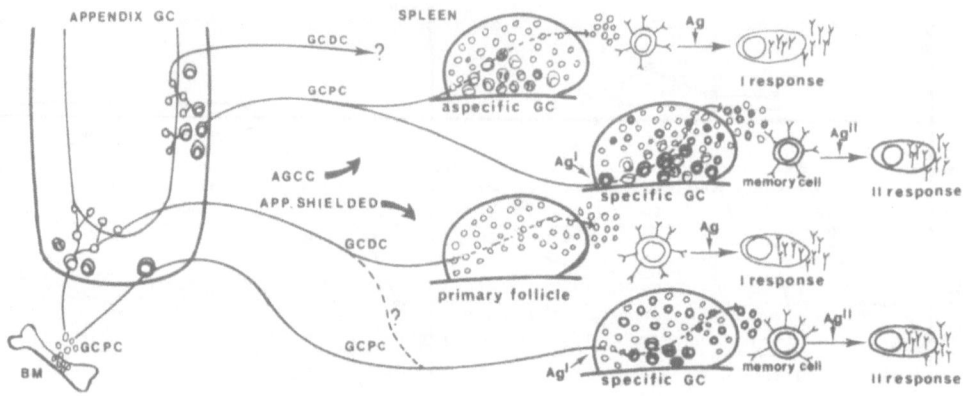

FIG. 4:   Possible B cell differentiation pathways in appendix GC.

CONCLUSION

The present results indicate that processing of B cells in germinal centers need not necessarily be a one way track involving maturation of immature bone marrow-derived cells into mature AFCP as was suggested on the basis of previous results (12). Fig.4 shows alternative or additional pathways, which are consistent with the results as presented above. At present, our efforts are focussed on characterizing the GCPC as present among AGCC.

REFERENCES

1.   Immunological Reviews 37 (1977).
2.   Cold Spring Harbor Symposia on Quantitative Biology vol. XVI (1977).
3.   Progress in Immunology III (1977).
4.   Parkhouse, R.M.E., Cooper, M.D., Immunol. Rev. 37 (1977) 105.
5.   Osmond, D.G., in: Stem cells of renewing cell population (1976) 195. Eds. A.B. Cairnie et al. Academic Press, N.Y.
6.   Metcalf, E.S., et al. Progress in Immunol. III (1977) 162.
7.   Strober, S., Progress in Immunol. III (1977) 183.
8.   Nossal, G.J.V., et al., Immunol. Rev. 37 (1977) 187.
9.   Kim, Y.B., Progress in Immunol. III (1977) 747.
10.   Gordon, H.A., Wostmann, B.S., Anat. Rec. 137 (1960) 65.
11.   Nieuwenhuis, P., et al., Immunology 26 (1974) 497.
12.   Nieuwenhuis, P., Keuning, F.J., Immunology 26 (1974) 509.
13.   Waksman, B.H., et al., Lab. Invest. 28 (1973) 614.

14.   Thorbecke, G.J., et al., Progress in Immunol. II vol. 3 (1974)
      25.

ACKNOWLEDGEMENTS

This study was supported by Fungo / ZWO (13-27-17).

THE INFLUENCE OF THE THYMUS UPON THE NUMBER AND CLASS DISTRIBUTION
OF IMMUNOGLOBULIN CONTAINING CELLS IN THE BONE MARROW AND OTHER
LYMPHOID ORGANS OF THE MOUSE

R. Benner, A. van Oudenaren, J.J. Haaijman, J. Slingerland-
Teunissen, Th. H. van der Kwast and E.A.J. Wolters

Dept. of Cell Biology and Genetics, Erasmus University,
Rotterdam, and Institute for Experimental Gerontology,
Organization for Health Research TNO, Rijswijk (ZH),
The Netherlands

INTRODUCTION

Due to the lack of mature T-cells, congenitally athymic (nude)
mice have severely decreased serum IgG and IgA levels, together
with normal or enhanced serum IgM levels (1-3). The cells responsible
for the synthesis of these immunoglobulins are demonstrable as
cytoplasmic immunoglobulin containing cells (C-Ig cells) by means
of immunofluorescence (4). C-Ig cell numbers in the spleen are
comparable in young and adult nude and heterozygous mice, whereas
the age-related increase of the C-Ig cell population in the other
lymphoid organs is retarded in nude mice (5). This is especially
true for the bone marrow, which contains the majority of all C-Ig
cells in thymus-bearing mice at adult age (5-7). In this paper the
effect of thymus transplantation was studied upon the number and
class distribution of C-Ig cells in spleen, bone marrow, mesenteric
lymph node and Peyer's patches of nude mice.

MATERIALS AND METHODS

Mice. Female and male nu/nu and nu/+ mice on a CBA and B10.LP
background were purchased from the Radiobiological Institute TNO,
Rijswijk (ZH), and the Central Institute for the Breeding of
Laboratory Animals TNO, Zeist, The Netherlands, respectively. During
the experiments the animals were maintained in laminar flow hoods.
Each experimental group consisted of 7 or 8 mice.

Thymus transplantation.   Single thymus lobes from neonatal
B10.LP mice were transplanted under the kidney capsule of 8-week-
old B10.LP nu/nu mice. The thymus donors were irradiated before
use with 300 rad in a Philips Müller MG 300 X-ray machine as
described previously (8). In Tables 1 and 2 thymus transplantation
is indicated as TH. Control nu/nu and nu/+ mice received a sham-
surgery.

Enumeration of C-Ig cells.   Cell suspensions of spleen, bone
marrow, mesenteric lymph node (LN) and Peyer's patches were prepared
as described previously (5). Cytocentrifuge preparations were made
according to Vossen et al. (9). The technique for the visualization
of C-Ig cells by means of immunofluorescence and the way of calculation of the total number of C-Ig cells per organ have also been
described in detail in previous papers (5,6). In Tables 1 and 2
the figures represent the arithmetic mean ± 1 standard error of the
mean.

Conjugated antisera.   A fluorescein conjugated goat antiserum
directed against mouse immunoglobulins (Nordic Immunological Laboratories, Tilburg, The Netherlands) was used to determine the total
number of C-Ig cells per slide. The Ig class distribution of the
C-Ig cells was determined by using combinations of rhodamine and
fluorescein labelled goat antisera specific for the Fc part of IgM,
IgG and IgA, respectively. These antisera and conjugates were
prepared, purified and generously supplied by Dr. J. Radl and Miss
P. van den Berg from the Institute for Experimental Gerontology TNO.
The antisera fulfilled all specificity criteria described previously
(5).

RESULTS

The total number of cells containing cytoplasmic immunoglobulin
(C-Ig cells) in spleen, bone marrow, mesenteric lymph node and
Peyer's patches is presented in Tab. 1 for both nu/nu and nu/+ mice
of 8 and 40 weeks of age. As reported previously (5) C-Ig cell
numbers in the spleen of nu/nu and nu/+ mice were comparable, whereas
the figures for bone marrow, mesenteric lymph node and Peyer's
patches were several times higher in the nu/+ mice. Transplantation
of 300 rad irradiated neonatal thymus tissue under the kidney capsule
of 8-week-old nu/nu mice could restore this C-Ig cell deficiency
(Tab. 1). This result suggests that the retarded development of the
immunological activity in nude mice (5) is not directly genetically
determined, but is due to the absence of a functioning thymus.

The immunoglobulin class distribution of the C-Ig cells in
spleen, bone marrow, mesenteric lymph node and Peyer's patches of
the 40-week-old mice is presented in Tab. 2. These profiles were

TAB. 1:   Effect of Thymus Transplantation upon the Number of C-Ig
Cells in Various Lymphoid Organs of Nude Mice and their Heterozygous
Littermates

Organ	Age	C-Ig cells x 10^{-3}/organ		
	(weeks)	nu/nu	nu/nu + TH	nu/+
Spleen	8	122±4	–	130±23
	40	140±16	277±40	159±67
Bone marrow	8	48±4	–	292±47
	40	288±27	805±83	1023±142
Mesenteric LN	8	3.5±0.7	–	29±6
	40	1.5±0.4	80±22	19±4
Peyer's patches	8	2.0±0.3	–	18±2
	40	0.3±0.1	8.6±1.3	6±2

obtained from the same mice that were used in Tab. 1. The selection
in the presented combinations of heavy chains is inherent to the
combinations of antisera we employed. It should be noted that the
specificity of the fluorescent conjugates is corroborated by the
fact that in a number of specimens no cells could be detected
containing more than one Ig class.

In the spleen, bone marrow and mesenteric lymph node of nu/nu
mice C-IgM cells were preponderant, while in the Peyer's patches of
nu/nu mice C-IgA cells were the most frequently occurring C-Ig
cells. In all lymphoid organs of nu/+ mice studied, the percentage
of C-IgM cells was much lower than in nu/nu mice. The total number
of C-IgG and C-IgA cells together tended to be more numerous on a
per cent basis in bone marrow, mesenteric lymph node and Peyer's
patches than in spleen. Transplantation of thymus tissue under the
kidney capsule of nu/nu mice restored the class distribution of the
C-Ig cells to that characteristic for nu/+ mice (Tab. 2).

                            DISCUSSION

The bone marrow is an important site of antibody production
in mice. This follows from a number of studies using both thymus-
dependent (10,11) and thymus-independent (12,13) antigens. After
primary immunization with thymus-dependent antigens only minor
numbers of antibody-producing plaque-forming cells (PFC) are to be
found in the bone marrow (10,11). After a second injection of the

TAB. 2:   Effect of Thymus Transplantation upon the Class Distribution of C-Ig Cells in Various Lymphoid Organs of Nude Mice and their Heterozygous Littermates

Organ	Mice	% of C-Ig cells				
		IgM	IgG	IgA	IgM+IgG	IgM+IgA
Spleen	nu/nu	83+3	7+3	2+1	3+1	5+3
	nu/nu + TH	26+3	32+8	25+11	11+2	6+3
	nu/+	31+7	29+1	22+9	16+3	2+1
Bone marrow	nu/nu	69+4	15+5	6+2	1+0.4	9+4
	nu/nu + TH	16+6	32+7	26+7	18+7	8+3
	nu/+	20+7	28+11	39+18	12+7	1+1
Mesenteric LN	nu/nu	52+6	17+2	25+7	6+3	0.6+0.6
	nu/nu + TH	16+3	43+11	38+12	3+1	0.4+0.3
	nu/+	17+5	40+13	38+11	4+1	1+0.5
Peyer's patches	nu/nu	34+4	11+3	54+5	1+1	0
	nu/nu + TH	36+1	41+4	21+5	2+1	0.5+0.2
	nu/+	29+7	42+3	25+8	4+1	0.2+0.2

same antigen, however, the number of PFC in the bone marrow can rise to a level which surpasses the total number of PFC in all the other lymphoid organs together (10,11).   Immunization with the thymus-independent antigen Escherichia coli lipopolysaccharide (LPS) induces bone marrow antibody formation not only during the secondary, but also during the primary response (12,13).   Concerning the total of all immunoglobulin containing cells (C-Ig cells) in mice, the majority of these cells is located in the spleen at a young age, whereas during ageing the bone marrow becomes the major site of localization of C-Ig cells (5-7).   We have suggested (6,7) that the gradually increasing importance of the bone marrow as site of C-Ig cells represents an adaptation of the individual mice to their antigenic environment.   The more an individual ages, the more often a given antigenic challenge will have been encountered previously. Consequently, during ageing secondary type responses will go to prevail, involving antibody formation in the bone marrow (10,11).

In nude mice thymus-dependent immune responses are deficient (12,14), but antibody formation in the spleen to thymus-independent antigens is normal (13,15).   Young adult B10.LP nu/nu mice were found to be deficient as regards anti-LPS PFC responses in the bone marrow, whereas the splenic anti-LPS PFC response was normal or enhanced (13).   This was found to be associated with the presence of relatively small numbers of C-Ig cells in the marrow of these mice (Tab. 1). During ageing C-Ig cell numbers in the bone marrow of nude mice become as high as in their heterozygous littermates (5), indicating a retarded development of the immunological activity in nude mice. Transplantation of thymus tissue under the kidney capsule of nude mice restored the C-Ig cell number in the bone marrow to a level which is normal for nu/+ mice (Tab. 1). This result suggests that the retarded development of immunological activity in nude mice is not directly genetically determined, but is due to their lack of normal thymus function.

Several immune functions which are deficient in nude mice restore after thymus transplantation or injection of H-2 compatible T cells (2,14,16). Usually it takes quite a long period for complete recovery, if ever reached (16). Here we show that C-Ig cell numbers and their Ig class distribution were normal in the various lymphoid organs at 32 weeks after thymus transplantation (Tables 1 and 2). At that moment the mesenteric lymph node contained 35+3% T cells, which is almost half the figure which was found in the heterozygous littermates (64+4%). The absolute number of T cells in the mesenteric lymph node of nude mice with a thymus transplant was also about half of that found in the heterozygous controls (data not shown). Apparently full quantitative recovery of the T cell population is not required for the appearance of normal C-Ig cell numbers and normal Ig class distribution.

Presently we are investigating the kinetics of the Ig class distribution of the C-Ig cells in the bone marrow and the other lymphoid organs of nude mice after thymus transplantation.

REFERENCES

1. Bloemmen, J., Eyssen, H., Eur. J. Immunol. 3 (1973) 117.
2. Pritchard, H., Riddaway, J., Micklem, H.S., Clin. exp. Immunol. 13 (1973) 125.
3. Bankhurst, A.D., Lambert, P.H., Miescher, P.A., Proc. Soc. Exp. Biol. Med 148 (1975) 501.
4. Hijmans, W., Schuit, H.R.E., Hulsing-Hesselink, E., Ann. N.Y. Acad. Sci. 177 (1971) 290.
5. Haaijman, J.J., Slingerland-Teunissen, J., Benner, R., van Oudenaren, A., Immunology, in press.
6. Haaijman, J.J., Schuit, H.R.E., Hijmans, W., Immunol. 32 (1977) 427.
7. Haaijman, J.J., Hijmans, W., Mech. Ageing Develop. 7 (1978) 375.
8. Benner, R., Meima, F., van der Meulen, G.M., Cell. Immunol. 13 (1974) 95.
9. Vossen, J.M.J.J., Langlois van der Berg, R.E., Schuit, H.R.E., Hijmans, W., J. Immunol. Methods 13 (1976) 71.
10. Benner, R., van Oudenaren, A., Cell. Immunol. 19 (1975) 167.
11. Hill, S.W., Immunol. 30 (1976) 895.

12. Benner, R., van Oudenaren, A., Immunol. 30 (1976) 49.
13. Benner, R., van Oudenaren, A., Haaijman, J.J., Immunol. in
     press.
14. Wortis, H.H., Clin. exp. Immunol. 8 (1971) 305.
15. Manning, J.K., Reed, N.D., Jutila, J.W., J. Immunol. 108 (1972)
     1470.
16. Loor, F., Kindred, B., Hägg, L.B., Cell. Immunol. 26 (1976) 29.

ACKNOWLEDGEMENTS

     We thank Dr. J. Radl and Miss P. van den Berg most sincerely
for making us available the purified fluorescent conjugates specific
for the Fc part of the different Ig classes. Furthermore, we thank
Prof. Dr. O. Vos and Prof. Dr. W. Hijmans for their continuous
support, and Mrs. Cary Meijerink-Clerkx for typing the manuscript.

SUMMING-UP

J.L. Gowans

Medical Research Council

20 Park Crescent, London W1N 4AL, England

Fleming was remarkably ahead of his time in regarding the lymphoid organs as dynamic structures. He did not picture germinal centres as permanent entities but as elements which arose and disappeared in response to changing demand. Further, he anticipated the discovery of lymphocyte recirculation by suggesting that lymphocytes might enter lymph nodes from the blood stream. His observations and speculations provided an admirable background for today's session on the origin of germinal centres and on the traffic of lymphocytes.

The origin and function of germinal centres has yet to be firmly established but the current view is that they are derived from cells which arise in the bone marrow and that they produce either B lymphocytes or antibody-forming plasma cells. They are thought to arise only as a consequence of antigenic stimulation. These views were supported by the work of Gastkemper et al who recorded the appearance of germinal centres in irradiated rats reconstituted with cells from normal donors. They made the interesting observation that the transfer from B rats of either bone marrow cells or of thoracic duct lymphocytes only led to the appearance of germinal centres if T lymphocytes were simultaneously given. Thus the precursors of germinal centres are present in both bone marrow and (surprisingly) in thoracic duct lymph but T help appears to be necessary for their expression. It was also confirmed that germinal centres only appeared if antigen was included in the restorative inoculum.

Circumstantial support for the idea of T dependence in the formation of germinal centres came from two other studies reported in this session. De Sousa et al found that B mice given Ly1 T lymphocytes developed larger germinal centres than those given Ly2,3 lymphocytes, while Reske-Kunz et al noted the ill-development of germinal centres in immuno-deficient mutant hr/hr mice in which there is an age-dependent proportional decrease in Ly1 cells. Thus the T cell subset involved in the formation of germinal centres may have been identified.

It is not clear whether Ly1 T cells are a constituent of germinal centres (although this appears unlikely (1)) or whether the presumed interaction between B and T cells which leads to their formation occurs deeper in the lymph node cortex where both varieties of lymphocyte emerge from the blood by way of the post-capillary venules. It is also not clear whether germinal centres always arise in a pre-determined location, although a technique for the isolation of germinal centres devised by Smithyman et al highlighted the complex vascular tree to which the centres are normally attached. This led to the suggestion that germinal centre sites are a permanent anatomical feature although the centres themselves only appear after antigenic stimulation.

These advances in our knowledge of germinal centres emphasize the difficulty of studying the origin and function of the organised elements within lymphoid tissue in contrast to the relative ease with which the performance of isolated lymphoid cells can be analysed in vitro.

The rapid turnover of lymphocytes in the blood is known to be due to a continuous reciruclation of cells from the blood to the lymph by way of the lymph nodes (2). Both B and T lymphocytes have been shown to recirculate (3), although they come to occupy different anatomical zones within the lymph nodes and the spleen (4), and both migrate from the blood by way of the post-capillary venules (1,3). The papers contributed to the current session were concerned particularly with the migratory step across the post-capillary venules in lymph nodes.

It has long been realised that there is an element of specificity in the passage of lymphocytes from the blood into the lymph nodes. Other leucocytes do not migrate across the post-capillary venules unless the nodes are inflamed (5) and traffic of lymphocytes across the fine blood vessels in peripheral tissues is extremely small by comparison. Certain pathological conditions are an exception to this rule and striking fluxes of lymphocytes have been observed through experimental hydronephrotic kidneys and through subcutaneous granulomata (6). The lamina propria of the normal small intestine may also be the site of a larger traffic of cells than was hitherto supposed (7). Little information is yet available about possible differences in the migratory patterns of lymphocyte subsets, although de Sousa et al have made a beginning by their observation that Ly 2, 3 cells migrate into the B cell areas of mouse lymph nodes.

The passage of lymphocytes from the blood into the lymph nodes involves two steps: first, the adherence of lymphocytes to the high-walled endothelium of the post-capillary venules and second, the migration through the endothelium into the lymph node. Butcher et al have shown that whatever the nature of the complementary structures which determine adherence, they are not strictly species specific. Rat and mouse lymph node and spleen cells were shown to migrate with equal efficiency into mouse lymph nodes in vivo and in an ingenious technique by which the adherence of lymphocytes to post-capillary venules in frozen sections of tissue can be observed in vitro, lymphocytes from both species were found to adhere with equal efficiency to the venules. On the other hand, chicken and human lymphocytes adhered much less well to the endothelium in the in vitro test and failed to migrate into the lymph nodes in vivo. Thus the lack of phylogenetic restriction is not absolute.

Previous work has shown that the surface components on lymphocytes which determine their predilection for the endothelium of the post-capillary venule are sensitive to treatment by trypsin (8) but not to neuraminidase (8) or Concanavalin A (9). Two studies reported in this session again distinguished adherence from migration in experiments in which lymphocytes were pre-treated with either cyto-chalasin or colchicine. Both Anderson et al and Smith and Ford have shown that the pre-treatment of rat thoracic duct lymphocytes with cytochalasin in vitro considerably decreased the subsequent migration of the treated cells after transfusion into syngeneic recipients. Although the treated cells failed to enter the lymph nodes, they were observed in auto-radiographs adhering to the endothelium of post-capillary venules. The implication of these studies is that inter-ference with the cytoplasmic contractile proteins of lymphocytes by treatment with cytochalasin did not affect the recognition structures on the lymphocyte surface but inhibited their motility and power to migrate into the nodes. Pre-treatment with colchicine, which disrupts microtubules and consequently may affect the organisation of surface membranes, reduced the accumulation of lymphocytes in the lymph nodes. Important controls are necessary before these experiments can be interpreted. Thus, the experiments with cytochalasin can be accepted because it was shown that the decrease in lymph node uptake was not associated with any increase in hepatic uptake showing that the cells were not severely damaged by pre-treatment; and, more importantly, that the decreased lymph node uptake was accompanied by a persistence of the transfused cells in the blood stream. In other words, the transfused cells were available for uptake into the nodes but were prevented from doing so by their pre-treatment. On the other hand, Smith and Ford showed that pre-treatment with colchicine led to an accumulation of the transfused cells in the lungs of the recipient with little evidence of their release into the blood. Thus, the failure to observe migration into the lymph nodes could have been due to the lack of cells in the blood and not to any intrinsic failure to adhere and migrate.

The aspect of lymphocyte recirculation which requires more attention is the search for its functional significance. The original suggestion that it provided a means by which sub-populations of specifically reactive lymphocytes could be recruited into regional lymph nodes following antigenic stimulation is supported by a number of experiemtns which have demonstrated that such specific selection of lymphocytes does take place in vivo. However, the major analysis of lymphocyte function has been carried out in vitro where efficient antibody responses can be initiated and carried to completion with small numbers of lymphoid cells and where it does not appear necessary to reproduce the essentials of lymphocyte recirculation either numerically or anatomically. Recirculation provides an attractive basis for regional selection among a heterogeneous pool of cells and provides the opportunities for cellular interactions among lymphocytes in vivo. The powerful analyses on in vitro systems which in recent years have illuminated so many aspects of cellular immunology need now to take account of the complex life history which lymphocytes enjoy in vivo.

REFERENCES

1.   Nieuwenhuis, P., Ford, W.L. Cellular Immunol. 23 (1976) 254.
2.   Gowans, J.L., Knight, E.J. Proc. Roy. Soc. B (London) 159 (1964) 257.
3.   Howard, J.C. J. exp. Med. 135 (1972) 185.
4.   Howard, J.C., Hunt, S.V., Gowans, J.L. J. exp. Med. 135 (1972) 200.
5.   Marchesi, V.T., Gowans, J.L. Proc. Roy. Soc. B (London) 159 (1964) 283.
6.   Smith, J.B., McIntosh, G.H., Morris, B. J. Path. 100 (1970) 21.
7.   Husband, A.J., Gowans, J.L. J. exp. Med. (1978) In press.
8.   Ford, W.L., Sedgley, M., Sparshott, S.M., Smith, M.E. Cell. Tissue Kinet. 9 (1976) 351.
9.   Smith, M.E., Sparshott, S.M., Ford, W.L. Exp. Cell Biol. 45 (1977) 9.

SESSION   A 2

IMMUNOLOGICAL FUNCTION
OF CELL SURFACE STRUCTURES

CHAIRPERSONS:

J.J. Marchalonis

R.M.E. Parkhouse

INTRODUCTION - THE IMMUNOGLOBULIN-LIKE T CELL RECEPTOR PROBLEM

John J. Marchalonis and Jane M. Moseley

Cancer Biology Program, NCI Frederick Cancer Research

Center, Frederick, Maryland 21701, U.S.A.

No problem in modern immunology has been more frustrating and controversial than that of the nature of the receptor for antigen on T lymphocytes. Since T cells, like antibodies and B cells, exhibit exquisite specificity for antigen, it is reasonable to propose as Ehrlich first did more than 80 years ago that the cell surface antigen receptor must be antibody (1). A good deal of experimental support was obtained for this concept in the late 60's and early 70's (reviewed in 2), but the hypothesis was not universally accepted because evidence from various approaches indicated that the T cell receptor, if an immunoglobulin (Ig), could not be identical to the known serum isotypes (3,4). However, a precedent for Igs associated only with the plasma membrane was set by the discovery of the IgD-like molecule of murine B cells (3,5-7) which does not occur in serum. It is not surprising that surface Ig molecules, which exist in a hydrophobic environment, differ from their serum counterparts, which exist in an aqueous miliue.

In this brief review, we shall analyze recent data supporting the minimal hypothesis that the T cell receptor for antigen is an Ig which shares variable (V) region-combining sites with circulating antibodies, but represents a distinct isotype which occurs in association with the T cell surface.

DO T CELLS POSSESS AND SYNTHESIZE IG?

Recent evidence in support of this hypothesis has come from the three following experimental approaches.

1.   The use of antisera directed against the V region-combining
sites (idiotypes) of antibodies (8-10).

2.   The use of mammalian antibodies to demonstrate surface Igs on
all lymphocytes of lower species (11,12), i.e. the principle of
"phylogenetic distance".

3.   The converse application of the phylogenetic distance principle
in which avian antibodies have been used to show Ig on mammalian T
and B cells (13-16).

Previous data, based upon use of mammalian antisera directed
against light chain and Fd region determinants, have been reviewed
(4,17). Mammalian antisera usually do not react with T cells in
direct binding studies such as immunocytofluorescence (2,3,5), but
have allowed the isolation of an Ig-like molecule from the surface
of these cells by several workers (3,4,18-24).

Some workers tend to discount the presence of Ig on T cells
because of a) the difficulty in demonstrating Ig by immunofluorescence
or autoradiography and b) the reported difficulty in isolation of Ig
(5,6). Recent studies have reported that surface Ig can be directly
visualized by fluorescent antibody or autoradiographic techniques on
mammalian T cells (13-16) if chicken antisera are used. Figure 1
illustrates the binding of purified chicken antibodies specific for
murine (Fab')$_2$, fragments to mouse T and B cells as visualized by
immunoelectronmicroscopy. Rigorous specificity controls were performed and the results indicate that murine T cell Ig crossreacts
with IgM (13) and Fab-region determinants (15,16,25). The chicken
antisera which stained human T cells were specific for the Fab
portion of human IgG (14). In a detailed series of studies, purified
chicken antibodies to the (Fab')$_2$ fragment of mouse IgG were shown to
bind only to lymphocytes and no evidence was obtained that binding
occurred to alloantigens or carbohydrate moities (15,16,25). In
lower vertebrates virtually all lymphocytes, including thymus lymphocytes, express and resynthesize IgM-like molecules detectable by
fluorescent antibody techniques (11,12). The apparent difficulty in
isolation of T cell Ig reflects the often confirmed observation that
the solubility of this molecule in detergents differs from that of B
cell surface Ig (4). This problem has been discussed at length elsewhere (4) and I will state only that various investigators have now
isolated surface Ig of thymocytes or T cells of man (26,27), mouse
(3,4,19-23), rat (18), pig (24), goldfish (12), bream (28) and carp
(29). In most cases, the extraction conditions routinely used for B
cells (e.g. 0.5% or 1% Nonidet P-40) were inadequate for quantitative
isolation of T cell surface Ig. Receptors bearing the idiotype of
circulating antibodies directed against alloantigens have been
demonstrated on T cells by both indirect functional assays (9,10) and
direct autoradiography by using labelled anti-receptor antibody.
Although it is possible that Ig V regions might be associated with

non-Ig C regions, this conjecture is not supported by observations
that the idiotypic markers studied show linkage with the arrays of
Ig heavy chain genes, and not elsewhere, e.g. within the major
histocompatibility complex. Moreover, an isolated idiotype-bearing
T cell surface receptor of the rat has a heavy chain of apparent
mass approx. 70,000 daltons (9). As will be noted below, T cell Ig
isolated using more conventional antisera has a heavy chain of
comparable nominal mass.

Thus, we can conclude that thymocytes or T cells of vertebrate
species ranging from teleost fish to mammals bear a surface molecule
which is antigenically related to serum Ig. Evidence supporting the
hypothesis that T cells synthesize surface Ig is as follows: a) T
cell receptors for antigen (30) and Ig-like components (31) are shed
and reappear, b) T cell Ig of lower species which is directly
visualized also caps, is shed and reemerges (11,12,32) and c) monoclonal T lymphoma cells synthesize Ig in vitro (33). In addition, T
cells contain relatively large amounts of mRNA specifying κ chains
(34,35). An observation which has generated questions regarding the
source of T cell Ig is the finding of receptors for pentameric IgM
on some human T cells (36) and reports of passive IgM on activated
murine T cells (37). These observations do not militate against the
results of phylogenetic studies, T lymphoma biosynthetic experiments
and studies employing avian antibodies.

IS T CELL IMMUNOGLOBULIN SPECIFIC FOR ANTIGEN?

Affirmative answers to this question have been obtained by the
use of antisera to Igs to inhibit the binding of antigen by T cells
(2,3) and by isolation of surface Ig from specifically activated T
cells and the demonstration that the molecules bound specifically to
the activating antigen (2,3,38). A possible drawback to inhibition
experiments is that Ig might not itself be the receptor, but might
be closely associated with the true receptor on the cell surface.
However, Roelants et al. (30) have reported evidence for an intimate
association between Ig and antigen, because the two molecules co-cap
on the T lymphocyte surface. Direct evidence showing the codistribution of antigen and Ig on antigen-binding T cells is given by
DeLuca et al. (this Symposium). Another objection is the question
of the source of the T cell Ig. Roelants et al. (30) have shown
that T cell receptor Ig caps off and re-appears, an observation
considered sufficient to establish that B cells synthesize their
surface Igs (39). This observation has been confirmed by other
workers (31). The argument that the isolated antigen-specific Ig
of activated T cells was made by B cells or plasma cells is challenged
because T cell Ig differs in physical and functional properties from
serum or B cell surface Ig. Moreover, monoclonal T lymphoma cells and
embryonic thymus rudiments free of B cells or plasma cells (40) synthesize and express "Ig T-type" molecules.

Comparative studies of the antigen-recognition question have shown that thymus lymphocytes and putative T cells can synthesize Ig (see 41 for review), all antigen-binding lymphocytes of amphibians and teleosts (41-43) including putative helper cells (43) can be inhibited by antisera made against circulating IgM immunoglobulin, and antigen and Ig codistribute on goldfish and carp thymocytes (44).

The use of "anti-receptor" antibodies has allowed direct verification of the hypothesis that surface receptors possess combining sites either identical or very similar to those found on circulating antibodies of comparable specificity. However, criticisms have been levelled at the anti-receptor (anti-idiotype) results and at the use of more "conventional" antibodies made against serum Ig; for example, what is the source of the idiotype-bearing molecule on T cells? A formally similar rebuttal of this objection has been made; e.g. apparently pure T cell populations express idiotypic determinants and the molecules bearing them on T cells are distinct from B cell surface Ig (9,10).

Thus, the evidence suggests strongly that surface molecules bearing Ig V regions and sharing some other antigenic determinants with Igs are involved in specific antigen recognition by T cells.

IS T CELL IG IDENTICAL TO SERUM ANTIBODIES OR B CELL SURFACE IGS?

The short answer to this question is no! Recent evidence from all three approaches under discussion indicates that T cell Ig, although cross-reactive with IgM using some antisera, can be distinguished from IgM and other serum antibodies by physicochemical, antigenic and functional criteria. From a functional standpoint, murine T cell Ig can serve as a collaborative factor in T/B cooperation, whereas serum IgM cannot (45). Ig of monoclonal, continuously cultured T lymphoma cells can block specific T/B cooperation, presumably by competing with specific T cell Ig for sites on macrophages (46), whereas myeloma proteins of various classes are ineffective (47). Consistent with these observations are the reports that T cell surface Ig, either alone (48) or complexed with antigen (20), binds to macrophages; whereas B cell surface Igs do not. These findings suggest that T cell Ig differs from IgM and "IgD" in its Fc region.

Antigenic data supporting this conclusion have recently been reported (49). Evidence from this laboratory indicates that antisera specific for Fc region determinants of μ chains do not react with T cell Ig produced by T lymphoma cells. T cell Ig heavy chains can be isolated, however, through a cross-reaction directed against Fd determinants.

Physicochemical differences were reported between IgM (T) and IgM (B). First, the two molecules differ in solubility properties in non-ionic detergents (4). Second, polyacrylamide gel electrophoresis in sodium dodecyl sulfate (SDS) under conditions of high resolution shows that the T cell Ig heavy chain migrates slightly but significantly faster than does μ of B cells or serum μ (23). This observation holds for murine T cell Ig of fetal thymus rudiments, T lymphoma cells and adult thymus, human thymus, and goldfish thymus. Third, the intact state of T cell Ig apparently differs from the usual structure of the Ig molecule which is comprised of two pairs of light chains and heavy chains linked together covalently by disulfide bonds. This model can be written L-s-s-H-s-s-H-s-s-L. Ig isolated from rat T cells expressing idiotype-bearing receptors directed against histocompatibility antigens has an "intact" mass of approx. 150,000 daltons under dissociating, but non-reducing, conditions rather than the 200,000 daltons characteristic of "7S" IgM (50). Upon reduction, heavy chains of mobility comparable to μ chains was found. However, no polypeptides comparable to light chains were apparently present. These results raised the possibility that T cell receptor Ig was a unique molecule; not only did it represent a new isotype, but it lacked conventional light chains. Genetic studies in the mouse showed that the gene specifying the T cell receptor mapped within the heavy chain gene cluster. Such analysis could not be performed for light chains, however, because no allotypic variants of mouse light chains have been reported. The apparent lack of light chains might be explained on the following grounds: a) light chains did not label under the conditions used: many heavy chains of myeloma proteins label disproportionately (51); and/or b) light chains are not covalently linked to the heavy chains and can be lost during isolation. Precedent for this possibility exists among "classical" Igs such as certain IgA subclasses of man (52) and mouse (53) where the α chains are disulfide bonded to one another, but not to the light chains. We would emphasize that a strong case for the presence of light chains in the T cell receptor can be made as follows: a) anti-light chain sera are the best blockers of antigen-specific T cells (2), b) T cells contain appreciable amounts of mRNA encoding κ chains (35), and c) all studies isolating T cell Ig using conventional antisera have demonstrated the presence of light chains (Gabison and Berke -- this symposium -- provide further evidence for light chains on T cells). Some workers, however, reported that the light and heavy chains of T cell Ig were not covalently associated (4,19,49).

Recent studies from this laboratory (49) have employed Ig produced by monoclonal T lymphoma cells to analyze the structure of this molecule. It was found that a) intact T lymphoma Ig migrates on SDS gels as a protein of nominal mass 150,000 daltons; it migrates substantially faster than does the 7S IgM isolated from B cell surfaces. b) Free light chains are found. Use of certain antisera allows isolation of IgT heavy chain in the absence of light chain and

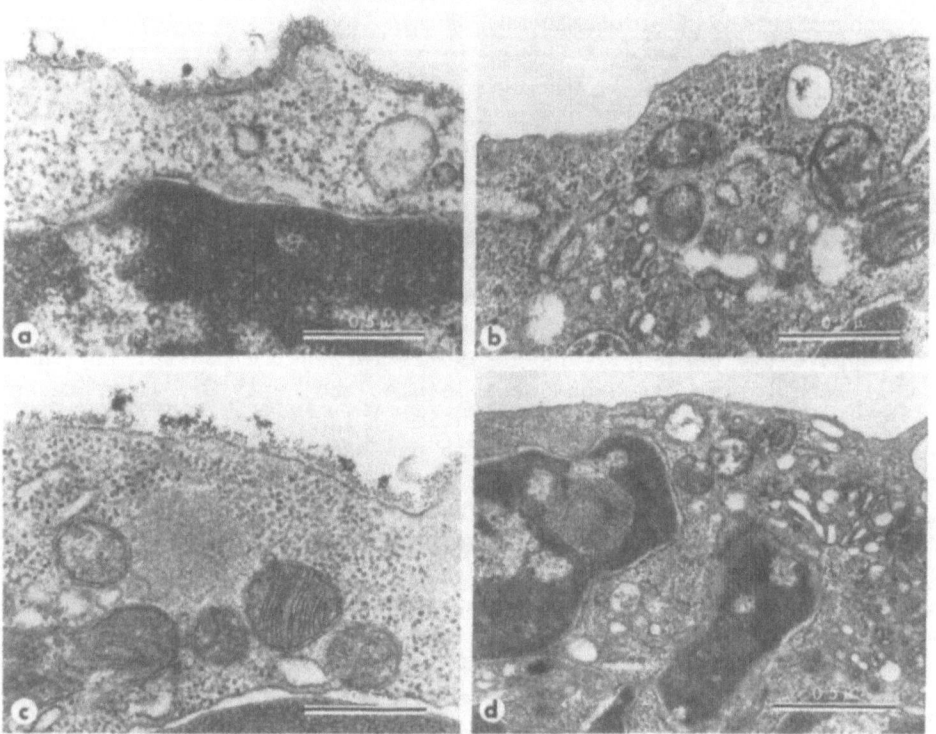

FIG. 1:   Visualization by transmission immunoelectronmicroscopy of
surface immunoglobulins on murine thymus lymphocytes and "nude" spleen
lymphocytes using chicken antibodies to mouse Fab. (a) T cell from
C57BL thymus reacted with chicken anti-Fab followed by ferritin-
labeled rabbit antibody to chicken IgY. (b) T cell from C57BL thymus
reacted with normal chicken IgY followed by ferritin-labeled rabbit
anti-chicken IgY. (c) B cell of nu/nu spleen reacted with rabbit anti-
mouse Fab followed by ferritin-labeled rabbit anti-chicken IgY. (d) B
cell reacted with normal chicken IgY followed by ferritin-labeled
rabbit anti-chicken IgY. Note the layer of ferritin immediately
external to the plasma membrane in (a) and (c). Binding of chicken
anti-Fab was abolished by absorption with insolubilized κ -chains
or IgG. (Courtesy of C. Bucana and L. Hoyer).

vice versa. c) IgT heavy chain migrates slightly ahead of serum μ
chain. Parallel results for the size of intact T cell Ig have been
reported for surface Ig of T lymphoma cells (33) and for fetal murine
thymus anlagen grown in culture (40). Some previous analyses of the
mass of human and murine T cell Ig were made by gel filtration under
gentle conditions (26) which probably would not have disrupted the
hydrophobic interactions holding light and heavy chains together. We
(Moseley and Marchalonis, unpublished) have also found that some
preparations of T lymphoma Ig contain very low levels of light chains
and consist predominantly of the heavy chain dimer. Based upon all
the results discussed in this section, we would suggest that T cell
Ig exists in the form (L) H-ss-H (L), where the brackets indicate a
lack of covalent association.

Figure 2 shows the T cell Ig heavy chain isolated from ^{125}I-
labelled culture fluid in which the monoclonal BALB/c T lymphoma
WEHI 22 had been grown and the same molecule biosynthetically
labelled with ^{3}H-leucine. The heavy chain migrates significantly
faster than μ chain, but is considerably slower than γ chain. The
isolated T cell heavy chain was compared with non-Ig molecules and
polypeptide chains of myeloma Igs by analysis of peptides produced
by cleavage with CNBr and by trypsin. Analysis of tryptic peptides
by two-dimensional mapping indicated that the heavy chain was clearly
distinct from viral glycoprotein gp71, bovine serum albumin and β_2-
microglobulin. It showed an overall resemblance, but not an identity
to the μ chain of MOPC 104E myeloma. More detailed comparisons of
radioiodinated tryptic peptides of WEHI 22 heavy chain and corresponding peptides of μ (from MOPC 104E), γ (from normal mouse IgG)
and α (from MOPC 315) were performed by simultaneous resolution of
double-labelled peptides by ion-exchange chromatography. As shown
in Figure 3, WEHI 22 heavy chain is markedly distinct from γ chain
in its peptide profile, but shares a number of peptides with μ and
α chains. We suggest that T cell Ig represents a new isotype
associated with the T cell surface and emphasize that detailed amino
acid sequence data are required to delineate precisely the degree of
similarity between this molecule and known serum and B cell surface
isotypes.

CONCLUSIONS

We have briefly outlined the main points resulting from three
approaches recently applied in investigations of the T cell receptor
for antigen. The overall conclusion gleaned from these studies is
that the antigen receptor on T cells is an Ig which shares V regions
with serum antibodies but differs from these as well as B cell 7S
IgM-and IgD-like molecules in its heavy chain C region. The minimal
hypothesis also gains strong support from analyses using "anti-
receptor" antibodies, antisera to Ig Fab fragment determinants and

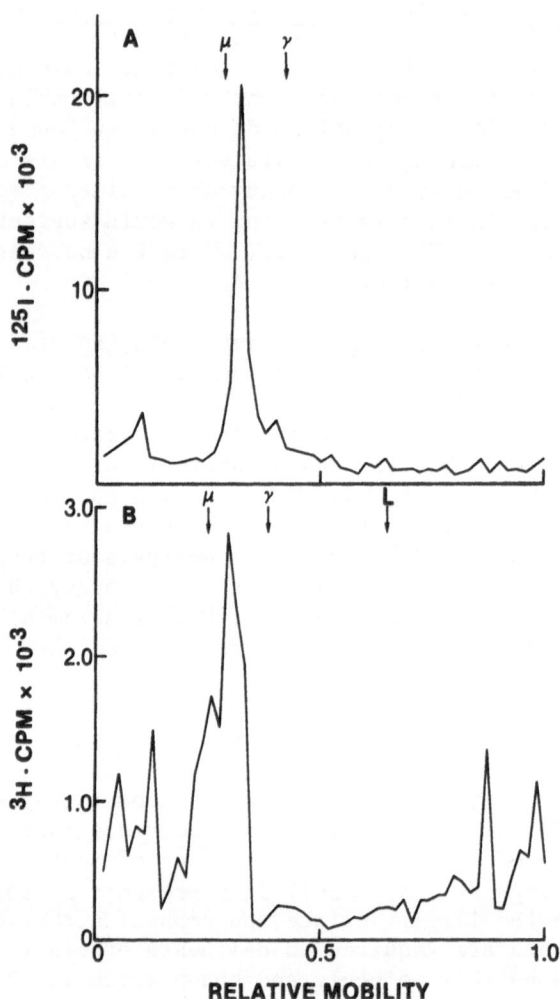

FIG. 2:   A.   Profile on 10% SDS polyacrylamide gel of purified heavy
chain of WEHI 22 immunoglobulin isolated from iodinated culture fluid
by extraction using immunoadsorbent directed against murine IgG.   B.
Profile on 10% SDS polyacrylamide gel of heavy chain of WEHI 22 immunoglobulin biosynthesized by uptake of ^{3}H-leucine and isolated by coprecipitation with chicken anti-Fab Ig plus goat anti-chicken Ig. (Courtesy
of J. Decker).   Arrows indicate the positions at which standard μ, γ
and light chains migrate.

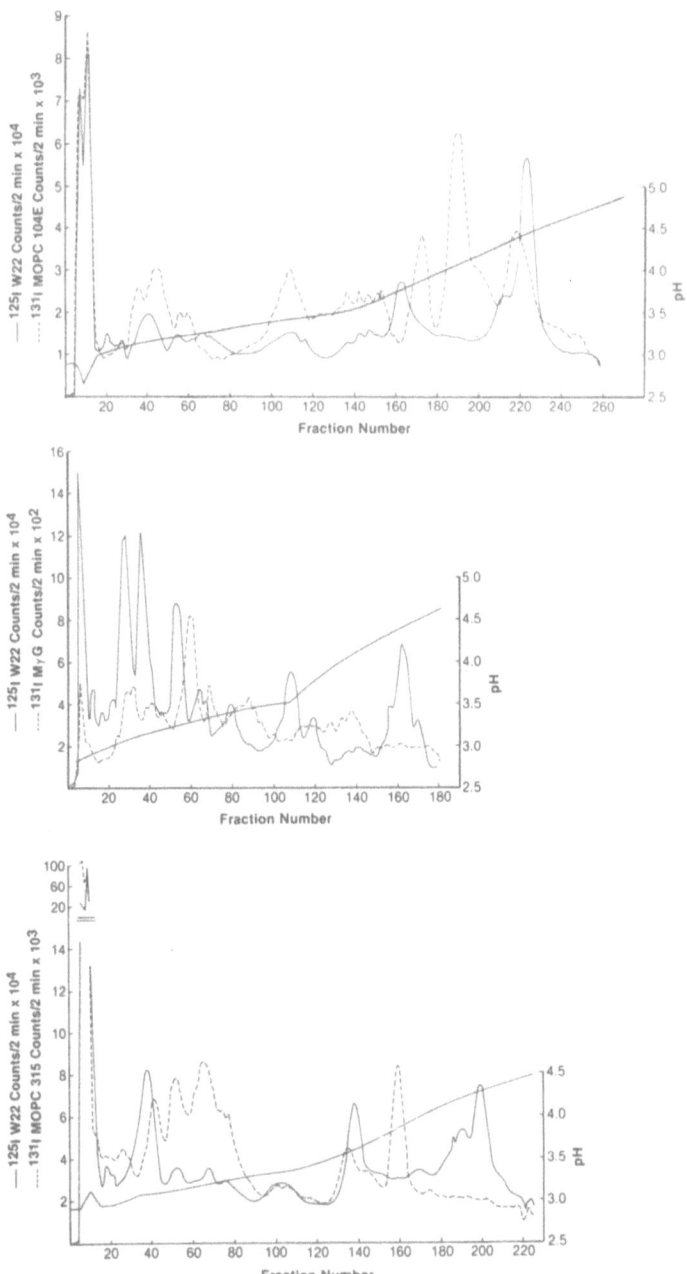

FIG. 3:   Comparison of the tryptic peptides of ^{125}I WEHI 22 heavy
chain ——— with: [131]I MOPC 104E μ ---- upper panel;   [131]I MɣG - ɣ
---- center panel and ^{131}I MOPC 315 - α---- lower panel.   Peptides
were eluted from Dowex 50W X 2 cation exchange resin at 40°C with a
pyridine acetate gradient from 0.02 M pyridine pH 3.0 to 0.2 M
pyridine pH 5.0.   4 ml fractions were collected.

phylogenetic studies of surface Igs. Other lymphocyte surface molecules are involved in regulation of immune responsiveness, but it is doubtful whether they function in primary antigen recognition (54). Evolutionary considerations (41) suggest that the T cell heavy chain probably diverged from serum μchain prior to the divergence of the ancestors of mammals and bony fishes. At this time, many investigators have presented information on the nature of the T cell receptor and further progress in this area will no doubt include detailed structural analysis of the molecule.

REFERENCES

1.   Ehrlich, P. Proc. Roy. Soc. B. 65 (1900) 424.
2.   Warner, N.L. Adv. Immunol. 19 (1974) 67.
3.   Marchalonis, J.J. Science 190 (1975) 20.
4.   Cone, R.E. Prog. in Immunol. 3 (1977) 47.
5.   Vitetta, E.S., Uhr, J.W. Science 189 (1975) 47.
6.   Abney, E.R., Parkhouse, R.M.F. Nature (Lond.) 252 (1974) 600.
7.   Goding, J.W., Warr, G.W., Warner, N.L. Proc. Natl. Acad. Sci. U.S.A. 73 (1976) 1305.
8.   McKearn, T.J. Science 183 (1974) 94.
9.   Binu, H., Wigzell, H. Contemp. Top. Immunobiol. 7 (1977) 113.
10. Rajewsky, K., Eichmann, K. Cont. Top. Immunobiol. 7 (1977) 69.
11. DuPasquier, L., Weiss, N., Loor, F. Eur. J. Immunol. 2 (1972) 366.
12. Warr, G.W., DeLuca, D., Marchalonis, J.J. Proc. Natl. Acad. Sci. U.S.A. 73 (1976) 2476.
13. Hämmerling, U., Pickel, H.A., Mack, C., Masters, D. Immuno-chemistry 13 (1976) 533.
14. Jones, V.E., Greaves, H.E., Orlans, E. Immunology 30 (1976) 281.
15. Szenberg, A., Marchalonis, J.J., Warner, N.L. Proc. Natl. Acad. Sci. U.S.A. 74 (1977) 2113.
16. Marchalonis, J.J., Warr, G.W., Bucana, C., Hoyer, L., Szenberg, A., Warner, N.L. In: Regulation of the Immune System, Genes and the Cells in Which They Function. Acad. Press, N.Y. 295 (1977).
17. Marchalonis, J.J., Warr, G.W. In: Basic Immunological Mechanisms in Cancer. Marcel Dekker, Inc., N.Y. In press (1978).
18. Misra, D.N., Ladoulis, C.T., Gill, T.J., III., Byzin H. Immuno-chemistry 13 (1976) 613.
19. Moroz, C., Lahat, N. Cell. Immunol. 13 (1974) 397.
20. Rieber, E.P., Riethmüller, G. Z. Immun. Forsch. 147 (1974) 262.
21. Boylston, A.W., Mowbray, J.F. Immunology 27 (1974) 855.
22. Gabison, D., Bergman, Y., Haimovich, J., Berke, G. Transplant. Proc. 9 (1972) 741.
23. Haustein, D., Goding, J.W. Biochem. Biophys. Res. Commun. 65. (1975) 483.
24. Chavin, S.I. Biochem. Biophys. Res. Commun. 61 (1974) 432.

25. Warr, G.W., Marton, G.A., Szenberg, A., Marchalonis, J.J. Immunochemistry. In press (1978).
26. Marchalonis, J.J., Cone, R.E., Atwell, J.L. J. Exp. Med. 135 (1972) 956.
27. Moroz, C., Hahn, J. Proc. Natl. Acad. Sci. U.S.A. 70 (1973) 3716.
28. Clem, L.W., McLean, W.E., Shankey, V.T., Cuchens, M.A. Dev. Comp. Immunol. 1 (1977) 105.
29. Fiebig, H., Ambrosius, H. In: Phylogeny of Thymus and Bone Marrow-bursa Cells. Elsevier/North Holland, Amsterdam 195 (1976).
30. Roelants, G.E., Ryden, A., Hagg, L.B., Loor, F. Nature (Lond.) 267 (1974) 106.
31. DeLuca, D., Miller, A., Sercarz, E. Cell. Immunol. 8 (1975) 286.
32. Emmerich, F., Fichter, R.F., Ambrosius, H. Europ. J. Immunol. 5 (1975) 76.
33. Haustein, D., Marchalonis, J.J., Harris, A.W. Biochem. 14 (1975) 1826.
34. Rabbitts, T.H., Forster, A., Smith, M., Gillawe, S. Europ. J. Immunol. 7 (1977) 43.
35. Storb, U., Hager, L., Putnam, D., Buck, L., Farin, F., Clagget, J. Proc. Natl. Acad. Sci. U.S.A. 73 (1976) 2467.
36. Moretta, L., Ferrarini, M., Durante, M.L., Mingari, M.C. Europ. J. Immunol. 5 (1975) 565.
37. Hudson, L., Sprent, J. J. Exp. Med. 143 (1976) 444.
38. Feldmann, M., Cone, R.E., Marchalonis, J.J. Cell. Immunol. 9 (1973) 1.
39. Unanue, E.R., Karnovsky, M.J. Transplant. Rev. 14 (1973) 184.
40. Haustein, D., Marchalonis, J.J., Harris, A.W., Mandel, T.E. In: Leukocyte Membrane Determinants Regulating Immune Reactivity. Acad. Press. N.Y. 205 (1976).
41. Warr, G.W., Decker, J.M., Marchalonis, J.J. Immunol. Commun. 5 (1976) 281.
42. Edwards, B.F., Ruben, L.N., Marchalonis, J.J., Hylton, C. Adv. Exp. Med. Biol. 64 (1975) 397.
43. Ruben, L.N., Warr, G.W., Decker, J.M., Marchalonis, J.J. Cell. Immunol. 31 (1977) 266.
44. DeLuca, D., Warr, G.W., Marchalonis, J.J. Europ. J. Immunol. In press (1978).
45. Feldmann, M. In: The Lymphocyte: Structure and Function, Marcel Dekker, N.Y. 279 (1977).
46. Stocker, J.W., Marchalonis, J.J., Harris, A.W. J. Exp. Med. 139 (1976) 785.
47. Feldmann, M., Boylston, A., Hogg, M.N. Europ. J. Immunol. 5 (1975) 429.
48. Cone, R.E., Feldmann, M., Marchalonis, J.J., Nossal, G.J.V. Immunol. 26 (1974) 49.
49. Moseley, J.M., Marchalonis, J.J., Harris, A.W., Pye, J. J. Immunogen. 4 (1977) 233.
50. Binz, H., Wigzell, H. Scan. J. Immunol. 5 (1976) 559.
51. Seon, B.K., Pressman, D. Immunochem. 13 (1976) 407.

52. Jerry, L.M., Kunkel, H.G., Grey, H.M. Proc. Natl. Acad. Sci.
     U.S.A. 65 (1970) 557.
53. Warner, N.L., Marchalonis, J.J. J. Immunol. 109 (1977) 657.
54. Marchalonis, J.J., Morris, P.J., Harris, A.W. J. Immunogen. 1
     (1974) 63.

ACKNOWLEDGEMENT

    This research was sponsored by the National Cancer Institute
under contract no. N01-CO-75380 with Litton Bionetics, Inc.

ISOLATION AND PARTIAL IDENTIFICATION OF IMMUNOGLOBULIN FROM T CELLS

Aleksander Szenberg

The Walter & Eliza Hall Institute of Medical Research
Post Office, Royal Melbourne Hospital
Victoria, 3050, Australia

Publication No. 2465

INTRODUCTION

We have reported previously (1,2) that antibody produced in fowls against mouse IgG (Fab)$_2$ fragments binds to a substance on mouse, rat and guinea pig thymocytes, T cells and cultured mouse thymoma cells. Specificity of this antibody was directed against κ chains, strongest binding occurring with κ chains connected to the Fd fragment (1,3). Using this antibody preparation we attempted to isolate and characterize the receptor molecule.

MATERIALS AND METHODS

Antisera. Fowl antibody to mouse IgG (Fab)$_2$ fragments was prepared and purified as described previously (1). Rabbit antibody to mouse IgG was prepared by injecting 2 mg of IgG in CFA* into multiple sites intramuscularly. The animals were boosted with the same dose of antigen in IFA* 3 weeks later and serum collected 8-10

---

*   CFA, Complete Freund adjuvant; DMEM, Dulbecco modified Eagle's medium; EDTA, Ethylenoliaminetetra acetic acid, disodium salt; IFA, Incomplete Freund adjuvant; MEM, Minimal essential medium; PAGE, Polyacrylamide gel electrophoresis; PBS, Mouse tonicity phosphate buffered saline pH 7.3 containing EDTA(20 mM) and sodium azide(0.01%); PMSF, Phenylmethylsulfonylfluoride; SDS, Sodiumdodecyl sulfate; SPF, Specific pathogen free.

days after the second injection. The antibody was purified by
absorption and elution from mouse IgG-Sepharose column. Monospecific antisera to mouse γ, μ and α chains were a gift from Dr. J.
Goding. Mouse IgG and IgM myeloma proteins were obtained from
Litton Bionetics.

Immunoglobulin preparations. Mouse IgG was prepared by
absorbing mouse serum on Staphylococcus A-protein-Sepharose column
(4) (Pharmacia) and elution with 2.5M guanidin chloride Fowl Ig was
prepared from serum by sodium sulfate precipitation (5).

Immunoabsorbent columns. Proteins were conjugated to CNBr-
activated Sepharose 4B (Pharmacia), approximately 15 mg of protein
per gr. of dry sepharose. The gel columns were equilibrated with
PBS* and before use washed with 3 volumes of Glycine-HCl buffer
pH 2.3 and with 3 volumes of 2.5M guanidin chloride. No detectable
amount of protein could be eluted from the columns.

Analytical techniques. Immunoelectrophoresis was performed
in a standard way on agarose slides in barbitone buffer pH 8.6.
PAGE* was performed in 10% SDS* gels using non-reduced or 2 ME
reduced samples.

Cultured thymoma lines. WEHI 22.1 and WEHI 7.1 thymomas (6)
were cultured in roller bottles containing appr. 500 ml of medium.
The medium used was DMEM* containing 10% FCS. The cultures were
harvested when the cell density reached $2-3 \times 10^6$/ml, usually after
3-4 days.

Preparation of activated T cells. (a) CBA thymocytes were
treated with anti Ia^k serum and complement (7), the damaged cells
removed (8) and 50×10^6 cells injected i.v. into 800 rad irradiated
(CBAXC57BL) hybrids (9). The donors and recipients were 8-10 weeks
old and were obtained as SPF* from our animal breeding facilities.
After 4 days, the spleens of the recipients were removed under sterile
conditions, cell suspensions prepared and the cells incubated from
6-8 hr in MEM* containing 10% FCS and 10mM HEPES. (b) Concanavalin
A activated thymocytes. Mouse thymocytes were cultured in tubes at
3×10^6 cells/ml, in MEM with 5% of FCS and 5µg/ml of Con A in 10%
CO_2 in air. After 48 hr the medium was replaced completely and
culture continued for another 2 days.

Preparation of thymocyte and thymoma cell derived immunoglobulin.
The cultured cells were separated from the medium by centrifugation
(400 g 5 min). The cells were lysed with NP40, 0.05% (8) on ice and
the lysates added to the culture fluid. To prevent proteolytic
activity, EDTA* was added to 20 mM and PMSF* to 1mM concentration.
The culture fluids were concentrated where necessary by pressure
dialysis (Amicon ultrafiltration cells) to appr. 150 ml. After

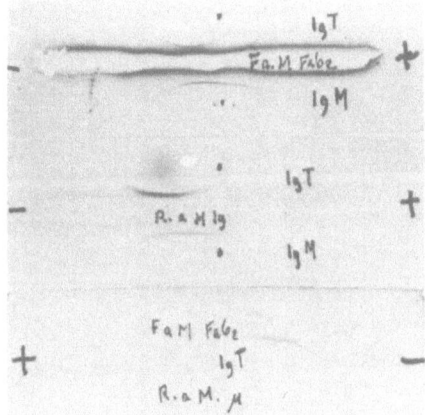

FIG. 1:   Immunoelectrophoretic analysis. IgT-immunoglobulin from
WEHI 22.1 thymoma cells;   F.aM Fab$_2$-Fowl antibody to mouse IgG
(Fab)$_2$; R a.M.Ig-Rabbit antibody to mouse Ig. IgM – mouse myeloma
IgM. R a. M.μ- Rabbit antibody to mouse μ chain.

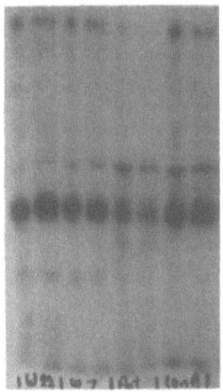

FIG. 2:   10% reduced SDA PAGE.

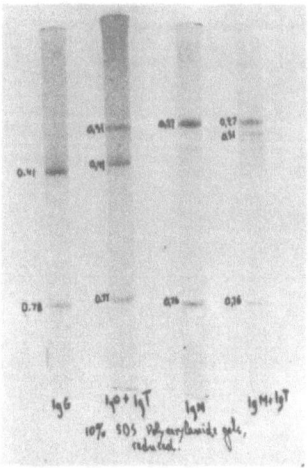

FIG. 3:   Reduced and non reduced 10% SDS PAGE of proteins from
following sources;   W22 – WEHI 22. 1 thymoma;   W7 – WEHI 7.1
thymoma;   Act – spleens from CBA thymocyte injected into irradiated
(CBAXC57BL) hybrid;   Con A;   Concanavalin A stimulated thymocytes.

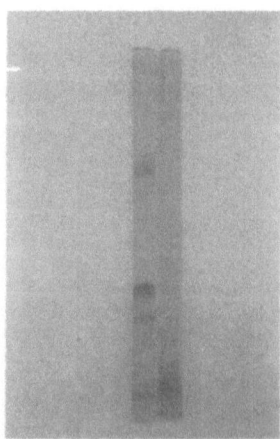

FIG. 4:   10% reduced SDS PAGE;   Protein from WEHI 7.1 thymoma.
Left;   absorbed and eluted from fowl a. mouse (Fab)$_2$ antibody column;
Right;   absorbed and eluted from fowl Ig column.

concentration, the culture fluid was passed through fowl anti mouse (Fab)$_2$ immunoabsorbent column, the column washed with PBS until no protein eluted with 2.5M guanidin chloride.

Protein containing eluate was immediately passed through a G25 Sephadex (Pharmacia) column to remove guanidine, and the eluate concentrated by pressure dialysis to 1-2 ml. The eluates were monitored with ISCO Model UA5 absorbence monitor and collected in 5 ml fractions. Final protein estimation in concentrated samples was made by measuring optical density at 280 nM in Gilford spectrophotometer. Absorption co-efficient of 1.4/mg/ml/cm was used to convert the absorbence value into mg. protein.

RESULTS

The average yield of protein from thymoma culture fluid and cell lysate of 1 x 10^9 cells and 500 ml medium, averaged over 25 runs was appr. 0.9 mg. Protein obtained from thymocytes was appr. 20-30 μg per irradiated spleen, and 20-25 μg per 10^8 Con A stimulated cells. The protein obtained from WEHI 22 tumor cells showed in immunoelectrophoresis against both fowl and rabbit anti mouse sera, typical immunoglobulin arc migrating slightly faster than IgM (Fig.1). No precipitation arc was produced with anti μ , γ or α sera, indicating that a different type of heavy chain was obtained from T cells.

PAGE results (Fig.2) show clearly that protein from all 4 sources possesses heavy and light chains. In the same autoradiograph a contamination of the major protein present – T cell immunoglobulin (IgT) with albumin and probably actin is revealed.

Fig.3 shows the relative mobility of the IgT heavy chain in relation to mouse myelomas IgG and IgM. IgT heavy chain migrates faster than μ and slower than γ . The light chains migrate exactly with the serum immunoglobulin light chains. The apparent molecular weight of the IgT heavy chains calculated from such gels is appr. 65,000.

Several control experiments have been performed to ensure that the results presented above are not artefacts. The only source of protein in the culture media besides the cells themselves is FCS. 500 ml of medium without cells was incubated for 4 days and then run through the fowl antibody to mouse (Fab)$_2$ column. Amount of protein bound to the column was appr. 50 μg – appr. 5% of the protein yield obtained from medium in which cells have been cultured.

To establish that not just any fowl immunoglobulin could bind proteins released by cultured thymoma cells, an immunoabsorbent column was prepared with fowl serum Ig from which natural antibodies reacting with mouse Ig had been removed by passage through a mouse IgG immunoabsorbent. Natural antibodies to other cell components of the mouse lymphocytes were present. A batch of WEHI 7 culture medium and cell lysate was passed through this column and an immunoabsorbent column of fowl anti mouse (Fab)$_2$ antibodies. Protein eluates from both columns were measured; fowl Ig column bound 0.39 mg of protein, whereas specific column bound 1.67 mg of protein.

On PAGE in reducing conditions the eluate from fowl a. mouse antibody column showed clear protein lines migrating like Ig light and heavy chains and some proteins around the end of the gel. The eluate from fowl Ig column the light and heavy chain lines were not visible (Fig.4). Fig.2 shows that even under non-reducing conditions some separation of light and heavy chains did take place. The results presented above indicate that our protein preparations contain at least 70% of immunoglobulin. Immunoelectrophoretic analysis of protein preparations from T cells against rabbit (anti - fowl immuno-globulin) serum gave negative results.

DISCUSSION

The existence of immunoglobulin and the identity of the antigen receptor on the surface of T cells has been the subject of a prolonged controversy which has been recently reviewed by Cone (11). In the last few years evidence has been accumulating of the presence of immunoglobulin heavy chains on the surface of T cells, but light chains have not been found (12,13).

We have shown previously (1,2) that a substance reacting with anti light chain antibodies is present on T cells. Now we have identified this substance on an Ig molecule (IgT) containing both light and heavy chains. The heavy chain seems to differ in molecular weight from μ and γ chains and seems to be antigenically different from μ, γ and α. The bond between the light and heavy chains of IgT seems to be largely non-covalent and the molecule is often broken up by 2.5M guanidin chloride used in elution from the columns. From the relative intensity of light and heavy chain lines on PAGE it seems that the separated light chains are more susceptible to further degradation, possibly by proteolytic enzymes. This finding may explain why only heavy chains have been detected till now on T cells. It will also predict that establishing of biological activity of the separated molecule may be very difficult unless less harsh method of isolation can be found.

The question presents itself as to whether the discovery of immunoglobulin on rodent T cells is limited to these species. Immunoglobulin has been detected on amphibian (14) and fish (15) thymocytes, using mammalian antisera. In unpublished experiments we have produced fowl antibodies to human $(Fab)_2$ fragments, and did not show that this antibody binds to human peripheral lymphocytes and to appr. 90% of monkey thymocytes.

It seems that the presence of immunoglobulin on T cells is a general phenomenon covering lower vertebrates and as widely distant mammalian species as mice and men.

SUMMARY

Using fowl anti mouse $(Fab)_2$ antibody, a protein has been collected from culture fluid and cell lysates of thymoma cells and stimulated thymocytes. This protein did show an immunoglobulin arc on immunoelectrophoresis against abovementioned antibody and against rabbit anti mouse Ig serum. No precipitation lines have been produced by mono-specific anti-mouse γ, μ and α sera.

On reduced PAGE heavy and light chains were present. Mobility of the heavy chain was between μ and γ chains and its apparent molecular weight was calculated at appr. 65,000 daltons. The light chain mobility corresponded to mouse serum κ chains.

REFERENCES

1. Szenberg, A., Marchalonis, J.J., Warner, N.L. Proc. Nat. Acad. Sci. (U.S.A.) 74 (1977) 2113.
2. Marchalonis, J.J., Bucana, Cora, Hoyer, L., Warr, G.W., Hanna, M.G., Szenberg, A. Science 199 (1978) 433.
3. Warr, G.W., Morton, Gabrielle, Szenberg, A., Marchalonis, J.J. Submitted for publication (1978).
4. Goding, J.W. J. Immunological Methods 13 (1976) 215.
5. Benedict, A.A. In Methods in Immunology and Immunochemistry Vol. 1 (Eds. Williams, C.A., Chase, M.W.) p. 229 (1967).
6. Harris, A.W., Bankhurst, A.D., Mason, Sally, Warner, N.L. J. Immunol. 110 (1973) 431.
7. Nossal, G.J.V., Pike, B.L. J. Immunol. 120 (1978) 145.
8. Von Boehmer, H., Shortman, K. J. Immunol. Methods 2 (1972-3) 293.
9. Sprent, J., Miller, J.F.A.P. Nature New Biology 234 (1971) 195.
10. Cone, R.E., Hoessli, D., Rosenstein, R.W. Immunochemistry 14 (1977) 345.
11. Cone, R.E. Progress in Immunology 3 (1977) 47.
12. Binz, H., Wigzell, H. Scand. J. Immunol. 5 (1976) 559.
13. Rajewsky, K., Eichman, K. Contemp. Top. Immunobiol. 7 (1977) 69.

14. Du Pasquier, L., Weiss, N., Loor, F. Eur. J. Immunol. 2 (1972)
     366.
15. Warr, G.W., Decker, J.M., Marchalonis, J.J. Immunol. Commun.
     5 (1976) 281.

ACKNOWLEDGEMENTS

I am grateful to my colleagues: Drs. Anders, Burgess, Harris,
Miller and Nossal for helpful discussions and advice; Mrs. Uren
for performing the cultures; Mr. Pye for radiolabelling proteins;
Miss Beal for competent technical assistance.

This work has been supported by a grant from the National
Health and Medical Research Council, Canberra.

CODISTRIBUTION OF ANTIGEN AND Fab DETERMINANTS ON THYMIC ANTIGEN-

BINDING CELLS

D. DeLuca, G.W. Warr and J.J. Marchalonis

Cancer Biology Program, NCI Frederick Cancer Research

Center, Frederick, Maryland 21701, U.S.A.

INTRODUCTION

In spite of the fact that thymus-derived lymphocytes (T cells) bind antigens specifically (1), interaction between the surface receptor and antigen on these cells has not been directly visualized as it has been for bone marrow-derived lymphocytes (B cells) (2-4). Several investigators have recently established that avian antibodies specific for mammalian Ig bind to T cells, as well as to B cells, and that this binding is demonstrable by immunofluorescence (5-8). If the T cell surface components visualized by avian anti-mammalian Ig are involved in primary immune recognition, these components should be coincidentally distributed with antigen on the surface of ABL from thymus.

In this communication, we present results of studies designed to test this question. Our experiments involved the simultaneous localization of Ig and antigen using two immunofluorescence labels, fluorescein and rhodamine. Our studies were performed using thymus

---

Abbreviations used in this paper: ABL, antigen-binding lymphocyte(s); CAM(Fab')$_2$, chicken anti-mouse (Fab')$_2$ fragments; DMSO, dimethyl sulfoxide; FCS, fetal calf serum; FITC, fluorescein isothiocyanate; HBSS, Hanks balanced salt solution; HSF, horse spleen ferritin; Ig, immunoglobulin(s); KLH, keyhole limpet hemocyanin; MHC, major histocompatibility complex; NCG, normal chicken globulin; PBS, phosphate buffered saline; RACG, rabbit anti-chicken globulin; RAMG, rabbit anti-mouse globulin; TRITC, tetramethyl-rhodamine isothiocyanate; NMγG, normal mouse gamma globulin.

TAB. 1:   Frequency of Antigen-binding Cells in Thymus and Spleen
of Mice

Organ	Antigen-binding Cells (ABC)/10^3 Cells $\pm$ S.D.		
	KLH	HSF	MYO
Thymus (BALB/c)	13 $\pm$ 4	8 $\pm$ 3	8 $\pm$ 4
Thymus (C3H)	5	2 $\pm$ 0	3 $\pm$ 1
Spleen (BALB/c)	26	16	22 $\pm$ 1

lymphocytes from unimmunized mice and specifically purified chicken
antibodies raised against the (Fab')$_2$ fragment of IgG isolated from
normal mouse sera (6,7). Additional studies with anti-Thy-1.2 and
anti-H-2^d sera were performed to demonstrate the T cell nature of
ABL, and to provide contrasting patterns of distribution of antigen
and non-Ig surface markers.

MATERIALS AND METHODS

Five μl of rhodamine-labeled antigen (in 5 x 10^{-2} $\underline{M}$ NaN$_3$) was
added to 50 μl of a 95% viable cell suspension from BALB/c or C3H
mice (giving a final antigen concentration of approximately 500 μg/ml
for about 10^7 total cells and 5 x 10^{-3} $\underline{M}$ NaN$_3$) for 1 h at 0°C in HBSS
+ 5% FCS. Then, a 1:20 dilution of anti-BALB/c serum, 1:20 anti-
Thy-1.2 serum, or 1:10 CAM(Fab')$_2$ was added to the cells while in
the presence of antigen for an additional hour at 0°C. After two
washes with either 5 ml of HBSS plus FCS, or with 1 ml of 100% FCS,
the cells were resuspended in 100 μl HBSS plus 5% FCS and incubated
with a 1:20 dilution of the appropriate developing reagent [RACG
(FITC) or RAMG(FITC)] for another hour at 0°C before a final washing
was done as before. Cells were then fixed in 1% p-formaldehyde in
0.1 $\underline{M}$ cacodylate buffer, pH 7.0. In order to slow cell motion, a
drop of pelleted cell suspension was mixed with a drop of 90%
glycerin in PBS on a glass slide, before being covered with a
coverslip.

Observation, counting and photography of ABL were accomplished
with a Zeiss photomicroscope III equipped with a fluorescence epi-

TAB. 2:   Frequency of Anti-Thy 1.2-bearing Cells and $H-2^d$-bearing Cells in Mouse Thymus

| Organ | % Total Lymphoid Cells $\pm$ S.D. | | | |
	RAM Ig	NCG	Anti-Thy 1.2	Anti-$H-2^d$
Thymus (BALB/c)	0.5	<1.0	99	84 $\pm$ 1
Thymus (C3H)	<1.0	0.3	84 $\pm$ 2	-

illuminator III RS containing the standard filter set plus an additional GG 475 cut-off filter to prevent ultraviolet excited autofluorescence. An HBO 200/4 mercury lamp was used for fluorescence excitation. GAF 500 color slide film was used with the microscope's camera set for spot reading and an ASA rating of 1000 (31 DIN) for FITC and phase contrast exposures, and 3400 ASA (37 DIN) for TRITC exposures. Photos of TRITC-ABL stained with the various FITC-antisera were taken in the order, TRITC, FITC, TRITC, then phase contrast. The bracketed exposures were done to ensure that cell movement had not occurred between the first and second exposures. The developed films were coded and examined under a magnifying glass to determine if antigen spots and antiserum spots were coincident.

RESULTS

The frequencies of ABL are presented in Tab.1. The frequencies of Thy 1.2 positive cells, $H-2^d$ positive cells, and CAM(Fab')$_2$ positive cells, as well as the frequencies of cells positive for the control sera (RAMG and NCG) are given in Tab.2. Spleen cells from BALB/c mice are also shown as controls for antigen binding and CAM(Fab')$_2$ reactivity.

ABL detected in our thymus cell populations are:

1.   Thy 1.2 positive,

2.   H-2 positive, and

3.   positive for CAM(Fab')$_2$ staining.

Only a small proportion of ABL (10% of KLH and MYO and no HSF ABL)

TAB. 3:   Inhibition of Thymic ABL by Anti-Ig Sera and Unlabeled
Antigen

		ABC/10^3		
	Inhibitor	KLH	HSD	MYO
Exp. #1	CAM(Fab')$_2$	0.9	0.9	0.9
	CAM(Fab')$_2$ ads NMɣG	8.9	9.4	7.5
	10 mg/ml HSF	14.3	0.9	4.9
	10 mg/ml MYO	9.7	9.8	1.7
Exp. #2	None	20.4	8.0	13.3
	10 mg/ml KLH	4.7	9.7	14.5

are weakly positive for RAMG (FITC) binding (and thus, might be
classified as B cell contaminants).

The data presented in Tab. 3 demonstrate that CAM(Fab')$_2$ added
before antigen prevents binding of labeled antigen by ABL. Prior
incubation of the CAM(Fab')$_2$ with mouse Fab fragments reverses this
inhibitory effect. It should be pointed out that immune complexes
made when the CAM(Fab')$_2$ was absorbed with mouse Fab, which were
left in the reaction mixture with the cells plus antigen, were not
responsible for antigen inhibition by binding to Fc receptors. Tab.
3 also presents data which indicate that an excess of unlabeled
antigen added before labeled antigen specifically inhibits ABL
detection.

The distribution of antigen spots vs. anti-Thy 1.2, anti-H-2^d,
or CAM(Fab')$_2$ spots was compared on coded photographs of randomly
selected ABL for each of the three antigens. Typical fluorescent
patterns found are shown in Fig.1. A cell was scored as having
coincident antigen and antiserum spots only if all antigen spots
coincided with antiserum spots. If any antigen spots were found
not to correspond to antiserum spots, the cell was scored as having
noncoincident spots. Some cells had patched antigen superimposed
on smooth rings for test antiserum. Such cells were scored as
questionable.

The combined data on the codistribution of antigen and antisera
to Thy 1.2, H-2^d and murine (Fab')$_2$ fragments are presented in Tab.4
These data show that antigens bound to thymic ABL coincide with
antiserum to (Fab')$_2$ fragments, but not with antisera to H-2^d and
Thy 1.2 determinants. Some of the noncoincident ABL seen when anti-
H-2^d serum and anti-Thy 1.2 serum were used did have a few antigen-
antiserum coincident spots, but they also had spots which were not
coincident.

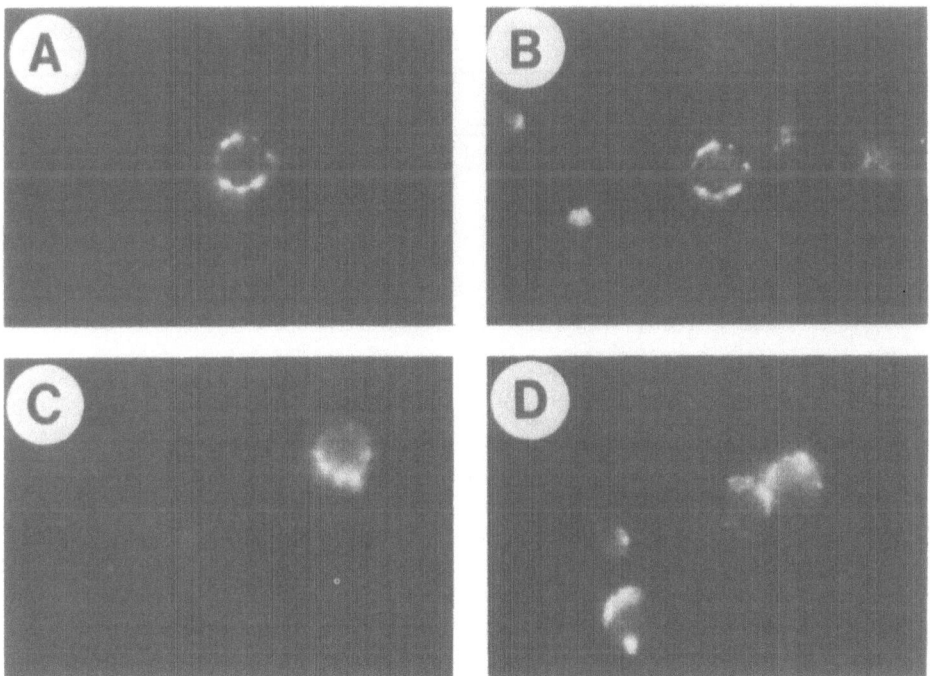

FIG. 1:   Codistribution of TRITC labeled KLH (A) and CAM(Fab')$_2$
followed by FITC-labeled rabbit anti-chicken Ig (B) on BALB/c
thymic ABL.   Lack of codistribution of TRITC-KLH (C) and anti-H-2^d
serum plus FITC rabbit anti-mouse Ig (D) on BALB/c thymic ABL

DISCUSSION

The results of this study are:

1.   ABL in the thymuses of unimmunized mice bear markers for Thy-
     1.2, for the appropriate H-2 specificity, and for Fab deter-
     minants.

2.   Most thymic ABL are not B cells since they bear the Thy-1.2
     alloantigen, and lack surface Ig when rabbit anti-Ig reagents
     alone are used.

3.   Antigen patches on thymic and splenic ABL show a strict
     correspondence with Fab determinants.

TAB. 4:   Patch Coincidence of Cell Surface Markers and Antigen

Organ	Antibody	Antigen								
		KLH			HSF			MYO		
		Co	?	Non-Co	Co	?	Non-Co	Co	?	Non-Co
Thymus	Anti-Thy 1.2	1	0	16	0	0	5	0	3	11
Thymus	Anti-H-2^d	0	5	14	0	2	7	0	1	7
Thymus	Anti-$(Fab')_2$	12	0	0	22	0	0	6	0	0
Spleen	Anti-$(Fab')_2$	25	0	0	15	0	0	12	0	0

4.   Patches of antigen on thymic ABL did not show a strict correspondence with Thy-1.2 determinants and H-2^d determinants.

The lack of codistribution for antigen and anti-Thy-1 serum was expected and agrees with the results of Loor and coworkers who found that anti-Thy-1 and antigen do not cocap (9). Similarly, the codistribution between antigen and anti-$(Fab')_2$ provides direct evidence to support the indirect data of Roelants et al. (10), which indicates that anti-Ig incubation of T-ABL under capping conditions results in capping of antigen.

However, we did not see a strict correspondence between H-2 determinants and antigen on thymic ABL. Such a result would have suggested that both Ig and MHC products play a role in antigen recognition by antigen-specific cells, an idea that might help explain the large collection of data which indicate that surface Ig is present on T cells (1,7,10,11-17), and that the mouse MHC is involved in immune responsiveness (18-20). In spite of the fact that our anti-H-2^d antiserum recognizes both H-2 and Ia determinants, it may be possible that it does not recognize the specific I-region gene product involved in the recognition of the antigens tested. Since a number of ABL did show some antigen spots which codistributed with H-2 determinants, it may be possible that Ig molecules can be weakly associated with H-2 molecules in the presence of antigen to form a complex involved in antigen-specific activation of lymphocytes (21).

Although the correspondence of antigen patches and CAM$(Fab')_2$ on the surface of ABL does not conclusively prove that Ig is the primary receptor for antigen, it does establish that $(Fab')_2$ determinants, unlike Thy-1.2 and H-2^d determinants, are at least in close proximity to the antigen receptor. A lack of correspondence between antigen and Ig determinants would, however, have been very difficult to reconcile with the concept that surface Ig is involved in T cell antigen recognition.

REFERENCES

1. Warner, N.L., Adv. Immunol. 19 (1974) 67.
2. Raff, M.C., Feldmann, M., de Petris, S., J. Exp. Med., 137 (1973) 1024.
3. Nossal, G.J.V., Layton, J.E., J. Exp. Med.143 (1976) 511.
4. Ashman, R.F., Immunol. 26 (1973) 539.
5. Hämmerling, U., Mack, C., Pickel, H.G., Immunochem. 13 (1976) 525.
6. Szenberg, A., Marchalonis, J.J., Warner, N.L., Proc. Natl. Acad. Sci. U.S.A. 73 (1977) 2113.
7. Marchalonis, J.J., Bucana, C., Hoyer, L., Warr, G., Hanna, Jr. M.G., Szenberg, A., Science 199 (1978) 433.
8. Jones, V.E., Graves, H.E., Orlans, E., Immunol. 30 (1976) 281.
9. Loor, F., Roelants, G.E., The Immune System: Genes, Receptor, Signals, (E. Sercarz, A.R. Williamson and C. Fred Fox eds), p. 201 Academic Press, New York and London (1974).
10. Roelants, G.E., Forni, L., Pernis, B., J. Exp. Med. 137 (1973) 1060.
11. Hämmerling, G.J., McDevitt, H.O., J. Immunol., 112 (1974) 1726.
12. Marchalonis, J.J., Science, 190 (1975) 20.
13. Haustein, D., Goding, J.W., Biochem. Biophys. Res. Commun. 65 (1975) 483.
14. Boylston, A.W., Mowbray, J.F., Immunol. 27 (1974) 855.
15. Cone, R.E., Brown, W.C., Immunochem. 13 (1976) 571.
16. Gabison, D., Bergman, Y, Haimovich, J., Berke, G., Transplant. Proc. 9 (1977) 741.
17. Moroz, C., Lahat, N., Cell. Immunol. 13 (1974) 397.
18. Krammer, P., Eichmann, K., Nature (London) 270 (1977) 733.
19. Benacerraf, B., McDevitt, H.O., Science 175 (1972) 273.
20. Paul, W.E., Benacerraf, B., Science 195 (1977) 1293.
21. Marchalonis, J.J., Contemp. Top. Mol. Immunol. 5 (1976) 125.

ACKNOWLEDGEMENTS

This research was sponsored by the National Cancer Institute under contract no. N01-CO-75380 with Litton Bionetics, Inc.

ONTOGENY OF SPONTANEOUS ROSETTE FORMING CELLS IN MICE

E.J. Steele

Ontario Cancer Institute

500 Sherbourne Street, Toronto, Canada M4X 1K9

INTRODUCTION

Lymphocytes binding autologous (or syngeneic) erythrocytes in vitro have been reported to occur in a wide range of animal species (1-6). High auto- (and allo-) RFC frequencies (10-20%) have been reported for man, pigs, rabbits, mice and rats (4-6). Auto- and allo-RFC may have immunological significance. Thus Bach and co-workers (7) have shown that auto-RFC isolated from the spleens of adult thymectomized mice mediate a GvH reaction in normal syngeneic mice. Owen et al (8) have demonstrated that allo-rosetting rat T cells appear to be the precursors of allo-reactive cells in mixed leukocyte cultures.

The presence of self recognizing lymphocytes in outwardly normal animals could suggest that the recognition of "self" may be positively selected for during ontogeny (cf. 9,10) but since gross manifestations of autoimmune disease are rarely seen it implies that the effector functions of such cells are normally suppressed in vivo (cf. 7). As the spontaneous rosette system of recognition may be relevant to our ideas on the somatic generation of the specificity repertoire (Jerne, 11) the aim of this study was to describe the ontogeny of RFC against a panel of different erythrocytes (syngeneic, allogeneic and xenogeneic). The main finding has been that the repertoire of naturally occurring RFC's in mice is orientated in both time and space towards self or closely related erythrocytes. This pattern is similar for both thymus and spleen. In addition, a portion of the splenic auto-RFC's seem to mediate this binding via conventional Ig receptors.

TAB. 1: Comparison RFC frequencies between foetal and adult thymocytes.

CBA/H Thymocytes	Erythrocyte tested							
	CBA/H	C57Bl	Balb/c	A.TL	SJL/J	Rat	GP	Horse
Foetus (18 day gest.)	38	26 (.7)*	20 (.5)	3 (.08)	4 (.1)	10 (.3)	<.5 (<.01)	<.3 (<.01)
Adult (10 wk)	39	33 (.8)	23 (.6)	16 (.4)	16 (.4)	4 (.1)	6 (.2)	<.3 (<.01)

* Frequency relative to syngeneic RFC.

MATERIALS AND METHODS

These are described in detail elsewhere (12). CBA/H and CBA/J mice were used as sources of lymphocytes. Erythrocytes were taken from various mouse strains (see Results) and from the rat, guinea pig (GP), horse and sheep. Female CBA mice were mated with males of the same strain and the day a vaginal plug was detected was taken as day 0 of gestation; birth occurred at day 19. Pooled single cell suspensions of thymus or spleen were made from at least two adult mice and up to 20 for foetuses. Rosettes were determined by mixing 0.05 ml lymphocytes (4-6 x 10^6/ml) in Hank's BSS + 5% FCS with 0.05 ml 1.6-2% erythrocytes (washed 3 x in saline), centrifuged (200 x g, 3 min, 25°C) and incubated at 4°C (1-3 hrs). Pellets were gently resuspended and lymphocytes stained with crystal violet (1 volume, 0.08% in saline). 150-1000 lymphocytes were counted (haemocytometer) and a rosette scored as any cell with 4 or more adhering erythrocytes. RFC counts were determined at least in duplicate (average standard error of the mean between duplicates $\leq$ 10%). RFC counts are expressed either as the percentage of total lymphocytes forming rosettes or as RFC frequency against test rbc:RFC frequency against syngeneic rbc. The latter normalizes for day-to-day variation in absolute RFC frequencies and allows ready comparisons within the data.

RESULTS AND DISCUSSION

Thymocytes and spleen cells from normal CBA mice were found routinely to form spontaneous rosettes at high frequency (1-40%) against syngeneic, allogeneic and some xenogeneic erythrocytes. Initial studies in adult mice (Tab.1) revealed a hierarchy of RFC's

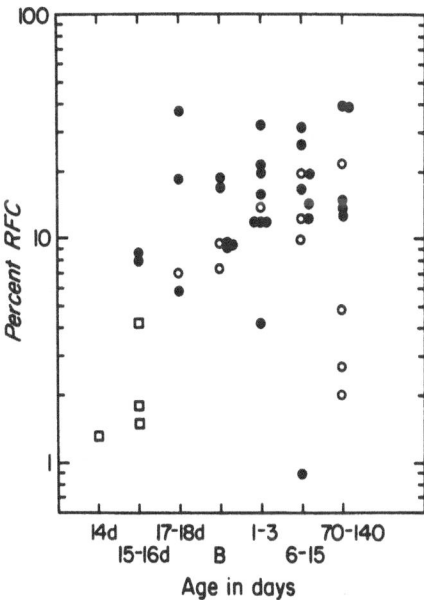

FIG. 1:   Ontogeny of syngeneic RFC.   Foetal liver (□), thymus (•)
and spleen (o).   Each point represents a given cell pool.   Results
summarized from 18 experiments.

in the order auto- $\geq$ allo- $\geq$ xeno-RFC, i.e., it appeared to correlate with the phylogenetic distance between mouse lymphocytes and
the target erythrocytes.   Syngeneic RFC are present very early in
ontogeny (Fig.1) at least by day 14 of gestation in foetal liver
($\sim$ 1%), days 15-16 in thymus ($\sim$ 8%) and days 17-18 gestation in
spleen ($\sim$ 7%).   The pattern of "self preference" generally extended
back into foetal life but changes in relative RFC numbers were
commonly found (Tab.1).   In some cases RFC types low to undetectable
in the foetal period occurred at high frequency in the adult (A.TL,
SJL/J, GP);   in other instances RFC's abundant in the foetus declined
into adulthood (rat).   These changes are seen more clearly in Figure
2.   Whilst some allo-rosettes are present at high frequency in the
foetus (C57B1, and to lesser extent Balb/c) others are low to
undetectable at this time becoming evident at birth or shortly after
(A.TL, SJL/J).   Amongst xeno-RFC some are present early (rat) whilst
others appear - and then sporadically - in neonatal (guinea pig) and
adult life (horse, sheep).   Changes such as these suggest a dynamic
developmental process governing the composition of the spontaneous
RFC repertoire.

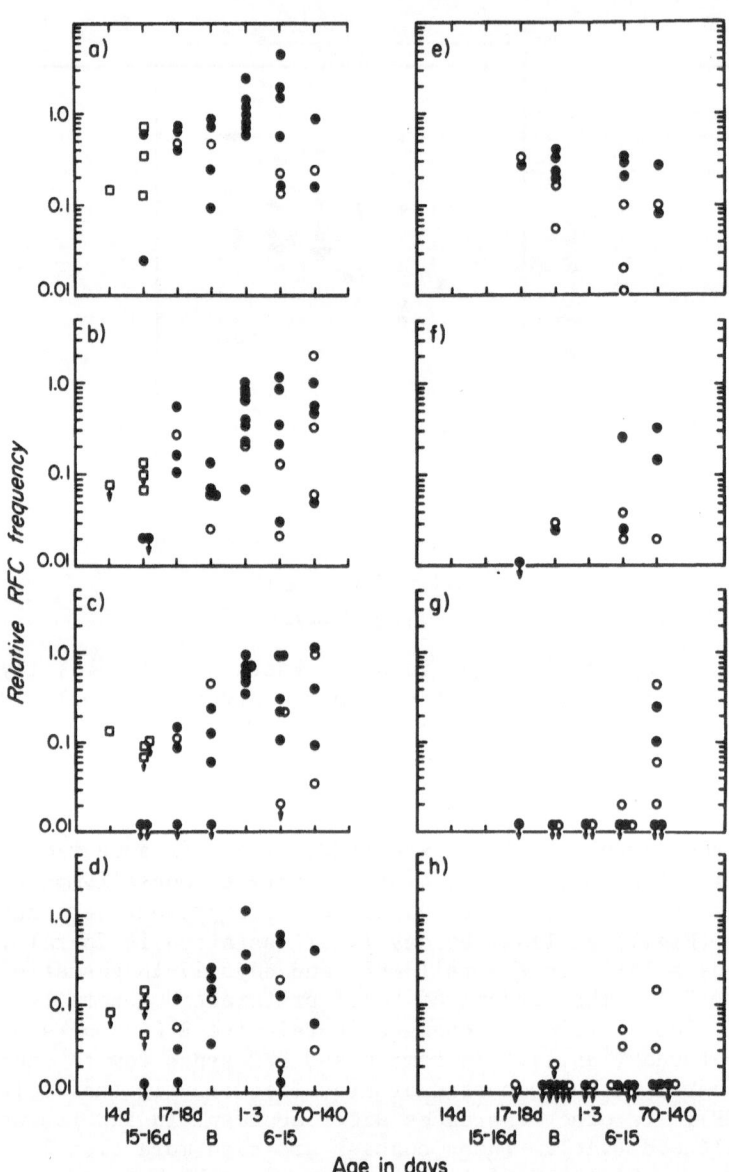

FIG. 2: Ontogeny of allo- and xeno-RFC. Determined on same cell populations as Fig.1. Results expressed as relative RFC (Materials and Methods). Foetal liver (□), thymus (●) and spleen (o). Erythrocytes were (a) C57Bl (b) Balb/c (c) A.TL (d) SJL/J (e) Rat (f) Guinea pig (g) Horse and (h) Sheep.

TAB. 2:   Properties of splenic auto-RFC's.

		% RFC	
Experiment	Treatment	Mrbc	Ig+
1. Spleen	Control	22	59
	Ig$^+$ cells removed	9	3
Thymus	Control	47	2
	Ig$^+$ cells removed	44	2
2. Spleen	Control	12	47
	Capped with $\propto$MIg	6	7
	T cells removed	12	77
	T cells removed then capped with $\propto$MIg	3	7

The properties of auto-RFC in spleen were studied (Tab.2). If cells bearing Ig are removed by depleting cells forming rosettes (on Ficoll gradients) with Srbc coated with the IgG fraction of sheep anti-mouse Ig (12), we observe a substantial decline (59%) in auto-RFC. This treatment applied to thymocytes was without effect. When T cells are killed by a rabbit anti-mouse brain + C' (provided by Dr. R. Gorczynski, 13) and dead cells removed on Ficoll gradients, little change in auto-rosette frequency is seen although it causes an enrichment for Ig$^+$ cells. If spleen cells are treated with sheep-$\propto$MIg (absorbed with CBA erythrocytes) under capping conditions (14), and washed, a 50% reduction in auto-RFC's is observed; an even better effect (75% reduction) is seen if T cells are first removed. Treatment of thymocytes with anti-Ig under capping conditions had no effect on auto-rosette numbers (data not shown). These results show that (a) Ig$^+$ and Ig$^-$ spleen cells form auto-RFC, (b) some of the auto-RFC in the Ig$^-$ fraction are formed by T cells and (c) a large fraction of the Ig$^+$ B cells mediate auto-rosettes via conventional Ig receptors. The failure of Ig$^+$ cell removal or capping with anti-Ig to affect auto-rosettes by thymocytes is consistent with the fact that the T cell antigen receptor does not bear determinents recognized by standard anti-Ig sera (15).

Although it is difficult to resolve whether the spontaneous rosette phenomenon reflects a true immunological recognition system or not (cf. well known capacity of human T cells to rosette Srbc), it is clear that the recognition system in mice is orientated towards self and closely related erythrocytes in both time and space. Further the B cell auto-rosettes in spleen appear to bind autologous erythrocytes via conventional Ig molecules. As outlined above, if the system does have immunological relevance it would likely comprise a mixture of effector and suppressor cells. The self orientation of the recognition would be consistent with Jerne's theory (11) and his model would predict that the binding affinity for self should be lower than for non-self. This question was not examined in this study.

The concept that the recognition capacity of the normal immune system is orientated towards self components is supported by several independent lines of evidence. The most intriguing recent example is the way T killer cells recognize virus infected target cells (16) or targets bearing minor-histocompatibility differences (17). Here the T cell recognition is restricted by self antigens coded in the major histocompatibility complex. Recent experiments show that the anti-self component of the dual recognition is acquired in ontogeny by a self antigen learning process dictated by the H-2 haplotype of the host in which the T cells differentiates (9). More recently it has been shown that this education appears dictated by the H-2 haplotype of the host's thymus epithelium (10).

These experiments are consistent with the present findings and the hypothesis preferred would be that the self orientation of the spontaneous rosette phenomenon is the result of a self antigen learning (selection) process operating on both T and B lymphocytes beginning early in foetal and neonatal life. Indeed there is evidence at the level of natural antibody formation that a high proportion of ongoing or potential Ig secreting B cells in normal mice produce antibody specific for bromelain treated mouse erythrocytes - depending on the organ examined between 1% to $\geq$ 50% of Ig secreting cells are BrM specific (18). Recent experiments suggest that the antigens exposed by bromelain treatment are shared by naturally occurring self components associated with the gastro-intestinal tract (19). These stomach autoantigens become expressed after birth, probably as a result of normal digestive processes, and appear to play an important role in educating early B cells to immune competence (19).

REFERENCES

1. Micklèm, H.S., Asfi, C. in: Morphological and Functional Aspects of Immunity. K. Lindahl-Kiessling, C. Alm and M.C. Hanna (eds.), Plenum Press, New York, p. 57 (1971).
2. Charreire, J., Bach, J.-F. Proc. Nat. Acad. Soc. U.S.A. 72 (1975) 3201.
3. Gluckman, J.-C., Gattegno, L., Cornellot, P. Eur. J. Immunol. 5 (1975) 301.
4. Baxley, G., Bishop, G.B., Cooper, A.G., Wortis, H.H. Clin. Exp. Immunol. 15 (1973) 385.

5. Sandelands, G., Gray, K., Cooney, A., Browning, J.D., Anderson, J.R. Lancet i (1974) 27.
6. Kolb, H. Immunology 33 (1977) 859.
7. Carnard, C., Charreire, J., Bach, J.-F. Cell. Immunol. 28 (1977) 274.
8. Owen, F.L., Stux, S.V., Nisonoff, A. J. Immunol. 118 (1977) 909.
9. Bevan, M.J. Nature 269 (1977) 417.
10. Zinkernagel, R.M., Callahan, G.M., Klein, J., Dennert, G. Nature 271 (1978) 251.
11. Jerne, N. Eur. J. Immunol. 1 (1971) 1.
12. Steele, E.J., Cunningham, A.J. Manuscript submitted (1978).
13. Gorczynski, R.M. J. Immunol. 112 (1974) 533.
14. Schreiner, C.F., Unanue, E.R. J. Exp. Med. 143 (1976) 15.
15. Rajewsky, K., Eichmann, K. Contemp. Top. Immunobiol. 7 (1977) 69.
16. Zinkernagel, R.M., Doherty, P.C. J. Exp. Med. 31 (1975) 23.
17. Bevan, M.J. Nature 256 (1975) 419.
18. Steele, E.J., Cunningham, A.J. Nature, in press (1978).
19. Steele, E.J., Cunningham, A.J. Proceedings of the VI International Conference on Lymphatic Tissues and Germinal Centers in Immune Reactions, Kiel (1978).

ACKNOWLEDGEMENTS

The author is grateful to Dr. A.J. Cunningham for critical discussions and to Sue Fordham for her dedicated technical assistance. Freda Sochasky is thanked for her patience in preparation of the manuscript.

MULTIPLE Ig CLASSES ON RABBIT B LYMPHOCYTES

Bert J.E.G. Bast, Ria Manten-Slingerland, Rudy E.
Ballieux and David Catty[1]

University Hospital Utrecht, the Netherlands

[1]Department of Experimental Pathology, University of
Birmingham, England

INTRODUCTION

In man and mice the two main classes of lymphocytes (T and B
cells) have extensively been studied. Less information is available
regarding lymphocyte subpopulations in the rabbit. The presence of
an IgD homologue on rabbit B cells has not yet been documented (1).
Knowledge regarding isotypes on the surface of B lymphocytes is
limited, compared to (isotype non-linked) a and b allotypes (2,3,4).
We have studied surface immunoglobulin (s-Ig) of rabbit lymphocytes
under conditions ensuring the endogeneous origin of these proteins.
This involved pronase stripping of s-Ig and subsequent regeneration
at 37°C incubation.

MATERIALS AND METHODS

Animals.   The rabbits used in this study were female outbred
Flemish Giants and New Zealands, obtained from the local breeder.
They were homozygous (hom.) or heterozygous (het.) for the allotypes
a (marker on the VH of all Ig classes) and d (located on the Fdγ
domain).

Conjugates.   IgG was isolated from the antisera used and all
IgG fractions (with the exception of anti d11) were pepsin digested.
Purified (Fab')₂ fragments (after Sephadex G 150 elution and protein
A Sepharose 4B absorption) were conjugated with Fitc and/or Tritc,

resulting in conjugates with molar F/P ratio's ranging from 1,8 - 4,5. Results of specificity tests, inclucing the Defined Antigen Substrate Spheres (DASS) (5), cytoplasmic staining of rabbit bone marrow cells, absorption studies, population studies and double marker studies are described elsewhere extensively (6). The data presented in this paper are limited to results obtained with Fitc or Tritc conjugates of heterologous anti IgM, IgA anti Fc γ and anti Fab antisera and of homologous anti d11 and anti a1 antisera. These conjugates all met the desired specificity and strength in fluorescence.

Lymphocyte preparations. The isolation procedure (sedimentation in 1% gelatine, followed by Ficoll Hypaque centrifugation, yielding a > 90% lymphoid cell suspension), pronase treatment and overnight incubation of rabbit PBL has been described earlier (7). Lymphocytes (10^6 x 50 μl) were incubated with 50 μl of the conjugate dilution (ranging from 1/8 - 1/64) under non-capping conditions ($1^o/_{oo}$ NaN3, 4°C) washed with Earles BSA (1%) (containing NaN3) and eventually treated with a second conjugate under similar conditions. Wet preparations were examined on a Leith Orthoplan (63 x Phaco objective, 4 x eyepieces). An HBO 100 lamp was used as an epi-iluminator whereas for specific Fitc and Tritc illumination blocks K and M (Ploemopak II) respectively were used.

RESULTS

The percentage of Ig bearing lymphocytes in rabbit PBL was determined in single incubation experiments (Tab. 1).

TAB. 1:   s-Ig on rabbit PBL;   single incubation

Anti:	Fab	a1 (Hom.)	IgM	IgA	IgG(Fc)	IgG(d11) Hom.	Het.
Mean + 1 s.d.:	38+6	41+7	34+7	6+2	0.4+0.3	32+3	15+10
N. of Expts. :	36	9	55	18	15	5	10

Having established the endogeneous origin of the s-Ig studied and particularily of IgG, experiments were performed in which lymphocytes were incubated sequentially with Fitc and Tritc conjugates. In every combination 150-1200 lymphocytes, positive for one conjugate, were examined for the presence of the other marker (3-12 expts.). Control experiments in single incubation revealed that no inhibition did occur in these combinations. At first Fab or a1 positive lymphocytes were studied in double

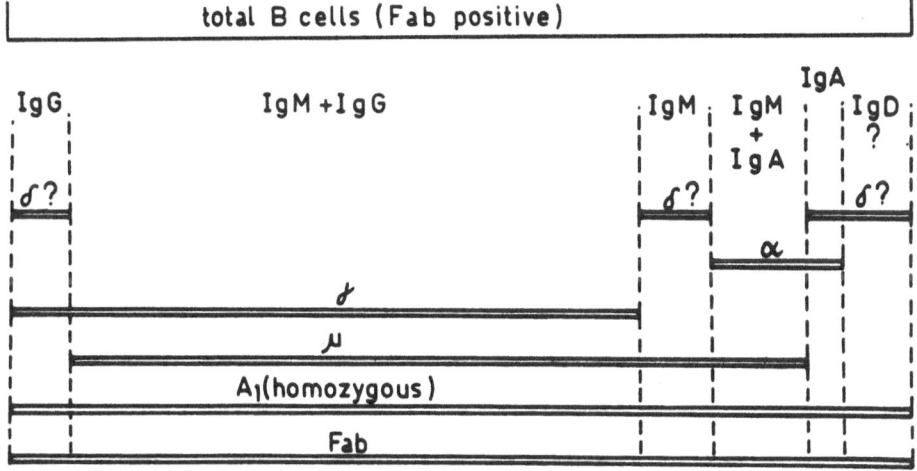

FIG. 1

incubation experiments using anti IgM or IgA. Furthermore, double
staining was carried out using anti Fab and anti al allotype
conjugates. A complete overlap was found of al and Fab positive
lymphocytes. IgM and IgA bearing lymphocytes are a major respectively minor subpopulation of the B cells. To investigate further
interrelationships between different isotypes double incubations
were done, using anti IgM, IgA and dll conjugates. It was found
that almost all IgA and IgG bearing lymphocytes were IgM positive
too,. only scarcely cells were seen bearing exclusively IgA or IgG.
IgG and IgA bearing lymphocytes are major respectively minor subpopulations in IgM bearing cells. No lymphocytes were found
bearing both IgG and IgA (see Fig. 1).

DISCUSSION

     Using experimental conditions ensuring the endogeneous origin
of s-Ig, we examined the occurence of different isotypes (IgM and
IgA) or isotype related allotype (dll on Fd-IgG) on rabbit B cells
(Fab or al positive in al homozygous rabbits). Control experiments
revealed that after pronase treatment all s-Ig determinants were
stripped from the cell. The specificity of the conjugates, the
interrelationship with T cell markers and further proofs of absence
 of absorption of IgG in vivo or in vitro is documented elsewhere
(6). We were able to find IgG positive lymphocytes, but only using
an anti Fdγ reagent, as described by Pernis (4). The entire Fcγ
domain is probably buried in the membrane or at least is inacces-
sible.

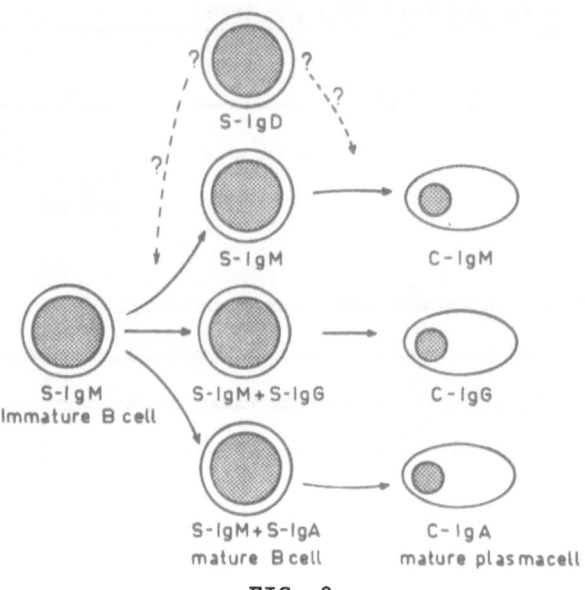

FIG. 2

The sum of all s-Ig positive PBL was greater than the total
number of B cells so double bearers must exist. This was tested
in combination experiments with anti μ, anti α and anti dll. In
dll heterozygotes half of the IgM positive lymphocytes were dll
positive too; in homozygous rabbits this overlap was even greater.
A smaller part of the IgM bearing cells is IgA positive too. On
the other hand, almost all IgG and IgA bearing lymphocytes are a
subpopulation of the IgM cells. On the basis of the obtained
percentages we could calculate that 91±10% is positive for IgM,
IgG or IgA.

Our results may suggest the presence of some "non IgM, IgA,
IgG" B cells (s-IgD), but to the rather high statistical error no
proof could be obtained. However, in view of the major IgG/IgM
overlap it can be argued that "s-IgD" in the rabbit (if present) in
the differentiation process does not develop in between IgG and
IgM (fig. 2). This does not conflict with the Parkhouse/Cooper
model (1), but is in contrast to models describing the sequential
appearance of IgM, IgD and IgG (Vitetta and Uhr (8), Pernis (9)).
We did not find any IgA and IgG double bearing lymphocytes. This
finding also fits very well in the Parkhouse/Cooper model of

different pathways: $\quad IgM < {IgG \atop IgA}$, in contrast to former models of
sequential development: IgM → IgG → IgA.

SUMMARY

Rabbit PBL were studied regarding the presence of different classes of s-Ig, under experimental conditions, ensuring the endogeneous origin of these proteins. About 40% of the lymphocytes are B cells (Fab positive and a1 positive in a1 homozygous rabbits). IgG positive lymphocytes could be found, but only using an anti d11 conjugate (allotype located on the Fdγ region of IgG). Anti Fcγ conjugates were negative. Most of the B cells are IgM positive, most of these IgM cells however were also positive for either IgG or IgA. No lymphocytes were found bearing both IgG and IgA. Careful analysis of the percentages of various isotypes found on B cells suggests that some "IgD" positive lymphocytes could be present. Results are discussed in relation to B cell differentiation.

REFERENCES

1. Parkhouse, R.M.E., Cooper, M.D., Immunol. Rev. 37 (1977) 105.
2. Molinaro, G.A., Bessinger, B.A., Gilmahi-Sachs, A., Dray, S., J. Immunol. 114 (1975) 908.
3. Jones, P.P., Cebra, J.J., J. Exp. Med., 140 (1974) 966.
4. Pernis, B., Forni, L., Amante, L., J. Exp. Med., 132 (1970) 1001.
5. Dalen, J.P.R. van, Knapp, W., Ploem, J.S., J. Immunol. Meth. 2 (1973) 383.
6. Bast, E.J.E.G., Catty, D., Ballieux, R.E. et al. Rabbit T and B cells in membrane fluorescence and rosette formation. Manuscript submitted.
7. Bast, E.J.E.G., et al. Fc receptors for antigen bound IgG on rabbit lymphocytes. Manuscript submitted.
8. Vitetta, E.S., Uhr, J.U., Immunol. Rev. 37 (1977) 50.
8. Pernis, B., Immunol. Rev. 37 (1977) 210.

ACKNOWLEDGEMENTS

This work was supported by Fungo/ZWO grant 13-40-12. Our thanks are due to Dr. J. Urbain, Université Libre de Bruxelles for a generous gift of anti a1 antiserum.

C3 RECEPTORS AND MEMBRANE COMPLEMENT COMPONENTS ON LYMPHOCYTES JOINTLY CAUSE BINDING OF EAC

M.P. Dierich and B. Landen

Institute for Medical Microbiology,

Augustusplatz, D-65 Mainz, West Germany

Binding of EAC1423 to C3 receptor positive lymphocytes is a temperature dependent event (1). This phenomenon was thought to be sufficiently explained by the fact that C3 receptors had to move laterally and to form clusters to enable the C3 receptor cell to bind complement coated erythrocytes (EAC1423) to its surface (2). Recently, it was shown that lymphoid cells coated with exogenous C3 (e.g. Raji-C3) formed rosettes with EAC142 (3). This complement-dependent bridge formation was dependent on the lymphocyte-bound C3 and the erythrocyte-bound C42 enzyme. Therefore it was investigated whether in addition to the lateral movement also an enzymatic activity was responsible for the temperature dependence of rosette formation between EAC1423 and complement receptor cells such as Raji cells.

It could be clearly shown that diisopropylfluorophosphate (DFP) suppressed rosette formation at concentrations of 0.01 mM up to 40%. By decaying the C42-enzyme of EAC1423 the rosette formation potential of these cells was reduced like by treatment with DFP. Upon reconstitution of the C42 enzyme by adding back C2 the rosetting potential was restored, suggesting that C42 was the acting enzyme.

Searching for the substrate of this enzyme led us to treat Raji cells with varying concentrations of IgG-anti C3 and for control with unrelated IgG. Only by IgG-anti C3 the Raji cells' rosette formation capacity with EAC1423 was reduced. To test whether this reduction was due to blockade of C3, the natural substrate of C42, or if it was due to steric hindrance of the C3 receptors on the Raji cells, binding studies with E^{tan}-C3 (tannic acid treated E, coated with $C3^{hum}$) were performed with Raji cells treated with various sera. Anti-C3 serum had no effect. In contrast, treatment of Raji cells with an antiserum directed against C3 receptor molecules isolated from human serum was well capable of inhibiting Raji cells to form rosettes with E^{tan}-C3. Rosette formation with EAC1423 was only partially inhibited.

From these data we conclude that rosette formation of EAC1423 with C3 receptor cells is a two step event depending on the inter-action of C3b/C3d with C3 receptors and in addition on the action of the C42-enzyme on membrane-bound (endogenous) C3.

REFERENCES

1. Lay, W.H., Nussenzweig, V. J. Exp. Med. 128 (1968) 991.
2. Dierich, M.P., Reisfeld, R.A. J. Exp. Med. 142 (1975) 242.
3. Dierich, M.P., Landen, B. J. Exp. Med. 146 (1977) 1484.

ACKNOWLEDGEMENT

This study was supported by the DFG, SFB 107, A5.

C3 AND C5 COMPETE FOR THE SAME BINDING SITE ON COMPLEMENT RECEPTOR CELLS

M.P. Dierich and B. Landen

Institute for Medical Microbiology,

Augustusplatz, D-65 Mainz, West Germany

Cell-cell contact can be mediated by C3, which is bound by its labile binding site (LBS) to C3 acceptors like on EAC1423b (1), in that the C3b's stable binding sites (SBS1 and SBS2) attach to C3 receptors on C3 receptor positive cells (CR$^+$C) thus performing C3 dependent rosette formation (2-4).

In addition, uncleaved C3 can induce cell-cell interaction in an alternative fashion, when bound first to C3 receptor carrying cells via its stable binding site SBS 1 (competent for C3b). Cleavage of this receptor bound C3 by C42 or even an unspecific protease on EAC142 or another cell results in liberation of the C3b's labile binding site and subsequent attachment of the latter to C3 acceptors on the protease carrying cell. This phenomenon has been called bridge formation (5). This bridge formation occurs not only via C3 but also via C5 as could be demonstrated by incubation of C5-coated Raji lymphoblastoid cells with EAC142 (5).

When C3 and C5 have been found to be structurally homologous (6) and when C5 was shown to enhance phagocytosis of complement coated erythrocytes by human granulocytes (7), the possibile identity of the receptors for C3 and for C5, respectively, was tested.

E^{tan}-C5(tannic acid treated sheep erythrocytes coated with C5) form rosettes with C3 receptor positive cells, but not with cells lacking C3 receptors. Binding of E^{tan}-C5 to Raji cells was clearly dependent on the amount of C5 incubated with E^{tan}.

Pretreatment of the CR$^+$C with soluble C3 or C5 (20 min, 37°C) at various concentrations inhibited this binding. These findings are in agreement with the observation that Raji cells, after incubation with soluble C5 (20 min, 37°C) showed a decreasing percentage of rosette formation with EAC1423b as well as with EAC1423d and with E^{tan}-C3. Taken together this indicates that C3 and C5 competed for the same binding site on CR$^+$C. Additional evidence for the identity of the receptors for C5 and for C3 comes from the fact that antisera, directed against C3 receptor material in human serum were able to inhibit the attachment of E^{tan}-C3 as well as of E^{tan}-C5 to Raji cells.

The immune adherence reaction is also inhibited by C5. Since Raji cells are supposed to carry only C3d receptors (8) while E^{hum} have only C3b receptors and as both types of cells were affected by C5, one would consider binding of C5 to both types of receptors corresponding to the binding behaviour of C3 (9).

REFERENCES

1.   Bokisch, V.A., Dierich, M.P., Müller-Eberhardt, H.J.   Proc. Nat. Acad. Sci. USA 72 (1975) 1989.
2.   Lay, W.H., Nussenzweig, V.   J. Exp. Med. 128 (1968) 991.
3.   Ross, G.D., Polley, M.J., Rabellino, E.M., Grey, H.M.   J. Exp. Med. 138 (1973) 798.
4.   Theofilopoulos, A.N., Bokisch, V.A., Dixon, F.J.   J. Exp. Med. 139 (1974) 696.
5.   Dierich, M.P., Landen, B.   J. Exp. Med. 146 (1977) 1484.
6.   Müller-Eberhard, H.J.   Ann. Rev. Biochem. 44 (1975) 697.
7.   Segerling, M., Opferkuch, W.   Fed. Proc. 35 (1976) 273.
8.   Ross, G.D., Tack, B.F., Rabellino, E.M.   Fed. Proc. 37 (1978) 1270.
9.   Dierich, M.P., Pellegrino, M.A., Ferrone, S., Reisfeld, R.A. J. Immunol. 112 (1974) 1766.

ACKNOWLEDGEMENT

This study was supported by the DFG, SFB 107, A5.

INHIBITION OF C3b AND C3d RECEPTOR ACTIVITY BY XENOANTISERA

PREPARED BY IMMUNIZATION WITH CELL-BOUND C3 RECEPTOR PROTEIN

J. Gerdes, U. Klatt, H. Stein and H. Herrmann

Institute of Pathology, University of Kiel

2300 Kiel, W. Germany

Receptors for complement fragment 3b (C3b receptors) and/or 3d (C3d receptors) have been demonstrated on various human cell populations, namely, erythrocytes (E_{hu}), platelets, granulocytes, monocytes, renal glomerular cells, liver cells, and lymphocytes (8). There are several indications that C3 receptors play an important role in various biological processes, such as immunophagocytosis (5,6), clearance of immune complexes (4), antibody triggering (7), and the germinal center reaction (2,9,10); but the different functions of C3 receptors are far from clear. Antibodies capable of blocking C3 receptors would thus be useful tools for studying the biological functions of C3 receptors in various in-vivo and in-vitro systems.

MATERIALS AND METHODS

For the immunoabsorption of receptor proteins, erythrocyte-antibody-complement complexes (EAC_{6def}) were prepared with serum from C6-deficient rabbits (the rabbits were a generous gift from Professor K. Rother, Heidelberg, Germany). Sheep erythrocytes (SRBC) were coated with antibodies of a crude anti-SRBC serum at a just subagglutinating titre and incubated in freshly drawn serum of C6-deficient rabbits. As indicator cells (IgM-EA) we used trypsinized SRBC, which were coated with the IgM fraction of an anti-SRBC serum at a just subagglutinating titre. The coating of IgM-EA with purified complement components (Cordis, Miami, Florida, USA) was carried out according to Stein et al. (10), resulting in EAC3b. An aliquot of the EAC3b was converted to EAC3d by using purified C3b inactivator (Cordis, Miami, Florida, USA). Tonsil cell membranes

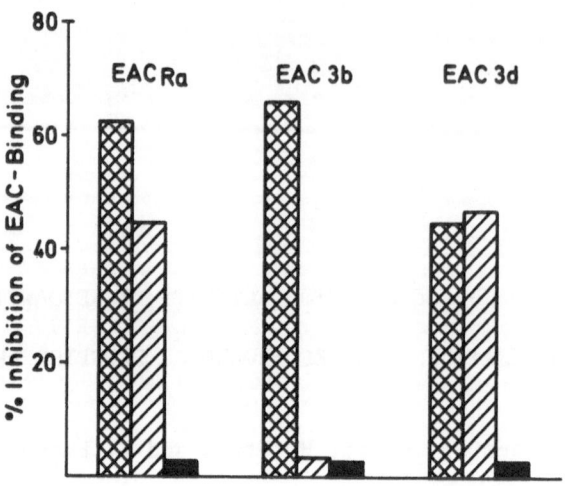

Inhibition of EAC binding to tonsil cells by a diluted (1:40) anti-C3
receptor serum before absorption (⬚), after absorption with human
erythrocytes (⬚), and after absorption with human tonsil cells (⬛)

FIG. 1

were prepared with the nitrogen cavitation method and differential
centrifugation as described by Ferber et al. (3). C3 receptors were
solubilized from the 20,000 g pellet by means of the method of Dierich
and Reisfeld (1).

5 x 10^8 EAC_{6def}/ml were incubated in a diluted receptor-active
potassium bromide membrane extract. The resulting complexes
(EAC_{6def}-C3 receptors) were washed three times in TC-199 medium
(Difco Lab., Detroit, Michigan, USA). The binding of C3 receptor
proteins to EAC_{6def} was tested with a rosette inhibition assay,
carried out according to Dierich and Reisfeld (1).

Rabbits were immunized once a week with EAC_{6def}-C3 receptors.
The antisera obtained from the animals were heat-inactivated and
exhaustively absorbed with SRBC, glutaraldehyde-insolubilized human
serum polymer, and human brain tissue homogenate. Specific
absorptions were carried out with human erythrocytes (E_{hu}) and tonsil
cells. The sera were tested for specific reactivity to C3 receptors
by means of the rosette inhibition assay and the EAC agglutination
inhibition test. Different dilutions of the antisera were mixed in
microtitre plates with 25 μl C3 receptor-enriched membrane extract.
After incubation for 40 minutes at 37°C, 25 μl EAC suspension
(1 x 10^8 cells/ml) were added to each dilution. The plates were

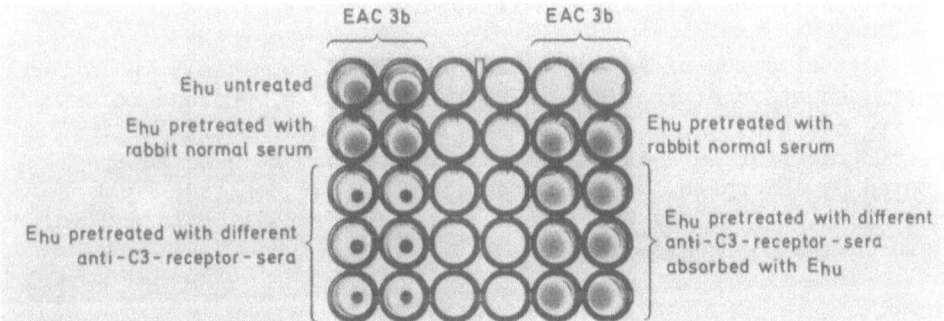

<u>FIG. 2:</u>   Inhibition of immunoadherence by means of pretreatment of
<u>human</u> erythrocytes (E_{hu}) with an anti-C3 receptor serum.

agitated for 5 minutes and incubated at 37°C. The agglutination
patterns were read after 60-90 minutes.

     As controls we used normal rabbit serum, C6-deficient rabbit
serum, sera obtained from rabbits that were immunized with EAC_{6def},
and sera obtained from rabbits that were immunized with SRBC
preincubated in C3 receptor-enriched membrane extract.

RESULTS AND DISCUSSION

     Different dilutions of antisera obtained from rabbits immunized
with EAC_{6def} incubated in C3 receptor-enriched membrane extract
(anti-C3 receptor sera) and different dilutions of the control sera
were tested for their activity against C3 receptors by means of the
EAC agglutination inhibition assay and the EAC rosette inhibition
assay. The anti-C3 receptor sera inhibited EAC3b agglutination at
dilutions of up to 1:128 and EAC_{6def} agglutination at dilutions of
up to 1:256, whereas the control sera did not inhibit. The anti-C3
receptor sera also showed strong inhibition of EAC binding to tonsil
cells (Fig.1) and the control sera showed no inhibition. The
capacity of the anti-C3 receptor sera to inhibit (a) EAC agglutination by solubilized C3 receptors and (b) EAC binding to tonsil
cells could be completely removed by absorption of the sera with
human tonsil cells. Absorption of the anti-C3 receptor sera with
E_{hu} caused a total removal of the capacity to inhibit EAC3b binding
to tonsil cells, whereas the inhibitory effect on EAC3d rosette
formation was not changed (Fig.1). These findings show that the
antisera we obtained were operationally specific and directed against
the binding site of the C3 receptor molecules. Furthermore, the
results indicate that the anti-C3 receptor sera could be made

operationally specific for C3d receptors.

Agglutination of E_{hu} with EAC3b could be completely inhibited by preincubation of E_{hu} in anti-C3 receptor sera, whereas it was not inhibited by the control sera (Fig.2). The capacity of the anti-C3 receptor sera to inhibit agglutination could be fully removed by absorption of the sera with E_{hu}. We conclude from these results that the C3b receptor of human tonsil cells and E_{hu} share common antigenic sites.

REFERENCES

1.   Dierich, M.P., Reisfeld, R.A., J. Immunol. 114 (1975) 1676.
2.   Dukor, P., Bianco, C., Nussenzweig, V., Proc. nat. Acad. Sci. (Wash.) 67 (1970) 991.
3.   Ferber, E., Resch, K., Wallach, D.F.H., Imm, W., Biochim. biophys. Acta (Amst.) 266 (1972) 494.
4.   Gelfand, F.C., Frank, M.M., Green, J., J. exp. Med. 142 (1975) 1029.
5.   Huber, H., Polley, M.J., Linscott, W.D., Fudenberg, H.H., Müller-Eberhard, H.J., Science 162 (1968) 1281.
6.   Mantovani, B., Rabinovitch, M., Nussenzweig, V., J. exp. Med. 135 (1972) 780.
7.   Möller, G., Coutinho, A., J. exp. Med. 141 (1975) 647.
8.   Müller-Eberhard, H.J., in: Textbook of Immunopathology, Vol.1, pp.45-74. Miescher, P.A., Müller-Eberhard, H.J., Eds., New York-San Francisco-London: Grune & Stratton (1976).
9.   Stein, H., Immun. Infekt. 4 (1976) 52 and 95.
10. Stein, H., Siemssen, U., Lennert, K., Brit. J. Cancer 37 (1978) 520.

MODULATION OF THE IMMUNE RESPONSE BY PRETREATMENT OF ANTIGEN WITH

COMPLEMENT

W. Opferkuch, W. Horn, F. Falkenberg and S.H.E. Kaufmann

Institute of Medical Microbiology, Ruhr-University

Bochum, D-4630 Bochum, West Germany

The only information on the participation of the complement system in the immune response is based on experiments with cobra venom treated mice and chicken (1,2). In these experiments, it was shown that C3 depleted mice were not capable of reacting normally to an antigenic stimulus. However, cobra venom treatment before immunization most probably does not only deplete the animals of C3, but has in addition other unpredictable consequences.

In contrast to this experimental approach, we wanted to know whether the modification of a cellular antigen (SRBC) with antibody and complement in vitro yields information on the influence of the complement system on the immune reaction. For this purpose, sheep erythrocytes were treated stepwise with antibody (either IgG or IgM) and individual purified complement components. 2×10^8 SRBC per mouse prepared in this manner were used for immunization. The immune response was measured by the Jerne-plaque-technique (direct and indirect plaques) (3,4).

Fig.1 shows the kinetics of plaque formation after immunization with 2×10^8 cells in NMRI mice. Either untreated SRBC (E) or SRBC pretreated with IgM antibody and lysed by complement (EIgM*) were used as antigen. It can be seen that the number of plaque forming cells (PFC) was 10 times lower using complement lysed cells for immunization.

In order to evaluate the contribution of individual complement components to the observed suppression of the immune response, SRBC were treated either with IgG or IgM antibody (Fig.2). While IgG antibody alone led to the expected suppression, IgM antibodies

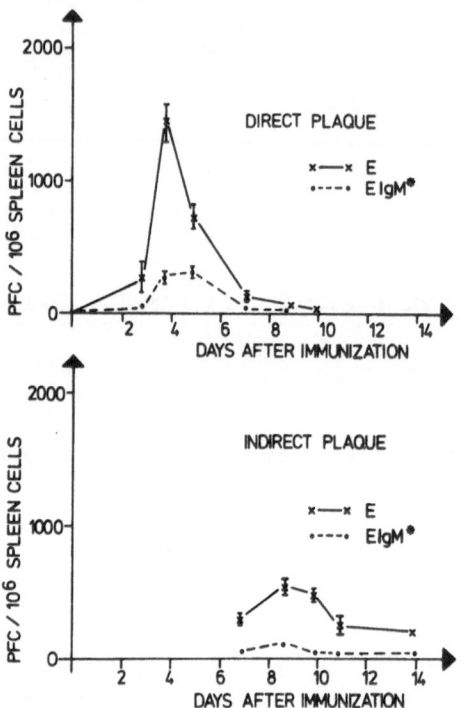

FIG. 1:   Kinetics of the generation of plaque-forming cells after immunization. Upper part: direct plaques; lower part: indirect plaques. The plaque formation after immunization with SRBC (E x——x) or with SRBC treated with IgM-antibody and complement (EIgM* ●---●) was determined.

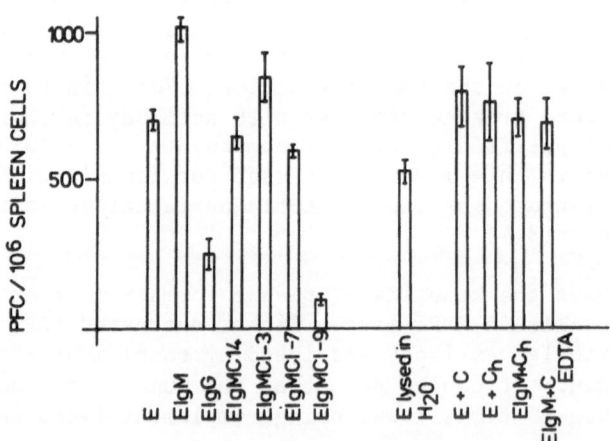

FIG. 2:   Influence of complement intermediates on antibody formation. The number of plaque-forming cells determined on day 4 after immunization.

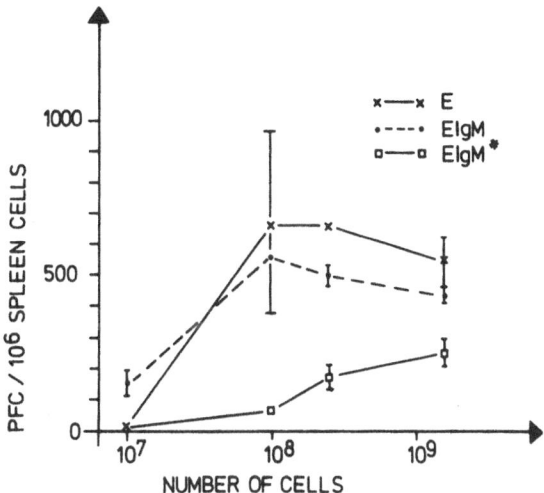

Fig. 3:   Dose-response curve was estimated after immunization with
varying amounts of cells on day 4.   SRBC (E x———x), SRBC treated
with IgM antibody (EIgM) or SRBC treated with IgM antibody and
complement (EIgM*) were used as antigen.

showed no effect on the anti-SRBC response. Stepwise treatment of
EIgM with C1 and C4, C1 - C3, or C1 - C7, did not lead to a significant change in comparison with E and EIgM. However, treatment with
C1 - C9 significantly reduced the immune response. As controls, SRBC
lysed with water, SRBC treated with fresh serum or with heat inactivated complement as well as EIgM treated with heated or EDTA inactivated complement, induced normal immune responses, thus demonstrating
that C9 is the critical component for the suppressive action.

    The dose response curve shows that increasing amounts of antigen
(2×10^9 cells/mouse) did not compensate the suppressive effect
(Fig.3).

    The experiment shown in Fig.4 was done to rule out whether
antigenic competition exerted by the xenogenic material (namely
rabbit anti-SRBC and guinea-pig complement) in the mouse was the
cause of the observed suppression. From the figure it can be seen
that E* rat (prepared with rat anti-IgM-SRBC and rat complement)
leads to a suppressed immune response in both species, rat and mouse.
Since rat complement is hemolytically highly active in contrast to
mouse serum, the response to EIgM alone was suppressed in rats
probably due to in vivo lysis, but not in mice.

    The results of the experiments clearly show that activation of
C9 on the red cell surface is necessary to induce complement mediated
immune suppression. Antigenic competition was ruled out by the use
of autologous reagents. Three hypotheses are offered:

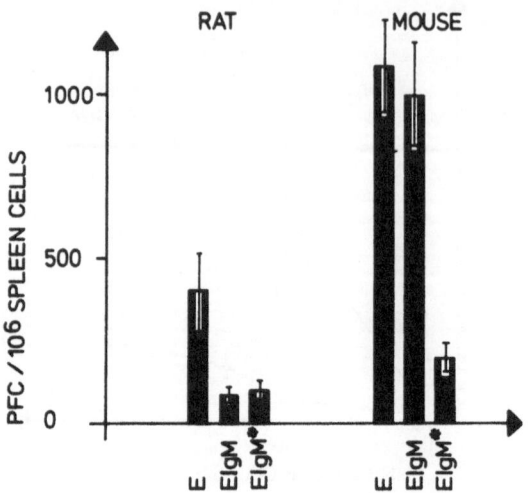

<u>FIG. 4</u>:   Influence of treatment of SRBC with rat IgM-antibody and
rat complement on the antibody formation in rat and mouse. The
plaque-forming cells were estimated on day 4 after immunization.

1.   The cell membrane of complement lysed SRBC is antigenically
modified in such a way that a different antibody population is
induced that cannot be tested with intact SRBC.

2.   Complement treated SRBC induce suppressor cells.

3.   The interaction of complement treated SRBC with T lymphocytes
is impaired.

This perspective is supported by the fact that in a case of genetical
C3 deficiency in man no impairment of the antibody production was
observed (5). On the basis of our data, one might speculate that
immune response depression in cobra venom treated mice is not caused
by C3 depletion but rather by generation of an excess of circulating
C3 - C9 complexes.

REFERENCES

1.   Pepys, M.B. Transplant. Rev. 32 (1976) 92.
2.   Nielsen, K.H., White, R.G. Nature 250 (1974) 234.
3.   Jerne, N.K., Nordin, A.A. Science 140 (1963) 405.
4.   Wortis, H.H., Taylor, R.B., Dresser, D.W. Immunology 11 (1966)
      603.
5.   Alper, C.A., Colten, H.R., Rosen, F.S., Rabson, A.R., McNab,
      G.M., Gear, J.S.S. Lancet 2 (1972) 1179.

CHARACTERIZATION OF AN IgG-Fc RECEPTOR PROTEIN ISOLATED FROM HUMAN

B-PROLYMPHOCYTIC AND B-CHRONIC LYMPHOCYTIC LEUKEMIA CELLS

[1]J. Thönes and [2]H. Stein

[1]Institute of Biochemistry and [2]Institute of Pathology,

University of Kiel, 2300 Kiel, West Germany

With the exception of antibody-dependent cellular cytotoxicity
(18) and immunophagocytosis (11), the biological role of Fc receptors
is still largely unclear. Since knowledge of the physicochemical
properties of Fc receptors might open up new possibilities for
elucidating other biological functions of Fc receptors and the
relationship between these receptors and other membrane proteins (6),
several attempts have been made to define the physicochemical
structure of the Fc receptor molecules. The studies performed so
far, however, have not yielded consistent data. In particular, the
molecular weight estimated by various authors (3,5,8,16,19,21) varied
from 15,000 to 130,000 daltons. These inconsistent estimates of the
molecular weight might reflect actual structural heterogeneity of Fc
receptors (9) on different types of cells or from different species,
or they might be just technical artifacts.

In an attempt to clarify this question, we isolated cell membranes from Fc receptor-positive cells of a B-type prolymphocytic
leukemia and two B-type chronic lymphocytic leukemias by means of
the nitrogen cavitation method (14) and differential centrifugation
(7). The membranes were solubilized with various media.

Abbreviations: EA = erythrocytes coated with antibodies. EAC =
erythrocyte-antibody-complement complex. EDTA = ethylenediamine-
tetraacetic acid. IEF = isoelectric focusing. ME = 2-mercapto-
ethanol. NP40 = Nonidet-P 40. PBS = phosphate-buffered saline.
pI = isoelectric point.

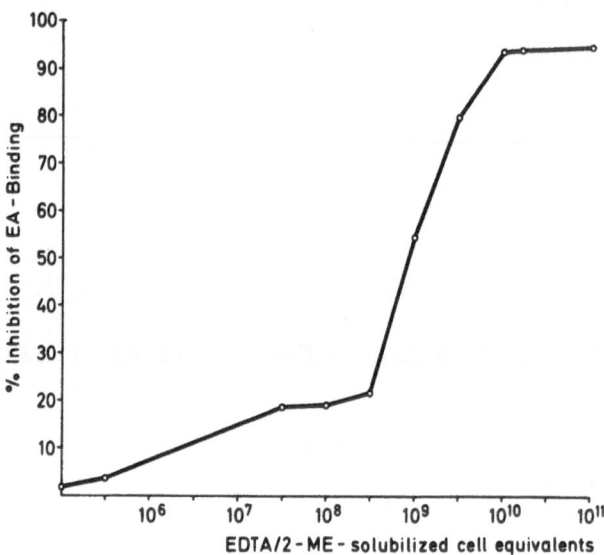

FIG. 1:   Membrane solubilisate inhibition of binding of ox EA to
prolymphocytic leukemia cells. The membranes isolated from 10^5 –
10^{11} leukemic cells ("cell equivalents") were solubilized in 80 mM
EDTA, 50 mM 2-mercaptoethanol, and 20 mM Tris/HCl, pH 7.3, for 20
minutes at 4°C and centrifuged at 105,000 g for 60 minutes. The
supernatant was dialyzed to PBS. Ox EA was pre-incubated in
increasing amounts of dialysate, washed twice, and rosetted with
leukemic cells. The dialysate showed a dose-dependent inhibition
of rosette formation.

RESULTS AND DISCUSSION

    After solubilization of isolated and iodinated (15) membranes
of leukemic cells with a mixture of EDTA and 2-mercaptoethanol
(EDTA/ME), preincubation of ox EA with increasing amounts of lysate
caused increasing inhibition of the binding of the preincubated ox
EA to leukemia cells (Fig.1). Absorption of the membrane solubilisates with an excess of ox EA, but not of uncoated ox erythrocytes,
removed the capacity of the membrane solubilisates to inhibit the
binding of preincubated ox EA to leukemia cells. This finding shows
that the EDTA/ME membrane solubilisates contained molecules that
were capable of binding to complexed IgG and were therefore possible
candidates for Fc receptor molecules.

    To isolate and to determine the molecular weight of the solubi-
lized molecules with the assumed Fc receptor-like activity, radioiodinated EDTA/ME lysates were incubated with IgG aggregates (1) and
coprecipitated with an anti-IgG serum. As shown in Figure 2, SDS
electrophoresis of the coprecipitate revealed a single peak, with an
apparent molecular weight of 28,000 daltons. Reduction and alkylation

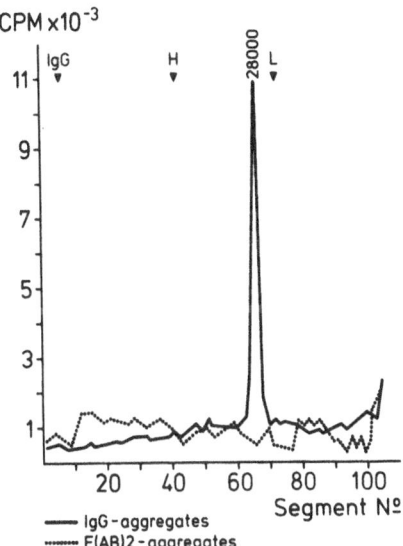

FIG. 2:   SDS electrophoresis of iodinated membrane proteins
solubilized with EDTA/ME and isolated by coprecipitation with IgG
aggregates (—) and F(ab')$_2$ aggregates (...). SDS electrophoresis
was performed by the method of Laemmli (13).

did not affect the relative mobility of this protein, showing that it
consists of a single polypeptide chain. When F(ab')$_2$ aggregates (17)
were used, no peak at all could be precipitated, indicating the Fc
region specificity of the protein solubilized with EDTA/ME.

     Significant amounts of Fc receptor protein were solubilized
only with a mixture of EDTA and ME (Fig.3). With EDTA or ME alone,
no, or only very small amounts of Fc receptor protein were solubilized.
This suggests that divalent cations and disulfide bridges are
involved in the linkage of the Fc receptor protein to the cell membrane.

     In contrast to solubilized C3 receptors, which strongly agglu-
tinate EAC (20), even concentrated EDTA/ME lysates did not aggluti-
nate ox EA heavily coated with IgG. This suggests that the Fc
receptor protein we solubilized has only one binding site.

     Solubilization analyses with NP40 yielded quite different
results. As shown in Figure 4a, electrophoresis of coprecipitates
isolated from NP40 lysates with IgG aggregates usually produced six
main peaks, with apparent molecular weights ranging from 115,000 to
15,000 daltons. It is thought that the 28,000 dalton component
corresponds to the Fc receptor-like protein isolated with EDTA/ME.
It is remarkable, however, that a fundamentally similar electro-

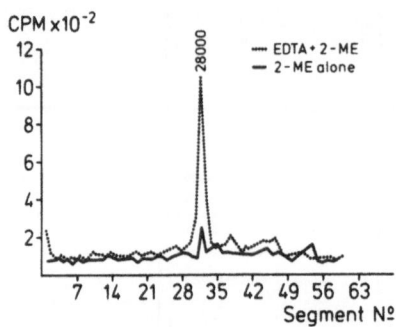

<u>FIG. 3:</u>   SDS electrophoresis of aggregated IgG coprecipitates
obtained from iodinated membranes solubilized with EDTA/ME (...)
and ME alone (—).

phoretic pattern was obtained with $F(ab')_2$ aggregates. We were not
able to isolate molecules from NP40 lysates with strict specificity
to the Fc region of IgG. Our conclusion about this finding is that
NP40 liberates proteins that can be bound to $F(ab')_2$ aggregates
(10,11) and are not solubilized by EDTA/ME.

It remains to be investigated why similar proteins were isolated
from NP40 lysates with IgG and $F(ab')_2$ aggregates. We assume that
the six proteins represented in the SDS pattern are associated in
situ in a complex, which contains one or more proteins with binding
affinity to aggregates of IgG and/or $F(ab')_2$. In detergent extracts
this heterogeneous complex precipitates with IgG and $F(ab')_2$ aggregates as a single entity (4). The complex is reduced to its individual protein components when the precipitates are prepared for SDS
electrophoresis.

After dialysis of EDTA/ME lysates to oxygenated PBS supplemented
with protease inhibitors and coprecipitation of the dialysed material
with IgG aggregates, SDS electrophoresis performed under non-reducing
conditions displayed two new peaks: a large one with an apparent
molecular weight of 115,000 daltons and a smaller one with 18,000
daltons (Fig.4b). The 115,000 dalton protein could be readily
dissociated into 28,000 dalton components in the presence of ME. The
Fc receptor protein isolated with EDTA/ME was thus shown to form
tetramers in the absence of ME. The 115,000 dalton protein precipitated from NP40 lysates might be a tetramer of the 28,000 dalton Fc
receptor protein.

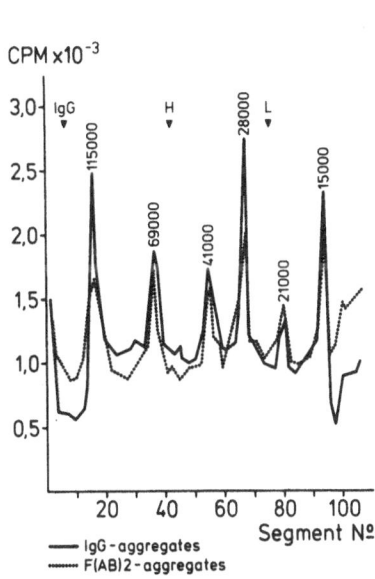
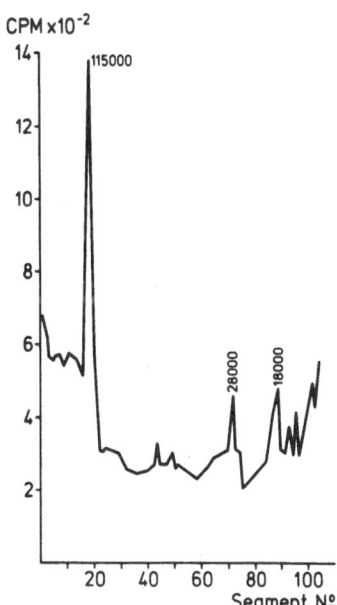

FIG. 4 a and b:

(a) SDS electrophoresis of iodinated membrane proteins solubilized with 0.1% NP40 in 20 mM Tris/HC1, pH 7.3, and isolated with IgG aggregates (—) and F(ab')$_2$ aggregates (...).

(b) SDS electrophoresis of EDTA/ME-solubilized, iodinated membrane proteins coprecipitated with aggregated IgG after exhaustive dialysis to oxygenated PBS supplemented with protease inhibitors.

The IEF pattern of total EDTA/ME membrane solubilisates is shown in Figure 5a. Twelve distinct peaks are discernable. One major peak with a pI of 5.5 was missing after absorption of the lysate with IgG aggregates followed by precipitation with an anti-IgG serum (Fig.5b). The missing peak with a pI of 5.5 could be recovered by IEF of the coprecipitates (Fig.5c).

We conclude from the data presented here that the Fc receptor molecule we isolated from leukemic B cells consists of a single polypeptide chain, with an apparent molecular weight of 28,000 daltons and a pI of 5.5. This structure appears to have only one binding site, and its linkage to the cell membrane might be mediated by divalent cations and disulfide bridges. It tends to aggregate to tetramers in the absence of ME and might be expressed on the cell membrane in the form of tetramers.

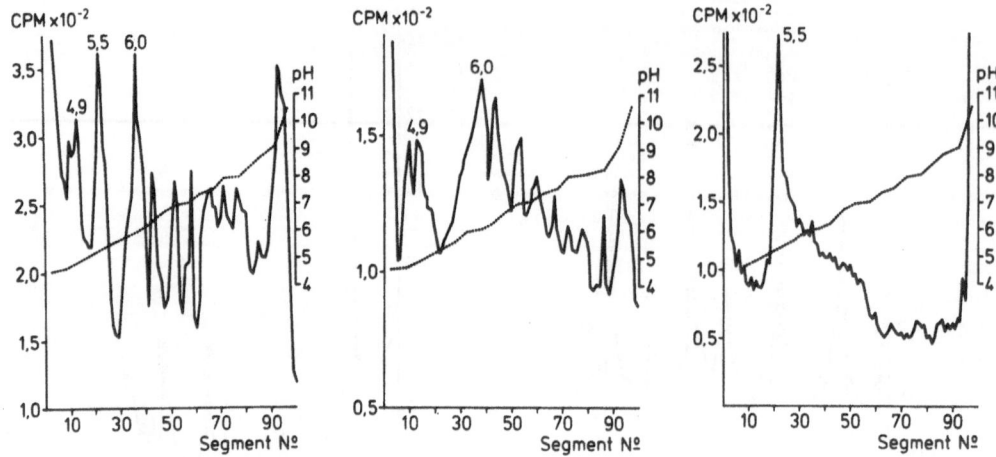

FIG. 5 a-c: IEF pattern of:

(a)   total EDTA/ME solubilisates of iodinated membrane proteins,

(b)   EDTA/ME solubilisates of solubilized and iodinated membrane proteins after absorption with IgG aggregates, and

(c)   coprecipitates obtained from (b).

IEF was performed in 5.5% polyacrylamide gels containing 6 M urea with ampholines in a pH range of 3.5 - 10 by means of a slight modification of the method of Bouman et al. (2).

REFERENCES

1.   Augener, W., Grey, H.M.   J. Immunol. 105 (1970) 1024.
2.   Bouman, H., et al.   FEBS Lett. 64 (1976) 201.
3.   Bourgeois, A., et al.   Eur. J. Immunol. 7 (1977) 691.
4.   Callahan, G.N., Allison, J.P.   Nature 271 (1978) 165.
5.   Cooper, S.M., Sambray, Y.   J. supramol. Struct. 6 (1977) 591.
6.   Dickler, H.B. et al.   J. exp. Med. 146 (1977) 1678.
7.   Ferber, E., et al.   Biochim. biophys. Acta (Amst) 226 (1972) 494.
8.   Frade, R., Kourilsky, F.M.   Eur. J. Immunol. 7 (1977) 663.
9.   Grey, H.M., et al. in: Cold Spring Harbor Symposion on Quant. Biol. (1977).
10.   Hofman, F., et al.   J. Immunol. 119 (1977) 2209.
11.   Huber, H., et al.   Science 162 (1968) 1281.
12.   Johnson, P.M., et al.   Immunology 28 (1975) 797.
13.   Laemmli, V.   Nature 227 (1970) 680.
14.   Manson, L.A. in: Transplantation Antigens, Chapt. 9 (1972).
15.   McConnahey, P.J., Dixon, F.J.   Int. Arch. Allergy 29 (1966) 185.

16. Molenaar, J.L., et al. Eur. J. Immunol. 7 (1977) 230.
17. Nisonoff, A., et al. Arch. Biochem. Biophys. 89 (1960) 230.
18. Perlmann, P. in: Clinical Immunobiology, Vol. 3, Academic
     Press, New York (1975).
19. Räsk, L., et al. Nature 257 (1975) 231.
20. Stein, H. unpublished data.
21. Wernet, P., Kunkel, H.G. in: Histocompatibility Testing,
     Munksgaard, Kopenhagen (1975) p. 731.

ACKNOWLEDGEMENTS

This work was supported by the Deutsche Forschungsgemeinschaft,
SFB 111/D7.

We thank Mrs. Karen Jenßen for skillful technical assistance.

ANTISERA CAUSE ALTERATIONS IN MORPHOLOGY AND ENZYME ACTIVITY IN THE PLASMA MEMBRANE OF RAT THYMOCYTES

U. Hurtenbach, V. Speth, E. Ferber and H.C. Bauer

Max-Planck-Institut für Immunbiologie

Stübeweg 51, D-78 Freiburg, W. Germany

INTRODUCTION

Binding of a ligand to its specific lymphocyte receptor induces interaction of lymphoid cells with each other. Such receptor - ligand interactions have shown to initiate plasma membrane (PM) alterations which might trigger immune reactivity (1). Various authors report about the effect of mitogens on PM (2). We investigated the early steps of rat thymocyte stimulation, using antisera directed against different surface structures. The advantage of antibodies as stimulation agents instead of the widely used plant lectins are, that antibodies are more physiological, and the role of certain cell interaction determinants can be investigated by specific antibodies.

In parallel to the effect of antisera on the activities of the PM enzymes alkaline phosphatase (AP) lysolecithin acyltransferase (AcTF) and γ-glutamyl transferase (γ-GT), scanning microscopy pictures of the antisera treated cells were taken to monitor eventual changes in cell shape.

MATERIALS AND METHODS

The procedure of alloantisera induction has been described elsewhere (3). For induction of α-MHC antiserum, MHC-congenic L.BN rats were immunized with Lewis lymphocytes and L.WP rats were injected with L.BD $\underline{V}$ lymphocytes. For non-MHC alloantisera, BN recipients were injected with L.BN lymphocytes, which are identical in their MHC but differ in the minor histocompatibility complex.

TAB. 1:   Effect of xenosera on activity changes of PM enzymes in
Lewis rat thymocytes.

	Alkaline phosphatase	γ-Glutamyl-transferase	Lysolecithin-acyltransferase
Control (normal rabbit serum)	spec. act. in n mole $\times$ mg^{-1} $\times$ min^{-1}		
	7.76	4.17	3.49
	100%	100%	100%
α-TC	142%	94%	198%
α-TC DA thymocytes absorbed	165%	113%	213%
α-TC Lewis RBC absorbed	184%	102%	253%
α-TC-PM	111%	75%	182%

Means from 3-9 single experiments are given.

Xenoantibodies were induced according to the same immunisation
schedule as described in ref.3.   Rabbits received 5×10^9 Lewis thymus
cells, or thymus membrane vesicles, which had been prepared out of
8-10 thymi by the N_2 cavitation method (4), emulsified in FCA.   The
antibody titers were estimated by dextran hemagglutination test.
The titers of all antisera ranged between 1:2048 and 1:4096.

Thymi from 8-12 week old Lewis rats were cut into pieces, and
cell suspension was prepared in cold phosphate buffered saline (PBS)
using a loose fitting glass homogenizer and adjusted to 1×10^8 cells/
ml.   Incubation with the antisera and mitogen was done in HEPES
buffered Dulbecco's modified Eagles medium pH 7.3 (1 hour, 37°C).

The ionophore A 23187, a gift of Dr. Robert Hamill, Eli Lilly
Company, Indianapolis, IN, U.S.A., was dissolved in DMSO.   The final
concentration of DMSO in the incubation mixture did not exceed more
than 1%.

A crude plasma membrane fraction was prepared by an osmolytic
method which is described in detail in ref. (5).   Protein concentrations and enzyme activities were determined according to Ferber
et al. (6).   Electron optical studies were performed by scanning
technique which has been described in detail elsewhere (7).

TAB. 2:   Effect of alloantisera and mitogens on activity changes
of PM enzymes in Lewis rat thymocytes.

	Alkaline phosphatase	-Glutamyl-transferase	Lysolecithin-acyltransferase
Control	spec. act. in n mole x mg^{-1} x min^{-1}		
	7.76	4.17	3.49
	100%	100%	100%
normal rat serum	114%	112%	152%
α-H-1[1]	156%	161%	218%
α-non H-1	120%	109%	200%
α-H-1[d]	113%	138%	N.D.
ConA (10 µg/ml)	167%	117%	120%
A 23187 (1 µM)	154%	40%	156%
A 23187 + α-H-1[1]	190%	100%	276%

Means from 3-9 single experiments are given.

RESULTS AND DISCUSSION

    In the first set of experiments, Lewis rat thymocytes were
incubated with xenoantisera, raised in rabbits against Lewis
thymocytes. Tab.1 shows an increase of AP and AcTF activities by
the antisera, whereas γ-GT remains unaffected. Preabsorption of the
antiserum on thymocytes of the DA rat strain, in order to eliminate
antibodies against public specificities of the rat species, increases
also the γ-GT activity and even potentiates the AP and the AcTF
activities of Lewis thymocytes. This effect is even stronger on the
AP and the AcTF, when the antiserum had been preabsorbed on Lewis
red blood cells (RBC). This procedure eliminates antibodies against
SD antigens. Preabsorption of α-Lewis thymocyte antiserum on Lewis
thymocytes completely abrogates enzyme activities.

    Previous experiments have shown that preparation of PM vesicles
enriched the activities of membrane enzymes 10-20 fold (8). Therefore
we tested if antibodies against plasma membrane vesicles further

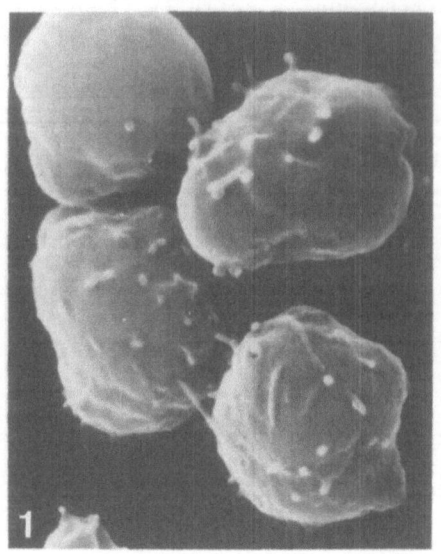

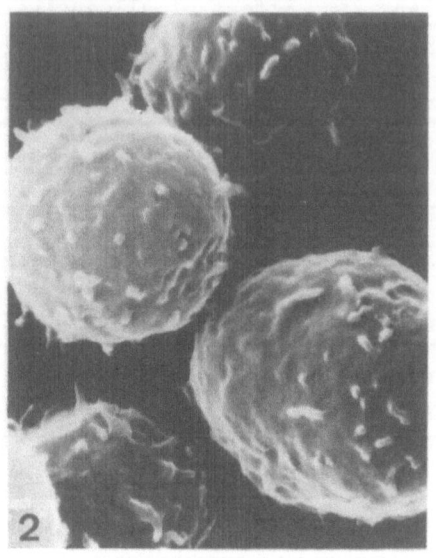

FIG. 1:   Normal rabbit serum.   FIG. 2:   ∝-MHC antiserum.

enhance PM enzyme activities. Surprisingly, addition of ∝-plasma
membrane antiserum (∝-TC-PM) diminishes enzyme activities, compared
to the effect of antiserum against whole thymocytes, and strongly
suppresses the γ-GT activity.

In a further set of experiments we investigated the effect of
antisera directed against determinants of the major histocompatibility complex (MHC) of the Lewis strain.

The increase of the AP, AcTF and γ-GT activities, demonstrated
in Tab.2, seems to be specific and might be due to antibodies
directed against MHC antigens: only congenic L.BN-∝-Lewis lymphocyte alloantiserum, which recognizes the relevant H-1^l antigen of
Lewis thymocytes, is effective. L.BN-∝-L.BD $\overline{V}$ alloantiserum,
directed against H-1^d antigen affects enzyme activities of Lewis
thymocytes significantly less, thus indicating a specific effect of
antibodies on PM enzyme activation. Moreover, BN-∝-L.BN alloantiserum, which is directed only against the minor histocompatibility
antigens of the Lewis strain, acts marginally on the AP and the
γ-GT, however, activates the AcTF. Activation of the PM enzymes
also takes place after incubation with the ionophore and ConA. An
additional effect was reached when cells were incubated with the
ionophore plus the ∝-MHC antiserum.

An explanation of these phenomena may be given by electronoptical

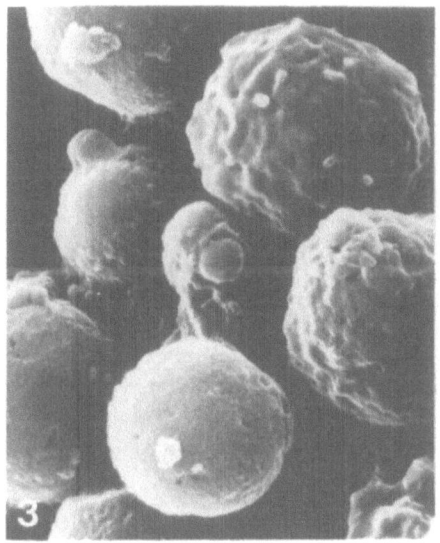   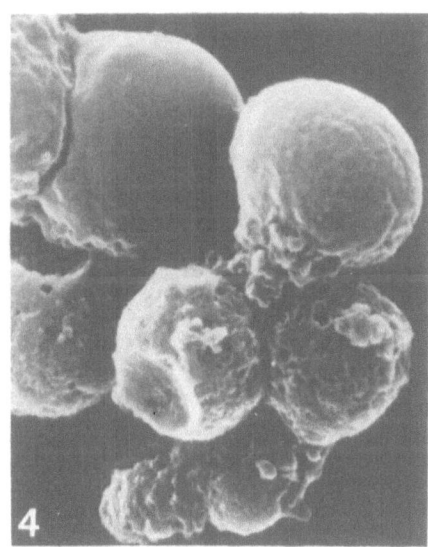

FIG. 3:   ∝-TC antiserum.   FIG. 4:   ∝-TC-PM antiserum.

pictures. Thymocytes, which had been incubated with ∝-TC-PM antiserum have quite an abnormal outlook (Fig.4). They are rounded,
show many microextrusions and have a more or less damaged plasma
membrane. Cells treated with the ∝-TC antiserum (Fig.3) do not
have such abnormal cell shapes, but are quite different in outlook
compared to the controls treated with normal serum (Fig.1). In
contrast, thymocytes treated with the absorbed xenosera (unpublished
observation) as well as those incubated with ∝-H-1[1] antiserum
(Fig.2), look rather normal, except that they are more rounded and
possess some more microextrusions than the controls. The outlook
of these cells indicates more membrane perturbation than membrane
damage.

     The most interesting result of these studies is that only
specific ∝-MHC antibodies cause strong activation of all PM enzymes.
This is consistent with the fact that only specific ∝-MHC antiserum
may induce a blast transformation, but not antibodies against minor
histocompatibility antigens (9). However, binding of large amounts
of antisera leads to membrane perturbation and finally to membrane
damage.

REFERENCES

1.   Lauf, P.K., Biochim. Biopyhs. Acta. 415 (1975) 173.

2. Ling, N.R., Kay, J.A., Lymphocyte stimulation. North Holland
    Publ. Springer Verlag, New York (1975).
3. Wekerle, H., Eshhar, Z., Lonai, P., Feldman, M., Proc. Nat.
    Acad. Sci., USA 72 (1975) 1147.
4. Ferber, E., Resch, K., Wallach, D.F.H., Imm, W., Biochim.
    Biophys. Acta. 266 (1972) 494.
5. Bauer, H.C., Ferber, E., Golecki, J., Brunner, G., Hoppe
    Seyler's Z. Biol. Chemi. 358 (1977) 1177.
6. Ferber, E., Reilly, C.E., Resch, K., Biochim. Biophys. Acta.
    448 (1976) 143.
7. Polliack, A., Normal, transformed and leukemic leukocytes.
    Springer Verl. Berlin, New York (1977).
8. Monneron, A., a'Alayer, J., J. Ce. Bio. 77 (1978) 232.
9. Hurtenbach, U., Ernst, M., Wekerle, H., in prep. (1978).

MODULATION OF CELL MEMBRANE ANTIGENS DURING DIFFERENTIATION OF RAT T-LYMPHOCYTES

R. Arndt, Rosemarie Stark and H.-G. Thiele

Abteilung für Immunologie, I. Med. Universitätsklinik

Hamburg-Eppendorf, W. Germany

INTRODUCTION

The aim of the experiments presented here was to trace the differentiation pathway of thymic lymphocytes to peripheral T-lymphocytes in serological and molecular terms. For this purpose the rat has the advantage over the mouse that in this species that antigenic structure being the predominating one on the surface membrane of thymus lymphocytes i.e. the thymus brain antigen, is practically not expressed on peripheral T-lymphocytes (1,2).

MATERIALS AND METHODS

All tissues and cells were from inbred DA-rats/Han or CBA/J Han. Treatment of lymphocytes and solubilized membrane fractions with soluble or sepharose-bound neuraminidase was performed as described by Stark et al. (3). Antisera against thymus lymphocytes (AThy-Ly), surface Ig negative lymph node lymphocytes (ALN-Ly^{Ig-}), and rat-brain (ABS) were raised in rabbits (3); anti-AKR Thy-1.1 antibodies were produced in CBA mice (4). AThy-Ly and ALN-Ly^{Ig-} were absorbed with packed DA-rat erythrocytes and with glutaraldehyde fixed liver membrane fractions (100,000 x g sediment) before use. Solubilization of Thy-Ly, neuraminidase treated Thy-Ly (Thy-Ly^{Neur}) and LN-Ly membranes and chromatography on LKB AcA 54 was performed in sodium deoxycholate (3,5). The schedule of quantitating analytical absorption analyses of the different antisera with various cell types or solubilized membrane fractions and testing the remaining cytotoxicity on different targets are described previously in detail (1).

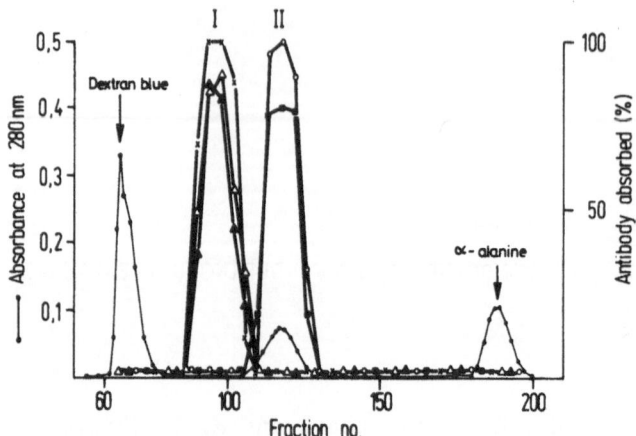

FIG. 1:   Absorption of various antisera with solubilized and chromatographed Thy-Ly membrane fractions (sodium deoxycholate, AcA 54), x———x AThy-Ly, target Thy-Ly;   △———△ ABS, target mouse Thy-Ly; ▲———▲ AThy-1.1, target Thy-Ly;   o———o ALN-Ly^{Ig-}, target LN-Ly^{Ig-}; ■———■ AThy-Ly, target LN-Ly^{Ig-}.

RESULTS AND DISCUSSION

By serial dilutions of AThy-Ly it became obvious that the lysis titre for Thy-Ly exceeded that one for LN-Ly^{Ig-}. A reversed cytolysis pattern was observed when ALN-Ly^{Ig-} was used instead. As may be seen from Table 1 LN-Ly had a 16 fold higher absorbing capacity for ALN-Ly^{Ig-} than Thy-Ly (target LN-Ly^{Ig-}). These findings indicate that ALN-Ly^{Ig-} detects antigenic structures, which are strongly expressed by T-lymphocytes but less by thymus-lymphocytes. By analytical absorptions of AThy-Ly and ALN-Ly^{Ig-} (target LN-Ly^{Ig-}) with solubilized and chromatographed Thy-Ly membrane fractions an antigen having an apparent molecular weight of 21,000 could be identified (Fig.1, Peak II). This antigen differs in molecular and serological terms from the well defined thymus brain antigen (Fig.1, Peak I) and the histocompatibility antigen AgB. That this structure represents indeed a major antigen of T-lymphocytes was confirmed by analytical absorptions of ALN-Ly^{Ig-} and AThy-Ly with solubilized and chromatographed membrane fractions of LN-Ly. Again a major antigen with an apparent molecular weight of 21,000 could be detected under the chosen conditions (Fig.2). To elucidate whether the higher absorbing capacity of LN-Ly compared to that of Thy-Ly (Tab.1) was due to increased de novo synthesis or to an improved accessibility of the antigen under study, Thy-Ly and LN-Ly were subjected to neuraminidase treatment. Remarkably, the absorbing capacity of Thy-Ly was raised 6-7 fold, while LN-Ly showed only slight

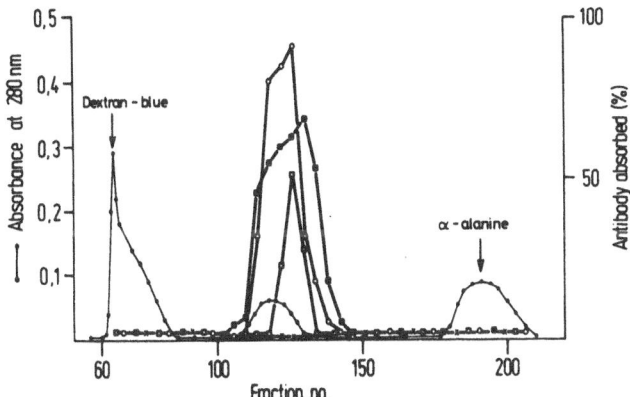

<u>FIG. 2</u>:   Absorption of various antisera with solubilized and chroma-
tographed LN-Ly membrane fractions (sodium deoxycholate, LKB AcA 54),
x———x AThy-Ly, target Thy-Ly;   o———o ALN-Ly^{Ig-} target LN-Ly^{Ig-};
■———■ AThy-Ly, target LN-Ly^{Ig-};   □———□   ALN-Ly^{Ig-}, target
Thy-Ly.

increase of the absorbing capacity (Table 1). After solubilization
and chromatography of neuraminidase treated Thy-Ly membranes the
21.000 daltons antigen exhibited a seven fold higher absorbing
capacity than that derived from untreated Thy-Ly (Table 2). Since
solubilization alone did not enhance the antigenicity the minor
absorbing capacity of the antigen is not a consequence of its
arrangement within the plasma membrane. The additional finding
that the absorbing capacity was enhanced after treatment of the
solubilized 21.000 daltons antigen from Thy-Ly with sepharose bound
neuraminidase is in good accordance with the suggestion that neuraminidase improves the accessibility of the antigenic determinants
by direct cleavage of masking sialic acid residues from the molecule
itself.

The concept that enzymatic cleavage of cell surface glycoproteins
by neuraminidase may play an important role in antigenic remodelling
of the plasma membrane in course of the differentiation pathway of T-
axis lymphocytes in the rat is further supported by the finding that:

1.   this enzyme caused only a slight increase of the absorbing capacity of LN-Ly for ALN-Ly^{Ig-},

2.   a comparable increase of the absorbing capacity was observed
when Thy-Ly were incubated for 20 h (37°C) at pH 6.0 without addition
of neuraminidase.

TAB. 1:   Absorption capacity of Thy-Ly and LN-Ly before and after
neuraminidase treatment for ALN-Ly^{Ig-} (target LN-Ly^{Ig-}).

Cells used for absorption	Cells x 10^7 used to absorb 50% antibodies out of 1 ml ALN-Ly^{Ig-} (20%)	relative absorption capacity
Thy-Ly	40	0.06
Thy-Ly Neur	6.0	0.4
LN-Ly	2.4	1
LN-Ly Neur	1.2	2

$$\text{relative absorption capacity} = \frac{\text{LN-Ly x } 10^7 \text{ used for absorption}}{\text{cells x } 10^7 \text{ used for absorption}}$$

TAB. 2:   Absorption capacity of the 21,000 daltons antigen (combined
fractions after AcA 54 chromatography) from Thy-Ly before and after
neuraminidase treatment and LN-Ly for ALN-Ly^{Ig-} (target LN-Ly^{Ig-}).

cellular source	Quantities of solubilized material obtained from cells x 10^6 necessary to absorb 50% antibodies out of 400 µl ALN-Ly^{Ig-} (2.5%)	relative absorption capacity
Thy-Ly	35	0.1
Thy-Ly Neur	5.0	0.7
LN-Ly	3.5	1

$$\text{relative absorption capacity} = \frac{\text{LN-Ly x } 10^6 \text{ used for absorption}}{\text{cells x } 10^6 \text{ used for absorption}}$$

The fact that this remodelling effect could not be inhibited by
DFP and, moreover, was strongly dependent on acid pH suggests that
the antigenic remodelling by neuraminidase may be indeed an in vivo
function of this enzyme.

REFERENCES

1.   Arndt, R., Thiele, H.-G., Stark, R., Wottge, H.U., Müller-
      Ruchholz, W., Eur. J. Immunol. 7 (1977) 131.

2.   Acton, R.T., Morris, R.J., Williams, A.F.   Eur. J. Immunol. 4
      (1974) 598.
3.   Stark, R., Arndt, R., Hamann, A., Thiele, H.-G.   (1978) submitted.
4.   Reif, A.E., Allen, J.M.   J. Exp. Med. 120 (1964) 413.
5.   Arndt, R., Stark, R., Klein, P., Müller. A., Thiele, H.-G.   Eur.
      J. Immunol. 6 (1976) 333.

INTERACTIONS BETWEEN NEURAMINIDASE-TREATED LYMPHOCYTES AND LIVER CELLS

Hubert Kolb[1], Amelie Kriese[2] and Hans-Albert Kolb[2]

[1]Diabetes Research Institute, University of Düsseldorf,
D-4000 Düsseldorf, W. Germany

[2]Department of Biology, University of Konstanz,
D-7750 Konstanz, W. Germany

SUMMARY

Neuraminidase-treated rat lymphocytes and rat hepatocytes spontaneously aggregate when mixed in vitro. Adhesion between cells is due to stereo-specific interactions between a mammalian hepatic membrane lectin and galactosyl residues which are exposed on the lymphocyte surface after removal of sialic acid residues. The hepatic galactose specific lectin may play a role in the accumulation of recirculating desialylated lymphocytes in the liver.

INTRODUCTION

Neuraminidase-treated lymphocytes have an altered recirculation pattern, they do not home to lymphoid organs but are accumulated in the liver (1,2). We have found that asialo-lymphocytes and hepatocytes spontaneously aggregate in vitro. Adhesion between cells is mediated by stereo-specific cell contacts.

MATERIALS AND METHODS

Animals. Outbred rats were purchased from a local source.

Cells. Hepatocytes were isolated as described previously (3). The primary cell suspension was freed of most Kupffer cells by centrifugation three times at 20 g for 3 min. Electron microscopic analyses showed that more than 95% of cells isolated from the rat

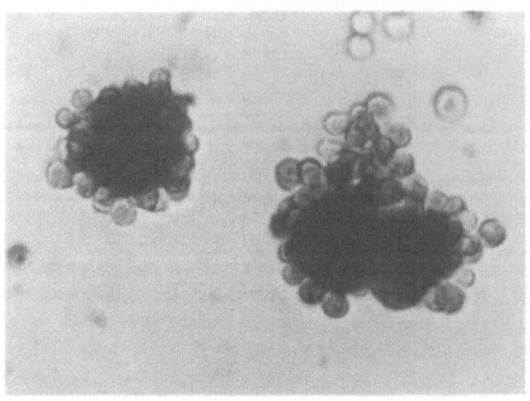

FIG. 1:   Hepatocytes are surrounded by a layer of lymphocytes.
Cells are stained with 0.5% crystal violet.

liver were hepatocytes and less than 3% were Kupffer cells. Cell
viability was between 85 and 90%. Lymphocytes were isolated from
spleen and thymus. Erythrocytes in the spleen cell preparation were
lysed by one wash in 0.83% NH_4Cl. Neuraminidase (Neuraminidase
vibrio cholerae, Behringwerke, Marburg, W. Germany) was added to
lymphocytes (2 x 10^8 cells/ml) at a concentration of 20 units per
ml. After incubation at 37°C for 30 min cells were washed three
times.

Cell interaction assay. Hepatocytes (5 x 10^4 cells in 50 µl)
and lymphocytes (5 x 10^6 cells in 50 µl) were incubated at 0°C for
2 hours. The sedimented cell mixture was shaken up and the percentage of lymphocyte binding liver cells was determined in a hemocyto-
meter by light microscopy. Lymphocyte adherence was considered
positive when 5 or more lymphocytes bound to a single hepatocyte.
The inhibitory acticity of mono- and disaccharides (Serva, Heidelberg,
W. Germany) was determined by preincubation of hepatocytes for 10
min at 0°C with the sugar. Preincubation of liver cells with inhibitors of ATP production (NaCN, NaN_3), with cytochalasin B and
colchicine (Serva) was performed for 30 min at 37°C.

RESULTS

When freshly prepared hepatocytes and neuraminidase-treated
lymphocytes were mixed, the formation of cell clusters could be
observed. Since the two cell types were mixed in a ratio of 1:100
aggregates had the appearance of rosettes, i.e. a single hepatocyte
was surrounded by a layer of lymphocytes (Fig.1). The majority of

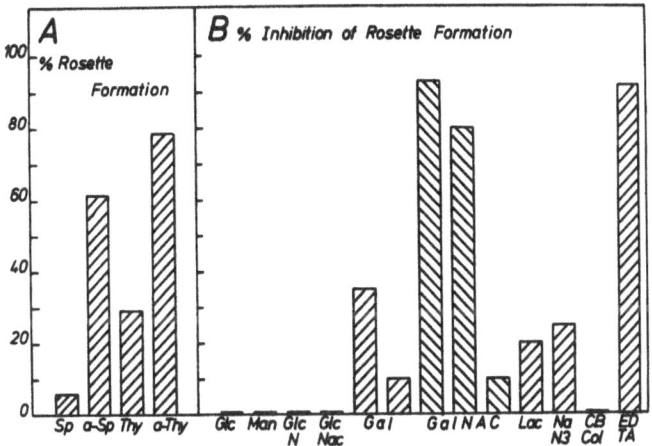

FIG. 2A: Sp, Thy :   Spleen, Thymus cells;   a-Sp, a-Thy : asialo-
Sp, -Thy.

FIG. 2B: Glc :   D-glucose 0.05 M;   Man :   D-mannose 0.5 M;   GlcN :
D-glucosamine 0.05 M;   GlcNAc : N-acetyl-D-glucosamine 0.05 M;   Gal :
D-galactose 0.05 M + 0.01 M;   GalNAc : N-acetyl-D-galactosamine
0.05 M + 0.01 M + 0.002 M;   Lac : lactose 0.05 M;   NaN$_3$ 0.01 M;   CB :
cytochalasin B 20 µg/ml;   Col :   colchisine 100 µg/ml;   EDTA 0.002 M.

rosettes consisted of 15-20 lymphocytes bound per hepatocyte. Similar
numbers of rosettes were found after incubation of test tubes at 0°C,
4°C, 22°C or 37°C. Splenic and thymic lymphocytes bound to hepatocytes to a similar degree after neuraminidase-treatment (Fig.2A).

We tested whether galactosyl groups which are exposed after
removal of sialic acid residues on the cell surface were involved in
binding. In Fig.2B it is shown that galactose related carbohydrates
were able to block specifically binding between hepatocytes and
asialo-lymhpocytes. N-Acetyl-galactosamine was the most potent
inhibitor with a 50% inhibition point at about 5 x 10^{-3} M. Cell
contacts between hepatocytes appeared to be of high affinity since
rosettes were formed within a few minutes.

Studies with inhibitors of ATP-production (NaN$_3$, NaCN) and
inhibitors of cell movement (cytochalasin B, colchicine) showed
that rosette formation was not an energy dependent process. No
rosettes however were formed when divalent cations were complexed
by the addition of EDTA (Fig.2B).

DISCUSSION

We have shown that adhesion between asialo-lymphocytes and hepatocytes is due to a hepatic carbohydrate binding protein. We have recently analysed cell contacts between hepatocytes and neuraminidase-treated erythrocytes and have found very similar binding characteristics (4). It has been shown previously by Ashwell and coworker (5) that hepatocytes in vivo are able to bind asialo-glycoproteins by a galactose specific protein, we believe that the same receptor is responsible for cell to cell contacts observed here. Hepatolectin - lymphocyte interactions may occur naturally after infection with microbes containing neuraminidase (6).

REFERENCES

1. Woodruff, J.J., Gesner, B.M., J. Exp. Med. 129 (1969) 551.
2. Freitas, A.A., de Sousa, M., Cell. Immunol. 22 (1976) 345.
3. Kolb, H.A., Adam, G., J. Membrane Biol. 26 (1976) 121.
4. Kolb, H., Schudt, C., Kolb-Bachofen, V., Kolb, H.A., Exp. Cell. Res. in press (1978)
5. Ashwell, G., Morell, A.G., Adv. Enzymol. 41 (1974) 99.
6. Woodruff, J.J., Woodruff, J.F., Cell. Immunol. 10 (1974) 78.

ACKNOWLEDGEMENTS

We thank Dr. C. Schudt for his help with the preparation of hepatocytes. This work was supported by the Deutsche Forschungsgemeinschaft, SFB 138.

IMMUNOLOGICAL CHARACTERISTICS OF NEO-ANTIGENS ON THE CELL SURFACE AFTER NEURAMINIDASE TREATMENT

R. Johannsen, H.H. Sedlacek and F.R. Seiler

Research Laboratories of Behringwerke A.G.

3550 Marburg/Lahn, West Germany

Blood cells from which sialic acid has been split off by Vibrio cholerae neuraminidase (VCN) differ markedly in their physiological behavior as well as in antigenicity when compared with untreated cells (1). In this respect the "cryptic" antigenic structures on the cell membrane which become uncovered by VCN-treatment have found particular interest especially with regard to tumorimmunotherapy (1,2,3). It has been shown that the antigenic structures which are revealed on lymphocyte membranes after VCN-treatment exhibit serological similarities to the T antigen (4) originally described by Thomsen (5) and Friedenreich (6). Naturally occurring cytotoxic antibodies against VCN-treated autologous cells have widely been used to elucidate the antigenic specificity of the neo-antigen (3, 4,7,8,9,10). The observations that after incubation with VCN cells retain detectable amounts of the enzyme on their surface (11,12,13) and that the naturally occurring antibodies show serological specificity for VCN (8,10) led to the assumption that the bacterial neuraminidase might be involved in the cytotoxic reaction as a membrane-bound exogenous neo-antigen.

In the present paper the serological results are discussed in connection with experiments to stimulate human lymphocytes in vitro with enzymatically active and inactive VCN. The results provide further evidence that the altered reactivity of VCN-treated lymphocytes in serological and cell-mediated systems can at least partly be attributed to surface-attached VCN.

TAB. 1:   Absorption of cytotoxic antibodies against VCN-treated
lymphocytes.

2×10^8 cells or 0.3 ml sedimented tissue homogenate were suspended
in 1 ml of antiserum at the highest dilution producing 70-100% lysis
of VCN-treated target lymphocytes and incubated for 1 h at room
temperature.

	% absorption		
buffy coat cells	0	-	10
melanoma cells	0	-	10
CLL cells	0		
fetal tissue homogenates	0		
VCN-treated erythrocytes	90	-	100
VCN-treated lymphocytes	90	-	100
VCN-treated fetal tissues	80	-	100
latex-bound VCN	95	-	100

Frequency and specificity of naturally occurring antibodies against VCN-treated lymphocytes

Using a two-step cytotoxicity test, complement-dependent cytotoxic antibodies against VCN-treated lymphocytes could be demonstrated in about 48% of young healthy adults, 43% of aged persons,
39% of patients with multiple sclerosis, 30% of tumor patients and
in none of the newborns tested (8). All sera were negative with
untreated lymphocytes and showed comparable titers with VCN-treated
lymphocytes of allogeneic and xenogeneic donors (8). Absorption
studies using antisera at the highest dilution producing 70-100%
lysis of VCN-treated target lymphocytes were performed with a
variety of untreated and VCN-treated cells and latex-bound VCN
(Tab.1). Only VCN-treated cells as well as latex-bound VCN were
able to absorb the antibodies. Control experiments with cytotoxic
HLA isoantibodies have shown that both enzymatically active and
inactive VCN-latex preparations selectively adsorbed the naturally
occurring antibodies but not isoantibodies (12).

Blastogenic response of human lymphocytes to VCN

To investigate the stimulatory capacity of VCN on human lymphocytes, cells were either cultured for 6 days together with VCN-
pretreated autologous lymphocytes or in the presence of 6.5 to 0.065
mU of added VCN (14). The results are summarized in Tab.2. In
agreement with the results of other groups (15,16,17) we found that

TAB. 2:   Spontaneous blastogenic response of human lymphocytes to
VCN after six days of culture.   (SI = stimulation index)

| Experiment | VCN (mU) | number of responding donors according to SI | | |
		< 2	2-5	> 5
A + VCN	65	7	5	0
	6.5	29	14	5
	0.65	27	18	3
A_{VCN} + A	$65/10^6$ cells			
	15 min 20°C	21	2	4

only some of the human donors responded sppntaneously to enzyme
while others did not: Of 48 donors 19 (40%) and 21 (44%) showed
a blastogenic response when their lymphocytes were cultured in the
presence of 6.5 and 0.65 mU VCN respectively.   Under these conditions
no positive reactions could be observed with the rest of the donors.
In comparison, experiments with VCN-treated lymphocytes to stimulate
untreated autologous lymphocytes (A_{VCN} + A) revealed that only 6 of
27 donors (22%) showed a positive response.

We have published previously (14) that the VCN-induced lymphocyte stimulation shows a striking similarity in the kinetics with
antigen-induced responses, i.e. the maximum of thymidine-incorporation
occurs after 6 to 8 days of culture and is dependent on the dose of
antigen applied and the state cell-mediated immunity of the cell donor
as well.   In addition, as is shown in Tab.3, the stimulating capacity
of VCN is independent from the enzymatic activity: Untreated
enzymatically active as well as heat-inactivated (100°C) VCN are
both stimulatory.   Moreover, partly inactivated VCN which has been
heated to 50° or 70°, appears as a stronger stimulant than the
untreated fully active enzyme.   This finding can possibly be explained
by a decrease of cell toxicity or an increase in immunogenicity due
to aggregation of enzyme molecules.

DISCUSSION

In the serum of 30-48% of adult human donors naturally occurring
complement dependent cytotoxic antibodies against VCN-treated lymphocytes can be demonstrated.   The antibodies react with VCN-treated
cells, to which VCN remains attached after enzyme treatment, as well as

TAB. 3:   Lymphocyte stimulation induced in vitro by untreated
enzymatically active VCN, or VCN heated to 50°, 70° and 100°C
respectively: 0.1 ml of VCN preparation was added to 1 ml cultures
containing 3 x 10^5 human lymphocytes in RPMI 1640 + 20% human serum.
0.075 μCi ^{14}C-thymidine is added on day 5, cells are harvested on
day 6 to estimate thymidine incorporation. Results are expressed
as stimulation indices.

		VCN			
donor	untreated	10 min 50°	10 min 70°	60 min 70°	10 min 100°
HR	40.2	12.6	37.2	19.5	14.1
LK	5.4	10.1	–	7.0	2.6
KG	2.1	13.8	8.4	5.7	6.9
AK	1.5	2.8	3.5	3.1	2.2
HE	1.6	1.8	2.0	–	1.9
HS	1.2	1.4	0.7	–	0.9

with VCN-coated latex beads or soluble VCN. Moreover, lymphocytes
of up to 44% of human adults undergo blast formation in the presence
of enzymatically active and inactive VCN, while the residual 56% do
not respond. These findings strongly support the assumption that
VCN is involved in the cytotoxic and lymphocyte-defined reactions
as a relevant antigen. It is not known whether VCN as an exogenous
neo-antigen is identical or crossreacting with the described cryptic
membrane antigen (T antigen) which becomes uncovered by VCN-treatment.
It remains to be proven whether the VCN molecule contains structures
which cross-react with unmasked autologous determinants. In this
respect oligosaccharides containing ß-D-galactosyl nonreducing end
residues are of particular interest because on the basis of carbohydrate inhibition studies these compounds have been found as an
integral part of the unmasked neo-antigen (9). Studies are presently
performed in our institute to find out whether these types of carbohydrates are constituents of VCN.

REFERENCES

1.   Sedlacek, H.H., Seiler, F.R., Schwick, H.G., Klin. Wschr. 55
      (1977) 199.
2.   Bekesi, J.G., Holland, J.F., Roboz, J.P., Medical Clinics of
      North America 61 (1977) 1083.
3.   Rogentine, G.N., J. Nat. Cancer Inst. 54 (6) (1975) 1307.
4.   Reisner, E.G., Transplantation 19 (1975) 357.
5.   Thomsen, O., Z. Immunitätsforschung 52 (1927) 85.

6.   Friedenreich, V., Levin and Munksgaard, Copenhagen, pp. 1-138
     (1930).
7.   Rosenberg, S.A., Rogentine, G.N., Nature New Biology 239 (1972)
     203.
8.   Johannsen, R., Sedlacek, H.H., Behring Inst. Mitt. 55 (1974)
     209.
9.   Rogentine, G.N., Plocinik, B.A., J. Immunol. 113 (1974) 848.
10. Johannsen, R., Sedlacek, H.H., Schmidtberger, R., Schick, H.J.,
     Seiler, F.R., J. Nat. Cancer Inst. in press.
11. Sedlacek, H.H., Seiler, F.R., Behring Inst. Mitt. 55 (1974) 254.
12. Lüben, G., Sedlacek, H.H., Seiler, F.R., Behring Inst. Mitt. 59
     (1976) 30.
13. Petitou, M., Rosenfeld, C., Sinay, P., Cancer Immunol. Immuno-
     ther.2 (1977) 135.
14. Johannsen, R., Sedlacek, H.H., Seiler, F.R., Proc. Symp. "Immuno-
     therapy of Malignant Diseases", Vienna, Nov. 9-10 (1977) in press.
15. Lundgren, G., Simmons, R.L., Clin. Exp. Immunol. 9 (1971) 915.
16. Han, T., Transplantation 14 (4) (1972) 514.
17. Flye, M.W., Reisner, E.G., Amos, D.B., J. Surgical Res. 15 (1973)
     96.

ACKNOWLEDGEMENTS

The work presented here has been performed in the Research
Laboratories of Behringwerke AG with the interest and support of
Prof. H.G. Schwick. The authors thankfully acknowledge the
skillful technical assistance of Karin Kanzy, Gudrun Muth-Naumann
and Christine Teuter.

CARBOHYDRATE INCORPORATION INTO GLYCOCONJUGATES OF MOUSE THYMOCYTES

DURING CON A STIMULATION - INVOLVEMENT OF TWO SUBPOPULATIONS

R.V.W. van Eijk and P.F. Mühlradt

Gesellschaft für Biotechnologische Forschung mbH

Mascheroder Weg 1, D-3300 Braunschweig, W. Germany

INTRODUCTION

Upon activation by antigens or mitogens lymphocytes undergo a series of metabolic and morphological changes (1). In previous studies we showed that biosynthesis of glycoconjugates and DNA follows a biphasic time pattern in Con A stimulated mouse thymocytes (2,3). Incorporation rates went through a first maximum, at 5-15 h, a minimum around 20 h, and a late, second maximum at 30-40 h of cultivation. Two hypotheses which may explain this phenomenon were tested:

1. The incorporation maxima represent two consecutive (cell cycle) related events, involving one Con A responsive cell population.

2. Two subpopulations of thymocytes are involved responding at different times to the Con A stimulus.

The murine thymus contains at least two different cell populations, a major one comprising 85-95% of total cells, which is sensitive to hydrocortisone, bearing high Thy.1 alloantigen, low H2 histocompatibility antigen and TL antigen, and a minor subpopulation, which is resistant to hydrocortisone, bearing low Thy.1 and high H2 antigen (4).

We report in this communication that both subpopulations respond to a Con A stimulus by synthesis of glycoconjugates and DNA after different times of mitogen stimulation.

TAB. 1:   Rate of labelling of DNA, glycolipids and glycoproteins
in Con A stimulated mouse thymocytes. Effects of hydroxyurea (H.U.).

| Time of pulse | Addition | Incorporation per culture (4 x 10^{6}cells) | | |
		^{3}H-thymidine	^{14}C-galactose into glycolipid	^{3}H-fucose into glycoprotein
(h)		(cpm)	(cpm)	(cpm)
5-15	None	17330	188	338
	5 mM H.U.	291	184	280
	Con A	37695	617	1004
	Con A, 5 mM H.U.	239	537	720
15-25	None	843	161	245
	5 mM H.U.	217	143	220
	Con A	6005	479	560
	Con A, 5 mM H.U.	240	408	425
30-40	None	280	117	290
	5 mM H.U.	75	84	275
	Con A	22784	1518	1310
	Con A, 5 mM H.U.	148	1275	1150

MATERIALS AND METHODS

To obtain hydrocortisone resistant thymocytes, CBA/J mice were
injected i.p. with 0.5 mg dexamethasone sodium phosphate and the
thymi were removed two days later. Thymocytes were cultivated at
4 x 10^6 or 1 x 10^7/ml in serum-free RPMI 1640 medium and stimulated
with 0.6 µg and 1.0 µg Con A/ml respectively. Labelled precursor
D- [1-^{14}C] galactose, L- [1,5,6,^{3}H]-fucose or [methyl-^{3}H]-
thymidine were added at a final concentration of 5 µCi/ml, 5 µCi/ml
and 1 µCi/ml respectively at the indicated times and for the stated
duration. DNA synthesis was measured by determining ^{3}H-Thymidine
incorporation into TCA precipitates, glycolipid synthesis by counting
^{14}C-galactose incorporation into chlorophorm-methanol extractable
material (80% of this label appears in the glycolipid fraction (3)),
and glycoprotein synthesis by measuring fucose incorporation into
TCA precipitates (fucose labels only glycoproteins in this system
(2)).

TAB. 2: Rate of labelling of DNA, glycolipids and glycoproteins in Con A stimulated thymocytes. Effect of hydrocortisone (H.C.) treatment of mice.

Time of pulse	Treatment of mice	Addition to culture	Incorporation per culture (4×10^6 cells)		
			^3H- thymidine	^{14}C- galactose into gylcolipid	^3H-fucose into glycoprotein
(h)			(cpm)	(cpm)	(cpm)
5-15	None	None	14128	176	371
	H.C.	None	14222	165	308
	None	Con A	35074	596	1103
	H.C.	Con A	14773	410	634
15-25	None	None	925	141	284
	H.C.	None	3931	139	304
	None	Con A	5833	436	622
	H.C.	Con A	15941	846	875
30-40	None	None	322	83	261
	H.C.	None	1534	95	241
	None	Con A	21623	1592	1240
	H.C.	Con A	68618	2593	2199

RESULTS AND DISCUSSION

Synthesis of glycoconjugates in the absence of DNA synthesis

To test whether the biphasic incorporation rates in untreated cultures were due to cell replication, glycoconjugate synthesis was measured in the absence of DNA synthesis (Tab.1). 5 mM hydroxyurea reduced ^3H-thymidine uptake to the level of control cultures, while synthesis of glycoconjugates as measured by ^{14}C-galactose incorporation into total glycolipids and ^3H-fucose incorporation into glycoproteins remained unaffected by hydroxyurea. These results indicate that :

a)   biosynthesis of glycoconjugates occurs independently of DNA synthesis and

b)   the biphasic incorporation rate is not due to cell replication.

Effects of hydrocortisone treatment on Con A stimulation of DNA and glycoconjugate synthesis

There was no Con A stimulation of early DNA synthesis in hydrocortisone resistant thymocytes. In contrast, the late response was clearly enhanced. Similarly early Con A-induced glycoconjugate synthesis was markedly depressed in hydrocortisone resistant cells. The increased incorporation rate at 30-40 h as compared to that of control cells is to be expected from the higher survival rate of hydro-cortisone resistant cells (5). The results strongly suggest that the early response is due to the major hydrocortisone sensitive population, whereas the late response is caused by the minor hydro-cortisone resistant population (Tab.2).

REFERENCES

1.   Wedner, H.J., Parker, C.W., Progress in Allergy 20 (1976) 195.
2.   van Eijk, R.V.W., Mühlradt, P.F., Eur. J. Biochem. 78 (1977) 41.
3.   Rosenfelder, G., van Eijk, R.V.W., Monner, D.A., Mühlradt, P.F., Euro. J. Biochem. 83 (1978) 571.
4.   Shortman, K., von Boehmer, H., Lipp, J., Hopper, K., Transpl. Rev. 25 (1975) 163.
5.   Hopper, K., Shortman, K., Cell. Immunol. 27 (1976) 256.

ARE ENDOGENOUS C-TYPE VIRUSES PHYSIOLOGICALLY REQUIRED FOR THE REGULATION OF THE HUMORAL IMMUNE RESPONSE?

G. Schumann, R.H. Gisler, A.F. Brownbill and Ch. Moroni

Research Department, Pharmaceuticals Division, CIBA-GEIGY Ltd., and Friedrich Miescher-Institut, CH-4002 Basel, Switzerland

INTRODUCTION

Over the last few years, we have studied the induction of endogenous C-type viruses from normal mouse lymphocytes. We found that some B-cell mitogens (LPS, LP, PPD) were powerful virus inducers whereas T-cell mitogens were not (1-6). Similar results from other investigators supported this conclusion (7-9). These studies revealed a difference between lymphoid subpopulations with respect to virus induction in that virus could only be induced from B cells (3).

The fact that the virus inducing B-cell mitogens LPS, LP and PPD also induce B cells to differentiate into immunoglobulin-secreting end cells led us to hypothesize that virus induction may be physiologically required for the regulation of differentiation of antibody-producing lymphocytes. We have therefore recently tested the effect on the humoral immune response of an antiserum directed against LPS-induced endogenous xenotropic C-type virus (10). This antiserum was immunosuppressive in vivo and in vitro. Virus absorption studies confirmed the viral specificity of this effect (10,11). Surprisingly, the serum interferes with early events of the immune response and has no effect when injected 24-48 h after antigen administration. The immunosuppressive effect was found in all mouse strains tested irrespective of their pattern of virus expression (11).

EXPERIMENTAL DESIGN AND RESULTS

We have previously shown that preincubation of mouse spleen cells with antiviral serum reduced the number of plaque-forming cells

TAB. 1:   Effect of preincubation of T cells, B cells and macrophages with antiviral and control serum in the three-cell-mosaic culture (12).

| Cells cultured: | | | Spleen[d] | PFC/10^6cells[e] | % Inhibition |
B[a]	T[b]	M[c]			
–	–	–	+	480	
–	–	–	+(AS)	140	71
+	–	+		0	
+	+	–		0	
+	+	+		840	
+(CS)	+	+		794	
+(AS)	+	+		494	38
+	+(CS)	+		1016	
+	+(AS)	+		464	55
+	+	+(CS)		770	
+	+	+(AS)		750	3

a 4×10^7 glasswool-filtered congenic nu/nu Balb/c lymph node cells were preincubated for 45 min at 37°C in 1 ml medium containing 50 µl control serum (CS) or antiserum (AS), washed twice and cultured at a density of 4×10^6 cells/ml culture.

b   As above, but 5×10^5 cortisone-resistant Balb/c thymus cells/ml culture.

c   As above, but 3×10^5 non-filtered 1000 R-irradiated Balb/c adherent peritoneal macrophages/ml culture.

d 8×10^6 Balb/c spleen cells/ml culture.

e   Direct plaque-forming cells (PFC) secreting immunoglobulin against sheep red blood cells were determined 5 days after stimulation of mosaic cultures with SRBC. Cell recovery from various cultures did not differ significantly. The values shown are the means of triplicate cultures.

in Mishell-Dutton cultures (11; Tab.1). Here we tested this antiserum on lymphoid subpopulations using the three-cell-mosaic culture method (12) in order to gain information on which cell type is the target of this immunosuppressive serum. In this system, Balb/c cortisone-resistant thymus cells (enriched T cells), Balb/c adherent peritoneal macrophages and Balb/c nu/nu lymph node cells (enriched B cells) are

TAB. 2:   Effect of preincubation of spleen cells with antiviral and control serum in the mixed lymphocyte culture (MLC).

| Mixed lymphocyte culture[a] | | | cpm/culture | |
Responder cell	Stimulator cell	-	CS	AS
Balb/c SC	-	338	995	314
Balb/c SC	C57B1 SC 800 R	24441	24322	27039

[a] 4×10^7 Balb/c spleen cells (SC) were preincubated for 45 min at 37°C in 1 ml medium containing 50 µl control serum (CS) or antiserum (AS), washed twice and added to 0.2 ml mini-cultures (Linbro plates) at a density of 2.5×10^5 cells/culture. The culture medium consisted of medium RPMI 1640, 8% fetal bovine serum, penicillin, streptomycin and 20 mM HEPES-buffer. To each MLC 2.5×10^5, 800 R-irradiated C57B1 spleen cells (SC) were added as stimulators and cultured for 4 days. Cultures wre labeled with ^{3}H-thymidine 16 h before harvesting. Trichloroacetic acid-precipitable radioactivity was determined after collection of samples with a semi-automated multiple sample harvester.

individually isolated and then mixed. Optimal antibody production against sheep red blood cells can only occur if the three subpopulations are co-cultured in optimal concentrations. Preincubation of T cells and B cells, but not of macrophages, with the antiviral serum (preparation see ref. 10 and 11) resulted in a significant reduction of plaque-forming cells. Control serum (preparation see ref. 10 and 11) used in a parallel series of tests was ineffective, indicating that the antiviral serum interacts with helper T cells as well as B cells (Tab.1).

To test whether this serum interferes also with cell-mediated immune responses, we preincubated Balb/c spleen cells with the antiviral serum and assayed them in mixed lymphocyte cultures and T-cell mediated lympholysis (Tabs. 2 and 3).

In neither system could immunosuppression be detected. Furthermore, addition of the antiserum directly to the mixed lymphocyte cultures had no effect in either system, indicating that viral antigens are not expressed during the generation phase of killer T cells and MLC-reactive cells (data not shown).

TAB. 3:   Effect of preincubation of spleen cells with antiviral and control serum in the T-cell mediated lympholysis (MLC-CML)[a].

Killer: Target ratio	% Specific lysis $\pm$ SEM Responder cells preincubated with:		
	−	CS	AS
200 : 1	70.1+3.6	65.4+3.0	64.2+3.6
40 : 1	50.4+2.0	48.1+3.8	46.7+2.5
8 : 1	21.4+3.6	17.6+2.6	16.8+1.2
1.6 : 1	4.7+1.6	6.3+1.7	4.1+0.8

[a]   2 ml medium RPMI 1640 + 20 mM HEPES-buffer containing 8×10^7 Balb/c spleen cells and 100 µl control serum (CS) or anti-serum (AS) were preincubated for 45 min at 37°C. After washing the cells once, MLC was performed by culturing 4×10^6 preincubated Balb/c spleen cells with 4×10^6 750 R-irradiated C57Bl spleen cells in a total volume of 4 ml. After 6 days of culturing, T-cell mediated lympholysis (CML) was carried out using ^{51}Cr-labeled concanavalin A-stimulated C57Bl lymph node target cells as described elsewhere (13).

DISCUSSION

These results demonstrate that viral antigens recognized by our antiserum are located on two well defined lymphoid subpopulations, namely helper T cells and antigen-reactive B cells. Supporting evidence for this result was recently presented by other workers who demonstrated the viral glycoprotein gp71 on helper T cells and antibody-forming B cells (14).

Since F(ab')$_2$ fragments of the antiserum are equally effective in immunosuppression (data not shown), one can postulate that this serum does not act by a cytotoxic effect but by blocking of receptor-like structures on T helper cells and antigen-reactive B cells. Two explanations can be given: blocking of viral antigens could lead to a steric hindrance of a functional receptor structure or, alternatively, viral antigen itself represents a receptor-like structure necessary for the generation of a humoral immune response. At present, our data cannot distinguish between these two explanations.

REFERENCES

1.   Moroni, Ch., Schumann, G., Nature 254 (1975) 60.
2.   Moroni, Ch., Schumann, G., Robert-Guroff, M., Suter, E.R., Martin, D., PNAS 72 (1975) 535.

3. Schumann, G., Moroni, Ch., J. Immunol. 116 (1976) 1145.
4. Moroni, Ch., Schumann, G., Virology 73 (1976) 17.
5. Morini, Ch., Schumann, G., J. Gen. Virol. 38 (1978) 497.
6. Schumann, G., Moroni, Ch., Virology 79 (1977) 81.
7. Greenberger, J.S., Phillips, S.M., Stephenson, J.R., Aaronson, S.A., J. Immunol. 115 (1975) 317.
8. Phillips, S.M., Stephenson, J.R., Greenberger, J.S., Lane, P.E., Aaronson, S.A., J. Immunol. 116 (1976) 1123.
9. Phillips, S.M., Stephenson, J.R., Aaronson, S.A., J. Immunol. 118 (1977) 622.
10. Moroni, Ch., Schumann, G., Nature 269 (1977) 600.
11. Schumann, G., Moroni, Ch., J. Immunol. (1978) in press.
12. Gisler, R.H., Dukor, P., Cell. Immunol. 4 (1972) 341.
13. Perren, B., Schumann, G., Gisler, R.H., Dukor, P., Transplantation 17 (1974) 392.
14. Wecker, E., Schimpl, A., Hünig, T., Nature 269 (1977) 598.

ACKNOWLEDGEMENTS

The excellent technical assistance of Elisabeth Edelmann, Nicole Martin and Véronique Rigo is gratefully acknowledged.

PLATING INHIBITION ASSAY (PIA): A NEW TEST FOR CELL MEDIATED CYTOTOXICITY

K. Ulrichs, K.-M. Kuhlencordt and W. Müller-Ruchholtz

Department of Immunology, Institute of Hygiene and

Microbiology, University of Kiel, Kiel, West Germany

The microcytotoxicity assay (MCA) of Takasugi and Klein, well established for testing cell-mediated immunity in the mouse, is however much less effective in the rat, showing far more unspecified cytolysis and less sensitivity. We therefore developed a new test system, the plasting inhibition assay (PIA). In this in-vitro test, T effector lymphocytes, increasingly with their strength of sensitization, prevent the plating of suspended target fibroblasts, i.e. their ability to adhere to surfaces such as the bottom of Terasaki microtest plates.

The essential procedures of this method, as compared with the MCA, are described in Figure 1. Results are documented in Figures 2 and 3, comparing the two test systems and using both, rat and mouse cell systems: In terms of E/T PIA is shown to be about 125 times more effective than the MCA in the rat cell system while only about 25 times in the mouse cell system. Furthermore, PIA does not appear to be restricted by unspecific cytolysis. The effector lymphocytes were identified as T cells. The specificity of target cell kill was examined against a third party strain. After 3 h incubation in the hanging drop, target cell fibroblasts, though functionally inactivated, were still viable (as shown by trypan blue exclusion). It may be mentioned that also tests for specific blocking serum factors can be performed.

Conclusions: (1) Inhibition of fibroblast adherence to surfaces is a much more sensitive and precise test to detect sensitized T lymphocytes than reduction of adhering fibroblast target cells as e.g. in the MCA. (2) This principle appears to be effective with mouse and still more with rat cell systems.

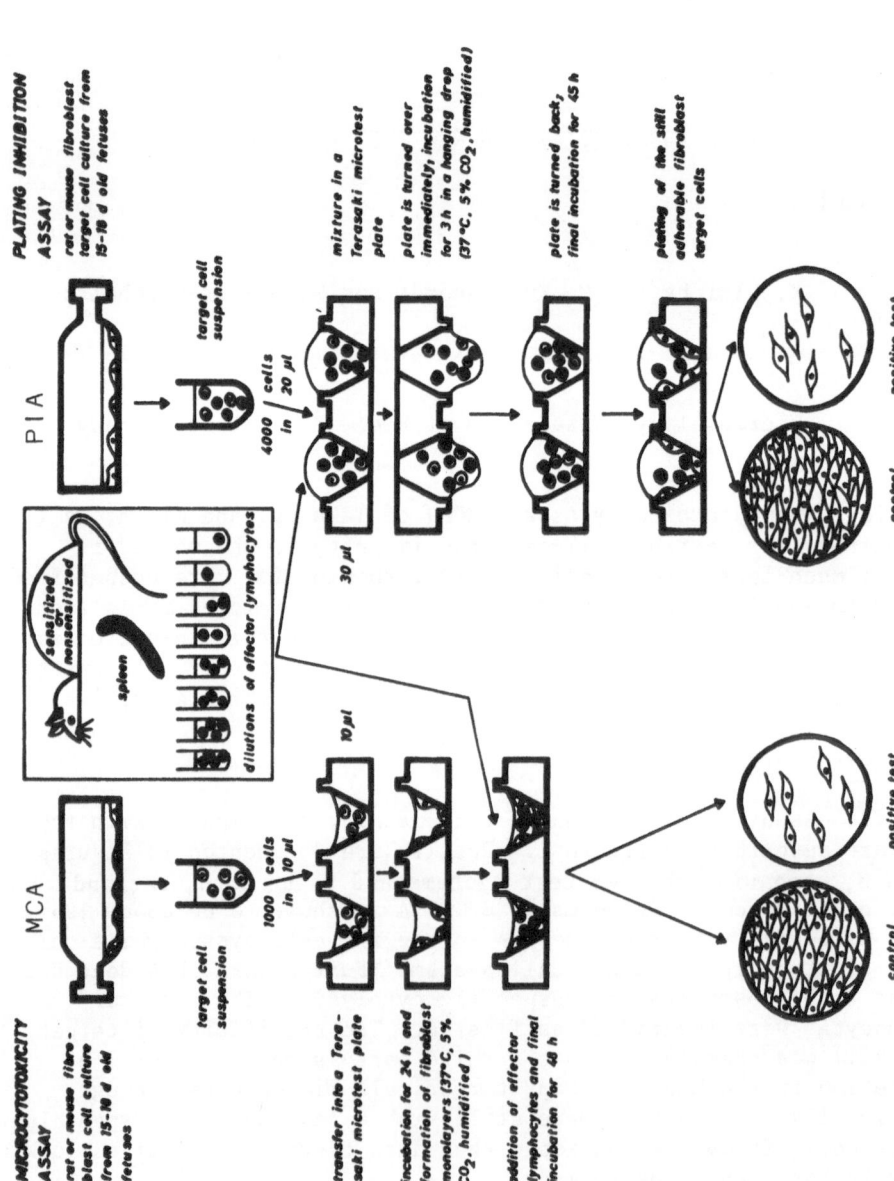

FIG. 1: Methodical procedure of PIA compared with the MCA.

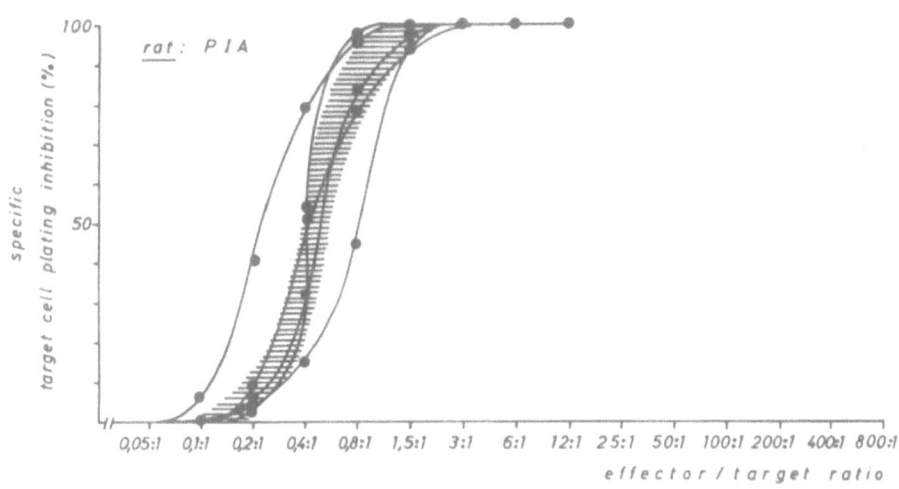

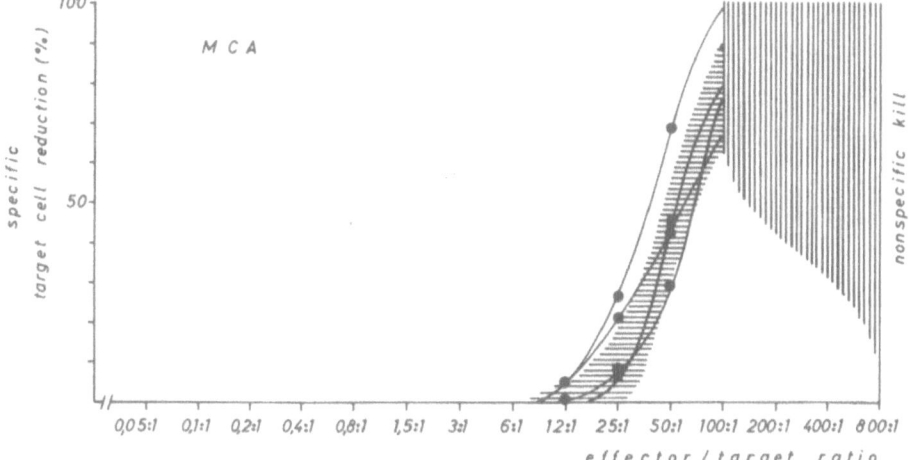

FIG. 2:   Comparison of PIA with MCA in the rat sensitization:
10^8 CAP(RT 1^c) spleen cells i.p. into LEW (RT 1^c), 8 d before
lymphocyte preparation; target cells: CAP fibroblasts; no. of
exp.: PIA: 27 tests with lymphocytes of indiv. rats in 5 groups;
MCA: 27 tests with lymphocytes of indiv. rats in 4 groups; the
curves represent the means of the groups; the striped area indicates the representative range of variability of one group.

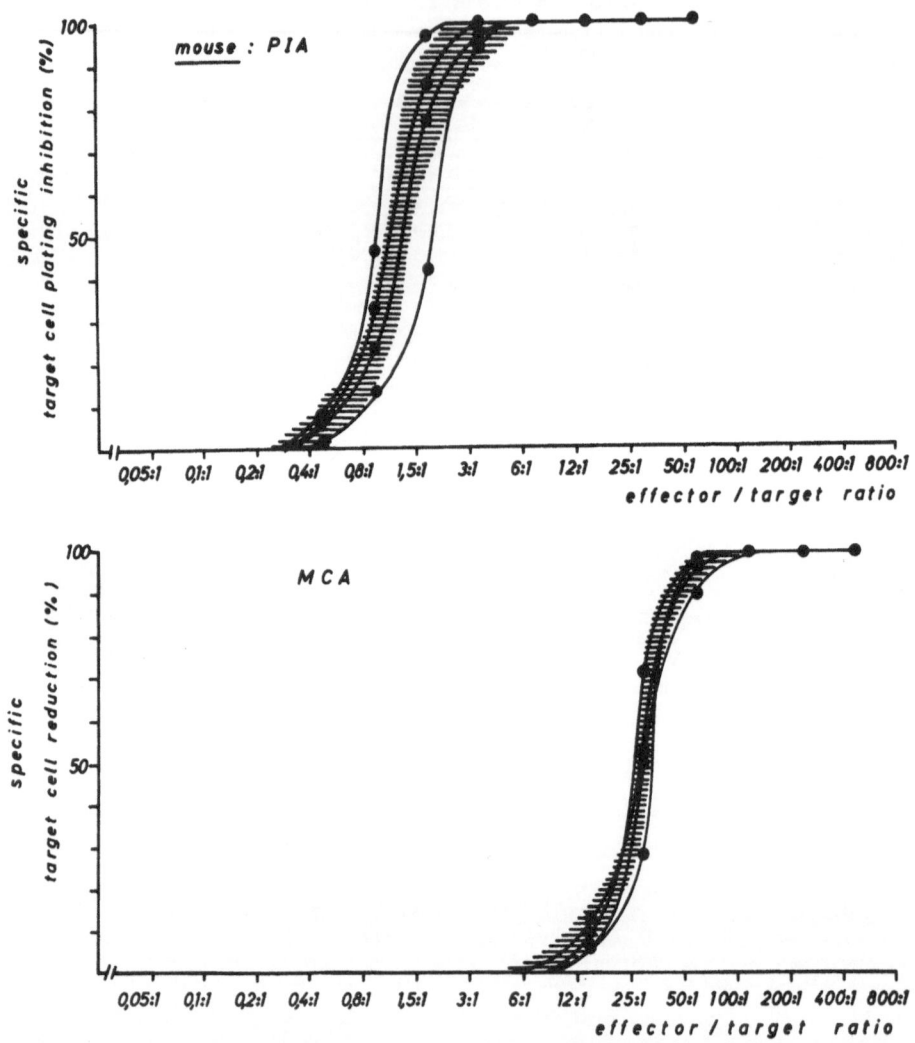

FIG. 3:   Comparison of PIA with MCA in the mouse sensitization:
5×10^7 C3H(H-2^k) spleen cells i.p. into C57(H-2^b), 8 d before
lymphocyte preparation; target cells: C3H fibroblasts; no. of
exp.: PIA: 21 tests with lymphocytes of indiv. mice in 4 groups;
MCA: 23 tests with lymphocytes of indiv. mice in 4 groups; the
curves represent the means of the groups; the striped area indicates the representative range of variability of one group.

SUMMING UP - LYMPHOCYTE RECEPTORS

R.M.E. Parkhouse

National Institute for Medical Research

Mill Hill, London, NW7, UK

A key question in biology is the regulation of gene expression following interaction of cells with hormones, drugs, antigens and other cells. In most cases the critical event is combination between the biologically active effectors and specific receptor molecules in the cell membrane. It is therefore of the utmost importance that such receptor molecules be isolated and identified, the long term aim being to explain in molecular terms the alteration of cell phenotype following the primary event of receptor-ligand interaction.

The process of transduction that follows the so-called "first message" of receptor-ligand interaction leads to development of the "second message", which is the intracellular signal that initiates the observed phenotypic change. The exact way that this is done is only understood in the most general of terms. For example, with small molecules such as acetylcholine there is presumably a conformational change in the receptor. In other systems, such as antigen receptors, it is very likely that receptors must be aggregated. At this initial stage of the transduction process, however, it is possible to imagine that the conformationally changed, or aggregated, receptor either acts directly or indirectly upon the system that generates the second message, be it a change in the activity of a membrane bound enzyme (e.g. adenyl cyclase) or in membrane permeability to a given ion. For example, a receptor could conceivably interact indirectly with a channel forming protein or enzyme via a membrane element only when in combination with its appropriate ligand. Alternatively, the receptor-ligand complex could directly activate production of the "second message".

Turning from the general to the specific, we may now enquire as to the state of our knowledge in the case of lymphocytes. The short answer is that we are incredibly ignorant. In some cases, like the B-lymphocyte, we can define both receptor and ligand (surface immuno-globulin (sIg) and antigen; Fc receptors and aggregated Ig). In others we know what is the ligand, but the receptor is undefined e.g. mitogen receptors, antigen receptor of T-lymphocyte, complement recep-tors. Conversely, there are cases like the Thy-1 antigen of the T-cell membrane, a glycoprotein very well studied and yet without any assigned function. Finally, there are a range of lymphocyte membrane proteins which appear as bands on SDS gels, and to date lack both a name and an assigned function.

In view of this general level of ignorance, it is hardly sur-prising that our knowledge of the process of transduction is insig-nificant, and this is so even in the most well studied case, that of the sIg of B cells. Indeed Coutinho and Möller have even argued that the function of sIg is merely to collect antigen for presentation to a postulated mitogen receptor (1). Although the weight of evidence argues against their view, this does nonetheless indicate our general ignorance. On the credit side, however, we can take some pleasure in reflecting that there is a great deal of work to be done in this field, and that all the interesting questions remain to be answered. What is the molecular nature and function of Fc and complement recep-tors? Why are there multiple classes of sIg (e.g. IgM and IgD) on one B-lymphocyte, and do sIgM, sIgG, sIgA and sIgD deliver unique and different signals to the cells which bear them? What is the basis of T cell recognition and its associated phenomenon of MHC restriction, i.e. do T cells recognise MHC products and antigens as one entity or separately? How is cell collaboration, be it positive (help), nega-tive (suppression) or for antigen presentation (macrophages) control-led and regulated at the level of receptor-ligand interactions? Work around these basic questions will undoubtedly form the basis for many future meetings devoted to the topic of "Immunological function of cell surface structures".

REFERENCES

1.   Coutinho, A., Möller, G. Scand. J. Immunol. 3 (1974) 133.

SESSION   A 3

IMMUNOLOGICAL   TOLERANCE

(SUPPRESSION/DELETION)

CHAIRPERSONS:

J.R. Batchelor

W. Müller-Ruchholtz

INTRODUCTION

W. Müller-Ruchholtz

Department of Immunology, Institute of Hygiene and

Microbiology, University of Kiel, Kiel, West Germany

How should dividing lines be drawn between specific responsiveness ("turn-on") and specific unresponsiveness ("turn-off")? This
may be asked in view of the long-standing basic observation that
nature cannot afford unlimited reactions of any type and that also a
response to an antigen becomes limited sooner or later by a "turn-
off".

A physiologist could probably help to explain these relationships by talking about feedback inhibition and making three statements:
1) according to a rather old physiological dogma, every "turn-on"
requires and implies "turn-off"; 2) under appropriate conditions,
lack of further responsiveness may be induced at almost any stage of
responsiveness; and 3) the resulting suppression of responsiveness
may reach almost any extent.

Our knowledge about the immunoregulatory network has, therefore,
necessarily led to the notion of suppression in relation to immunological tolerance. However, we should be aware of the danger of including here any feedback inhibition since some authors end up
inadvertently considering immunotolerance as a regular element within
any sensitization response. In other words, I am afraid we should be
very concerned about the ability of a suppressive mechanism under
study, to really induce specific non-reactivity that can also be
observed in vivo. I would suggest that we keep this in mind throughout the forthcoming session when talking about immunotolerance.

At least some of the various suppressive mechanisms will be
discussed mainly during the second part of the session. Synoptically,
the suppressive "turn-off" may be called "reactive" since it is based

on humoral and/or cellular reactive entities which evolved as reaction
to the antigen which can be studied in vitro and transferred in vivo.
It may be opposed to the "active turn-off" which is implied in the
classical notion of true non-reactivity.

The fundamental necessity of protection against immunological
self-destruction may well require other regulatory systems, being
more basic and only supported by the "reactive turn-off" of suppressors'good suppression (or even: only temporarily accompanied by
suppressive phenomena). Whether these other regulatory systems act
through cell elimination, through stripping-off of their antigen
receptors or receptor blockade by antigen is open to discussion, and
we are glad to have many outstanding scientists with us who will
probably discuss this mainly during the first part of the session.

How clearly do our experimental conditions allow us to find out
what happens in nature? Let me briefly discuss this with regard to
the stem cell problem: It is generally accepted that the immunologically differentiated organism, not only in the adult but already
to a large extent at birth, necessarily has both, less or more
differentiated lymphoid cells of limited survival time and stem cells
which will provide the future immunological potential. (Remember
that B type lymphocytes can already be shown in the 12-day-old mouse
embryo.) Only very early in ontogeny would we be dealing with stem
cells only. There we would most clearly meet the conditions under
which a regulation becomes purely antigen-driven rather than co-
determined by the kind of reaction within a less or more established
immunoregulatory network. But how can we collect enough of such
cells early enough in intrauterine life to do experiments with them?

Nevertheless, several observations, particularly those following
intrauterine LCM virus infections or neonatal injections of large
doses of alloantigens in mice and especially those reported by Sir
Gus Nossal (see below), have provided good evidence for the predominance of an "active turn-off" in the immature immunological
system. But in adults we hardly know what happens under conditions
in which antigens, such as histocompatibility antigens, are present
before new lymphoid cells with reactivity against them start to
differentiate, though there it may be most interesting.

This problem became a major interest of our own group when a
methodologically new approach allowed us to perform combined in vitro/
in vivo experiments in the adult. The methodology evolved from quite
different studies, aiming at the serological analysis of xenogeneic
anti-lymphocyte serum and showing that it contained various antibodies
against a variety of lymphoid cell surface antigens, most of which
are shared by other cells. We succeeded in eliminating the anti-stem
cell-antibodies maintaining cytotoxicity against all lymphoid cells.
In vitro incubation in such specified antiserum allowed the preparation
of lymphocyte-free stem cells from adult rat bone marrow as outlined

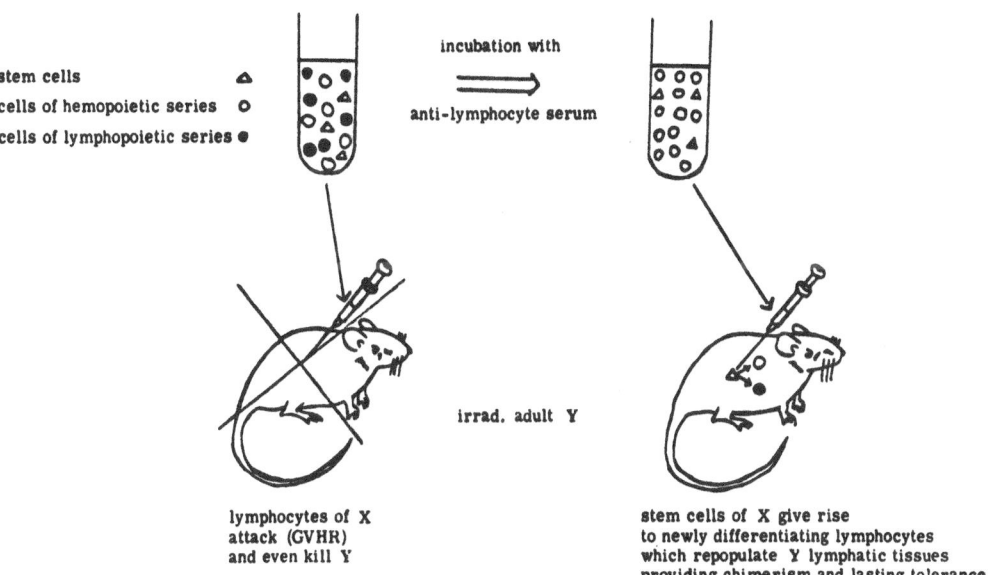

FIG. 1:   Stem cell chimerism: principles and approach.

in Fig.1: Adult bone marrow may be considered to contain three groups of cells, namely stem cells, cells of the various hemopoietic series and cells of the lymphopoietic series. Allogeneic transplantation into an irradiated rat usually leads to fatal, acute GVHR. A 45 minute 137°C incubation of this bone marrow in the antiserum eliminates quantitatively the lymphocytes, and now allogeneically grafted stem cells give rise to newly differentiating lymphocytes.

Only if this treatment also inactivated the lymphoid precursors, could the cells be successfully grafted in strongly and fully allogeneic recipients (recently even in xenogeneic recipients) which became chimeric and could be observed for long periods of time. Some of our recent data will be presented in this session by Dr. Müller-Hermelink and by Dr. Wottge.

All tests thus far have not yielded evidence for any reactivity, including suppressive, of the lymphatic offspring of the grafted stem cells against their foreign environment, whereas they appeared to be normally reactive against third party antigens. Summarizing the preliminary survey of these 11 tests (Table 1), it may be said that considering the possibility of different states of unresponsiveness in different lymphocyte subpopulations, we tested the afferent as well as the efferent limb, humoral and cellular reactivities, in vitro and in vivo.

TAB. 1:   Testing for specific nonreactivity of stem cell chimera
(preliminary survey).

1.   Specifically negative MLC with chimera responder lymphocytes

2.   No MLC suppression by chimera spleen cells

3.   Negative MCT (Takasugi-Klein):   no killer cells in spleen

4.   No MCT blockade by chimera serum factors

5.   Negative plating inhibition assay (PIA)

6.   No PIA suppression by chimera lymphocytes

7.   No PIA blockade by chimera serum factors

8.   Negative popliteal lymph node assay (POLNA)

9.   No POLNA suppression by chimera lymphocytes

10. No POLNA blockade by chimera serum factors

11. Specific sensitization of syngen. transferred normal
     lymphocytes

TAB. 2:   Group topics and authors of the session on immunotolerance.

Clonal abortion theory	Nossal
Stem cell manipulation	Müller-Hermelink Wottge
Regulatory role of auto-antigens	Singhal Steele
Regulatory role of ag.-ab. complexes	Klaus
Lymphatic tissue morphology of specific. non-react. organisms	Vainio
Suppressor cells	
1. Models for induction	Eisenthal Kaufmann
2. Characterization by surface markers etc.	Zan Bar
3. Characterization by CY	Droege l'Age-Stehr
4. Role in low zone tolerance	Heuer
Non-specific suppression	Jankovic Globerson Hanna

It may be pointed out that in this model the conditions clearly differ from the well-known model in which lymphoid cells of the adult may be taken and treated with antigen successfully (in terms of tolerance induction), but only if selected antigens had been prepared, e.g. human gammaglobulin by deaggregation. It may also be discussed how far the one or the other of these models reflects what happens in nature generally, not only exceptionally, e.g. with regard to auto-antigens.

In concluding this introduction, Table 2 is given to survey the group topics under which the papers of this session have been placed.

DIFFERENTIATION OF B CELLS AND THE CLONAL ABORTION THEORY

G.J.V. Nossal

The Walter and Eliza Hall Institute of Medical Research
Post Office, Royal Melbourne Hospital, Victoria 3050,
Australia

During the early years of research on immunological tolerance
(1), it was generally believed that induction of the phenomenon
could only be achieved in embryonic or very young animals, implying
a special susceptibility of immature lymphoid cells. A plausible
mechanism for tolerance emerged in 1957, when Burnet (2) postulated
his clonal selection theory, and ascribed tolerance to a deletion
of clones through contact between immature lymphocytes with their
corresponding antigen. This straightforward view of the problem
received a number of challenges during the 1960's. A watershed was
the discovery by Dresser (3) that small amounts of de-aggregated
proteins could induce tolerance in adult mice. A further complication
was the discovery of the helper function of T lymphocytes and the
demonstration that, in some tolerance models, tolerance was confined
to the T lymphocyte compartment (4). Then, when the important role
of suppressor T cells in antibody formation and immunological
tolerance became clear (5,6), the idea of clonal deletion as a
general explanation of tolerance lost favour in many quarters.

The aim of recent research in our laboratory (reviewed in 7,8)
has been to re-open the question of a special susceptibility of
immature cells to tolerance induction. We have concentrated on the
B lymphocyte. Furthermore, we have introduced the term clonal
abortion to describe more precisely the concept of a cell that reacts
to antigen with a negative signal because it is immature. The
implication is that if the cell were in the process of acquiring
receptors with reactivity to a "self" antigen, above a certain
threshold of avidity for a given concentration of "self" antigen, its
maturation into a mature functional B cell would be prevented.

Our attempts to gain experimental support for the clonal
abortion theory have fallen into four distinct phases. During the
first phase (9), we sought to reconstitute adult, lethally irradiated
mice with a source of cells lacking B cells but capable of generating
B cells following a lag of some 8 days. During the reconstitution
phase, we injected hapten-protein conjugates, acting as putative
tolerogens, into the adoptive hosts and demonstrated a reduction in
the capacity of the reconstituted animals to respond to the relevant
hapten following challenge with a T-independent antigen. The chief
interest of this study was that even potent antigens, such as DNP-
polymerized flagellin, could act as tolerogens for the maturing B
cells, while obviously immunizing mature B cells similarly transferred.

The second phase of the research moved to in vitro models of
tolerance induction, followed by assessment of B cell function on
adoptive transfer (10). Adult mouse bone marrow was chosen as the
B cell source. This model showed that the response capacity per
viable nucleated cell rose as bone marrow was cultured, and that low
concentrations of hapten-protein conjugates could abrogate that rise.
This was in line with the strictest interpretation of the clonal
abortion theory, as it appeared that cultures incubated with tolerogen
always maintained some residual capacity to respond. As bone marrow
is such a heterogeneous mixture of cells, at various stages of differentiation more rigorous assay methods were called for, which could
analyze the actual numbers of responsive B cells following putative
tolerogenesis.

During the third phase of our research (11,7) a two-stage tissue
culture approach was used. First, cells from immature or mature B
cell sources were incubated in bulk for various periods with putative
tolerogens. Then, the cells were harvested, washed, and distributed
at limit dilution in a microculture system (12) that allowed clonal
growth of individual hapten-specific B cells under the stimulus of
a T-independent antigen or a polyclonal B cell activator. This work
confirmed that both adult bone marrow and newborn spleen were readily
tolerized, but only when tolerogen acted for longer than 24 hr.

Shortly after this work was completed, we became aware of the
work of Metcalf and Klinman in a T-dependent cloning system (13,14).
This provided useful confirmation of the ready tolerizability of
immature B cells, but raised two related dilemmas for us. First,
their report stated that tolerance could be induced within 8 hr.
Secondly, they produced evidence suggesting that a given cell could
either be rendered tolerant or be triggered to yield an antibody-
forming clone depending on the nature of the signals reaching it.
Such an event would not be consistent with the clonal abortion theory
sensu strictu, as that theory invokes a postulated transition from
tolerizable but not immunizable to immunizable but not tolerizable.

We therefore embarked on the fourth phase of our work, designed to test the behaviour not just of unfractionated cells from heterogeneous sources containing many immature B cells, but rather of a selected subset of B cells, already Ig-positive but coming from a newborn mouse spleen (15).

Mice aged 3 to 5 days were killed in batches of 200, their spleens removed and a single cell suspension prepared. Then, cells with receptors specific for the hapten fluorescein (FLU) were separated on FLU-gelatin dishes according to the method of Haas and Layton (16). These FLU-specific B cells were then placed into micro-culture at limit dilution in the presence or absence of $FLU_{3.6}$-human gammaglobulin (HGG) acting as a tolerogen. After periods varying from 2 to 48 hr, the tolerogen was removed and either FLU-polymerized flagellin (FLU-POL) or E. coli lipopolysaccharide (LPS) was added. After a further 62-66 hr, the microcultures were harvested and analyzed for FLU-specific plaque-forming cells, allowing the number of clonable anti-FLU precursor cells to be determined through the use of Poisson statistics.

Using this selected set of cells, we were able to show that tolerance could be induced with far lower concentrations of tolerogen in the case of the newborn cells than when adult hapten-specific cells exhibiting a similar range of avidities for the hapten were cultured. In fact, with 24 hr exposure to tolerogen, a 50 per cent reduction in numbers of effective precursor cells was shown with $0.08\mu g/ml$ of $FLU_{3.6}$-HGG, versus $80\mu g/ml$ when adult hapten specific cells were used. There thus was a 1000-fold difference between adult and newborn B cells in their susceptibility to this tolerogen.

This result stood in contrast to the claim by Cambier et al. (17) that, for cells capable of responding to T-independent antigens, there was no major difference in tolerance-susceptibility between adult and newborn spleen. A feature of the work of this group has been the use of highly substituted hapten-protein conjugates. Accordingly, we studied the effects of FLU_{12}-HGG in our system. Interestingly, this proved to be a much more powerful tolerogen than $FLU_{3.6}$-HGG. For example, when it acted on unfractionated adult spleen cells for 24 hr, a 50 per cent reduction in responsiveness was induced, and about $0.5\mu g/ml$ achieved the same effect for hapten-gelatin fractionated cells. Nevertheless, newborn unfractionated cells of each type were 5 to 10 fold more sensitive still. These results suggest that the loss of capacity to be tolerized as cells mature is not absolute, but rather relative. Even with these powerfully tolerogenic antigens, the heightened susceptibility of newborn cells was demonstrated.

A further feature of this fourth phase of our work has been to show that tolerance, once induced, is stable to challenge with a

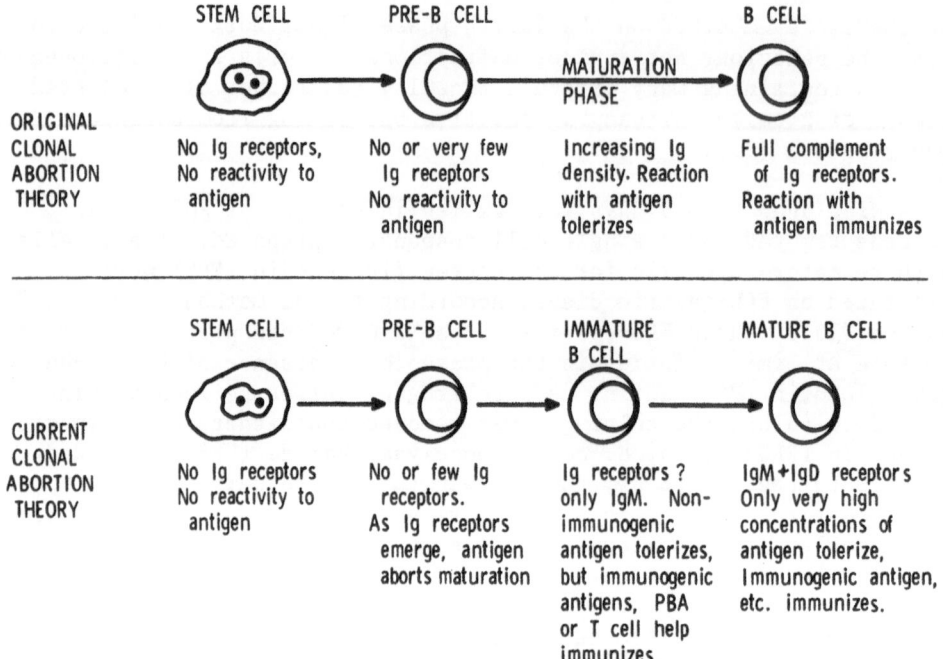

FIG. 1:   The clonal abortion theory restated.

polyclonal B cell activator such as LPS. It appears that tolerance
induction is accompanied by the accumulation of negative signals
inside the cell, and is not simply due to modulation or blockade of
B cell surface receptors for antigen.

Finally, we have investigated the effects of anti-μ antibodies
acting as a kind of "universal tolerogen". Two cloning systems have
served as the read-out, namely the 3-day T-independent liquid micro-
culture system and the agar colony system for B lymphocyte growth
(18). In respect of a) the heightened susceptibility of newborn B
cells to inhibition, and b) the relative concentration and time
parameters, the effects of anti-μ closely resembled those of tolerogen.
This means, of course, that B cells as a group can be studied, and
not just the small sub-set of B cells binding a particular hapten.
The finding offers many advantages for studies of the molecular basis
of tolerogensis.

SUMMARY AND CONCLUSIONS

In the light of the studies summarized here, we have had to
modify the clonal abortion theory as outlined in Fig.1. We now
believe that there are two distinct and separable phenomena in clonal
abortion. The first phenomenon, clonal abortion sensu strictu,

involves an abolition of the transition from surface Ig-negative to surface Ig-positive cells. From our earlier work, and particularly from the work of M.D. Cooper's group (e.g. 19), we believe this to require extremely low concentrations of Ig receptor-binding ligands. The second phenomenon describes the behaviour of Ig-positive B cells which are already capable of reacting to antigens and mitogens, but which still retain a certain immaturity. These cells can be immunized under some circumstances, but still retain a ready tolerizability when the antigen to which they are exposed lacks "Signal 2" properties (20) or when T cell helper factors are absent.

A final point to note is that even fully mature B cells can be switched off by antigen, but under circumstances of concentration and valency that are somewhat extreme.

REFERENCES

1. Medawar, P.B. Harvey Lectures 52 (1958) 144.
2. Burnet, F.M. Aust. J. Sci. 20 (1957) 67.
3. Dresser, D.W. Immunol. 4 (1961) 13.
4. Weigle, W.O., Chiller, J.M., Habicht, G.S. Transplant. Rev. 8 (1972) 3.
5. Gershon, R.K., Kondo, K. Immunol. 21 (1971) 903.
6. McCullogh, P. Transplant. Rev. 12 (1972) 180.
7. Nossal, G.J.V., Shortman, K., Howard, M., Pike, B.L. Immunol. Rev. 37 (1977) 188.
8. Nossal, G.J.V., Pike, B.L., Teale, J.M., Layton, J.E., Kay, T.W., Battye, F.L. Immunol. Rev. (1978) in press.
9. Nossal, G.J.V., Pike, B.L. In: Immunological Aspects of Neoplasia. E.M. Hersh, M. Schlamowitz (eds). Baltimore, Williams and Wilkins (1975b) p.87.
10. Nossal, G.J.V., Pike, B.L. J. exp. Med. 141 (1975) 904.
11. Stocker, J.W. Immunol. 32 (1977) 283.
12. Nossal, G.J.V., Pike, B.L. J. Immunol. 120(1) (1978) 145.
13. Metcalf, E.S., Klinman, N.R. J. exp. Med. 143 (1976) 1327.
14. Metcalf, E.S., Klinman, N.R. J. Immunol. 118 (1977) 2111.
15. Nossal, G.J.V., Pike, B.L. J. exp. Med. (1978) November.
16. Haas, W., Layton, J.E. J. exp. Med. 141 (1975) 1004.
17. Cambier, J.C., Vitetta, E.S., Uhr, J.W., Kettman, J.R. J. exp. Med. 145 (1977b) 778.
18. Metcalf, D., Nossal, G.J.V., Warner, N.L., Miller, J.F.A.P., Mandel, T.E., Layton, J.E., Gutman, G.A. J. exp. Med. 142 (1975) 1534.
19. Kearney, J.F., Klein, J., Bockman, D.E., Cooper, M.D., Lawton, A.R. J. Immunol. 120 (1978) 158.
20. Schrader, J.W. Europ. J. Immunol. 4 (1974) 20.

ACKNOWLEDGEMENT

    This work was supported by the National Health and Medical
Research Council, Canberra, Australia and by Grant Number AI-03958
from the National Institute for Allergy and Infectious Diseases,
U.S. Public Health Service.

PERMANENT ABOLITION OF REACTIVITY TO MAJOR HISTOCOMPATIBILITY

ANTIGENS REQUIRES ELIMINATION OF PRETHYMIC PRECURSORS

H.K. Müller-Hermelink[1], H.-U. Wottge[2] and W. Müller-Ruchholtz[2]

[1]Institute of Pathology and [2]Department of Immunology
University Medical School, D-2300 Kiel, W. Germany

INTRODUCTION

The major problem of allogeneic bone marrow (BM) transplantation is still the graft-versus-host reaction (GVHR), with its implications and consequences resulting from the high lymphocyte content of the BM graft. Of the various methodological attempts at achieving a complete elimination of lymphoid cells from BM and leaving the hemopoietic stem cells untouched, short-term in-vitro incubation of BM grafts in a specifically absorbed anti-lymphocyte serum (ALS) and complement was used in this study rather than physical separation of BM cells, since it has been postulated that antibodies against antigenic determinants on lymphocytes not shared by hemopoietic stem cells represent a better dissecting tool than cell size and density. After exhaustive absorptions with rat erythrocytes, peritoneal macrophages, and fetal liver cells, rabbit anti-rat lymphocyte serum (ALS) is able to eliminate all lymphoid-determined cells from BM, leaving hemopoietic stem cells undamaged (3).

The above observation was substantiated by the detailed analysis of radiation chimeras resulting from the transplantation of incubated BM cells in lethally irradiated syngeneic and strongly and fully allogeneic rats. The main characteristics were the following:

1.   Lethally irradiated recipients of incubated BM survived, whereas those receiving fresh BM died of acute GVHR within 3 weeks (Fig.1).

2.   Six weeks after transplantation of allogeneic BM cells incubated in ALS, even the thymus was repopulated similarly to syngeneic controls, whereas fresh allogeneic BM led to severe GVHR with complete

thymus atrophy. The histology of the thymus and lymph nodes was the
most sensitive sign of intercurrent GVHR. Using specific alloantisera, it has been shown that about half of the cells in BM and
lymphoid tissue originated from the donor and a stable cellular
chimerism was observed throughout the whole observation period of
more than a year.

3.   Skin graft experiments 6 weeks after BM transplantation showed
nonreactivity to donor strain skin and normal immunological reactivity
to third-party skin.

Several reports (4,5) have suggested that, instead of eliminating
all lymphoid cells, it might be sufficient to eliminate mature T cells
from BM to avoid GVHR. Most of these experiments were performed in
semi-allogeneic mouse combinations, in which GVHR after BM transplantation was of the chronic type and it was relatively easy to avoid
the lethal effects of GVHR (6). A generalization of these findings
would indicate that prethymic lymphoid precursors always adapt themselves in a "foreign" environment and become functionally incapable
of reacting against foreign major histocompatibility antigens (MHA).
Thus, the aim of this study was to answer the question of whether or
not prethymic lymphoid precursors in BM are irreversibly determined
to recognize foreign MHA.

MATERIAL AND METHODS

The basic methodology for the experiments has been published
in detail elsewhere (3). The results of BM transplantation were
compared after short-term incubation (37°C for 30 min) of donor BM
in ALS, either eliminating all lymphoid cells or leaving precursors
of T and B cells in BM unaffected. As "anti-lymphocyte serum",
eliminating all lymphoid-determined cells from rat BM, we used rabbit
anti-rat lymphocyte sera exhaustively absorbed with rat erythrocytes,
peritoneal exudate cells, and fetal liver cells. "Anti-T cell serum"
was prepared by additional absorption of anti-lymphocyte serum with
spleen cells from B rats, i.e., adult thymectomized lethally irradiated
and BM-reconstituted animals.

Rats of two strongly histoincompatible inbred strains were used
(LEW (RT1^1 as recipient) and CAP (RT1^C as donor)). The incubation of
donor BM in ALS plus fresh rat serum as the source of complement was
performed at equicytotoxic titers (determined with rat thymocytes).
At different times, but mostly 6 weeks after transplantation, the
lethally irradiated and reconstituted rats were examined for signs of
GVHR by determination of survival rates and morphological examination
of lymphoid tissues.

RESULTS

Survival Rates

Fig.1 shows the data for lethally irradiated BM recipients.
Preincubation of donor BM in anti-lymphocyte serum led to 100%
survival of the recipients. On the other hand, only 30% of the
recipients survived 6 weeks after preincubation of donor BM in
anti-T cell serum in this strongly allogeneic system. The survival
curve for lethally irradiated BM recipients shows a similar decline
to that of recipients of fresh allogeneic BM, delayed by about 3
weeks.

Morphological Evaluation

The thymus of recipients of BM incubated in anti-lymphocyte
serum was well reconstituted, with a lymphocyte-rich cortex and
clear cortico-medullary differentiation, 6 weeks after BM transplantation. In contrast, the thymus of recipients of BM incubated
in anti-T cell serum showed no restitution. The epithelial
structure of the thymus was almost free of lymphocytes (Fig.2).
Activated macrophages containing lipids and other ingested material
could be observed among epithelial cells. The widened perivascular
spaces at the cortico-medullary junction and the thymic capsule
contained a few lymphocytes, plasma cells, and macrophages. This
picture corresponds to the morphology of thymuses of animals
suffering from GVHR after transplantation of fresh allogeneic BM.

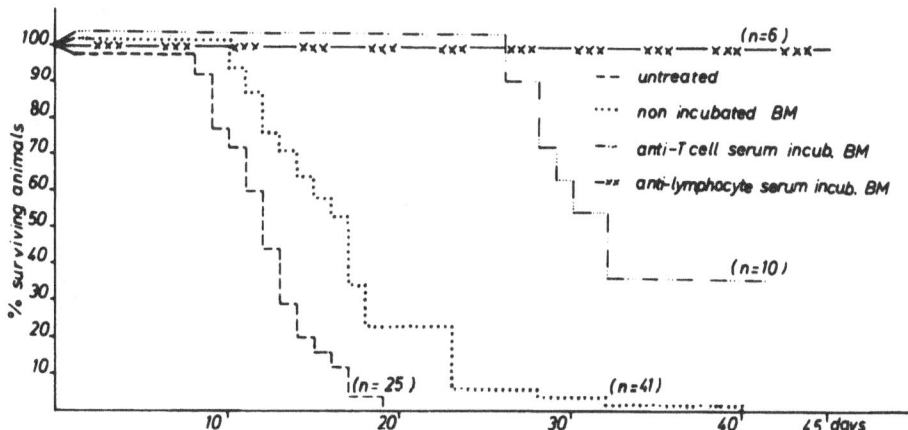

FIG. 1:   Comparison of survival rates of rats after lethal
irradiation and treatment with RT1-incompatible bone marrow
incubated in different antisera.

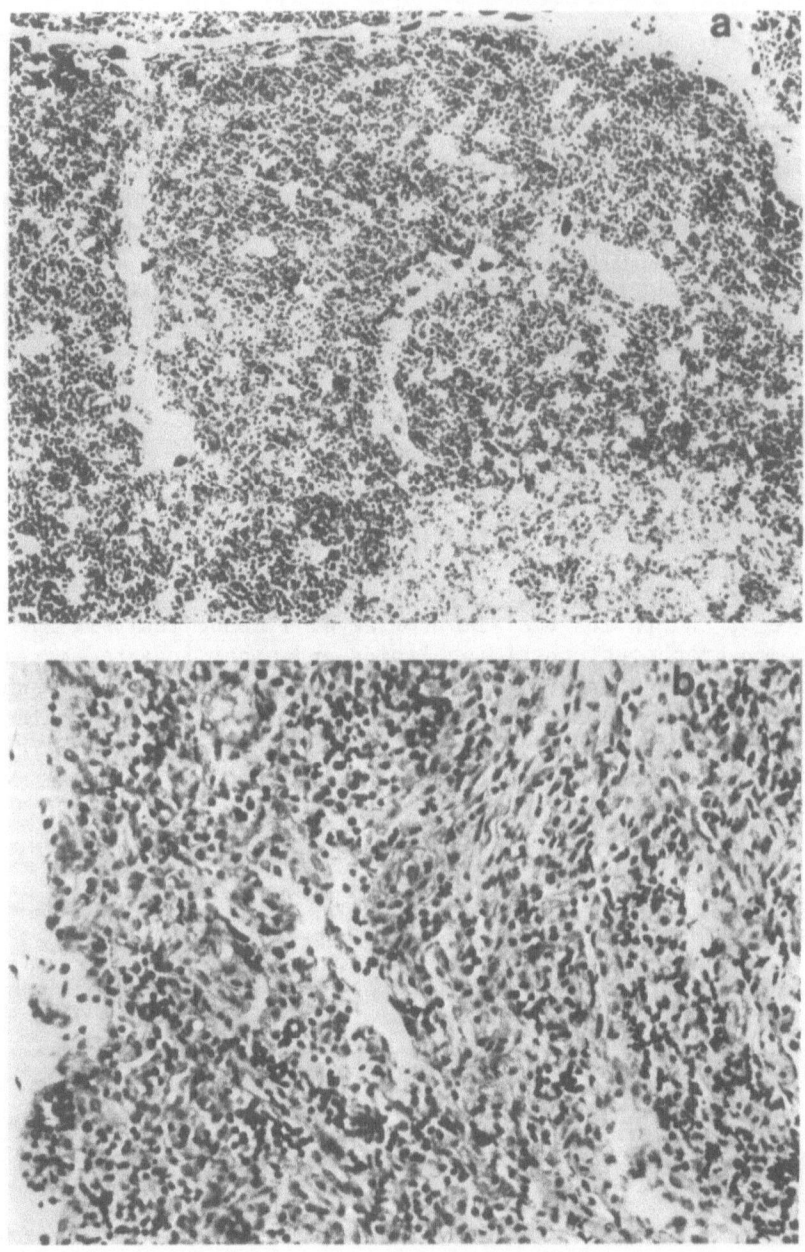

FIG. 2:   Morphology of thymus of lethally irradiated rats, 6 weeks
after treatment with allogeneic bone marrow (BM). (a) BM incubated
in anti-lymphocyte serum: normal restitution of the thymic cortex
and medulla. X 64. (b) BM incubated in anti-T cell serum: no
restitution as sign of GVHR. X 64.

The spleen of recipients of BM incubated in anti-lymphocyte serum showed an almost normal structure of the white pulp, with a densely populated periarteriolar lymphocyte sheath and a broad marginal zone. The red pulp was rich in hemopoietic cells. In contrast, recipients of BM incubated in anti-T cell serum showed no repopulation of splenic white pulp, although the red pulp displayed a similar number of hemopoietic cells. The iron content of splenic macrophages (Fig.3) of recipients of BM incubated in anti-T cell serum was much higher than that of recipients of BM incubated in anti-lymphocyte serum. In addition, erythrophagocytosis was seen in activated macrophages. This finding indicates hemolytic anemia, which could be confirmed by the direct Coombs test: it was strongly positive in recipients of BM incubated in anti-T cell serum, whereas recipients of BM incubated in anti-lymphocyte serum were negative.

The lymph nodes of recipients of BM incubated in anti-lympho-cyte serum were also well repopulated 6 weeks after transplantation. They showed developing germinal centers in the B-lymphocyte region of the cortex and a lymphocyte-rich paracortex. In contrast, recipients of BM incubated in anti-T cell serum showed expanded T cell areas, with activated macrophages, hemophagocytosis, and immuno-blasts. These findings also strongly suggest an ongoing GVHR.

CONCLUSION

The experiments presented here show that elimination of mature T cells from BM could not prevent GVHR after transplantation in fully (not only semi-) allogeneic, lethally irradiated recipient rats. A severe, but delayed and modified type of GVHR was suggested by (a) the fatal outcome of BM transplantation, (b) the described histological evidence of GVHR, and (c) Coombs-positive hemolytic anemia. In contrast to previous results obtained after short-term incubation of donor BM in anti-lymphocyte serum, eliminating all lymphoid cells in BM, the intervening GVHR in these experiments prevented the repopulation of lymphoid tissue, especially of the thymus.

Recent findings of Bevan (2) and Zinkernagel et al (7,8) sug-gested that in certain semi-allogeneic mouse models the thymic microenvironment is of great importance for the recognition of H2-self and associated antigens. Our findings indicate, however, that functional recognition of MHA is already irreversibly determined at the stage of prethymic precursor cells in rat BM. The results obtained with anti-lymphocyte serum for BM incubation, which eliminated all lymphoid cells, suggest that the step of self-tolerization occurs during early differentiation processes of the pluripotent hemopoietic stem cell to (T and B) lymphoid precursor cells. Differences in the MHA between lymphoid cells and the stable

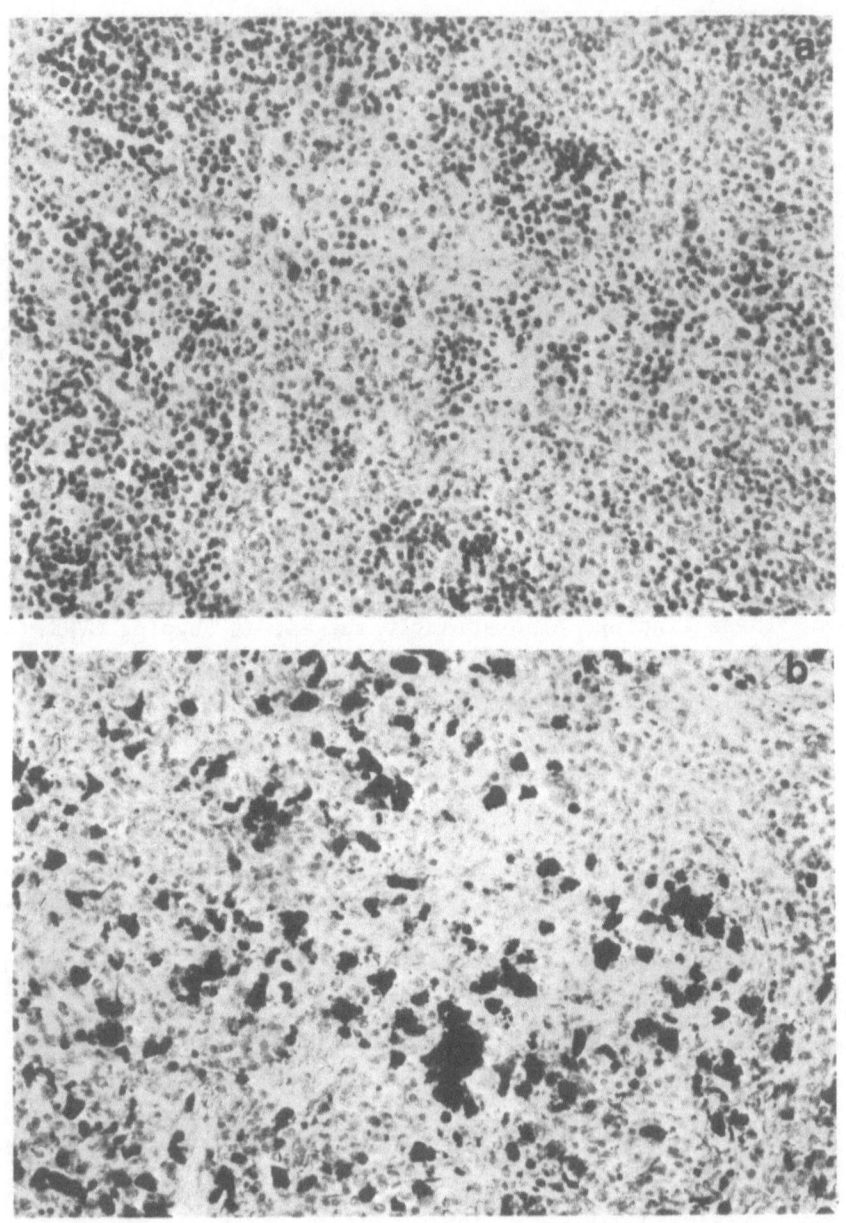

FIG. 3:   Demonstration of iron content in the spleens of lethally
irradiated rats, 6 weeks after treatment with allogeneic bone marrow
(BM). (a) BM incubated in anti-lymphocyte serum: macrophages of
white pulp contain almost no or only few iron particles. (b) BM
incubated in anti-T cell serum: increased iron content (black
patches) is a sign of GVHR-induced hemolytic anemia. Berlin blue
reaction, X 64.

microenvironment after this step of differentiation lead to the induction of severe GVHR. The presence of recognition structures on early lymphoid precursors, as demonstrated for prethymic precursor cells in rat BM by our experiments, has also been shown in early differentiating B cell precursors in neonatal mice (1).

The dependence of differentiation processes on identity between differentiating cells and microenvironment is peculiar to the lymphoid compartment, since differentiation of other hemopoietic cell systems (e.g., granulopoiesis and erythropoiesis) was not impaired in the allogeneic milieu.

Thus, establishment of long-lasting lymphoid chimerism by BM transplantation in the adult appears to require the elimination of all lymphocytes, including the prethymic precursors, from donor BM, so that the offspring of the pluripotent hemopoietic stem cell can adapt themselves within and become immunotolerant to an environment with different MHA.

REFERENCES

1. Accolla, R.S., Gearhart, P.J., Sigal, N.J., Cancro, M.P., Klinman, N.R. Eur. J. Immunol. 7 (1977) 876.
2. Bevan, M.J. Nature 269 (1977) 417.
3. Müller-Ruchholtz, W., Wottge, H.-U., Müller-Hermelink, H.K. Transplant. Proc. 8 (1976) 537.
4. Rodt, H., Thierfelder, S., Eulitz, M. Blut 25 (1972) 385.
5. Rodt, H., Thierfelder, S., Eulitz, M. Europ. J. Immunol. 4 (1974) 25.
6. Thierfelder, S., Rodt, H. Transplantation 23 (1977) 87.
7. Zinkernagel, R.M., Callahan, G.N., Althage, A., Cooper, S., Klein, P.A., Klein, J. J. Exp. Med. 147 (1978) 882.
8. Zinkernagel, R.M., Callahan, G.N., Althage, A., Cooper, S., Streilein, J.W., Klein, J. J. Exp. Med. 147 (1978) 897.

SURVIVAL AND IMMUNOLOGICAL RESPONSIVENESS OF RAT-MOUSE BONE MARROW CHIMERAS

H.-U. Wottge, H.K. Müller-Hermelink[1], and W. Müller-Ruchholtz

Dept. of Immunology/Institute of Hygiene and [1]Dept. of Pathology, University of Kiel, Kiel, W. Germany

Successful bone marrow transplantation (BMT) in an allogeneic donor-recipient combination can be achieved by eliminating all lymphocytes from donor BM. Our group has presented data showing that this, using a selectively lymphocytotoxic antiserum, leads to permanent hemopoietic chimerism without GVHR and to subsequent selective acceptance of skin grafts in a strongly and fully allogeneic rat strain combination (1,2). To determine whether the efficiency of this BM treatment is peculiar to the chosen model or whether its success is based on a more general principle, we tried to apply our protocol to a xenogeneic system with rats as donors and mice as recipients of BM.

MATERIAL AND METHODS

Animals: Twelve week old female C3H mice were used as recipients and irradiated with 950 rads from a ^{60}Co source. CAP rats were BM donors. Balb/c mice were donors of control skin grafts. Anti-lymphocyte-serum preparation and bone marrow treatment was done as described previously (1,3). Cellular chimerism was tested with a lymphocytotoxic mouse-anti-CAP-rat-serum in trypan blue dye exclusion test.

RESULTS

The first question to be answered was how long do lethally irradiated mice survive after treatment with bone marrow. As shown in Fig.1 most recipients of untreated BM died within 3 weeks, only

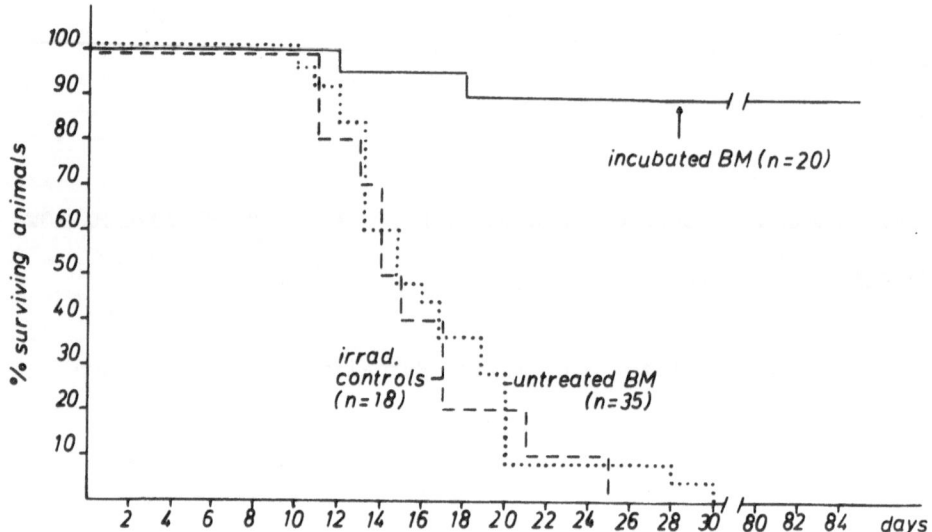

FIG. 1:   Comparison of survival rates of lethally irradiated C3H
mice after transplantation of differently treated CAP rat BM.

few survived longer and could be evaluated histologically. Recipient
mice of incubated BM survived the whole observation period (now 16
weeks).   The early death of some recipients of this group was caused
by untreated infections.

     The cause of death of recipients of untreated BM was GVHR. This
is shown in Fig.2. The thymus is atrophic and only few lymphocytes
can be seen in perivascular areas.   In lymph nodes the T-dependent
area is lymphocyte-deprived but activated macrophages are visible,
characteristically indicating GVHR.   In contrast the thymus of
recipients of incubated BM shows normal restitution with clearly
defined cortex and medulla.   Lymph nodes are repopulated normally
and germinal centers can be seen.

     The second question concerned lymphatic chimerism in the recip-
ients of incubated xenogeneic BM, as tested by cytotoxic mouse-
anti-rat lymphocyte-serum. The results are presented in Tab.1.   The
various tissues showed presence of BM donor cells. These preliminary
data, however, should be considered as lower limit figures because of
some remaining methodological problems.

     The third question concerned the immunological competence of
restituted animals, as tested by grafting skin of an H-2 incompatible

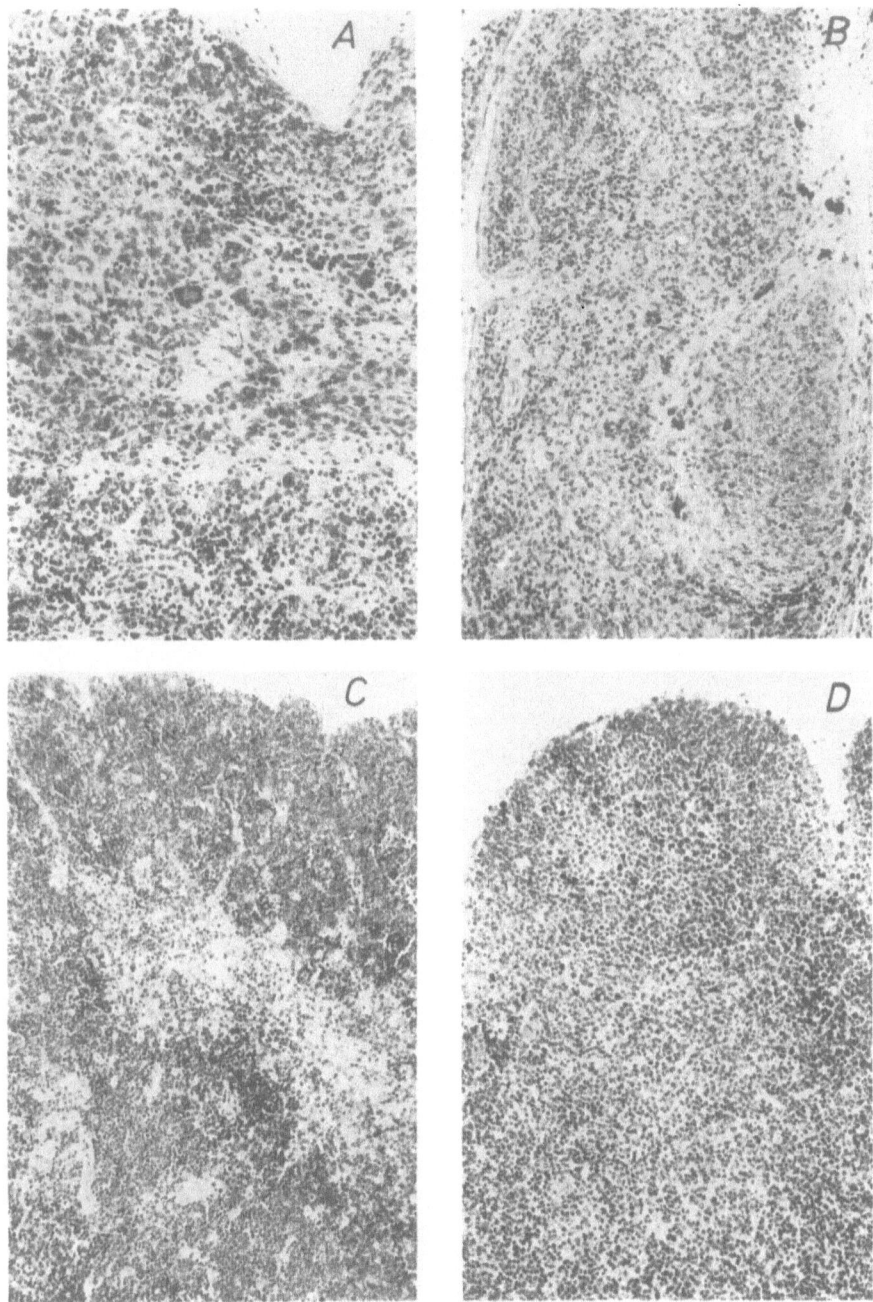

FIG. 2: Histology of thymus and lymph nodes of C3H recipients of untreated CAP BM (A,B) or of ALS-treated CAP BM (C,D) (day 42).

TAB. 1:   Percentages of donor cells (CAP rat) in xenogeneic BM
recipients (C3H mice, n = 12) tested by cytotoxic C3H-anti CAP serum.

	4 wks.	6wks.	8wks.
thymus	8 – 15	15 – 20	17 – 24
lymphnode	20 – 25	22 – 29	25 – 30
spleen	10 – 21	12 – 25	15 – 20
bone marrow	30 – 40	35 – 50	35 – 50

mouse strain 6 weeks after BM transfer. These allografts were
rejected normally (in 7 of 7 cases) compared to allografts of
normal mice (after 7-9 days). The grafting of skin of BM donor
origin was first laden with technical prolems since the nutrition
of the graft by the mouse appeared to be inadequate due to the
thickness of rat skin. This problem was solved some weeks ago by
using ear skin of the rat. These grafts appear to be visibly intact
in 12 of 12 cases throughout the forty-day observation period to
the present time.

CONCLUSIONS

     The manipulation of BM stem cells is an attractive approach to
influence the immunological responsiveness of an adult organism. As
mentioned it had been shown earlier in a strongly and fully allogeneic rat model that a lethally irradiated recipient was repopulated
by allogeneic BM freed from GVHR-inducing lymphocytes and their
precursors and that a roughly 50% chimerism was established concurrent with selective nonreactivity against BM donor skin. The
lymphatic offspring differentiating from the undamaged transferred
stem cells apparently adapted itself to the new surrounding. These
phenomena are now confirmed in the xenogeneic rat-mouse system
investigated, indicating that BM transplantation can be successfully
achieved not only across allogeneic histocompatibility barriers, but

even into a xenogeneic system, using the above procedure. The acute and lethal GVHR seen in recipients of untreated BM demonstrates clearly that the xenogeneic histocompatibility barriers are not weaker than the allogeneic, although the involvement of histocompatibility antigens different from the MHC cannot be excluded.

ACKNOWLEDGEMENTS

The authors wish to acknowledge the generosity of Prof. Gremmel for providing the facilities within his clinic to irradiate experimental animals, and the expert technical assistance of Mrs. Ch. Gronau.

REFERENCES

1. Müller-Ruchholtz, W., Wottge, H.-U., Müller-Hermelink, H.K. Transplant. Proc. 7 (1975) 859.
2. Müller-Ruchholtz, W., Wottge, H.-U., Müller-Hermelink, H.K. Transplant. Proc. 8 (1976) 537.
3. Müller-Ruchholtz, W., Wottge, H.-U., Müller-Hermelink, H.K. In: Advances in experimental medicine and biology, Vol. 66 Immune reactivity of lymphocytes p. 147 (1976).

THE CONTROL OF AUTOREACTIVE LYMPHOCYTES BY A RECEPTOR BLOCKADE

MECHANISM

John C. Roder, David A. Bell and Sharwan K. Singhal

The Dept. of Microbiology and Immunology and the Dept.
of Medicine, The University of Western Ontario
London, Ontario, Canada N6A 5C1

INTRODUCTION

The ability to discriminate self from non-self is perhaps one
of the most important biological mechanisms in the life cycle of the
vertebrates since the absence of such a mechanism would ultimately
lead to an autoimmune reaction and the subsequent death of the
organism during early stages of development. It is hoped that
investigations into the abnormal breakdown of this discrimination
during autoimmunity will lead to a clearer understanding of the
mechanisms controlling self-tolerance in normal animals and man.

Recent theories have focused on faulty immunoregulation as a
predisposing factor in the development of autoimmunity (1-4).
Defective induction or maintenance of self-tolerance could exist at
the level of the B cell (5), T cell (2) or both. Since tolerance
is transient and more difficult to achieve in B cells than in T
cells (6) most investigators have sought evidence to support the
hypothesis that a loss of tolerant or suppressor T cells allows
self-reactive B cells to respond. Several observations suggest
that active suppression may be involved in the maintenance of
tolerance to some autoantigens such as those found on erythrocytes
(1,5,7), lymphoid cell (8) or thyroglobulin (4) but other mechanisms
such as receptor blockade clearly play a role as well in preventing
autoreactivity against these (9) and other self-determinants (10-
12). In addition recent experiments with tetraparental mouse
chimaeras provides new evidence that autoreactive clones may be
eliminated during early development (13). This heterogeneity is not
unexpected since several control mechanisms (suppressor cells and
factors, receptor blockade, and clonal elimination) would clearly

have a selective advantage during evolutionary history in view of the lethal character of autoimmunity. Studies on the interaction between these various levels of control would be greatly facilitated by the development of in vitro models of autoimmunity. In the present report we summarize an in vitro system involving a loss of tolerance to DNA.

The findings suggest that many normal as well as autoimmune susceptible strains of mice possess autoantigen sensitive precursor lymphocytes, which may escape normal regulatory mechanisms in vitro and differentiate into autoantibody secreting cells. One mechanism controlling these cells may involve the suppression of B cell function by an auto-antigen mediated receptor blockade mechanism. In addition it is suggested that a re-evaluation of the general validity of the suppressor T cell theory of autoimmunity is in order since it cannot explain autoreactivity to all autoantigens.

RESULTS AND DISCUSSION

In a previous report we found that many normal (CBA, DBA, BDF, C57Bl, CFW) and autoimmune susceptible strains (NZB/NZW, Nude) of mice possess auto-reactive B cells which escape normal regulatory mechanisms in vitro and expand into clones of auto-antibody (IgM) secreting, plaque forming cells (PFC) specific for single-strand DNA (sDNA); in the absence of detectable DNA from endogenous ecotropic or xenotropic virus or from exogenous sources (10). It has recently been shown that the in vitro production of anti-thyrotrophin (TSH) receptor autoantibodies is augmented by mitogens (14) and polyclonal B cell activators may enhance the production of anti-DNA antibody in vivo (15). The anti-sDNA response reported here was also augmented by mitogens (10) but a significant response also occurred in the absence of mitogens or serum. In addition the anti-sDNA response did not require T cell or macrophage help. Although a superimmunogenic form of DNA excreted in these cultures cannot be ruled out as a potential immunogen the results suggest that the anti-sDNA response we detect in vitro represents a spontaneous loss of self-tolerance.

In the present report we have investigated the mechanisms which might control these autoreactive lymphocytes in vivo. In these experiments regulation of the anti-sDNA response may be accomplished in part by the antigen itself since the addition of small quantities of free sDNA to culture markedly inhibited the anti-sDNA response (10). As shown in Tab.1, small numbers of spleen cells were capable of specifically binding sDNA and removal of these cells prior to culture resulted in a greatly diminished anti-sDNA response on day 5. These precursors divide early in culture and can be eliminated by a "hot" thymidine, suicide technique. It seems possible therefore

TAB. 1:   Requirement for Antigen Binding Precursors and Cell
Division in the In Vitro Anti-sDNA Response.

Depletion of cells binding to[a]:	Anti-sDNA PFC/culture	% Depression	P value
-	1260+64	-	-
SRBC	1146+62	9	N.S.[b]
SRBC-sDNA	281+70	70	<.001
ficoll control	1280+21	0	N.S.
Treatment of cultures[c]			
None	610+92	-	-
Pulse	152+16	76	<.001
Pulse and block	490+24	20	<.05

[a]   Young (6 wk) B/W spleen cells were rosetted with SRBC, SRBC
coupled to sDNA or non-rosetted and then separated on ficoll-hypaque
gradients prior to culture. The number of anti-sDNA RFC/10^3
nucleated cells in the top of the gradient compared to the bottom
pellet or unseparated spleen cells were 1, 30 and 6 respectively.
Small amounts of sDNA (1.0 μg/ml) completely inhibited the formation
of anti-sDNA RFC.

[b]   N.S., non significant (p > .05).

[c]   After 24 hr, cultures marked pulse received 15 μ Ci of tritiated-
thymidine (23 Ci/mmole) and cultures marked block also received 100 μg
"cold" thymidine. After 48 hr, cultures marked only "pulse" also
received 100 μg thymidine.

that free sDNA added to culture might effectively block the expression
of these specific precursor cells by a receptor blockade mechanism
which has been proposed by others to account for certain forms of
tolerance (12,16,17). A number of observations support this hypothesis. Firstly, spleen cells incubated with sDNA for as little as one
hour and then washed extensively and cultured for 5 days, exhibited
a dose dependent depression of the anti-sDNA PFC response (Tab.2).
Secondly, the PFC response of these antigen blocked cells could be
restored to near normal levels by treatment with a combination of
DNase I and trypsin. Thirdly, most if not all receptor blockade
mechanisms have been shown to act on the B cell (12,16,17) and we
have found that macrophage depleted spleen cells from both B/W and
homozygous nude mice or adult thymectomized, lethally irradiated,
bone marrow reconstituted mice are readily suppressed by sDNA which

TAB. 2:   The Abrogation of sDNA Mediated Suppression with Trypsin
and DNase I.

Pre-treatment of spleen cells prior to culture[a]	Enzyme Treatment[b]	Anti-sDNA PFC/Culture[c]	P Value[d]
None	None	496+58	-
0.5 µg sDNA/ml, 1 hr	None	451+22	-
0.5 µg sDNA/ml, 24 hr	None	243+51	-
50.0 µg sDNA/ml, 1 hr	None	350+65	-
50.0 µg sDNA/ml, 24 hr	None	90+20	-
50.0 µg sDNA/ml, 24 hr	Trypsin (400 µg/ml)	375+39	<.001
None	Trypsin (400 µg/ml)	510+53	-

[a]   Young (6 wk) B/W spleen cells were incubated with sDNA,
harvested, treated with enzymes and placed in fresh medium for an
additional 4 days.

[b]   Cells were treated with varying concentrations of trypsin
together with a constant amount of DNase I (20 µg/ml).

[c]   Values represent the mean PFC + standard error of triplicate
or quadruplicate cultures assayed individually on day 5.

[d]   P value was compared to the group above.

suggests that the B cell might be the target of suppression in our
system as well. In addition, if sDNA-mediated suppression acted on
specific immunoglobulin receptors at the B cell surface then the
addition of small amounts of sDNA to culture should preferentially
shut off those cells possessing receptors of relatively high affinity
as predicted under the clonal selection theory (18). The PFC
remaining in these partially blocked cultures were indeed found to
be of lower avidity than PFC in unblocked cultures (Tab.3). In
addition the anti-sDNA were specific since they were not inhibited
by dsDNA or RNA.

     Another observation compatible with the receptor blockade
hypothesis was that large intact molecules of sDNA (approximately
10^7 daltons) were more effective in suppressing the anti-sDNA
response at high concentrations, than sDNA sheared into smaller
fragments (approximately 10^5 daltons) as reported previously (10).
This would be expected if receptor blockade operated by a cross-
linking of cell surface receptors since larger, polymeric molecules
would be capable of cross-linking a greater number of receptors.

TAB. 3:   The Specificity and Avidity of Anti-sDNA PFC.

Pretreatment of cultures[a]	Nucleic acid incorporated into plaquing system	Maximum % Inhibition (10 µg nucleic acid/slide)	Amount (µg) of nucleic acid required for 50% inhibition of anti-sDNA PFC
None	ssDNA (10^7 daltons)	100	0.005
	ssDNA (10^5 daltons)	100	0.01
	dsDNA (native)	17	> 50.0[b]
	RNA (3.5×10^4 daltons)	4	>50.0[b]
ssDNA	ssDNA (10^7 daltons)	94	0.2

[a]   Young B/W spleen cells were cultured 5 days in the presence or absence of 5 µg sDNA/ml. Harvested cells were assayed for anti sDNA PFC with or without varying concentrations of nucleic acid incorporated into the agarose.

[b]   The 50% inhibition level was not attained.

Although receptor blockade can explain the observations presented, it is not yet clear whether this blockade prevents B cell differentiation or rather inhibits the rate of antibody secretion as occurs in effector cell blockade (17).   It is probable that both of these mechanisms are operative since the anti-sDNA responses of cultures pulsed with sDNA and washed as early as day 1 is equally suppressed relative to cultures pulsed with sDNA as late as 4 hrs prior to assay on day 5 (10).

In addition to sDNA mediated suppression, certain cell types may also regulate the anti-sDNA response, in vitro. Thymocytes and splenic T cells but not bone marrow cells inhibited the in vitro anti-sDNA response whereas the anti-SRBC response was not suppressed (10). However, it was also found that old B/W thymocytes from overtly autoimmune mice, 7 mo of age, were equally capable of suppressing the anti-sDNA response compared to young B/W thymocytes, 6 wk of age, which suggests that a loss of suppressor T cells may not explain increasing autoreactivity to sDNA with age as proposed by others (19,20).

SUMMARY AND CONCLUSIONS

The present data together with the findings of others support the concept that autoreactive lymphocytes exist in normal individuals

TAB. 4:   The Cellular Target of sDNA Mediated Suppression.

Spleen Cell Source	Treatment of spleen cells prior to culture[a]	5 µg sDNA per culture	Anti-sDNA PFC/Culture	% Inhibition
B/W	None	−	800+63	−
B/W	None	+	500+30	38
B/W	Carbonyl iron	−	750+51	−
B/W	Carbonyl iron	+	200+25	74
B/W (ATxBM)[b]	None	−	910+90	−
B/W (ATxBM)[b]	None	+	591+46	36
homozygous nude	None	−	570+23	−
homozygous nude	None	+	325+41	43
homozygous nude	Carbonyl iron	−	550+16	−
homozygous nude	Carbonyl iron	+	218+35	61

[a]   Spleen cells were untreated or treated with carbonyl iron and a magnet to remove macrophages and then cultured 5 days with or without sDNA added.

[b]   Mice were adult thymectomized, lethally irradiated and reconstituted with 2×10^7 bone marrow cells alone or together with 10^8 thymocytes, 3 weeks prior to culture.

as well as those destined to develop overt manifestations of auto-immunity. Under the in vitro conditions described here, these autoreactive cells may differentiate into clones of autoantibody secreting lymphocytes. One mechanism controlling these cells may involve specific B cell inhibition by a receptor blockade mechanism. Further work is necessary to elucidate the relationship between these cellular and humoral controls.

REFERENCES

1.   Cunningham, A.J., Transpl. Rev. 31 (1976) 23.
2.   Bretscher, P., Hypothesis: Cellular Immunol. 6 (1973) 1.
3.   Allison, A.C., In "Immunological Tolerance: Mechanisms and Potential Therapeutic Applications". (Katz, D.H., Benacerraf, B., eds). Academic Press Inc. N.Y. p. 25 (1974).
4.   Rose, N.R., Bacon, L.D., Sundick, R.S., Transplant. Rev. 31 (1976) 264.
5.   DeHeer, D.H., Edgington, T.S., Transpl. Rev. 31 (1976) 23.

6.   Chiller, J.M., Weigle, W.O., Contemp. Topics Immunobiol. 1
     (1972) 119.
7.   Steinberg, A.D., Law, L.W., Talal, N., Arthritis Rheum. 13
     (1970) 369.
8.   L'Age-Stehr, J., Diamantstein, T., Nature 271 (1978) 663.
9.   Lord, E.K., Dutton, R.W., J. Immunol. 115 (1975) 1631.
10. Roder, J.C., Bell, D.A., Singhal, S.K., J. Immunol. (in press)
     (1978).
11. Borel, Y., Transpl. Rev. 31 (1976) 3.
12. Aldo-Benson, M., Borel, Y., J. Immunol. 116 (1976) 223.
13. Barnes, R.D., Wills, E.J., Lancet 20 (1976).
14. McLachlan, S.M., Smith, B.R., Petersen, V.B., Davies, T.F.,
     Hall, F., Nature 270 (1977) 447.
15. Izui, S., Kobayakawa, T., Zryd, M., Louis, J., Lambert, P.H.,
     J. Immunol. 119 (1977) 2157.
16. Klaus, G.G.B., Eur. J. Immunol. 6 (1976) 389.
17. Schrader, J.W., Nossal, G.J.V., J. Exp. Med. 139 (1974) 1582.
18. Siskind, G.W., Benacerraf, B., Adv. Immunol. 10 (1969) 1.
19. Allison, A.C., Denman, A.M., Br. Med. Bul. 32 (1976) 124.
20. Steinberg, A.D., Gerber, N.L., Gershwin, M.E., Morton, R.,
     Goodman, D., Chused, T.M., Hardin, J.A., Barthold, D.R.,
     In "Suppressor Cells in Immunity". (Singhal, S.K., Sinclair,
     N.R., eds.). Univ. of Western Ont. Press, London, Canada,
     p. 174 (1975).

STIMULATION OF NATURAL ANTIBODIES BY SELF ANTIGENS

E.J. Steele and A.J. Cunningham

Ontario Cancer Institute

500 Sherbourne Street, Toronto, Canada M4X 1K9

INTRODUCTION

The lymphoid organs of normal mice contain numerous background plaque forming cells specific for buried self antigens on mouse erythrocytes revealed by treatment with the proteolytic enzyme bromelain (1,2). We have documented elsewhere (3) the extent of this reactivity by measuring the number of B cells making αBrM antibody to the total number of B cells producing immuno-globulin (Ig) irrespective of specificity. The proportion of αBrM reactive B cells is very high – depending on the organ examined between 1% to > 50% of the ongoing or potential Ig secreting cells are BrM specific. This result is probably not unique. There are many reports showing that autoantibodies are a common occurrence in normal healthy individuals and include those specific for "buried" or "enzyme revealed" antigens on erythrocytes and lymphocytes, Ig molecules and reproductive organs (2,3). These facts have led us to suggest that much of the "natural" Ig synthesis of an animal is directed towards buried self components (3). Rather than deleting immuno-competent cells autoantigens of this type (at least) seem to prime them, contributing to the development of the immune repertoire. This paper documents the very significant effect which the BrM auto-antigen has on the developing immune system.

MATERIALS AND METHODS

CBA/J mice and outbred Swiss mice reared under conventional or germ free conditions were used. Haemolytic plaque assays (PFC) for antibody forming cells were determined (4) using as indicators,

TAB. 1:   Composition of background PFC specificities in different lymphoid organs of the mouse[a].

		Ig PFC per 10^6 cultured cells[b]	%Ig PFC with specificity for		
			BrM	S	S-TNP
	Foetal liver[c]	$50-5\times10^2$	<0.2	<0.2	13
	Neonatal spleen[d]	10^3-10^4	≤0.1	≤0.1	4.8
8-10 wk ♀	Spleen	2×10^4	1.4	0.1	1.9
	Thymus	10^2-10^3	2	<1	21
	Peyer's Patches	2×10^3	2.2	n.t.	3.5
	Peritoneal cells	10^4	36	n.t.	1.8
8-10 wk pregnant ♀	Spleen	2×10^4	0.3	0.2	1.2
	Thymus	4×10^3	0.7	1	36
	Peyer's Patches	2×10^3	<0.1	<0.1	5
	Peritoneal cells	10^4	87	<0.1	5.4
Outbred Swiss spleens	− Conventional	10^4	0.8	n.t.	3.1
	− Germ free	10^4	0.7	n.t.	2.2

[a]   Results summarized from 10 experiments. Outbred Swiss mice, conventional and germ free, obtained from Sprague Dawley. All other mice CBA/J obtained direct from Jackson Labs. or bred at the O.C.I.

[b]   Approx. numbers given with Log_{10} range where appropriate. All PFC assays in a given experiment determined at least on duplicate cultures.

[c]   Foetal livers days 17-18 gestation cultured for 3-5 days in presence 50 µg LPS. All other organs cultured with 10 µg LPS: 3 days for spleen, Peyer's patches and peritoneal cells and 4-5 days for thymus.

[d]   Neonatal spleens, ages ranging from newborn to 5 days.

bromelain treated mouse erythrocytes (BrM, 1), sheep erythrocytes (S) and trinitrophenylated S (S-TNP, 5). Total Ig secreting B cells (Ig PFC) were determined by a reverse plaque method (6) using S coated with sheep anti-mouse Ig and PFC developed with a rabbit anti-mouse Ig serum. Control experiments using class specific anti-Ig developers showed that most of the Ig PFC at the times assayed were due to IgM secretors (>70%). All "background" PFCs were determined after 3-5 days of culture in the presence of LPS - a poly-clonal B cell activator (7). Background PFC appearing in culture with LPS are termed "potential" antibody forming cells to distinguish from "ongoing" Ig secretors present in freshly collected lymphoid

TAB. 2:   Materials specifically absorbing mouse αBrM antibody.

Absorbing Material		HL titre (Log$_2$)*		Absorbing Material	HL titre (Log$_2$)	
		α BrM	αHrbc		αBrM	αHrbc
NIL		5.3	5.3	Foetal Stomach	5.5	5
BrM		<1	5.7	FS - pH4	4	5
Hrbc		4	<1	FS - Pepsin/pH4	<1	5
Mrbc		5	5	Ground Food Pellets	5	5
Mrbc - pH4		4	5.3	GFP - bromelain	6	n.t.
Mrbc - Pepsin/pH4		4	4	GFP - pH4	5	5
Stomach	Conventional	<1	5.6	GFP - Pepsin/pH4	5	4.5
	Germ free	<1	5.5			

*   Titres after two absorptions.

tissues (see 3). Cultures were 1 ml in plastic tubes (12 x 75 mm, Falcon, Oxnard, Ca., U.S.A.) containing 2-5 x 10^6 lymphoid cells, 10-50 µg LPS (from E. coli 0128:B12, Difco), 5 x 10^{-5} M 2-Mercapto-ethanol in α MEM medium plus 10% (v/v) foetal calf serum.

The naturally occurring "in vivo form" of the BrM antigen was searched for by a serological absorption assay using a high titre mouse αBrM serum (obtained from CBA/J mice stimulated 10 days previously with 50 µg LPS i.p.). Material for use in the absorption test was washed three times, mixed with the serum (1 volume to 5 volumes of serum) and placed at 4°C for 15 minutes. After centri-fugation the serum was usually absorbed again (Tab.1). The anti-BrM haemolytic titre (HL) was determined by diluting the serum serially in 2 fold steps and BrM erythrocytes and complement added. Titres were read after 1 hr at 37°C. For titration of the absorbing capacity of stomach of mice of different ages, 4 HL doses of mouse αBrM were abosrbed once with washed homogenized stomach ranging from 20% (v/v) to 0.16% (v/v). Absorbing capacity was expressed as the reciprocal of that amount of packed stomach causing 50% inhibi-tion of lysis.

RESULTS AND DISCUSSION

The antigenic history of B cells in normal animals is likely to be reflected in the proportions of lymphocytes making antibody of different specificities either at the time of sacrifice or after

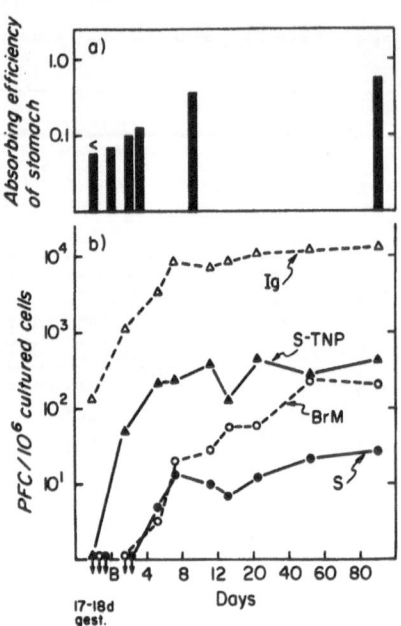

FIG. 1:   Ontogeny background PFC and BrM antigen.   (A)   Relative
absorbing efficiency of stomach from pools of mice of the ages
shown.   (B)   Background PFC determined day 3 of culture with 10 µg
LPS, on pooled spleens of mice of the ages shown.   Cultures contained
5×10^6 viable cells at day 0.

short term culture with a mitogen.   If the BrM antigen is an important stimulator we would expect a high proportion of the Ig produced
to be BrM specific.   As mentioned above, this seems to be the case
(Introduction and 3).   Recent results are shown in Tab.1.   It is
clear that a high proportion of Ig PFC are $\propto$BrM, especially in
peritoneal cell cultures (36-87%).   Note also that germ free mice
contain a similar proportion of $\propto$BrM PFC in their spleens ($\sim$1%)
as do their non-germ free controls - showing that $\propto$BrM background
PFC (and total Ig PFC) do not arise from chronic stimulation by
antigens of the normal microbial flora (see also 1,2).   In addition
background PFC against S are low in all tissues - 1/10 of the BrM
PFC level.

      As a comparison and control for BrM PFC we also determined the
numbers and organ distribution of background PFC against S-TNP -
commonly thought of as a non-specific indicator of Ig secretion
(Tab.1).   S-TNP reveals numerous PFC - which appear early in ontogeny
before $\propto$BrM or $\propto$S PFC (see also Fig.1) - ranging from relatively
low in some organs (e.g. peritoneum) to high in foetal liver, neonatal spleen (5-10%, c.f., 8) and very high in thymus (21-36%). These
interesting patterns suggest an influence of self antigens (although

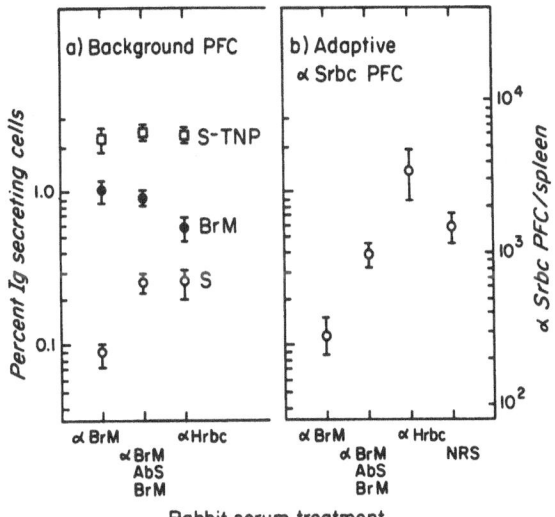

FIG. 2:   Effect of ∝BrM serum on the early B cell repertoire.
Serum was given at birth (10 µl and 20 µl per mouse i.p. for (a)
and (b) respectively). At day 10 individual mice were examined for
(a) background PFC: 5 x 10^6 spleen cells cultured for 3 days with
10 µg LPS,   (b) ∝Srbc response in spleen 4 days after challenge
with 0.1 ml 10% Srbc i.p. Arithmetic mean $\pm$ S.E.M. of 4-5 mice.

no formal proof is yet available that S-TNP mimic a self immunogen).
The fact that the numbers of ∝BrM and ∝S-TNP PFC vary widely in
ontogeny and between organs argues that they are not simply "non-
specific acceptors" for the same constant total of the Ig produced
(i.e. they detect two specific high frequency B cell subsets).

An attempt was made to look for the target organ(s) within the
mouse which contain the antigen(s) likely to stimulate anti-BrM PFC.
In this survey we used a quantitative absorption assay testing a
range of mouse tissues for their ability to specifically absorb
∝BrM haemolytic antibody. Two controls for specificity and possible
artifacts in the complement sources were included in the tests. Both
rabbit and guinea pig serum were used as complement sources. As a
specificity (and anti-complementary) control a primary CBA ∝ -horse
erythrocyte (Hrbc) serum was admixed with the CBA ∝ BrM serum to
give about the same HL titre as ∝BrM (Tab.2). Our first thought
was that artificially aged mouse erythrocytes should absorb ∝BrM.
These tests were negative. Various other organs were then tried
including heart, lung, liver, kidney, spleen, thymus, bone marrow,

peritoneal cells, testes, ovaries and brain – none of these showed
any consistent specific absorbing capacity. We finally tested
gastrointestinal tissues – these proved to be very active in specif-
cally removing αBrM antibody (stomach, small intestine and upper
large intestine all had this effect). Representative positive
results using washed homogenates of stomach, with the appropriate
controls, are displayed in Tab.2. It can be seen that (a) the BrM
antigen is associated with stomachs taken from conventional or germ
free mice – excluding the normal microbial flora as a source of the
antigen; (b) foetal stomach lacks the BrM antigen, but will express
it on a serologically detectable form if first treated with pepsin
and (c) ground food pellets treated or not with proteolytic enzymes
(bromelain, pepsin) show no absorbing capacity, making it unlikely
that food contains appreciable amounts of the antigen. These
results suggest that the naturally occurring form of the BrM
autoantigen appears after birth either as a result of some change
in the antigenic constitution of the gut or as a consequence of
normal enzymatic digestive processes acting on self components of
the gastrointestinal tract..

The ontogeny of the "BrM-gut" antigen as well as background
PFCs in spleen are compared in Fig.1. These results show that
both the naturally occurring form of the BrM antigen and the antibody response to BrM appear in ontogeny at about the same time
(i.e. within the first week of life). Note also that αS PFC emerge
about the same time as αBrM PFC and plateau at their adult levels
by day 7. BrM PFC however continue rising in number reaching adult
levels by 3-6 weeks.

An important question is whether the BrM-gut antigen, which
appears early in ontogeny, has any role in stimulating the development of cells reactive to foreign antigens? As our foreign antigen
we selected sheep erythrocytes. This was chosen because as it is
well documented that Srbc and BrM cross-react to varying degrees at
both the B and T cell levels (9-12) – this cross-reactivity is
particularly marked in those PFC appearing in peritoneal cell
cultures (9; Steele and Cunningham, unpublished). An additional
reason for choosing Srbc lay in the similar emergence kinetics of
αBrM and αS background PFC early in ontogeny (Fig.1b), suggesting
that αS PFC could be induced and/or controlled by the response to
the early appearing BrM-gut antigen (Fig.1a). This idea was tested
by treating newborn mice with rabbit anti-BrM serum (absorbed with
spleen, thymus and normal mouse erythrocytes). At day 10 of life
mice were examined for background PFC in spleen and their ability
to mount a response to sheep erythrocytes on in vivo challenge with
antigen (Fig.2). Control sera were normal rabbit serum (NRS) or
rabbit anti-horse rbc (αHrbc). It can be seen that Rb αBrM
depresses αS PFC backgrounds as well as the adaptive αS response
to antigen (3-5 fold). Both effects are removed by pre-absorbing

the serum with BrM, demonstrating a connection between two specificities, BrM and the capacity to respond to Srbc.

The main findings of this paper concern the high proportion of
Ig secreting cells which are BrM specific and the possibility that
the response to BrM plays a role in the development of the immune
repertoire. The results argue against the idea that all anti-self
reactive cells are deleted early in ontogeny, at least for this
class of self antigens. Instead the BrM-gut type self antigens
appear to play a positive role in priming the immune system (although
it is not proved that the gut antigen actually does the priming).
The concept that early B cells are positively educated to immune
competence by self components may be analogous to the observations
on the development of immune competence in T cells (13,14), one
interpretation of which is that T cell anti-self specificities are
acquired in ontogeny (13-15). In this case the relevant educating
self determinants appear to be MHC encoded antigens expressed in
thymus (14). For B cells, the educating antigens may be more
diffuse and less anatomically restricted. One important source may
be gut associated self components subjected to normal digestive
processes - resurrecting the idea of the gastrointestinal tract as
a mammalian equivalent of the avian Bursa of Fabricius. Another
source could be determinants on isologous Ig (16) possibly serving
an important stimulating role in network development (17).

REFERENCES

1.   Cunningham, A.J. Nature 252 (1974) 749.
2.   Cunningham, A.J. Transplant. Rev. 31 (1976) 33.
3.   Steele, E.J., Cunningham, A.J. Nature, in press (1978).
4.   Cunningham, A.J., Szenberg, A. Immunology 14 (1968) 599.
5.   Rittenberg, M.B., Pratt, K.L. Proc. Soc. Exp. Biol. Med. 132
     (1969) 575.
6.   Molinaro, G.A., Dray, S. Nature 248 (1974) 515.
7.   Möller, G. Transplant. Rev. 23 (1975) 126.
8.   Melchers, F., Anderson, J., Phillips, R.A. Cold Spring Harbor
     Symposium Quant. Biol. 41 (1977) 147.
9.   Pages, J., Bussard, A.E. Nature 257 (1975) 316.
10. Lord, E.M., Dutton, R.W. J. Immunol. 115 (1975) 1199.
11. Lord, E.M., Dutton, R.W. J. Immunol. 115 (1975) 1631.
12. Ramshaw, I.A., Eidinger, D. Nature 267 (1977) 441.
13. Bevan, M.J. Nature 269 (1977) 417.
14. Zinkernagel, R.M., Callahan, G.M., Klein, J., Dennert, G.
     Nature 271 (1978) 251.
15. Jerne, N.K. Eur. J. Immunol. 1 (1971) 1.
16. Dresser, D. Nature, in press (1978).
17. Jerne, N.K. Ann. Immunol. (Inst. Pasteur). 125C (1974) 373.

ACKNOWLEDGEMENTS

    The authors thank Dr. Reginald Gorczynski for stimulating
discussions, Marion Kennedy and Pat Heard for excellent technical
assistance and Freda Sochasky for her patience in preparing the
manuscript. This work was supported by the Canadian Medical Research
Council and by the National Cancer Institute of Canada.

THE ROLE OF ANTIGEN-ANTIBODY COMPLEXES IN GENERATING IMMUNOLOGICAL MEMORY AND AUTO-ANTIIDIOTYPIC IMMUNITY

G.G.B. Klaus

National Institute for Medical Research

Mill Hill, London NW7, U.K.

Considerable evidence has accumulated within recent years indicating that germinal centres are sites of B cell proliferation, and are probably the birthplace of B memory (B_M) cells (1). In addition, it is well-established that lymphoid follicles trap antigen-antibody complexes, which remain bound to follicular dendritic cells for long periods (2).

ROLE OF IMMUNE COMPLEXES AND C3 IN B_M DEVELOPMENT

We have been attempting to analyse the events that lead to B_M development in the germinal centre. Initially, we showed (3) that chronic C3 depletion of mice abrogated not only the antibody (Ab)-dependent localization of antigen (Ag) in lymphoid follicles, but also the generation of B_M cells (i.e. cells committed to make a secondary IgG response). This suggested that the development of B_M cells required the C3-dependent deposition of Ag-Ab complexes in lymphoid follicles, thus providing an Ag-specific B cell trap within the follicles (4).

Subsequent experiments showed that pre-formed immune complexes of dinitrophenylated-haemocyanin (DNP-KLH) with mouse anti-DNP or anti-KLH Ab were at least 100-fold more effective in priming B_M cells than soluble DNP-KLH, and at least as effective as Ag in conventional adjuvant (5). Optimal priming required complexes at equivalence or in Ag excess. The adjuvant effect was totally C3-dependent and operationally T cell-independent. Optimal priming required the integrity of the Fc portion of the Ab, although $F(ab')_2$ complexes

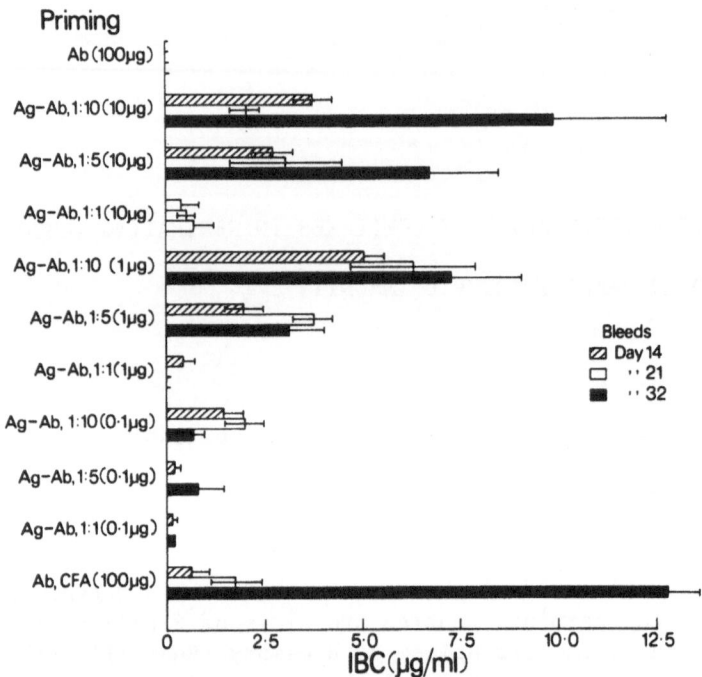

FIG. 1: Dose-response for the induction of autoantibodies to M315 by DNP-KLH-M315 complexes. BALB/c mice were given 0.1 - 10 µg DNP-KLH in complex with M315 (w/w ratios given) i.v. or M315 in Freund's complete adjuvant i.p. on Day 0. On day 21 all groups were boosted with 100 µg purified M315 i.p. IBC = idiotype-binding capacity, determined by double antibody radioimmunoassay.

were also effective. Finally, as predicted, complexes generated memory more rapidly than Ag in adjuvant.

IMMUNE COMPLEXES AND ANTI-IDIOTYPIC IMMUNITY

We reasoned that if Ab was so effective in generating memory to the Ag, perhaps it would also enhance auto-anti-idiotypic antibody formation. Preliminary studies have supported this concept (6). The Ab used in these experiments was M315, an IgA myeloma protein of BALB/c mice with anti-DNP antibody activity. BALB/c mice were injected intravenously with various doses of DNP-KLH-M315 complexes

TAB. 1:   Coexistence of anti-hapten and anti-idiotypic memory in mice primed with Ag-Ab complexes.

Priming[a]	Boost[b]	Indirect PFC/spleen: [c] Anti-DNP:	Anti-M315:
Ag-Ab (1:10)	Ag-Ab (1:10)	6,200	2,000
Ag-Ab (1:10)	Ag-Ab (1:5)	9,400	900
Ag-Ab (1:5)	Ag/Ab (1:10)	7,800	1,400
Ag-Ab (1:5)	Ag-Ab (1:5)	8,500	1,200
Ag-Ab (1:1)	Ag-Ab (1:10)	9,700	500
Ag-Ab (1:1)	Ag-Ab (1:5)	16,000	200
Ag	Ag-Ab (1:10)	1,100	50
Ag	Ag-Ab (1:5)	500	25

[a]   Groups of 4 BALB/c mice given 10 ug DNP_{172}-KLH-M315 complexes (Ag-Ab) (w/w ratio in brackets) i.v. on Day 0. Dose refers to amount of Ag given.

[b]   10 ug Ag-Ab given i.v. on day 21.

[c]   Assayed 5 days after boosting.

prepared at w/w ratios of Ag-Ab 1:1, 1:5 (equivalence) and 1:10. Three weeks later they were boosted with soluble M135. Fig.1 shows that 10 µg Ag-M315 in Ab excess elicited comparable anti-M315 antibody titres to 100 µg M315 in complete Freund's adjuvant. Even 100 ng Ag-M315 (1:10) induced a significant response. Complexes prepared at equivalence were less immunogenic, while those in Ag excess were essentially non-immunogenic. The idiotypic (Id) specificity of these antibodies has been described (6). BALB/c mice given purified M315 in adjuvant respond almost exclusively to idiotopes associated with the ligand-binding site of the antibody (7). However, mice given immune complexes respond to both site-associated and non site-associated idiotopes (6). The proportion of site-directed antibodies increases with increasing Ab-Ag ratio (not shown).

One might predict that Ag-Ab complexes would simultaneously prime for an antibody and an anti-Id response. Tab.1 shows the results of priming mice with complexes prepared at various ratios, following by boosting with Ag-Ab and assays for both anti-M315 and anti-DNP plaque-forming cells. All groups produced an anti-DNP IgG response, regardless of the Ag-Ab ratio used for priming. However, those primed with complexes in Ab excess also made a concurrent anti-M315 response.

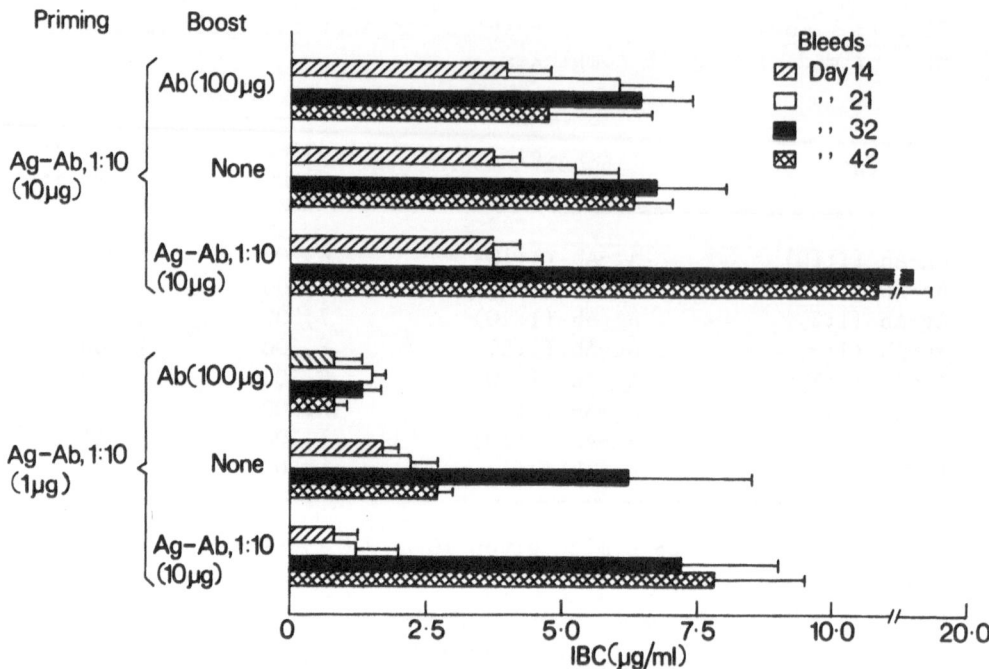

<u>FIG. 2</u>:   Effects of boosting with M315 or with DNP-KLH-M315
complexes. BALB/c mice were given 1 or 10 μg DNP-KLH-M315
complexes i.v. on day 0 (1:10 w/w ratio). On day 21 they were
boosted with either 100 μg M315 (Ab) or 10 μg DNP-KLH-M315 (Ag-Ab)
i.v. or nothing. IBC = idiotype-binding capacity (μg/ml serum).

An important question was whether DNP-KLH-M315 complexes
localized in lymphoid follicles, since M315 is an IgA antibody. We
have shown that they do (although rather weakly). This is presumably because M315 activates the alternative pathway of mouse C (in
preparation).

More recently, we have examined the nature of the lymphocyte
cooperation involved in the anti-Id response. Mice immunized with
isologous myeloma proteins have been shown to produce anti-Id T
helper (T_H) cells (8,9) which could presumably cooperate with anti-
Id B cells. Fig.2 shows the effects of priming mice with antigen-
M315 complexes, followed by a boost on day 21 with Ag-Ab, M315 or
nothing. It is evident that M315 boosted and unboosted groups had
very similar antibody titres on days 21 and 32, whereas those
boosted with Ag-Ab gave a true secondary response. In other words,
the increase in antibody titres in Fig.1 represents a slow primary
response.

TAB. 2:   Cooperation between anti-idiotypic B cells and antigen-specific T cells.

B cells primed with:[a]	KLH-primed spleen cells:[b]	Boost:[c]	IBC (μg/ml)[d]
Ag–Ab	+	Ag–Ab	43.3
Ag–Ab	+	Ab	0.36
Ag–Ab	–	Ag–Ab	2.0
Nothing	+	Ag–Ab	1.75

[a]   From BALB/c mice primed with 10 μg DNP-bovine serum albumin-M315 complexes (1:10 w/w Ag-Ab) 3 weeks previously and treated with anti-Thy 1.2 and C prior to transfer.

[b]   From mice given 100 μg alum-adsorbed KLH plus 10^9 B. pertussis 3 weeks previously.

[c]   20 x 10^6 of cells indicated transferred to irradiated (400R) mice boosted with 10 μg DNP-KLH-M315 (1:5) or 50 μg M315.

[d]   Idiotype binding capacity of recipient sera 10 days post transfer, determined by radioimmunoassay.

In the experiment in Tab.2 irradiated mice were given B cells from mice primed with Ag-Ab complexes, KLH primed spleen cells (as a source of T_H), and were either boosted with DNP-KLH-M315 complexes, or with M315. This combination of cells, when boosted with Ag-Ab gave a strong anti-Id response, while boosting with M315 alone was ineffective. Thus, KLH-specific T_H cells can cooperate with anti-M315 B cells to give an anti-Id response to immune complexes. It is not yet clear if this is the only form of cell cooperation which occurs in mice given complexes. Earlier experiments (5) suggested that complexes did not generate T_H as effectively as Ag in adjuvant. This is supported by more recent results (not shown) which demonstrate that priming mice with KLH (on alum) followed by priming and boosting with DNP-KLH-M315 substantially increases anti-Id antibody titres.

DISCUSSION

These results support the concept that Ag-Ab complexes (and C3) play a central regulatory role in the establishment of immunological memory to antigenic determinants and perhaps also to idiotypic determinants of the antibody. We assume that memory for both responses is initially established by similar mechanisms, commencing with follicular localization of complexes and followed by trapping of relevant B lymphocytes in the follicle.

The demonstration that immune complexes can readily generate auto-anti-Id responses is particularly relevant to network concepts of immunoregulation (10). Although it has been clearly shown that idiotypes are autoimmunogenic (11-13), the induction of autoanti-bodies to purified antibody generally requires hyperimmunizytion using potent adjuvants. For anti-idiotypic immunity to bear any relevance to homeostasis of the immune system, there must be a mechanism to render self-idiotypes autoimmunogenic during the course of an immune response. The generation of immune complexes provides such a mechanism. In addition, the finding that anti-idiotypic B cells can cooperate with antigen-specific T cells provides a further attractive mechanism for introducing auto-antiidiotypic immunity, since it bypasses the requirement for anti-idiotypic T cells.

REFERENCES

1. Thorbecke, G.J., Lerman, S.P.,in: The Reticuloendothelial System in Health and Disease (Reichard, Escobar and Friedman, eds) p.83 New York: Plenum Press (1976).
2. Nossal, G.J.V., Ada, G.L., Antigens, Lymphoid cells and the Immune Response. New York: Academic Press (1971).
3. Klaus, G.G.B., Humphrey, J.H., Immunology 33 (1977) 31.
4. White, R.G., Clinical Aspects of Immunol. (P.G.H. Gell, R.R.A. Coombs, P.J. Lachmann, eds) p.411 Oxford: Blackwell Pubs.(1975).
5. Klaus, G.G.B., Immunol. 34 (1978) 643.
6. Klaus, G.G.B., Nature 272 (1978) 265.
7. Sirisinha, S., Eisen, H.N., Proc. Nat. Acad. Sci. USA 68 (1971) 3130.
8. Janeway, D.A., Sakato, N., Eisen, H.N., Proc. Nat. Acad. Sci. USA 72 (1975) 2357.
9. Julius, M.H., Augustin, A.A., Cosenza, H., Nature 265 (1976) 251.
10. Jerne, N.K., Ann. Immun. Inst. Pasteur 125c (1974) 373.
11. Rodkey, L.A., J. Exp. Med. 139 (1974) 712.
12. Iverson, G.H., Nature 227 (1970) 273.
13. Sakato, N., Eisen, H.N., J. Exp. Med. 141 (1975) 1411.

GERMINAL CENTER FORMATION IN BSA-TOLERANT CHICKENS

Olli Vainio, Matti K. Viljanen and Auli Toivanen

Departments of Medical Microbiology and Medicine,

Turku University, SF-20520 Turku 52, Finland

SUMMARY

In chickens rendered neonatally tolerant to BSA the germinal center formation was significantly decreased after stimulation with BSA at the age of 3 weeks. At the breakdown of tolerance after the age of 6 weeks the IgG antibody formation recovered before the IgM production. Stimulation of tolerant birds with unrelated antigens resulted in slightly decreased antibody response but the germinal center formation was on the same level as in normal controls.

INTRODUCTION

Although it is well established that germinal centers are an essential part of an immune response, their biological role remains unknown. A number of authors have suggested that they are involved in the generation of immunological memory (1-4). Ada and Parish (5) propose that reaction of lymphocytes with antigen within the germinal centers might actually result in tolerance. On the other hand Cohen and Thorbecke (6) have demonstrated a lack of specific histological changes during immunological tolerance after stimulation with the tolerogen. Our own work indicates that germinal center formation is age-dependent and not necessarily related to the antibody production (7). To elucidate the role of germinal centers in the presence or absence of an immune response, we have followed their formation in neonatally tolerised and in normal chickens. The results indicate that during tolerance the germinal center generation after stimulation with the tolerised antigen is reduced.

MATERIALS AND METHODS

Experimental design: Chickens were rendered tolerant to BSA
at hatching. Groups of tolerant birds were immunised with BSA at 1,
3, 6 and 12 weeks of age. Ten days after the immunisation the
resulting anti-BSA antibodies and germinal centers were assessed.
As controls, tolerant unimmunised, and normal unimmunised or immunised birds were studied.

Chickens: White Leghorn chickens of line V (genotype $B^{15}B^{15}$)
from our own colonies were used throughout the study.

Tolerance induction: Tolerance to BSA was induced in newly-
hatched chickens by injecting one single dose of 1250 mg BSA/kg body
weight intraperitoneally.

Antigens and antigen stimulations: BSA (fraction V from bovine
plasma, Armour Pharmaceutical Company, Ltd., Eastbourne, England) was
used as antigen. Tolerant chicks were divided into four groups and
immunised with BSA as follows: first group at one week of age with
0.5 mg, second group at 3 weeks also with 0.5 mg, third group at 6
weeks with 2.5 mg, and fourth group at 12 weeks also with 2.5 mg of
BSA per bird intraperitoneally.

As unrelated antigens, sheep red blood cells (SRBC) in a dose
of 2×10^9 SRBC per bird, and phenol-killed Brucella abortus in a
dose of 6.4×10^9 organisms per bird were used and administered
intraperitoneally.

Antibody assays: A blood sample for antibody determination
was taken in each group ten days after immunisation with heparinised
syringes. IgM and IgG anti-BSA antibodies were measured by enzyme
linked immunosorbent assay (ELISA; a modification of our RIA method,
ref. 8) and the antibody concentrations were given as per cent of
the same standard plasma in each experimental group. Anti-SRBC and
anti-Brucella antibodies were titrated as described earlier (9).

Autopsies and microscopic examination: Ten days after the
immunisation the birds were killed with ether. The preparation of
the spleen samples was as described earlier (9). At microscopic
examination the number of germinal centers in three cross sections
was recorded. As a result, the arithmetic mean of the three was
used. Every sample was studied without any knowledge of the origin
of the sample.

Statistics: Student's t-test was used for statistical analysis.

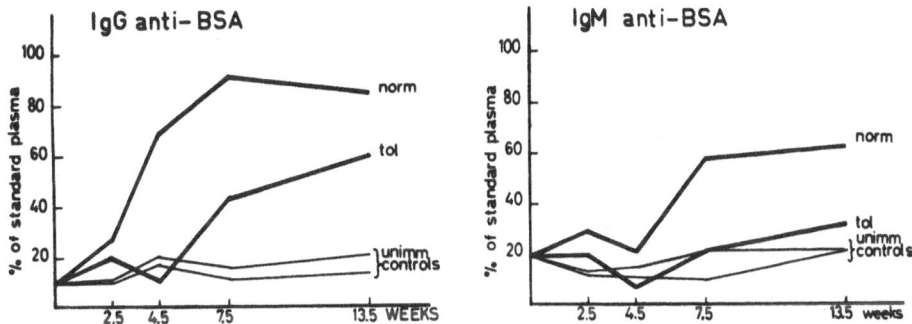

FIG. 1:   IgG and IgM anti-BSA antibody production in BSA-tolerant
and normal chickens.   Age in weeks at termination.

RESULTS

Persistence and breakdown of tolerance: IgG and IgM anti-BSA
antibody production in immunised BSA-tolerant and normal chickens
and in their unimmunised hatchmates is presented in Fig.1.   The neonatally tolerated birds were entirely suppressed to produce IgG
anti-bodies for the first three weeks after tolerance induction.
When immunised at 6 weeks of age they began to produce IgG antibodies, and at 12 weeks of age the antibody production had still
increased, but not yet to the normal level.   The unimmunised tolerant
and normal controls formed only negligible amounts of IgG and IgM
anti-BSA antibodies.

The inability to produce IgM antibodies in tolerised birds
persisted longer than observed for IgG antibodies.   At 6 weeks of
age tolerant birds did not form detectable IgM anti-BSA antibodies
and at 12 weeks the amount was still significantly less than in
normal immunised birds.

Germinal center formation in tolerant and normal chickens:
Germinal center formation in the spleen of tolerant and normal
chickens is demonstrated in Fig.2.   Very young birds, which were 1-
week-old when immunised, developed only on the average 1 to 3 germinal centers per cross section,no matter whether they were tolerised
or normal.   When the immunisation was carried out at three weeks,
there was a marked difference between tolerant and normal chickens.
Neonatally tolerated birds formed on the average 6 germinal centers
per cross section of the spleen after antigen stimulation, whereas
in normal immunised controls the corresponding figure was 16.   The
difference is statistically highly significant (P $<$ 0.001).   The
number of germinal centers in tolerant immunised birds was on the
same level as in unimmunised normal and tolerant controls.   At this

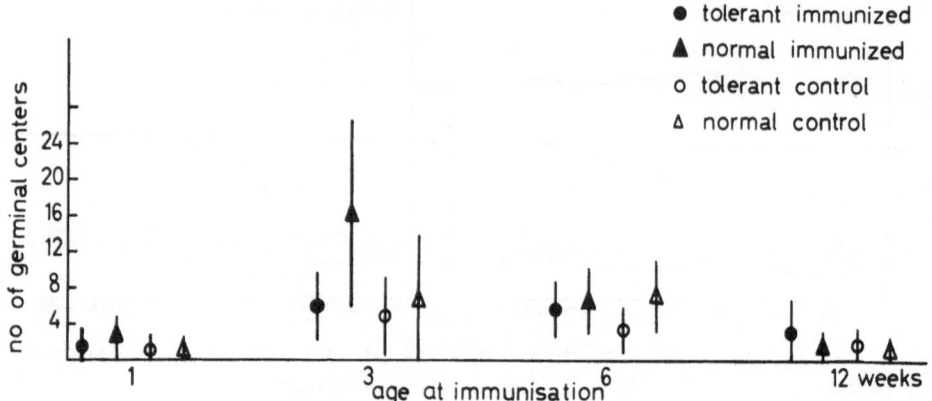

FIG. 2:   Germinal center formation in the spleen of BSA-tolerant
and normal chickens. Mean ± SD are given.

age the neonatally tolerated birds formed neither IgM nor IgG antibodies. After 6 weeks of age when the breakdown of tolerance
started, no difference in the number of germinal centers between
tolerant and control birds was seen. Thus when the breakdown of
tolerance starts, there is no suppression of germinal center formation in the spleen.

     The specificity of neonatally induced tolerance: To test the
specificity of BSA-tolerance, tolerant birds were immunised with
SRBC and Brucella. The antibody production against unrelated antigens in BSA-tolerant birds was only slightly decreased as compared
with normal controls and germinal center formation was as vigorous
as in normal controls (data not shown).

                              DISCUSSION

     Results obtained with different experimental conditions suggest
that formation of germinal centers after antigenic stimulation is
linked to the immunological memory (1-4). The present work was
triggered by the question how germinal centers, if related to memory,
are formed in chickens during neonatal tolerance. Earlier we have
demonstrated that their formation is strongly related to the age but
not necessarily to the antibody response (7). The present results,
in concert with those of Cohen and Thorbecke (6), demonstrate that
in tolerant birds, the tolerogen induces reduced germinal center
formation. Also White et al. (10) have shown poor antigen localization in germinal centers of tolerant birds. On the other hand, Ada

et al. (5) have suggested that germinal centers themselves are the actual site of tolerance generation. The question arises which one is the primary event: generation of tolerance or reduction in germinal center formation. In order to answer this question, further follow-up experiments have to be carried out.

REFERENCES

1. Thorbecke, G.J., Lerman, S.P. In: The Reticuloendothelial System in Health and Disease: Function and Characteristics, (S.M. Reichard, M.R. Escobar, H. Friedman, Eds.), Plenum Press, New York (1976) p.83.
2. Klaus, G.G.B. Immunology 34 (1978) 643.
3. Grobler, P., Buerki, H., Cottier, H., Hess, M.W., Stoner, R.D. J. Immunol. 112 (1974) 2154.
4. Vainio, O., Viljanen, M.K., Toivanen, A. Devel. Comparat. Immunol., in press.
5. Ada, G.L., Parish, C.R. Proc. Nat. Acad. Sci. USA 61 (1968) 556.
6. Cohen, M.W., Thorbecke, G.J. J. Immunol. 93 (1964) 629.
7. Toivanen, P., Toivanen, A., Molnár, G., Sorvari, T. Int. Archs Allergy Appl. Immunol. 47 (1974) 749.
8. Viljanen, M.K., Granfors, K., Toivanen, P. Immunochemistry 12 (1975) 699.
9. Toivanen, P., Toivanen, A. Eur. J. Immunol. 3 (1973) 585.
10. White, R.G., French, V.I., Stark, J.M. J. Med. Microbiol. 3 (1970) 65.

ACKNOWLEDGEMENTS

Supported by a contract with Association of Finnish Life Insurance Companies, and by grants from Emil and Blida Maunula Foundation and Finnish Medical Society Duodecim.

STUDIES OF ALLOSPECIFIC SUPPRESSOR CELLS IN CULTURE

A. Eisenthal, D. Nachtigal and M. Feldman

Department of Cell Biology, The Weizmann Institute

of Science, Rehovot, Israel

INTRODUCTION

Suppressor T lymphocytes are presumed to constitute an important regulatory mechanism of immune responses and a considerable body of information has been gathered concerning their role in humoral and cellular immunity, as well as in immune tolerance. However, very little is known as to the mechanism of suppressor cell induction on the cellular level, as well as to the cellular parameters of their function. The present study was undertaken in order to gain some insight into the respective cellular mechanisms, particularly concerning allospecific cellular responses. For a critical analysis of the relevant parameters, an experimental model was developed in which both the generation of suppressor cells and the assay of their subsequent suppressive function were studied in culture. We have reported on this in a previous publication (1), showing that allospecific suppressor T lymphocytes could be induced in vitro by stimulation of mouse thymus cells with allogeneic irradiated spleen cells. When this primary culture was harvested at an appropriate stage and transferred to a one-way mixed lymphocyte reaction, a significant suppression of thymidine incorporation could be demonstrated, as compared with control MLR. The prerequisite was that the responder cells be syngeneic with the thymocytes of the primary culture, and that the stimulator cells be syngeneic with its spleen cells. The following report provides additional information concerning the cellular parameters of suppressor cell generation and function.

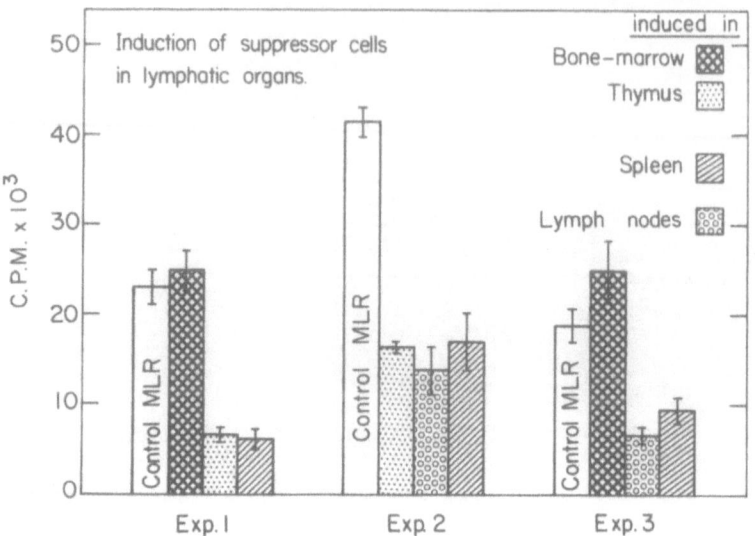

FIG. 1:   cpm in mixed lymphocyte reactions with and without addition of primed lymphoid cells.

RESULTS

Lymphoid organs comprising precursors of suppressor lymphocytes

We checked other lymphoid organs besides the thymus as potential sources of suppressor T cells. Spleen and lymph node cells were found to generate suppressors in culture similarly to thymocytes, while bone marrow cells were found to be ineffective in this respect (Fig.1).

We reported previously (1) that the efficiency of thymus cells as a source of suppressor lymphocytes decreased with the age of thymus donors. When this parameter was tested in spleen cells, however, the opposite was found true, namely, the efficiency of spleen cells for the generation of suppressor lymphocytes increased with the age of donor mice up to 60 days. This increase was independent of the presence of adherent cells (Fig.2).

Radiosensitivity of suppressor lymphocytes and of their precursors

Allospecific suppressor cells are known to be relatively radio-resistant (2). We observed, however, that this does not apply to their precursors. Thus, when we irradiated the primary cultures at

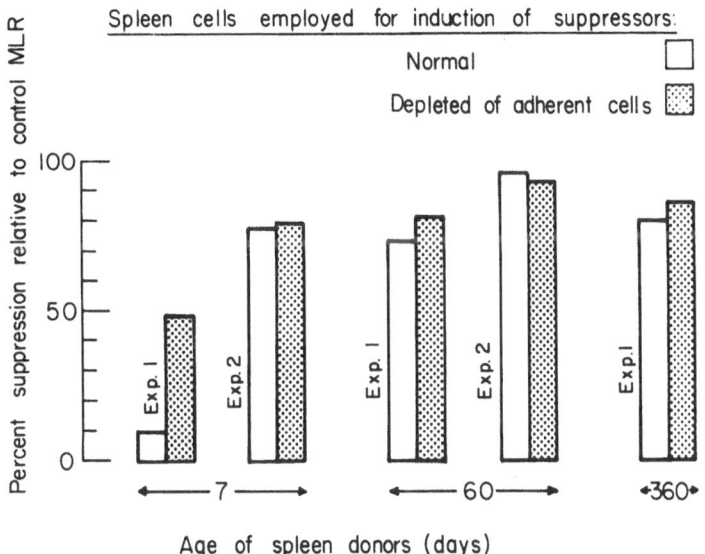

FIG. 2: Increase of suppressive capacity of mouse spleen with the age of spleen donors.

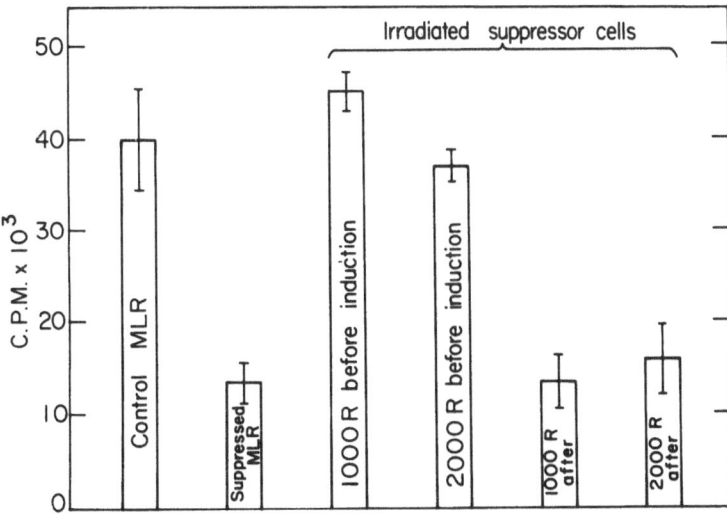

FIG. 3: The relative radioresistance of functional suppressor cells, as compared with their precursors.

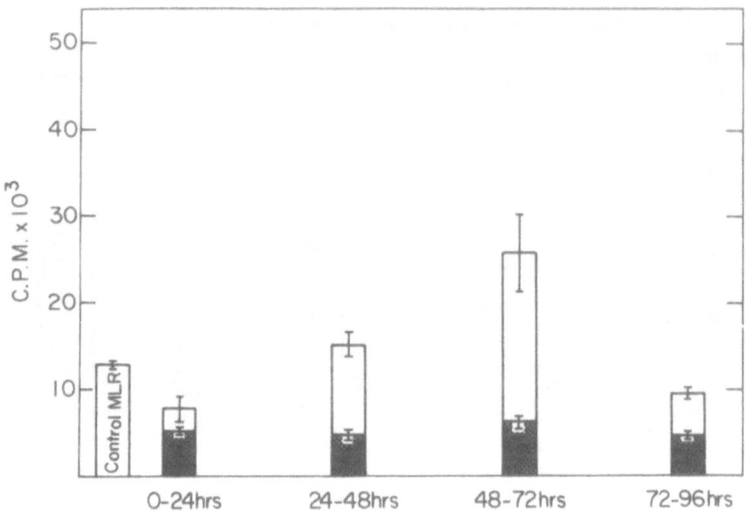

<u>FIG. 4</u>:   Effect of treating induction cultures with cytosine arabinoside on suppressor cell induction.

96 h, their suppressive capacity was not abrogated, while when irradiated at time zero, no suppressive effect could be demonstrated in addition to the MLR (Fig.3).

<u>Dependence of suppressor cell generation on cell replication and protein synthesis</u>

The radiosensitivity of suppressor cell precursors suggests that cell replication might be essential for the generation of suppressors in culture. This was verified more critically by pulsing with cytosine arabinoside at various stages after setting up the primary culture (Fig.4).

It is evident that pulsing from 48 to 72 h abolished entirely the suppressive effect and, moreover, brought about a potentiating effect instead. This finding suggests that sensitization in the primary culture induces both suppressive and potentiating cells, while what is actually measured is the balance between the two. It appears that the differentiation of those two cell populations runs along different kinetical courses, and thus, each can be demonstrated in predominance under appropriate conditions (1).

It could be shown in a similar manner that generation of

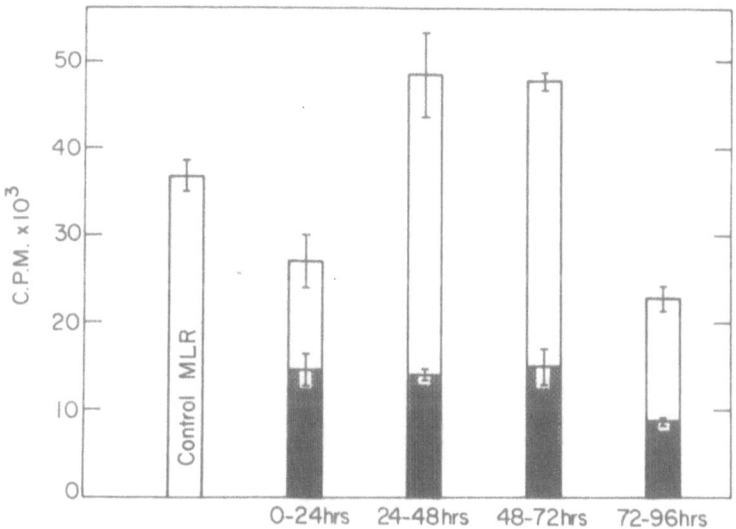

FIG. 5:   Effect of cycloheximide treatment on suppressor cell induction.

suppressor lymphocytes depends on protein synthesis as well. It was demonstrated by pulsing with cycloheximide at varying time intervals that a 24 h pulse at the 24-72 h stage of the induction culture will reverse suppression and generate potentiation (Fig.5).

Cell cooperation in generation of suppressor lymphocytes

It was reported in previous publications from our group that induction of tolerance to protein antigens, which was shown to be dependent on suppressor cells, was also dependent on the presence of cortisone-sensitive lymphocytes during the induction process (3, 4). We reported also that the generation of suppressor lymphocytes in culture required cortisone-sensitive lymphocytes as well (1). This finding was analyzed by employing cell separation with the aid of peanut lectin (peanut agglutinin, PNA). PNA has been shown to bind selectively to cortical type thymus cells, the immunologically incompetent, cortisone-sensitive T cells (6). With this technique a neat separation is possible between cortical type and medullar type cells from a suspension of thymocytes. When each fraction was sensitized separately in the induction culture, no suppressor cells were generated. When, however, the separated fractions were re-mixed in optimal proportions and put into an induction culture together, the mixture was again as effective as the starting cell suspension (Fig.6).

Thus, apparently, at least two cell types are required to interact during sensitization in order to generate suppressor lymphocytes.
Our preliminary findings suggest that the medullar type lymphocyte
may be the actual precursor of suppressor cells, while the cortical
type lymphocyte seems to be an accessory cell.

SUMMARY

Allospecific suppressor T cells can be generated by allostimu-
lating thymus, spleen and lymph node cells in culture. Bone marrow
cells do not yield suppressor lymphocytes. While the efficiency of
thymocytes for suppressor cell generation decreases with the age of
thymus donors, the efficiency of spleen increases with age.
Generation of suppressor lymphocytes depends on cell replication
and protein synthesis. The suppressor function as such does not
require cell replication. Induction of suppressor T cells in
culture requires cell to cell interaction of cortical type and
medullar type T cells.

REFERENCES

1.   Eisenthal, A., Nachtigal, D., Feldman, M., Cell. Immunol. 34
     (1977) 112.
2.   Sinclair, N.R.St.C., Lees, R.K., Missiuna, P.C., Fung, F.Y.,
     "Suppressor Cells in Immunity", ed. S.K. Singhal, N.R.St.C.
     Sinclair, The University of Western Ontario, 1975.
3.   Zan-Bar, I., Nachtigal,D., Feldman, M., Cell. Immunol. 17 (1975)
     202.
4.   Zan-Bar, I., Nachtigal,D., Feldman, M., Cell. Immunol. 17 (1975)
     215.
5.   Nachtigal, D., Zan-Bar, I., Feldman, M., Transplant. Rev. 26
     (1975) 87.
6.   Reisner, Y., Linker-Israeli, M., Sharon, N., Cell. Immunol. 25
     (1976) 129.

REGULATION OF DELAYED TYPE HYPERSENSITIVITY TO SHEEP RED BLOOD
CELLS: DEMONSTRATION OF SUPPRESSOR T CELLS AND A SOLUBLE
SUPPRESSOR FACTOR

S.H.E. Kaufmann and H. Hahn

Institutes of Medical Microbiology, Ruhr-Universität,

D-4630 Bochum, and Freie Universität Berlin, D-1000 Berlin

The regulation of an immune response proceeds via a complex
sequence of cellular interactions that involve both helper and
suppressor cells. The induction of a humoral or a cellular immune
response to sheep red blood cells (SRBC) is dependent on the dose
of antigen used for sensitization. It has been postulated that high
doses of SRBC induce suppression of delayed type hypersensitivity
(DTH) by either B cell-derived soluble immune complexes (1) or by
suppressor T cells (2,3). The studies summarized in this paper
provide evidence that suppressor T cells participate in the regulation of DTH induction to SRBC and a soluble factor of suppressive
activity can be obtained in vitro from spleen cells of anergic mice.

Suppression of DTH induction: (B6D2)F1 mice injected with 10^6
SRBC i.v. display DTH when challenged with 2.5×10^8 SRBC four days
later whereas no DTH reactions occur in mice injected with 10^9 SRBC
(Tab.1). Mice that receive the latter dose are therefore anergic
and when subsequently injected with 10^6 SRBC remain unable to develop
DTH reactions. The state of anergy is antigen-specific. Thus while
DTH induction to SRBC is suppressed by 10^9 SRBC, DTH to chicken red
blood cells (CRBC) can still be induced by an optimal dose of CRBC
(Tab.1). However, partial suppression is seen in SRBC-anergic mice
when an optimal dose of horse red blood cells (HRBC) is used for
sensitization, indicating partial cross-reactivity at the level of
suppression of DTH induction. Specific suppression of DTH in mice
given 10^9 SRBC lasts for at least eight weeks as was evident by their
inability to exhibit DTH after administration of 10^6 SRBC (Tab.2).

Transfer of suppression by T cells: Prospective donor mice
were rendered anergic and four days later their spleens removed.

307

TAB. 1:   Specific Suppression of DTH Induction[a]

Suppression (d-4)	Sensitization (d 0)	DTH (units)	Suppression (%)
nil	SRBC	15.8	0
SRBC	nil	2.3	85.4
SRBC	SRBC	3.1	80.4
nil	HRBC	14.4	0
SRBC	HRBC	7.0	51.3
nil	CRBC	8.7	0
SRBC	CRBC	8.0	8.0

[a]Mice were rendered anergic by 10^9 SRBC i.v. 4 days before sensitization with an optimal dose of SRBC, HRBC or CRBC, respectively(d_0). 4 days after sensitization mice were challenged with 2.5×10^8 SRBC, HRBC or CRBC.

TAB. 2:   Duration of Suppression[a]

Time of sensitization after injection of 10^9 SRBC (weeks)	DTH (units)		Suppression (%)
	anergic	normal	
0	2.8	12.2	77.0
1	4.2	13.4	68.7
2	3.2	9.1	64.8
3	2.9	11.7	75.2
4	1.8	10.5	82.9
5	2.2	11.3	80.5
6	4.8	8.9	46.1
7	3.9	9.7	59.8
8	3.3	12.5	73.6

[a]Mice were rendered anergic by injecting 10^9 SRBC and at the indicated times it was attempted to induce DTH with 10^6 SRBC. Challenge with 2.5×10^8 SRBC 4 days after injection of 10^6 SRBC.

5×10^7 glass wool nonadherent cells were transferred to normal recipient mice one hour before injecting a sensitizing dose of 10^6 SRBC. DTH induction was almost completely suppressed in recipients of cells from anergic donors (Tab.3). The suppressive cells are

TAB. 3: Transfer of Suppression by T cells[a].

Donor sensitization	Treatment of cells	Recipient DTH	Suppression (%)
nil	nil	12.0	0
10^9 SRBC (d-4)	nil	4.4	63.3
10^9 SRBC (d-8)	nil	10.2	15.0
10^9 SRBC (d-4)	anti Thy 1.2 + C	11.9	0.8
10^9 SRBC (d-4)	serum + C	5.0	58.3

[a]Donors were rendered anergic with 10^9 SRBC 4 or 8 days before cell transfer. DTH was induced in recipients with 10^6 SRBC immediately after transfer. Challenge with 2.5×10^8 SRBC 4 days after sensitization.

sensitive to anti Thy 1.2 serum plus complement (Tab.3). However, spleen cells collected eight days after injection of 10^9 SRBC from anergic donors did not transfer suppression, although DTH induction in donors was still suppressed at that time (Tab.3).

Therefore, suppressor T cells can be obtained only transiently from spleens of anergic mice. They either leave the spleen and act in the periphery, or they are short lived and suppression is mediated by a soluble long lasting factor.

Transfer of suppression by a soluble factor: A mixture consisting of the 10,000 g supernatant from sonicated spleen cells from anergic donors and glass wool purified viable spleen cells from normal donors was incubated and injected into normal mice. This mixture was capable of suppressing DTH induction (Tab.4). These data therefore indicate that spleen cells from anergic mice might contain (release?) a soluble factor capable of suppressing DTH induction.

Presence of effector T cells in anergic mice: Theoretically, suppression by 10^9 SRBC could block the formation of specific effector T cells or alternatively prevent their functioning in the periphery. In order to distinguish between these two alternatives, spleen cells from mice sensitized either with 10^6 or 10^9 SRBC were transferred to two groups of normal recipient mice on day 4 of the immune response. As shown in Tab.5, spleen cells from both types of donors transferred DTH reactions, provided the challenge dose was high enough (5×10^8 SRBC). This experiment indicates that specific effector T cells are generated in anergic mice, but are prevented from expressing DTH in the periphery.

TAB. 4:   Transfer of Suppression by a Soluble Factor[a]

Factor + cells transferred	DTH (units)	Suppression (%)
nil	14.7	0
factor from normal donors + cells from normal donors	13.6	7.5
factor from anergic donors + cells from normal donors	7.7	47.6

[a]Donors were rendered anergic with 10^9 SRBC 4 days before transfer. DTH was induced in recipients with 10^6 SRBC immediately after transfer. Challenge with 2.5×10^8 SRBC 4 days after sensitization.

TAB. 5:   Transfer of DTH with spleen cells[a]

Sensitization of donors	Donor DTH	Recipient DTH
10^6	18.2	10.3
10^9	7.7	9.7

[a]Donor mice were sensitized with 10^6 or 10^9 SRBC, respectively. In one group of donor mice DTH was elicited on day 4. 5×10^7 spleen cells of another group of mice were transferred into normal recipients and recipient's DTH elicited one day after transfer with 5×10^8 SRBC.

The data indicate that in addition to splenic suppressor T cells, other mechanisms are involved in suppression of DTH. A B cell-derived humoral suppressive factor has been shown by Mackaness et al. (1) to occur in anergic mice. The factor described by us appears to be different, however. The data in Tab.5 are in agreement with findings by Askenase et al. (5). They suggest that both suppressor T cells and effector T cells are generated in spleens of anergic mice, effector T cells being prevented from mediating DTH reactions in the periphery.

REFERENCES

1. Mackaness, G.B., Lagrange, P.H., Miller, T.E., Ishibahi, T., J. Exp. Med. 139 (1974) 543.

2. Askenase, P.W., Hayden, B.J., Gershon, R.K., J. Exp. Med. 141
    (1975) 697.
3. Ramshaw, I.A., Bretscher, P.A., Parish, C.R., Eur. J. Immunol.
    6 (1976) 674.
4. Julius, M., Simpson, E., Herzenberg, C.A., Eur. J. Immunol. 3
    (1973) 645.
5. Askenase, P.W., Hayden, B., Gershon, R.K., J. Immunol. 119
    (1977) 1830.

INDUCTION OF TOLERANCE TO DNCB-CONTACT SENSITIVITY IN GUINEA PIG FETUSES

L. Polak and C. Rinck

Pharma Research Department, F. Hoffmann-La Roche & Co.Ltd.

Basel, Switzerland

It has been demonstrated that tolerance to contact sensitivity, induced by intravenously injected hapten, is transferable by parabiosis from tolerant to normal partners (Polak 1975). In order to distinguish between cellular and humoral factors, the transfer of tolerance from pregnant guinea pigs to their fetuses was studied. In this species, low molecular weight substances (Sisk 1976) and some proteins, e.g. antibodies, are passing the placental barrier whereas cellular elements are retained.

In the first group of experiments, female strain 2-guinea pigs were tolerized by two intravenous injections of dinitrobenzene-sulfonic acid sodium salt (DNBSO$_3$) with a 14 day interval and two weeks later mated for 30 days with syngeneic males. One month after birth, both the mothers and the offspring were sensitized to dinitrochlorobenzene (DNCB) and challenged 14 days later. The reactions were evaluated 24 hours later according to an arbitrary scale from 0.5 to 2 (Frey & Wenk 1957).

In Tab.1, it is shown that the offspring of tolerant mothers became sensitized to the same degree as offspring of normal controls. This failure to transfer tolerance to fetuses during pregnancy supports the view that tolerance is mediated by a cellular mechanism such as suppressor cells rather than by humoral factors. Furthermore, this result indicates that a suppressor factor, which in guinea pigs is still hypothetical, either does not penetrate the placenta or loses its activity before the offspring are sensitized, i.e. during the first month after birth.

In further experiments, the possibility of inducing tolerance in fetuses by tolerization of the mothers during pregnancy was

TAB. 1

	Degree of contact sensitivity to		
	DNCB		OXA
	1.sens.	2.sens.	
Control mothers	$1.53\pm0.59(17)$	$2.60\pm0.55(17)$	n.d.
Their offspring	$1.43\pm0.50(45)$	$2.20\pm0.61(17)$	$1.85\pm0.75(10)$
Tolerant mothers	0 (23)	0 (23)	n.d.
Their offspring	$1.34\pm0.42(56)$	$2.42\pm0.56(12)$	$1.86\pm1.03(7)$

Figures in brackets represent the number of animals.

studied. For this purpose, guinea pigs in various stages of pregnancy were injected intravenously with 500 mg/kg $DNBSO_3$ and both the mothers and the offspring sensitized and challenged with DNCB one month after birth as described above. The age of the fetuses at the time of tolerization was calculated from the date of birth in view of the fact that pregnancy in guinea pigs lasts 68 days (Goy et al. 1957). Tolerization of fetuses through prenatal exposure to the tolerogen (feeding or intraperitoneal injection) was reported by Baer et al. (1958), and by Harber et al. (1962), but their results were criticized by Chase (1963) and by Lowney (1970) because the differences between the offspring of tolerogen-treated and control guinea pigs were too slight.

In Tab.2, it is shown that the offspring exposed to the tolerogen in the 10th week of fetal life (group 2) became completely tolerant to the first sensitizing attempt and reacted only marginally to the second one. Offspring exposed to the tolerogen one week earlier (group 3) became only partially tolerant, whereas in other groups where exposure took place earlier no tolerance could be detected, despite the successful tolerization of the mothers (group 9).

In order to establish the specificity of this tolerance, offspring from all groups were sensitized to oxazolon one week after the first challenge with DNCB and challenged 14 days later. Results presented in Tab.3 confirm the specificity of tolerance to DNCB-contact sensitivity, since the offspring tolerant to DNCB could become sensitized to an unrelated antigen (oxazolon) in the same way as controls.

TAB. 2

Fetuses tolerized at age of	Number of animals	Degree of contact sensitizing to DNCB	
		1.sens.	2.sens.
birth	3	1.00+0.53	1.67+0.76
10 weeks	13	0.15+0.24*	0.50+0.54*
9 weeks	13	0.65+0.43*	1.17+0.84**
8 weeks	17	1.38+0.70	n.d.
6 weeks	18	1.31+0.52	2.11+0.61
5 weeks	18	1.53+0.47	2.39+0.44
4 weeks	13	1.50+0.35	2.38+0.76
3 weeks	7	1.21+0.27	1.93+0.43
tol. mothers	23	0.14+0.22	0.41+0.69
offspring of normal mothers	45	1.43+0.50	2.20+0.61

Statistical significance: * $p < 0.001$; ** $p < 0.002$.

Since suppressor cells causing tolerance in the mothers cannot reach the fetuses, one has to accept that the tolerance of offspring was due to active tolerization in the fetal life. The tolerogen ($DNBSO_3$) was passing from the pregnant guinea pig to the fetuses via the placental communication. The failure to induce tolerance in fetuses before the 9th week of fetal life could be explained by their immaturity. This may apply to the development of either the vascular or the immunological system.

In order to find out whether the tolerogen reaches the fetuses, guinea pigs at different stages of pregnancy were injected intravenously with radiolabelled $DNBSO_3$ ($^3H-DNBSO_3$, spec. act. 50μCi/mg) and the radioactivity in the blood of offspring was estimated one month after birth. In Tab.4, it is demonstrated that radioactivity could be detected in the blood of guinea pigs exposed to the tolerogen in the 8th week of fetal life at the earliest.

Since guinea pigs exposed to the antigen at that time did not become tolerant, it is suggested that this was due to immunological immaturity rather than to insufficiently developed vascularization. Moreover, this result indicates that in offspring seeing the tolerogen earlier in their fetal life no functional tolerogenic depot was formed which would induce tolerance when the fetuses become immunologically mature. It is suggested that this takes place between the 54th and 61st day of fetal life.

TAB. 3

| Fetuses tolerized | Degree of contact sensitivity to | |
at age of	DNCB	OXA
10 weeks	0.15+0.24(13)	2.17+0.73(13)
9 weeks	0.65+0.43(13)	1.86+0.83(11)
<6 weeks	1.38+0.43(58)	1.86+1.17(14)
offspring of normal mothers	1.43+0.50(45)	1.85+0.75(10)

Figures in brackets represent numbers of animals.

TAB. 4

Fetuses tolerized at age of	Contact sensitivity to DNBC	^{3}H-DNBSO$_3$/50μl blood ng
9 weeks	0.65+0.43(13)	14.0+8.0(5)
8 weeks	1.38+0.70(17)	2.7+0.9(21)
<6 weeks	1.38+0.43(58)	0.1+0.4(9)
Mothers of fetuses tolerized at age of		
9 weeks	0 (2)	117.9+58.9(2)
8 weeks	0 (8)	52.7+38.1(8)
<6 weeks	0 (4)	18.7+ 6.8(4)

Figures in brackets represent numbers of animals.

SUMMARY

1.   Female guinea pigs made tolerant before pregnancy do not transfer tolerance to their offspring. This result favours the concept of cellular mechanism of tolerance.

2.   Guinea pig fetuses become tolerant when exposed to the tolerogen in the last two weeks of pregnancy. This is due to active tolerization by the tolerogen passing the placental barrier.

3. Fetuses exposed to the antigen earlier did not develop tolerance. This is due to immunological immaturity rather than to insufficiently developed vascularization. No functional active depot of tolerogen is formed.

4. Guinea pigs become immunologically mature between the 54th and 61st day of fetal life.

REFERENCES

1. Baer, R.L., Rosenthal, St. A., Hagel, B., J. Immunol. 80 (1958) 429.
2. Chase, M.W., La tolérance acquise et la tolérance naturelle à l'égard de substances antigéniques définies. Centre National de la Recherche Scientifique, Paris. p. 139 (1963).
3. Frey, J.R., Wenk, P., Int. Arch. Allergy 11 (1957) 81.
4. Goy, R.W., Hoar, R.M., Young, W.C., Anat. Rec. 128 (1957) 747.
5. Harber, L.C., Rosenthal, St. A., Baer, R.L., J. Immunol. 88 (1962) 66.
6. Lowney, E.D., J. invest. Derm. 54 (1970) 355.
7. Polak, L., J. Immunol. 114 (1975) 988.
8. Sisk, D.B., In: The Biology of Guinea Pigs, Eds. J.E. Wagner, P.Y. Manning, Academic Press, New York, San Francisco, London, p. 86 (1976).

SUPPRESSOR CELLS FOR IN VIVO CYTOTOXIC RESPONSES - REGULATION OF

THE IN VIVO ACTIVATION OF CYTOTOXIC T-LYMPHOCYTES BY SUPPRESSIVE CELLS

Wulf Dröge, Werner Süßmuth and Reinhard Franze

The German Cancer Research Center (DKFZ)

Im Neuenheimer Feld 280, D 69 Heidelberg, West Germany

ABSTRACT

A significant in vivo activation of cytotoxic T-lymphocytes (CTL) against trinitrophenyl (TNP)-modified autologous cells and of a DNA-synthesis response in the peripheral lymphnodes is observed in cyclophosphamide (CyP) treated mice after skinpainting with trinitrochlorbenzene (TNCB) or after injection of TNP-coupled spleen cells (TNP-Spl) into the footpads. The activation of these responses can be suppressed by the transfer of spleen cells or lymphnode cells from skinpainted normal mice, but not from skinpainted mice that had been pretreated with CyP. Suppressive activity is also induced by injections of TNP-Spl i.p. or trinitrobenzosulfonate (TNBS) i.v. Optimal activation of suppression occurs within 3 - 4 days. The suppressive activity is antigen-specific at least in respect to its activation.

Suppressor cells of this kind also suppress the induction of delayed hypersensitivity (DH) responses and the priming for in vitro secondary responses. However, these two responses are less sensitive to the suppression, and their in vivo activation is accordingly much less restricted with the in vivo activation of DNA-synthesis and primary CTL responses. DH and CMC memory can be activated by TNCB skinpainting without pretreatment with CyP.

INTRODUCTION AND DESCRIPTION
OF THE EXPERIMENTAL SYSTEM

The regulation of humoral responses by a special class of antigen-specific suppressor T-cells has been investigated extensively in

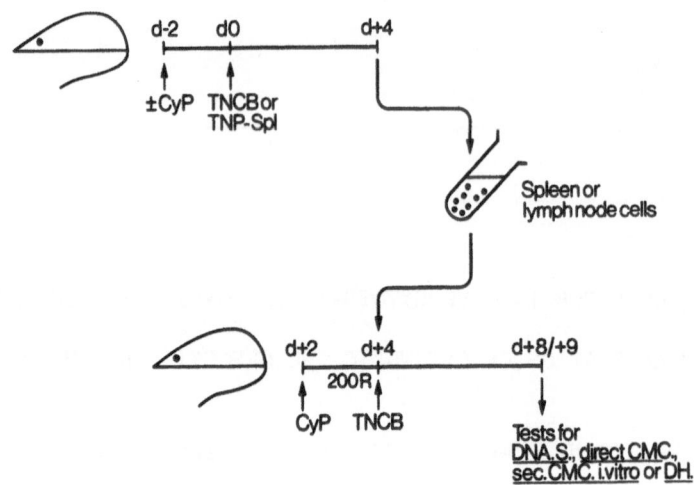

FIG. 1:   Experimental protocol of the tests for suppressive activity.
CyP treated or untreated donor mice were sensitized with TNBC or with
TNP-Spl i.p. (in some cases also with TNBS i.v.) and sacrificed 4
days later. Their spleen cells (usually 6 x 10^7) or lymph node cells
(2 x 10^7) were injected intraorbitally into CyP treated lightly
irradiated recipients, which were then sensitized with TNBC and tested
for DNA synthesis, direct CMC, secondary CMC in vitro or DH 4 or 5
days later.

various systems. These suppressor cells have the phenotype Ly-1^-2^+
(1-3), their induction is sensitive against the early effects of
adult thymectomy (4,5), and they produce antigen-specific suppressive
factors (6,7). At least one type of cell-mediated immune response,
namely the effector phase of DH was also found to be regulated by a
similar type of suppressor cells, which was also found to be sensitive
against the early effects of adult thymectomy (8) and which also can
generate antigen-specific suppressive products (9).

Another group of experiments provided evidence for another type
of suppressive cells to be involved in the regulation of the induction
of DH-responses and DNA-synthesis responses (10-16). These suppressor
cells were reported to have the phenotype Ly 1^+2^- (15) and their
activation was sensitive to pretreatment with CyP (12-14) but resistant to the early effects of adult thymectomy (13,14). Attempts of
different investigators to obtain suppressive factors from these
kinds of suppressor cells by sonication or by in vitro incubation
have failed (16) (J.F.A.P. Miller, personal communication) whether
these cells are mechanistically related to the Ly 1^+2^- suppressor
cells is not yet clear.

TAB. 1:   Activation of suppressive cells by skin painting with TNBC.

Treatment of the donors	CTL-activity	DNA-Synthesis x 10^{-3} CPM
TNBC skinpainting	8-1-0	47
none	22-5-0	121
no cells transferred	23-5-1	149

a)   6 x 10^7 cells of $C_3D_2F_1$ mice skinpainted with 6 mg TNCB 4 days previously were transferred intraorbitally into syngeneic recipients that were treated with 3 mg CyP 2 days before and with 200 R whole body irradiation 2 hours before transfer (see Fig.1). The recipients were then immunized by skinpainting with 6 mg TNCB and tested for CTL activity (killer: target cell ratios = 25.5 and 1) and DNA Synthesis 4 days later.

TAB. 2:   Activation of suppressor cells for the in vivo primary CTL response and primary DNA synthesis.

Treatment of the donors	CTL-activity		DNA synthesis (x 10^{-3} CPM)	
	- Cyp	+ Cyp	- Cyp	+ Cyp
3 mg TNBS i.v.	12-1-0		56	
TNP-Spl i.p. 3 x 10^8	12-2-0	30-8-1	45	146
none	46-16-3		206	218
no cells transferred	47-15-3	47-15-3	187	187

a)   Normal CBA donors (-CyP) or donors injected with 4 mg CyP i.p. (+CyP) received the indicated treatment 2 days later, and their spleen cells were transferred again 4 days later into CyP-treated syngeneic recipients (see Fig.1). The recipients were skinpainted with 6 mg TNCB immediately after the transfer and their lymph node cells were tested for CTL activity and DNA-synthesis 4 days later.

We have investigated the regulation of the in vivo induction of cytotoxic T-lymphocytes (CTL) against TNP-modified syngeneic cells. We found that this response is apparently regulated by a number of different suppressor-cells most of which are still poorly character-ized. A dominant role is played by a type of suppressor cell, which

TAB. 3:   Specificity of TNBS and DNBS activated inhibitory cells [a].

Treatment of the donors	Sensitization of the recipients	DNA-Synthesis $(x \ 10^{-3} \ CPM)$
TNBS	TNCB	20 (17-22)
	DNCB	67 (66-68)
DNBS	TNCB	111 (95-112)
	DNCB	12 (9 -14)
none	TNCB	98 (87-111)
	DNCB	84 (76-93)

[a]   The donors received 3 mg TNBS or 8 mg DNBS i.v. 4 days prior to the transfer (see Fig.1). The recipients were immediately sensitized with either TNCB or DNCB and tested for DNA synthesis 5 days later. The data indicate the median (lower and upper limits are given in brackets).

TAB. 4:   Suppression of different cell mediated immune responses.

	i.vivo CTL	DNA-S.	CMC-memory	DH
immun. donors	12-2-0	48	42-18-5	1.4(2,3)
normal donors	46-16-3	227	60-51-30	2.0(5,2)
no cells transferred	47-15-3	250	56-50-26	

Spleen cells from normal donors or from donors immunized with $1-3 \times 10^8$ TNP-Spl i.p. 4 days previously (Fig.1) were transferred into CyP-treated recipients. The DH-responses are indicated as ear-swelling indices. The data in brackets indicate the ^{125}JUDR-indices as measured by the procedure of Vadas et al. (19). The indices represent the values of the sensitized ear divided by the values of the unsensitized ear.

is essentially indistinguishable from the suppressor cells described in (10-16), e.g. ist induction is sensitive against pretreatment with the alcylating agent cyclophosphamide (CyP). We found that this suppressor cell affects the induction of the in vivo CTL-response more significantly than the induction of DH-responses. Some details about these suppressor cells are described here.

TAB. 5: Activation of different immunological functions in response to TNP-coupled autologous cells (schematic illustration).

Immunization	Suppressor cells -CyP +CyP	DNA S -CyP +CyP	CTL i.vivo -CyP +CyP	CMC memory -CyP +CyP	DH -CyP +CyP
TNP-coupled spleen cells i.p. 10^7	(+) -	- -	- -	+ +	+ +
10^8	+ (+)	- -	- -	- +	- +
Skinpainting 6 mg TNCB	(+) -	- +	- +	+ +	+ +

+   indicates strong activation of the corresponding function
(+)   indicates weak but still demonstrable activation
-    indicates the absence of demonstrable activity

THE DEMONSTRATION OF SUPPRESSOR CELLS
AND THE EFFECTS OF CYCLOPHOSPHAMIDE

The experimental system is outlined in Figure 1. It is based on the previous observations that normal mice produce no significant CTL-responses after immunization with TNP-coupled autologous cells (e.g. after skinpainting with TNCB), while significant CTL-activity can be obtained in vivo after immunization (especially after skinpainting) of CyP treated mice (17,18). We found on the other hand that skin-painting of normal mice (or injections of TNP-Spl i.p. or TNBS i.v.) generates suppressive activity in the spleen or lymphnode cells, which after transfer into CyP treated mice can inhibit the otherwise optimal response against TNCB (Fig.1) (Tabs. 1 and 2). It should be emphasized that these responses were only inhibited by cells from antigen treated donors and not from antigen inexperienced donors (Tabs. 1 and 2). And it was found that the activation of this suppressive activity is prevented by pretreatment of the donors with CyP (Fig.1) (Tab.2).

THE SPECIFICITY OF THE SUPPRESSION

For testing the specificity of the suppression, we took advantage of the fact that suppressor cells can also be activated by dinitro-benzosulfonate (DNBS) and that at least the DNA-synthesis response can also be measured after skinpainting with dinitrochlorobenzene (DNCB). Transfer experiments revealed that TNBS and DNBS activated suppressor cells inhibit preferentially the homologous DNA-synthesis response against TNCB and DNCB, respectively, with little or no cross reactivity (Tab.3). The results show that the suppressor cells are specific at least in respect to their induction. The experiment cannot exclude, that the antigen activated suppressor cells mediate non-specific suppressive effects after thay have been specifically restimulated in the recipient.

THE SUPPRESSIVE EFFECT ON OTHER
TYPES OF CELL-MEDIATED IMMUNE RESPONSES

It is well known that skinpainting with TNCB can activate DH-responses in normal mice without pretreatment with CyP (for example see (8,9)). Skinpainting or injections of TNP-Spl into the footpads can also activate memory cells for secondary in vitro cytotoxic responses without pretreatment with CyP (W. Suessmuth, unpublished observation). These observations indicate that both the DH and the memory responses are not affected by or at least less sensitive to the suppressor cells described above. Transfer experiments revealed that the antigen activated suppressor cells can indeed inhibit the inducation of DH and CMC-memory (Tab.4). The activation patterns of suppressor cells and the four types of cell-mediated immune responses, which are schematically summarized in Table 5, show that the activation profile of the suppressor cells on the one hand and the primary in vivo CTL and DNA-synthesis responses on the other hand are completely mutually exclusive, while the activation of CMC-memory and DH is only inhibited under conditions, which allow the most powerful activation of suppressor cells, that is after injection of 10^8 TNP-coupled spleen cells i.p. into mice not treated with CyP (Tab.5). These differences may reflect different effector cells with different sensitivities to the suppressor cells; but they can also be explained by possible differences in the sensitivities of the assays used.

REFERENCES

1.   Cantor, H., Shen, F.-W., Boyse, E.A. J. Exp. Med. 143 (1976) 1391.

2.   Feldmann, M., Beverly, P.C.L., Dunkley, M., Kontiainen, S. Nature 258 (1975) 614.

3.   Vadas, M.A., Miller, J.F.A.P., McKenzie, I.F.C., Chism, S.E., Shen, F.W., Boyse, E.A., Gamble, J.R., Whitelaw, A.M. J. Exp. Med. 144 (1976) 10.

4.   Basten, A., Miller, J.F.A.P., Johnson, P. Transplant. Rev. 26 (1975) 130.

5.   Nachtigal, D., Zan-Bar, I., Feldmann, M. Transplant. Rev. 26 (1975) 87.

6.   Taniguchi, M., Tada, T., Tokuhisa, T. J. Exp. Med. 144 (1976) 20.

7.   Kapp, J.A., Pierce, C.W., Benacerraf, B. J. Exp. Med. 145 (1977) 828.

8. Asherson, G.L., Zembala, M., Mayhew, B., Goldstein, A. Eur. J. Immunol. 6 (1976) 699.
9. Zembala, M., Asherson, G.L. Eur. J. Immunol. 4 (1974) 799.
10. Phanuphak, P., Moorhead, J.W., Claman, H.N. J. Immunol. 113 (1974) 1230.
11. Moorhead, J.W. J. Immunol. 117 (1976) 802.
12. Miller, S.D., Sy, M.S., Claman, H.N. J. Immunol. 7 (1977) 165.
13. Asherson, G.L., Wood, P.J., Mayhew, B. Immunol. 29 (1975) 1057.
14. Datta, U., Barnet, K., Asherson, G.L. Int. Arch. Allergy 50 (1976) 574.
15. Ramshaw, I.A., McKenzie, I.F.C., Bretscher, P.A., Parish, C.R. Cell. Immunol. 31 (1977) 364.
16. Droege, W., Suessmuth, W. Z. Immunitätsforsch. (Immunobiology) in press (1978).
17. Röllinghoff, M., Starzinski-Powitz, A., Pfitzenmaier, K., Wagner, H. J. Exp. Med. 145 (1977) 455.
18. Targart, V. Transplantation 23 (1977) 287.
19. Vadas, M.A., Miller, J.F.A.P., Gamble, J., Whitelaw, A. Int. Arch. Allergy 49 (1975) 676.

DEMONSTRATION OF CELL MEDIATED AUTOIMMUNITY AND INDUCTION OF A SUPPRESSIVE CONTROL MECHANISM

Johanna L'age-Stehr, Tibor Diamantstein and Hans Teichmann[*]

Klinikum Steglitz, Free University

1000 Berlin 45, W. Germany

In the last few years there is increasing evidence accumulating for the idea that tolerance to self-antigens is maintained by active suppressor mechanisms. Autoimmunity may thus arise not primarily as an effector cell abnormality but rather as a consequence of a defect in these control mechanisms (see 1,2 for review).

We would like to demonstrate here the induction of a specific suppressormechanism controlling the activity of autoreactive T-cells (T-ARC) in normal mice.

As reported earlier (3), 5-7 days after treatment of normal female inbred mice (AKR, BALB/c or C_3H) with a single high dose (125 mg/kg) of cyclophosphamid (CY) or a low dose of CY (20 mg/kg) and a blastogenic dose of lipopolysaccharide of E. coli (LPS), splenic T-cells can be isolated which, after s.c. injection into syngeneic recipients, will induce a massive recruitment and proliferation of lymphoid cells in the draining popliteal lymphnode (PLN) when measured 6 days after s.c. inoculation of the cells.   The PLN-enlargement following the injection of these autologous spleen cells is in the same order of magnitude as that which will be induced by s.c. inoculation of allogeneic spleen cells.

The detectability of the T-ARC in the spleen of CY-treated mice is only a transient phenomenon with a peak occuring at the 6th day after treatment. Spleen cells obtained from mice 8-9 days after CY-injection failed to elicit an increase of PLN-weight and of the

---

[*]in partial fulfillment of his doctoral thesis

TAB. 1:   Evidence for the Development of Specific Suppression of
the Activity of Autoreactive T-cells (T-ARC) in Cyclophosphamid
(CY) pretreated mice.

Cells injected s.c. into BALB/c mice:	PLN-Index in BALB/c mice			
	untreated	-6d CY	-8d CY	pretreated
3×10^6 T-ARC(BALB/c)	3.10 +0.18	3.52 +0.35	1.02 +0.18	
3×10^6 T-ARC(AKR)	3.42 +0.21	n.t.	3.36 +0.24	
3×10^6 BALB/c splenic T-cells	1.19 +0.12	n.t.	1.05 +0.05	
3×10^6 AKR splenic T-cells	3.39 +0.32	n.t.	3.27 +0.36	

T-ARC   =   nylon wool filtered spleen cells isolated from mice
               6 days after treatment with 125 mg/kg CY.
splenic   =   nylon wool filtered spleen cells of normal mice.
t-cells
PLN-   =   ratio of weight of draining over contralateral
index   popliteal lymphnode (6-8 mice per group).
n.t.   =   not tested.

content of nucleated cells in the nodes (PLN-index) when injected
into syngeneic recipients.

    The question arises, whether the failure to detect T-ARC in the
spleen 8 days after CY treatment was due to the development of a
specific control mechanism suppressing the activity of T-ARC by that
time. This hypothesis could be supported by several findings:

a)   Autologous T-ARC when injected into mice, which had been
treated 8 days previously with CY (125 mg/kg), did not elicit PLN-
enlargement, whereas the PLN-index following injection of allogeneic
spleen cells was similar in normal and in CY-pretreated animals (Tab.
1).

    These data indicate that the expression of T-ARC activity is
specifically suppressed in syngeneic CY-pretreated mice.

b)   When T-ARC were mixed prior to s.c. inoculation with either
nylon wool non-adherent spleen cells or serum obtained from mice 8
days after CY treatment, the PLN-index in normal syngeneic recipients

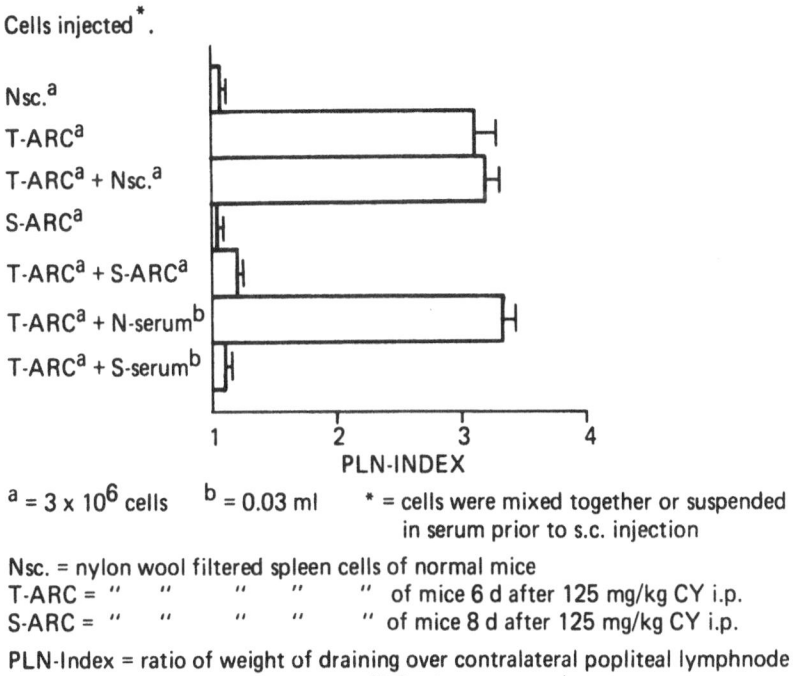

FIG. 1: Influence of Suppressor Mechanisms on EXPRESSION of the Activity of Autoreactive T-cells (T-ARC).

was reduced (Fig.1). These results also indicate that the expression of T-ARC activity is controlled by a suppressor mechanism – consisting of nylon wool non-adherent spleen cells and a serum factor – which becomes established after the transient appearance of T-ARC.

c) Intravenous injection of spleen cells from suppressed mice into normal syngeneic animals 1 hour prior to application of a T-ARC inducing dose of CY could abolish the induction or did mask the detectability of T-ARC in the spleens 6 days later. Injection of normal spleen cells or thymocytes prior to CY treatment had no effect on the induction of T-ARC. However, intravenous injection of normal spleen cells or thymocytes 1 day after CY application (a time interval which allows CY to become metabolized and renders

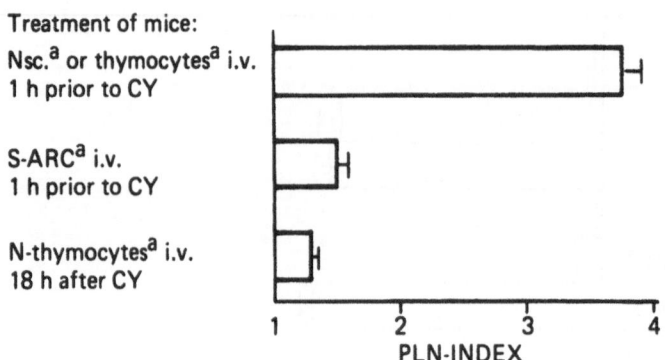

Treatment of mice:

Nsc.[a] or thymocytes[a] i.v.
1 h prior to CY

S-ARC[a] i.v.
1 h prior to CY

N-thymocytes[a] i.v.
18 h after CY

PLN-INDEX

[a] = 5 x 10^7 cells

PLN-Index = ratio of weight of draining over contralateral popliteal
            lymphnode in syngeneic recipients of 3 x10^6 T-ARC
            (6-8 mice/group)

T-ARC = nylonwool filtered spleen cells from mice 6 days after 125 mg/kg CY i.v.

S-ARC = spleen cells of mice treated 8 days previously with 125 mg/kg CY i.v.

Nsc. = Normal spleen cells

FIG. 2:   Influence of Suppressor cells on INDUCTION of Autoreactive
T-cells (T-ARC). Evidence for Different Sensitivity of Suppressor
Cell-Precursors and "Primed" Suppressor Cells to Cyclophosphamid (CY).

it ineffective to the inoculated cells) could suppress detectability
of T-ARC in the spleens at day 6 after CY treatment (Fig.2).   These
results suggest that in normal spleen cell- or thymocyte populations
only precursors of suppressor cells (S-ARC) for T-ARC activity are
present.   These precursors are CY sensitive and cannot prevent expression of already established T-ARC (Fig.1), whereas "primed"
specific suppressor cells of T-ARC are CY-resistant.

CY treatment in vivo damages mainly B-cell areas in the spleen
(4) whereas cell mediated immune reactions are even stimulated by
this alkylating agent (5), probably as a consequence to elimination
of suppressor cell precursors (6). We asked the question: what may
be the nature of the stimulus ("new" self-antigen?) for induction of
T-ARC and of the subsequent suppressor mechanism? Our working hypothesis is that blast-cells which form consequent to CY or LPS treatment express "new" antigens that are recognized and stimulate T-ARC

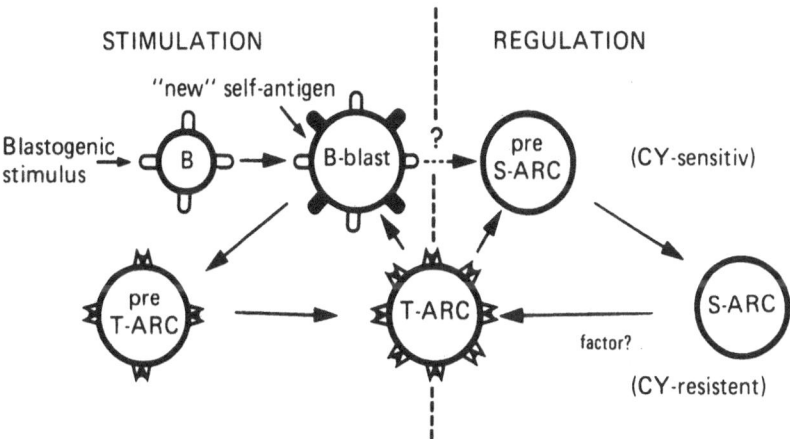

Fig. 3 Hypothetical Scheme of Induction and Suppression of
Autoreactive T-cells (T-ARC).Pre = Precursor,
S-ARC = Suppressor of T-ARC, CY = Cyclophosphamid)

FIG. 3: Hypothetical Scheme of Induction and Suppression of
Autoreactive T-cells (T-ARC). Pre = Precursor, S-ARC =
Suppressor of T-ARC, CY = Cyclophosphamid.

(7). Experiments with isolated splenic blastoid cells of this
regeneration phase show that these blastoid cells can induce T-ARC
as well as suppressor mechanisms when transferred i.v. into normal
syngeneic animals[++].

We suggest in the hypothetical scheme shown in Fig.3 that precursors of T-ARC will be stimulated first by "new" self-antigens
appearing at the surface of blastoid cells (e.g. differention
antigens, expression of endogenous virus genomes?). This stimulation
would then induce qualitative or quantitative changes of T-ARC which
will be the trigger for precursors of suppressor cells to develop a
mature CY-resistant suppressor mechanism controlling T-ARC activity
(network of idiotype-antiidiotype responses?). In normal animals
this dominant suppressor mechanism will prevent manifestation of
autoreactivity or autoimmune diseases. However, if the immune
system of animals is depleted on precursors of suppressor cells -
e.g., i) genetically like in NZB mice (2), ii) permanently as
after thymectomy (8), or iii) transiently by drug treatment like
CY or hydrocortisone (9) - any stimulus that will trigger precursors
of autoreactive cells may lead to manifestation of autoimmune phenomena.

[++] Johanna L'age-Stehr and Hans Teichmann unpublished observations.

REFERENCES

1. Waldmann, T.A., Broder, S., in: Progress in Clinical Immunology
    3. Ed. by R.S. Schwarz, Grune-Stratton, New York.
2. Talal, N., Steinberg, A.D., in: Current Topics in Microbiology
    and Immunology. Springer Verlag 64 79.
3. L'age-Stehr, J., Diamantstein, T., Nature 271 (1978) 663.
4. Turk, J.L., Poulter, L.W., Clin. Exp. Immunol. 10 (1972) 285.
5. Lagrange, P.H., Mackaness, G.B., Miller, T.E., J. Exp. Med.
    139 (1974) 1529.
6. Askenase, P.W., Hayden, B.J., Gershon, R.K., J. Exp. Med. 141
    (1975) 697.
7. L'age-Stehr, J., Diamantstein, T., Europ. J. Immunol. in press.
8. Carnaud, C., Charreire, J., Bach, J.F., Cell. Immunol. 28 (1977)
    274.
9. Nachtigeal, D., Zan-Bar, I., Feldman, M., Transplant. Rev. 26
    (1975) 87.

ACKNOWLEDGEMENTS

This work was supported by the Deutsche Forschungsgemeinschaft
(Habilitationsstipendium: La 388/1).

SUPPRESSOR T CELLS IN INDUCTION AND MAINTENANCE OF LOW ZONE TOLERANCE TO BOVINE SERUM ALBUMIN

R. Stumpf, J. Heuer and E. Kölsch[*]

Heinrich Pette-Institut für Experimentelle Virologie
und Immunologie an der Universität Hamburg

[*]Present address: Lehrstuhl für Immunologie, Hygiene
Institut, Westfälische Wilhelms-Universät, Westring 10,
4400 Münster, W. Germany

INTRODUCTION

Previous studies on the mechanism of low zone tolerance (LZT) using antigen phage fd have demonstrated the presence of suppressor T cells in tolerant mice (1-4). These suppressor T cells are activated at low doses of antigen not yet sufficient to trigger helper T cells. Probably unprimed helper T cells are then target of suppression (4). The experimental data allowed to discuss a model of LZT in which suppressor T cells could play a role in induction of LZT. Important for the validity of such a model is its generalization for other antigen systems.

Bovine serum albumin (BSA) is a classical antigen for the study of LZT (5). Here we report that it is possible to activate suppressor cells with low zone tolerogenic doses of BSA and that these suppressor cells persist in tolerant animals, though they decay upon adoptive transfer with a rate known for the fd system (4). We also discuss experiments intended to break LZT with antisera against I-J determinants.

MATERIALS AND METHODS

Male CBA/J mice (at least 5 mice per group) 10-12 weeks old at beginning of experiments were used. BSA was purchased from the Behring-Werke, Marburg (Lahn). For tolerance induction and priming

BSA was deaggregated by ultracentrifugation in a fixed angle head rotor (Beckman Rotor 65) for 3 hours at 140,000 g. The upper third of the supernatant was used. Its protein concentration was determined photometrically.

Mice were injected with 2.5 mg hydrocortisone (HC) (crystal suspension, Hoechst, Frankfurt) 2 days before the first tolerogenic treatment. The mice received then 7 consecutive daily intraperitoneal (i.p.) injections of 10 μg deaggregated BSA. For priming mice were also HC-treated but received 7 injections of 100 μg deaggregated BSA. Thus the dose of antigen but not its physical form is relevant for tolerance induction or priming (5). For immunisation we avoided use of adjuvans and injected 1 mg of heat-denatured BSA (c-BSA, ref.6) per mouse (i.p.). Antibody titers were assayed using the Farr-test (5). Adoptive transfers were done as previously described (4) except that recipient mice were irradiated with 200 r 4-6 hours before cell transfer. In contrast to the fd system, suppression is impossible upon adoptive transfer into unirradiated recipient mice.

LZT induction, antibody assay, and adoptive transfers using antigen phage fd, were as previously described (2,4).

Antisera with anti I-J activity were prepared in the following way. (C57Bl/6 x DBA/2) Fl hybrids were injected with 2 x 10^7 B10. A(5R) spleen and thymus cells in weekly intervals for 2 months. Anti I-J activity of this anti I-J, E antisera was assessed by its capacity to enhance 5-7 fold over normal the plaque forming cell response of CBA mice after an injection of 5 x 10^5 sheep red blood cells (SRBC) (7).

RESULTS AND DISCUSSION

The outline of BSA-LZT experiments is shown in Fig.1.

Groups of CBA mice received a single injection of HC, followed by seven daily injections of 10 or 100 μg BSA or saline (controls). They were then immunized by 2 injections of 1 mg c-BSA spaced by a 10 days interval. Antibody titers were assayed one week later (Fig. 1 test (1) and Fig.2 open bars (1)).

Animals treated with saline showed a primary, those treated with 100 μg BSA an enhanced response. Mice treated with 10 μg BSA were unresponsive. Ten weeks after the beginning of the experiment the animals were challenged again and it was verified that those, which had originally received 10 μg BSA still remained unresponsive. (Fig.1, test (3) and Fig.2 open bars (3)).

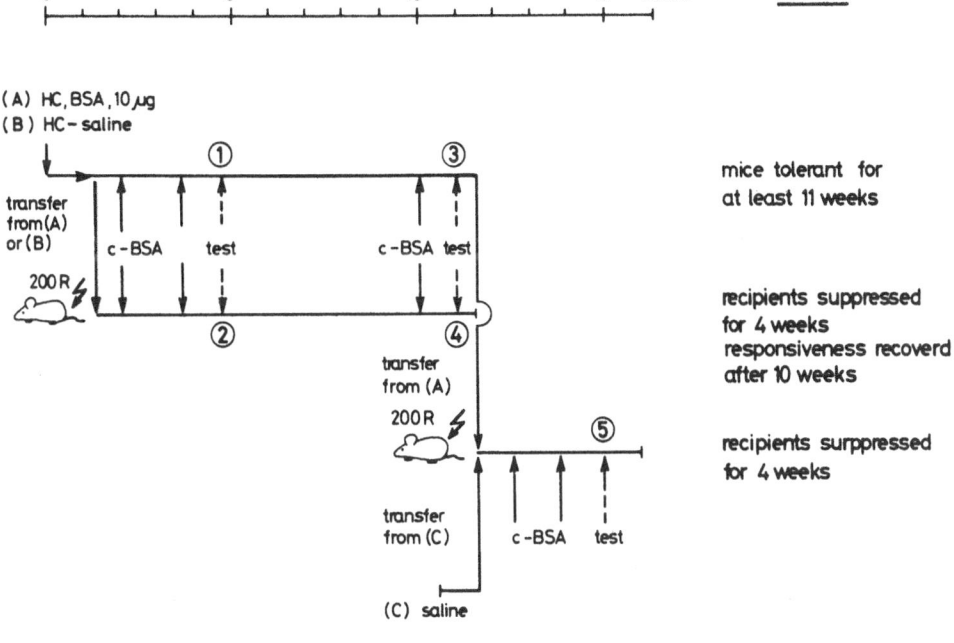

FIG. 1:   (see text for details)

Responsiveness at tests (1) - (5)

$(ABC_{33}$ (µg BSA/ml serum))

	"Saline" group	"10 µg BSA" group
(1)	7.4	<0.5
(2)	4.4	0.8
(3)	25.4	1.1
(4)	13.4	8.6
(5)	8.8	1.1

To test for suppressor cell activity spleen cells from donor
mice treated with HC and saline, 10 µg BSA or 100 µg BSA were
adoptively transferred into 200 r irradiated mice. These mice were
then immunized as described and tested 4 weeks after transfer.
At that time, mice which had received spleen cells from tolerogen
treated donors were suppressed (Fig.1, test (2) and Fig.2, dashed

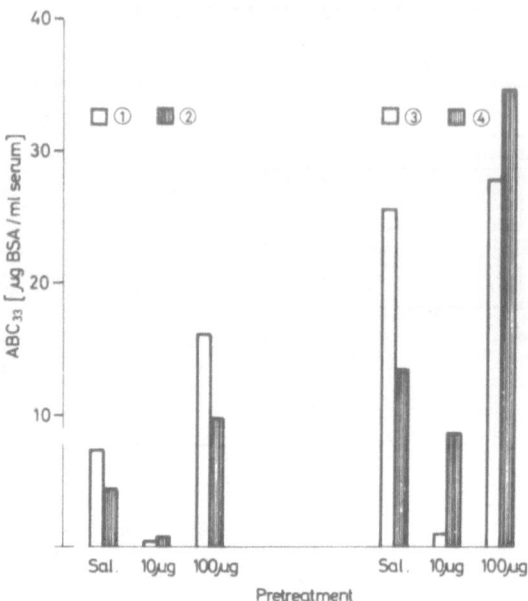

<u>FIG. 2</u>:   (see text for details)

bars (2)). However, when rechallenged and tested at the 11th week
those initially suppressed recipients had recovered from suppression
and showed a primary response (Fig.1 test (4) and Fig.2 dashed bars
(4)).

   At the same time it was tested whether the original groups of
tolerant donor mice still harboured suppressor cells. A new adoptive
transfer of donor spleen cells was made into recipients irradiated
with 200 r. They were then challenged twice and antibody titers
were determined. The response of recipient mice, which had received
spleen cells from donors tolerant for 11 weeks was suppressed (Fig.1
test (5)). This shows that suppressor cells are activated and
persist in BSA-low zone tolerant mice and can be demonstrated by a
suitable adoptive transfer. Persistence of suppressor cells in
tolerant mice is longer than expected from their half life estimated
in adoptive transfers.

   Based on the finding that anti I-J antisera can enhance the
plaque forming cell response to 5×10^5 SRBC (7) by presumably
blocking suppressor T cells, we tested the effect of such an antiserum (anti-I-J,E in this case) on BSA- and fd-LZT. A single
injection of 20 μl of anti I-J,E antiserum per mouse at the beginning
of tolerogenic treatment did not prevent induction of BSA- or fd-LZT
(Tab.1 & 2).

TAB. 1:   Effect of pretreatment with anti I-J,E on BSA-LZT

$(ABC_{33}$ (μg BSA/ml serum))

Treatment with	Mice injected before treatment with			
	normal mouse serum		anti I-J,E	
	group 1	group 2	group 1	group 2
HC, saline	5.8	27.0	17.9	31.3
HC, 10 μg BSA	0.5	0.8	4.0	0.4
HC, 100 μg BSA	40.4	69.6	26.9	33.1

Group 1:   After treatment challenges at days 7 and 17 with 1 mg
           c-BSA. Test one week later
Group 2:   After treatment challenges at days 7, 17 and 26 with
           1 mg c-BSA. Test one week later.
See text for further details.

TAB. 2:   Effect of pretreatment with anti I-J,E on phage fd-LZT
and adoptive transfer of suppressor T cells (K values of anti
fd sera).

Treatment of mice	non transfer groups	transfer groups
HC, saline + normal serum	12.0	8.1
HC, saline + anti I-J,E	9.4	9.9
HC, fd + normal serum	2.9	4.7
HC, fd + anti I-J,E	2.6	10.1

See text for further details.

In a preliminary experiment the same procedure abolished
suppressor T cell activity in adoptive transfer (Tab.2).

The experiments using antisera with anti I-J activity had been
designed to decide between suppression and deletion models for LZT.
However, use of these antisera might not be the proper method to
solve this issue:

1. A single injection of anti I-J antiserum might not remove the whole pool of suppressor T cells from tolerant animals.

2. Prolonged treatment with anti I-J antisera does not selectively affect suppressor- but also blocks T helper cell activity (unpublished results, see also ref.8).

At the present state of analysis there remains for two structurally very different antigens the strong correlation between dose of antigen which induces LZT and dose of antigen which activates suppressor cells. In addition persistence of suppressor cells in low-zone tolerant mice suggests a possible function in maintenance of LZT.

REFERENCES

1. Weber, G, Kölsch, E., Eur. J. Immunol. 3 (1973) 767.
2. Kölsch, E., et al., Transplant. Rev. 26 (1975) 56.
3. Heuer, J., et al., Eur. J. Immunol. 7 (1977) 769.
4. Stumpf, R., et al., Eur. J. Immunol. 7 (1977) 74.
5. Mitchison, N.A., Immunol. 15 (1968) 509.
6. Benacerraf, B., et al., Brit. J. Exp. Path. 38 (1957) 35.
7. Pierres, M., et al., Proc. Nat. Acad. Sci. USA 74 (1977) 3975.
8. Tada, T., et al., J. Exp. Med. 147 (1978) 446.

ACKNOWLEDGEMENTS

This work was supported by the Deutsche Forschungsgemeinschaft. The HPI is supported by HH and BmJFG.

CATION-INDUCED IMMUNOSUPPRESSION: THE EFFECT OF LITHIUM ON ARTHUS
REACTIVITY, DELAYED HYPERSENSITIVITY AND ANTIBODY PRODUCTION IN THE
RAT

B.D. Janković, Ljiljana Popesković and Katarina Isaković

Immunology Research Center, Vojvode Stepe 458,

Belgrade, Yugoslavia

ABSTRACT

Arthus reactivity and delayed skin sensitivity to bovine serum
albumin (BSA), and anti-BSA antibody production were markedly
impaired in female Wistar rats repeatedly injected with lithium
chloride.

INTRODUCTION

It is well known that lithium is capable of attenuating and
preventing recurrences of manic and depressive episodes in patients.
Although lithium interacts with many biological systems and affects
transports and cellular functions, including receptor processes,
cell membrane transports and enzyme activation, the mechanism of
its action is still unclear (1-4). Although there is an enormous
amount of literature on the biological role of lithium, systematic
experimental and clinical evaluations of the effect of lithium on the
immune system have not previously been conducted. The pilot study
described here yielded the first results on the relationship between
lithium and immune responses in the rat.

MATERIALS AND METHODS

Treatment of rats with lithium chloride (LiCl). Female 8-week-
old Wistar rats were injected intraperitoneally with LiCl, m.w. 42.20
(Barker Chemical Co., Phillipsburg, N.J.). In order to reach and

maintain an equilibrium between intake and excretion of lithium, rats
were treated with LiCl dissolved in saline for a period of 30 days.
One group of rats received 2 injections per day of 3 mEq/kg. of body
weight on day 4, 2 and 0 before immunization, and thereafter every
second day 1 injection of 3 mEq/kg. b.w. Another group was treated
in an identical manner with 5 mEq/kg. b.w., except that the first
injection after immunization was administered on day 8. Thus, the
"3 mEq/kg group" received 17 injections and the "5 mEq/kg group" 12
injections of LiCl. Controls were treated with saline alone. The
animals were carefully observed every day, and weighed on a standard
small-animal scale.

Immunization and skin-testing. The rats were immunized with
0.5 mg of bovine serum albumin (BSA) incorporated into complete
Freund adjuvant (5). The animals were skin-tested at 8 days, and
again at 16 and 25 days with 30 µg of BSA in 0.1 ml of saline.
Arthus reactions were read at 4 hours and delayed reactions at 24
hours (5).

Antibody determination. Serum samples were obtained 8, 16 and
25 days after immunization, and anti-BSA antibody titers determined
by a modified microhemagglutination technique (5).

Postmortem. Rats of all groups were autopsied at 30 days after
the beginning of treatment with lithium. Lymphoid and nonlymphoid
organs were inspected grossly, and taken for histological examination.

RESULTS

Body, spleen and thymus weights. Rats treated with saline of
LiCl did not show a failure to gain weight during the whole period
of experimentation (Tab.1). There were some statistically insignificant variations in the weights of spleens and thymuses (Tab.1).
All animals injected with lithium survived. Although different
somatic side effects may occur during lithium treatment (3), no
symptoms of lithium-poisoning were observed in rats used in this
study. However, in an additional experiment on Wistar and DA rats,
only 3 injections of 10 mEq/kg. b.w. induced a very high mortality
rate (77.7-81.2%). Histological changes in lymphoid and nonlymphoid
tissues of lithium-treated rats will be presented elsewhere.

Immune responses. Statistical evaluation of results (Student's
t test) showed that Arthus and delayed skin reactions to BSA were
significantly lower in rats injected with lithium (Tab.2). The
intensity ("mean score") of reactions was sharply reduced in lithium-
treated animals. As for antibody production, a striking decrease in
elaboration of BSA-specific IgM and IgG occurred on days 8 and 16,
but not on day 25 after immunization (Tab.3). According to these

TAB. 1:   Body and organ weights in rats treated with lithium.

Group	Mean (±SE) weight		
	Body (g)	Spleen*	Thymus*
Nontreated	236.7±4.9 (9)	369.0±16.9 (9)	149.5±11.1(9)
Lithium-treated			
with 3 mEq/kg	227.7±4.6(18)	334.6±21.5(18)	138.3±8.7(18)
with 5 mEq/kg	226.2±4.0(17)	330.4±15.2(17)	161.6±7.9(17)

Rats were weighed and sacrificed 30 days after the beginning of
treatment with lithium chloride or saline (nontreated controls), i.e.
26 days after immunization with BSA.

*mg/10 of body weight.

results, it seems that a prolonged treatment of rats with lithium
affected the immune inflamatory skin reactions more than the antibody-
producing capacity.

DISCUSSION

A number of apparent inconsistencies regarding the action of
lithium makes it impossible to avoid some speculative inferences
when considering the biological effects of lithium, and in particular
its involvement in immune mechanisms.

a)   Some immunological effects of Li^+ may result from a competition
for "receptor sites" on cell membrane between Li^+ and other physiological cations (Mg^{2+}, Ca^{2+}, Na^+ or K^+). Such a competition may
affect the conformational state of receptors on the lymphocyte
membrane, as has already been demonstrated for the neuronal membrane
(4). Besides, this competition may be accompanied by lowering or
blocking of conductibility of Na^+ and K^+ through their "channels" in
the cell membrane, or may antagonize the action of Mg^{2+} (6). Although
no specific Li-binding protein is known, the possibility remains that
lithium may combine with Ig molecules (or other receptors) on the
lymphocyte membrane.

b)   Lithium influences the turnover and metabolism of the biogenic
amines (7). Accordingly, lithium may affect biogenic amines which
are important for immune reactions, and certain immuno-mediators
(e.g. lymphokines).

TAB. 2:   Arthus and delayed skin reactions to BSA in rats treated with lithium.

Group	Mean (mm+SE) reaction			Degree of reaction (mean score)*		
	Days after immunization			Days after immunization		
	8	16	25	8	16	25
ARTHUS REACTIVITY						
Nontreated	12.9+1.5(10/10)	14.8+1.1 (9/9)	18.1+1.1 (9/9)	1.94	2.11	2.56
Lithium-treated with 3 mEq/kg	8.1+1.2(15/20) P< 0.001	12.9+1.6(16/19) P< 0.05	12.8+0.9(18/18) P< 0.001	0.95	1.39	1.18
with 5 mEq/kg	1.9+0.8 (4/18) P< 0.001	6.8+1.4(10/17) P< 0.001	6.9+1.4(10/17) P< 0.001	0.17	0.59	0.62
DELAYED HYPERSENSITIVITY						
Nontreated	13.7+1.8 (8/10)	14.8+1.3 (9/9)	15.6+1.1 (9/9)	1.50	1.89	1.56
Lithium-treated with 3 mEq/kg	5.5+1.3(10/20) P< 0.001	9.3+1.5(13/19) P< 0.01	6.6+1.2(12/18) P< 0.001	0.55	0.79	0.39
with 5 mEq/kg	3.4+1.0 (7/18) P< 0.001	3.3+1.2 (5/17) P< 0.001	3.2+1.2 (5/17) P< 0.001	0.29	0.21	0.24

In parenthesis: Nominator, number of rats with reactions; denominator, number of rats in group.
* Mean score: an arithmetic score reflecting an overall response was calculated for each group of rats,
depending on the degree of edema (Arthus reactions) and induration (delayed reactions) defined as follows:
negative = 0; + = 0.5; + = 1; ++ = 2; and +++ = 3 (an arbitrary scale)

TAB. 3: Circulating anti-BSA antibody in rats treated with lithium.

Group	Mean antibody titer ($\log_2\pm$SE)					
	Days after immunization					
	8		16		25	
	Pre-ME	Post-ME	Pre-ME	Post-ME	Pre-ME	Post-ME
Nontreated	5.0+0.4 (10/10)	2.1+0.2 (10/10)	5.2+0.1 (9/9)	4.7+0.2 (9/9)	6.5+0.3 (9/9)	6.1+0.2 (9/9)
Lithium-treated with 3 mEq/kg	2.9+0.3 (20/20) $P<0.001$	0.9+0.2 (11/19) $P<0.01$	4.2+0.2 (19/19) $P<0.01$	3.6+0.1 (19/19) $P<0.01$	6.0+0.1 (18/18) $P<0.05$	5.5+0.2 (18/18) $P<0.05$
with 5 mEq/kg	2.0+0.2 (18/18) $P<0.001$	0.6+0.1 (9/18) $P<0.001$	4.3+0.1 (17/17) $P<0.01$	3.7+0.2 (17/17) $P<0.05$	6.3+0.2 (17/17) $P<0.05$	5.8+0.2 (17/17) $P<0.05$

Pre-ME, before treatment with mercaptoethanol.
Post-ME, after treatment with mercaptoethanol.
In parenthesis: Nominator, number of rats with antibodies; denominator, number of rats in group.

c)   Lithium influences adenylate cyclase and c-AMP, and thus interferes directly with intracellular metabolic processes by activating or inhibiting enzymatic systems (8).

d)   Finally, lithium has many effects on hormonal functions. Lymphopenia which accompanies the administration of lithium may be caused by an increase of plasma cortisol (9). Mice treated chronically with LiCl developed lymphopenia (10). In any case, the role of lithium in immunity should be tested by further experiments.

REFERENCES

1.   Gershon, S., Shopin, B., eds.,"Lithium: Its Role in Psychiatric Research and Treatment". Plenum Press, New York (1973).
2.   Schou, M., Biochem. Soc. Trans., 1 (1973) 81.
3.   Johnson, S., in: Lithium Research and Therapy. (F.N. Johnson, ed) Academic Press, New York 533 (1975).
4.   Bunney, Jr., W.E., Murphy, D.L., Neurosci. Res. Prog. Bull, Vol. 14, No. 2 (1976).
5.   Janković, B.D., Waksman, B.H., Arnason, B.G., J. Exp. Med. 116 (1962) 159.
6.   Trautner, E.M., Morris, R., Noack, C.H., Gershon, S., Med. J. Australia, 2 (1955) 280.
7.   Bliss, E.L., Ailion, J., Brain Res. 24 (1970) 305.
8.   Smith, L.D., Kizer, D.E., Biochim. Biophys. Acta. 191 (1969) 415.
9.   Radomski, J.L., Fuyat, H.N., Nelson, A.A., Smith, P.K., J. Pharmacol. 100 (1950) 429.
10.   Perez-Cruet, J., Dancey, J.T., Experientia 33 (1977) 646.

ACKNOWLEDGEMENTS

Supported by Republic of Serbia Research Fund, Belgrade.

CHARACTERIZATION OF REACTIVE AND SUPPRESSIVE CELLS IN THE MOUSE

EMBRYONIC LIVER BY PEANUT AGGLUTININ (PNA)

A. Globerson, H. Rabinowich, T. Umiel, Y. Reisner and
N. Sharon
Departments of Cell Biology and Biophysics
The Weizmann Institute of Science
76100 Rehovot, Israel

INTRODUCTION

The mouse embryonic liver is known as a site of development of
B cells (1) and seems also to contain cells which can give rise to
T cells upon thymus influence (2-4). Recently we observed that the
embryonic liver cells can interfere with reactions of adult immunocompetent T and B cells (5,6) and it was thus suggested that
suppressor cells develop in this tissue. We therefore attempted
to characterize these suppressor cells and find out whether
suppression is exerted by cells separable from the potentially
reactive ones.

MATERIALS AND METHODS

Animals: Female and male (Balb/c x C57BL/6)F_1, Balb/c and
C57BL/6 mice supplied by the Weizmann Institute Animal Breeding
Center were used throughout this study, at the age of 2-3 months
or as embryos at the 19th day of gestation.

Cell preparation and separation: Liver cell suspensions were
prepared as previously described (7). Separation by peanut agglutinin (PNA) was performed as reported for suspensions of thymus
cells (8), emplozing 3 mg/ml PNA on samples of 4-5 x 10^8 cells.

Culture techniques: Mixed lymphocyte culture (MLC) technique
was examined, as reported in previous studies (10). The liver cells
were treated with mitomycin before they were added to the cultures
(10). Mitogen stimulation with concanavalin A (Con A, Miles Yeda,

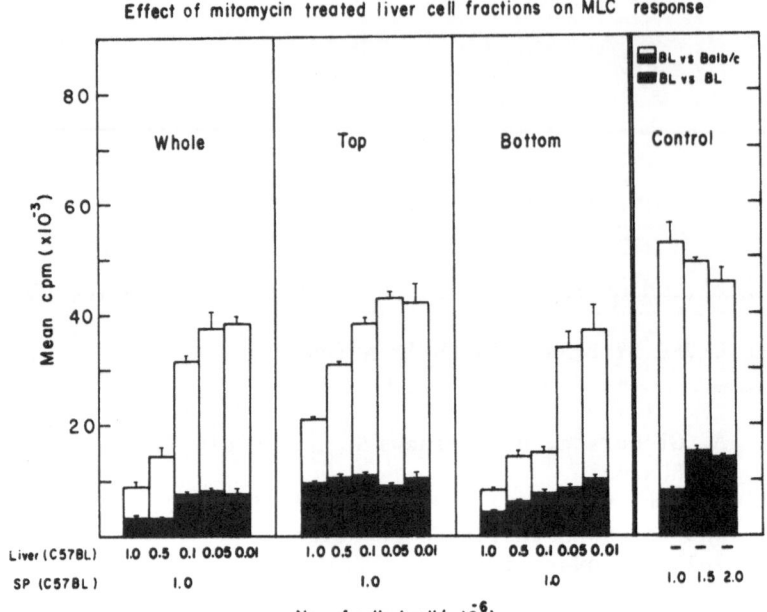

FIG. 1:   Suppression of C57BL vs. Balb/c MLC response by unseparated
and separated fractions of C57BL embryonic liver cells.

Rehovot), phytohemagglutinin (PHA, Wellcome Res. Labs., Beckenham,
England), lipopolysaccharide (LPS, E. coli O111:B4, Difco Labs.,
Detroit, USA) and Dextran sulfate (DxS, Pharmacia, Sweden), was
performed according to Rotter and Trainin (9). The results shown
in the figures represent mean ± S.E. values of triplicate cultures.

RESULTS AND DISCUSSION

We showed previously that embryonic and neonatal mouse liver
cells interfere with MLC response of adult mouse spleen cells (5).
In order to determine whether this suppression is exerted by mature
or immature cells in the liver, we employed PNA, which is known to
separate adult thymus cells (8) and bone marrow cells (11) into two
such populations. Hence, liver cells were separated by PNA into two
fractions containing the unagglutinated (PNA⁻) top of the separation
mixture and the agglutinated (PNA⁺) cells which settled at the
bottom of the separation test tube. These fractions, as well as
unseparated liver cells, were added to mixed lymphocyte cultures at
various cell doses. As shown in Fig.1, the intact liver cell
suspension suppressed the reaction, as shown previously (10). The
PNA⁺ ("bottom") fraction was more potent in suppression than the
PNA⁻ ("top"), as revealed from the effective cell doses in these
two groups.

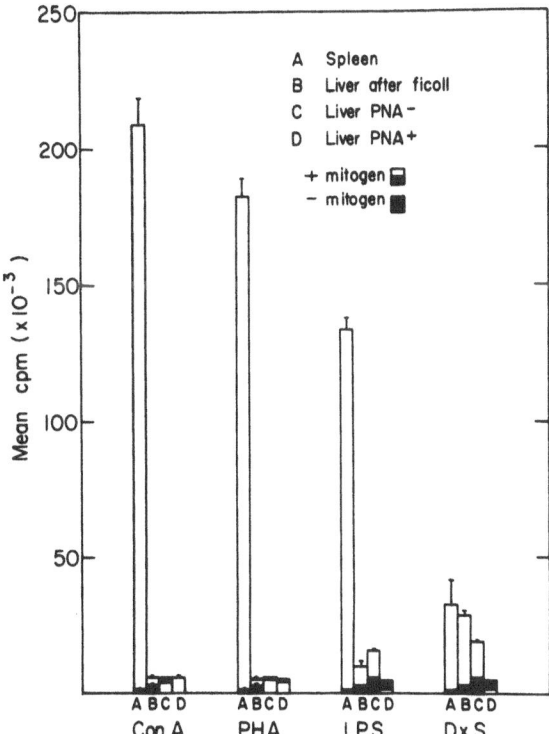

FIG. 2: Response of (Balb/c x C57BL)F_1 embryonic liver cells to mitogens.

Since this separation procedure resulted in a more efficient fraction of suppressor cells, we attempted to find out whether potentially reactive cells are located in the unagglutinable fraction. To examine this possibility, we employed a variety of T and B cell mitogens and examined the response of the separated cell populations, as compared to unseparated liver cells and to normal adult spleen cells as positive controls. As shown in Fig.2, reactivity of liver cells manifested only to the B cell mitogens (LPS and DxS) and not to the T cell mitogens (Con A and PHA), whereas the spleen cells reacted to all of them. These responses of the liver cells were expressed in the PNA$^-$ and not in the PNA$^+$ fractions.

In a parallel set of experiments we examined whether the response of adult spleen cells to these T and B cell mitogens is suppressed by the liver cells. Accordingly, unseparated as well as PNA and PNA$^+$ fractions were added to adult spleen cells stimulated with Con A, PHA, LPS and DxS, respectively. Control cultures were

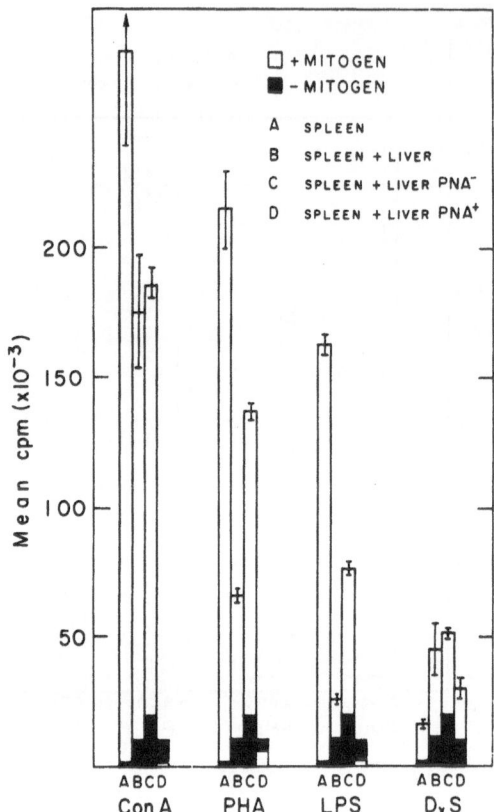

FIG. 3: Suppression of adult spleen cell response to mitogens by
embryonic liver cell preparations.

set up in parallel, without liver cells. It was found (Fig. 3) that
the responses to Con A, PHA and LPS were lower in cultures containing
the whole liver cell preparation and the PNA$^-$ fraction. Cultures
containing the PNA$^+$ cells did not manifest any response. It was of
interest to note that the response to DxS was not reduced in any of
these liver cell containing cultures. This may indicate that
interference with the responses does not stem from nonspecific
cytotoxic effect of the liver cell preparations.

Finally, we examined whether suppression occurs only if the
liver cells are applied to cultures concomitantly with mitogen
stimulation, or whether suppression may manifest also if the cells
are added at a later period. The experiment was thus repeated,
applying the liver cell preparations 24 h after stimulation of the
spleen cells with mitogens. As revealed from Fig.4, the PNA$^+$ cell

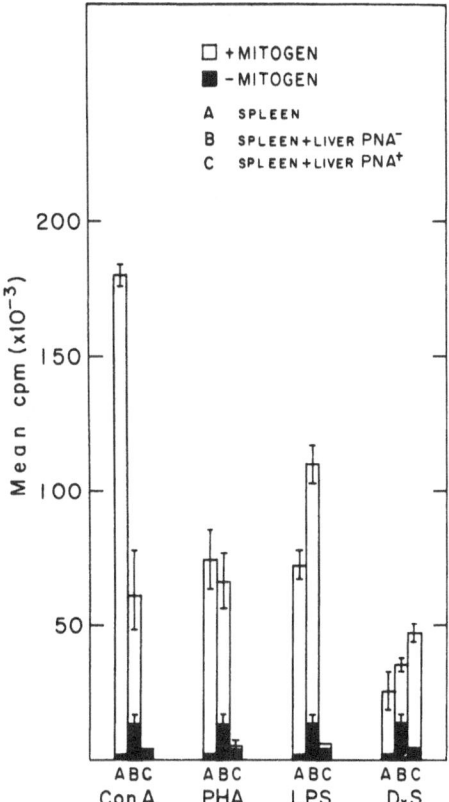

FIG. 4: Suppression of adult spleen cell response to mitogens by embryonic liver cell preparations added to culture 24 h after stimulation.

fractions suppressed the response in this case as in the previous experiment.

These results suggest that the major suppression by embryonic liver cells is exerted by a distinct cell population having a membrane sugar receptor D-galactose. It has been pointed out that such cells may be representing the less mature population (8,11). Whether indeed this procedure separates cells at different stages of maturation in the liver and whether a priori the reactive cells in the PNA⁻ fraction stem from cells which had the potential to suppress lymphocyte responses remains to be determined.

SUMMARY

Embryonic liver cells suppressed the MLC response of adult mouse spleen cells and reactivity to mitogens Con A, PHA and LPS. Suppression was exerted by cells agglutinated by PNA (PNA$^+$ cells). Cells reacting to LPS and to DxS were found in the nonagglutinated (PNA$^-$) cell fraction. The PNA$^+$ fraction did not react to DxS nor did it reduce the response of adult spleen cells to this mitogen.

REFERENCES

1. Owen, J.J.T., Cooper, M.D., Raff, M.C., Nature 249 (1974) 361.
2. Barnes, D.W.H., Loutit, J.F., Samson, J.M., N.Y. Acad. Sci. 120 (1968) 218.
3. Taylor, R.B., Brit. J. Expl. Pathol. 46 (1965) 376.
4. Globerson, A., Kirov, S.M., Parish,C.R. in: Immune Reactivity of Lymphocytes: Development, Expression and Control, M. Feldman, A. Globerson, eds., New York, Plenum, (1975) p.69.
5. Globerson, A., Zinkernagel, R.M., Umiel, T., Transplantation 20 (1975) 480.
6. Globerson, A., Rabinowich, H., Umiel, T., in:Developmental immunobiology, J.B. Solomon, J.D., Horton, eds., Amsterdam: Elsevier, (1977) p.331.
7. Umiel, T., Globerson, A., Differentiation 2 (1974) 169.
8. Reisner, Y., Linker-Israeli, M., Sharon, N., Cell. Immunol. 25 (1976) 129.
9. Rotter, V., Trainin, N., Cell. Immunol. 16 (1975) 413.
10. Umiel, T., Globerson, A., Trainin, N., Transplantation 24 (1977) 282.
11. Reisner, Y., Itzicovitch, L., Meshorer, A., Sharon, N., Proc. Nat. Acad. Sci. US (in press) (1978).

ACKNOWLEDGEMENTS

Partial support for these studies was provided by the Thyssen Foundation (A. Globerson) and the Bureau of the Chief Scientist, Israel Ministry of Health, Tel Aviv (T. Umiel). The skillful technical assistance of Ms. Rachel Gury and Ms. Ruth Goldman is gratefully acknowledged.

THE EFFECT OF ADJUVANT INDUCED SUPPRESSOR CELLS ON IN VITRO AND IN

VIVO LYMPHOCYTE RESPONSES

Nabil Hanna and David Nelken

Laboratory of Immunohematology
Hadassah University Hospital
Jerusalem, Israel

INTRODUCTION

Suppressor cells which are able to inhibit lymphocyte proliferative responses in vitro have been described in the spleens of mice injected with corynebacterium parvum (1) or bearing progressively growing tumors (2,3). In vitro studies have shown that such suppressor cells inhibit DNA-synthesis of both T and B lymphocytes and suppress immune responses which require cellular proliferation.

Based primarily on in vitro experimentation it was speculated that non-specific suppressor cells might play a significant role in regulating excessive lymphocyte proliferation in vivo and, when present in large numbers, they might cause generalized suppression of the host immune responses.

In the present work suppressor cells were induced by injection of $AL(OH)_3$ into mice and their effect on in vitro and in vivo immune reactions was studied.

MATERIALS AND METHODS

Mice were injected i.p. with 0.5 ml of $AL(OH)_3$. At various intervals thereafter spleens and lymph nodes were excised and single cell suspensions were prepared. Aliquats of 0.5×10^6 lymphoid cells were cultured in microculture wells in the presence of PHA or LPS for a total period of 72 hours. Twenty hours before harvest the cultures were pulsed with 1 μci of ^{3}H-thymidine and the amount of TCA-precipitable radioactivity was measured.

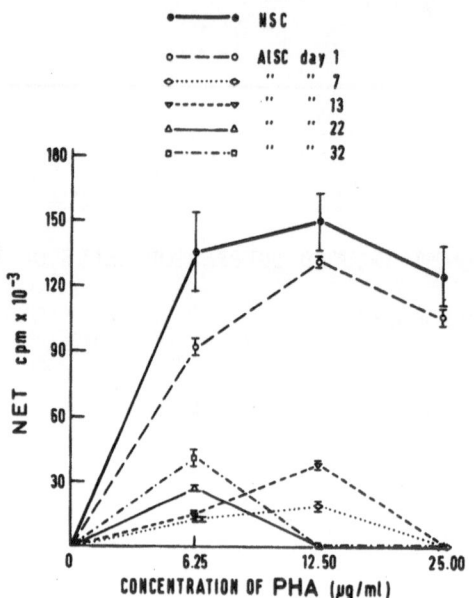

FIG. 1:   Thymidine uptake by PHA-stimulated spleen cells from
normal (NSC) and AL(OH)$_3$ treated (ALSC) mice.

Suppressor cell activity was assessed by mixing mitomycin-c
treated AL(OH)$_3$ induced suppressor cells with normal spleen cells
at the initiation of the cultures followed by pulsing, harvesting
and measuring the amount of incorporated ^{3}H-thymidine as above.

Adherent cells were removed by filtration through nylon wool
columns (4) and depletion of Fc-receptor bearing cells was done on
EA-monolayers (5).

The in vivo anti-SRBC plaque forming cell (PFC) response of
normal and AL(OH)$_3$ injected mice was measured 5 days after antigen
administration.

RESULTS AND DISCUSSION

In Fig.1 it is clearly shown that the in vitro mitogenic
responses of spleen cells obtained from mice injected i.p. with

TAB. 1:   PHA-stimulation of spleen cells from normal and AL(OH)$_3$ treated mice

	Net cpm per culture
Normal control - Unfractionated	168,000
- Nylon wool purified	170,000
AL(OH)$_3$ - Unfractionated	20,000
- Nylon wool purified	176,000
- Absorbed on EA/monolayer	135,000
Mixtures of equal numbers of normal spleen cells and mitomycin-C treated: [1]	
- Normal spleen cells	110,000
- AL(OH)$_3$ spleen cells	54,000
- AL(OH)$_3$ - nylon wool purified cells	131,000
- AL(OH)$_3$ - nylon wool adherent cells[2]	69,000
- Normal - nylon wool adherent cells[2]	139,000
- AL(OH)$_3$ - EA/monolayer adherent cells[3]	13,000

1.   Mitomycin-C 40 μg/10^7 cells/ml.
2.   Recovered by mechanical disruption and agitation of the nylon wool in medium.
3.   Eluted after lysis of the erythrocyte - monolayer by tris - ammonuim chloride.

AL(OH)$_3$ are markedly depressed. This low reactivity was detected very early after adjuvent administration and remained so for several weeks thereafter. The depressed response was found not to be due to inner functional defects in T or B lymphocytes nor to dilution of reactive cells by myeloid and other non-lymphoid cells present in spleens of AL(OH)$_3$ treated mice. Removal of nylon wool adherent cells caused a significant increase in the mitogenic response of spleen cells of the adjuvant treated groups. This enhancement might have resulted from T cell enrichment and/or removal of suppressor cells that actively inhibit the mitogen response of otherwise functional lymphocytes. However, in cocultivation experiments we were able to show that spleen cells from AL(OH)$_3$ treated mice do suppress the proliferative response of normal spleen cells, and that the adherent Fc-receptor bearing cells are responsible for this suppression (Tab.1). In these experiments the most potent suppressors were those eluted from the EA-monolayers. These suppressor cells appear to be similar to those described in tumor-bearing and C. parvum treated mice which were identified as activated mononuclear phagocytes (6,7).

TAB. 2:   Effect of AL(OH)$_3$ [1] on the induction of anti-SRBC PFC

		PFC/10^6 spleen cells	
		i.v.	i.p.
10^8 SRBC	Normal	208 $\pm$ 6	198 $\pm$ 8
	AL(OH)$_3$	355 $\pm$ 48 (170%)	9 $\pm$ 4 (5%)
10^9 SRBC	Normal	125 $\pm$ 21	294 $\pm$ 30
	AL(OH)$_3$	220 $\pm$ 26 (176%)	188 $\pm$ 11 (63%)

1.   AL(OH)$_3$ was injected i.p. 3-7 days before antigen injection.

Faced with the difficulty of relating the inhibition of lymphocyte responses in vitro to the regulation of lymphocyte proliferation
by suppressor cells in vivo, we tried to determine if suppressor
cells present in spleens of adjuvant treated mice suppress antibody
production against SRBC in vivo. The results of such an experiment
are summarized in Tab.2. It is obvious that the route of antigen
administration is of paramount importance in determining whether the
antibody response will be suppressed or enhanced. Intravenous
injection of 10^8 or 10^9 SRBC resulted in a strong PFC-response in
spleens of both normal and AL(OH)$_3$ treated mice. Moreover, adjuvant
induced enhancement was detected in the later group. On the other
hand, strong suppression was observed upon i.p. injection of 10^8
SRBC. However, this suppression was partially overcome by increasing
the antigen dose to 10^9 SRBC per mouse. This result might be
attributed to the destruction and elimination of antigen by the
highly active inflammatory cells induced locally by the i.p. injection
of AL(OH)$_3$ rather than to the inhibition of lymphocyte proliferative
response to antigen stimulation.

The present findings indicate that although splenic suppressor
cells are able to inhibit lymphocyte mitogen responses in vitro they
fail to exert any suppressive effect on the in vivo immune reactivity
of lymphocytes optimally stimulated with antigen. Therefore, we feel
that the immunological significance of suppressor macrophages, as
well as the in vivo relevance of in vitro mitogen reponses should be
carefully evaluated.

REFERENCES

1.   Scott, M.T., Cell. Immunol. 5 (1972) 459.

2.   Kilburn, D.G., Smith, J.B., Gorczynski, R.M., Eur. J. Immunol.
      4 (1974) 784.
3.   Fernbach, B.R., Kirchner, H., Bonard, G.D., Herberman, R.B.,
      Transplantation 21 (1976) 381.
4.   Julius, M.H., Simpson, E., Herzenberg, L.A., Eur. J. Immunol.
      3 (1973) 645.
5.   Kedar, E., Ortiz de Landazuri, M., Bonavida, B., J. Immunol.
      112 (1974) 1231.
6.   Kirchner, H., Muchmore, A.V., Chused, T.M., Hodden, H.T.,
      Herberman, R.B., J. Immunol. 144 (1975) 206.
7.   Scott, M.T., Cell. Immunol. 5 (1972) 469.

MIDDLE EAR TRANSPLANTATION: A NEW CONCEPT IN CLINICAL OTOLOGY

[1]J.E. Veldman, [1]A.J. Boezeman, [1]H.C. Overbosch, [1]G.A. Sedee, [1]Else Borsteilers, [2]W. Kuijpers, [2]P. van den Broek, [3]Thea M. Feltkamp-Vroom

[1]University Hospital, Utrecht, The Netherlands
[2]University Hospital, Nijmegen, The Netherlands
[3]Slotervaart Hospital, Amsterdam, The Netherlands

INTRODUCTION

Serious hearing impairment as a consequence of extensive excision of the chronically inflamed middle ear is still very common. After the introduction of tympanoplasty in 1952 a large variety of tissues and synthetic materials have been employed to repair this acquired defect in the sound conducting system (1,2,3).

During the past decade a new technique has been developed to establish an optimal anatomical and physiological reconstruction of the sound-conduction by the introduction of preserved allogenous tympanic membranes, ossicles and even tympano-ossicular block (4) (external ear skin manchet-tympanic membrane-ossicles).

Although the initial success rate varied, nowadays the results reported by some authors seem to reach the score obtained with isogenous tissue-grafts (5).

A very remarkable finding in allograft-tympanoplasty is the fact that no clear evidence of graft rejection has been reported in the literature. The lack of any immunological reaction to the human implant has been suggested to be due to a decrease or even total abolition of the antigens by the used preservatives (alcohol 70%, formadelyde 4%, Cialit ®*, 1:5000 solution)(6).

Although success or failure is highly dependent on the surgical

---

*   Sodium salt of an organomercuric compound.

INCUS TRANSPLANTATION (ORTHOTOPIC)

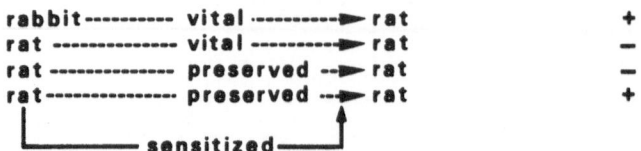

FIG. 1:   Experimental incus transplantation into middle ears of rats.

technique, secondary infection or recurrence of the middle-ear disease, also diminished immunogenicity or even the possibility of an active immunological interference - immunotolerance or immune-responsiveness, i.e. graft rejection - should be seriously considered as being the underlining explanation for both take and/or rejection of the implant. Experimental and clinical data support the idea that a particular state of immunological unresponsiveness may occur in this type of allografting, nowadays still performed without prior tissue-typing procedures or concomitant immunosuppression (7,8,9).

THE CONCEPT OF TOLEROGENESIS
IN MIDDLE EAR TRANSPLANTATION

Prior to developing this concept, one should first consider the problem whether the afferent and efferent loop of an immune response really exists in the middle ear complex. The following experimental data seems to be of crucial importance (Fig.1).

In rats vital xenogenous includes transplanted into the middle ear are rejected during a primary response. Vital allogenous incudes are accepted for observation periods up to two years, while vital or preserved allogenous incudes are definitely rejected within 2-3 weeks during a secondary immune response, i.e. when the recipients have been presensitized for donor alloantigens (6,10).

There is no reason to believe that vital allogenous tympano-ossicular bloc transplants (external ear manchet - tympanic membrane-ossicular chain) would act differently in the above mentioned experimental models. Moreover, although it seems very likely that prior preservation diminishes and probably also alters the antigenic structure of the allografts, it definitely does not abolish it.

Histological analyses of the regional lymph nodes in rabbits and rats draining the site of ectopic implantation of preserved allografts

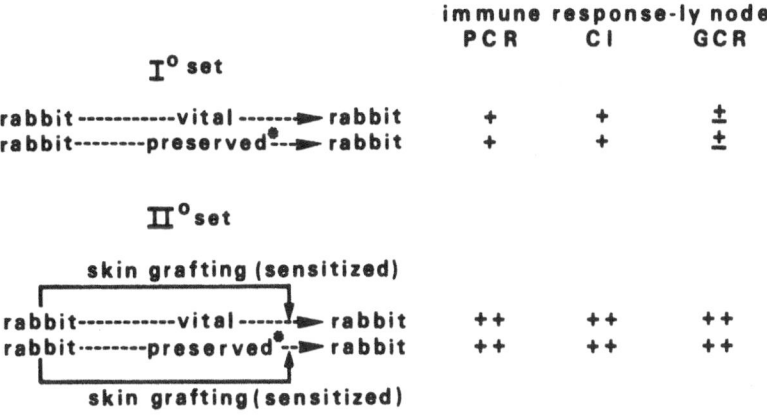

FIG. 2:   Antigenicity of tympanic membranes. Analyses of immune
response in draining lymph node (animal model).

*   alcohol 70% or formaldehyde 4%, pH 5.6 or Cialit ® 1:5000
solution.

of tympanic membrane, external ear skin or ossicles in a subcutaneous
pocket provoke a cellular immunity reaction in the thymus dependent
areas and a concomitant plasma cell and germinal centre reaction in
the non-thymus dependent areas, during a testing period of 5 days.

Furthermore, when the same experiments were performed on rabbits,
which were pre-sensitized by split-skin grafting, a strong second set
reaction was observed in the regional lymph nodes (Fig.2).

Histologically, no significant difference in reaction pattern
could be observed in the lymph node with the use of vital or preserved
allografts. In control experiments no second set reaction was
obtained, when tympanic membrane implantation was performed with a
second donor allograft. It can be concluded from these experimental
data that even after use of any of the mentioned preservatives, at
least part of the original antigenicity persists in the allografts.

From the reported clinical data no substantial evidence can be
derived, whether failures might be attributed to immunological graft
rejection. In our departments anti-leucocyte antibody titers in 8
patients, prior to allograft tympanoplasty and 1-3 months after
transplantation, were determined (none of the recipients had earlier
bloodtransfusion!) and all found negative. However, parallel findings
from our clinical cases in which the tympanic membranes were removed
because of recurrent "myringitis", 3 months-1 year after implantation

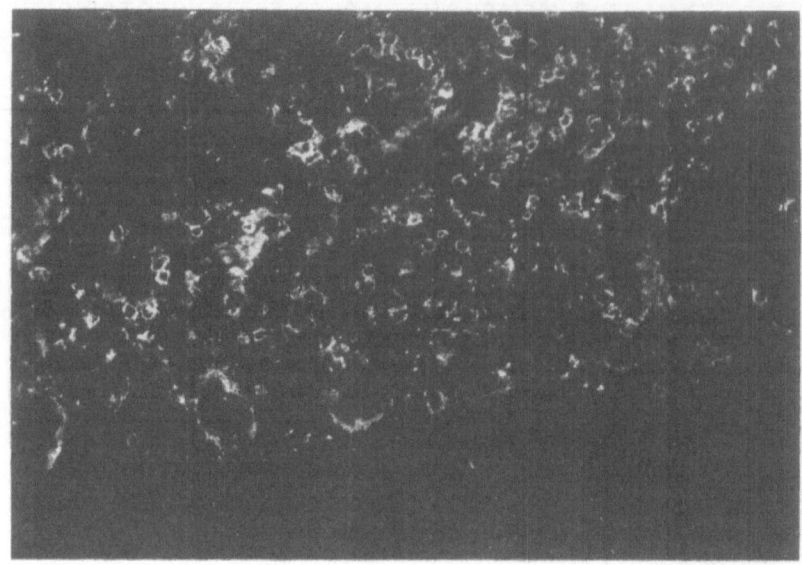

FIG. 3:   Tympanic membrane rejected. + 5 months after transplantation.   T-cell membrane fluorescence.

of preserved grafts, revealed that immunological interference cannot
be ruled out at all.

     Histological sections of these membranes showed the presence of
large accumulations of small lymphoid cells and mononuclear phagocytes, perivascularly and close to the lamina propria of the implants.

     Immuno-fluorescence studies of removed tympanic membranes failed
to show cytoplasmic fluorescence for any of the immunoglobulin classes.

     Hardly any B-cells could be detected in this tissue by immuno-
histochemical techniques, whereas T-cells, identified by a membrane
fluorescence technique with a specific anti-human T-lymphocyte antigen serum (11) were present in large numbers (Fig.3).

DISCUSSION AND CONCLUSIONS

     The findings, although not absolutely conclusive strongly suggest
that immune reactivity might interfere with implant failure in allograft tympanoplasty. Furthermore, the experimental data clearly
demonstrate that through the currently used preservatives of tympano-
ossiculair implants no total abolition of the antigenicity occurs.
Since second set reactions could be elicited, the preservation pro-

cedure seems to leave at least part of the original histoincompatibility. According to these observations it seems likely that immunological 'unresponsiveness' might also be an underlying factor in
implant acceptance.

In order to explain the mechanism which might account for the
absence of an immunological rejection in the majority of the otologic
tissue grafts, when transplanted orthotopically, the following data
have to be taken into consideration:

1.   A lack of antigenicity can be excluded;

2.   Experimental evidence about an adequately functioning afferent
and efferent immune loop does not make the hypothesis of the existence
of a special privilege conferred upon the graft by virtue of the
middle ear itself very solid;

3.   'Adaptation' of the graft within the recipient, the covering by
an epithelial layer on the outside of the eardrum and a mucosal lining
on the middle ear side – a similar phenomenon as has been suggested in
keratoplasty – can hardly be an explanation for non-immunological
interference on the host;

4.   The only remaining explanation seems to be the occurrence of
changes in the host which renders it unable to respond to the donor
histoincompatibility antigens or, if sensitized, to reject them.

The question whether in otologic tissue grafting immunotolerance
is functioning, is a challenging problem for further elucidation.
Clinical and experimental data support the idea that the middle ear
might be an immunologically privileged site for tolerance-inducation
in allograft-tympanoplasty.

REFERENCES

1.   Wullstein, E. Arch. Ohr., Nas., Kehlk. Heilk. 161 (1952) 422.
2.   Plester, D. Arch. Otolaryng. 78 (1963) 310.
3.   Cornish, C.B., Scott, P.J. Lancet ii (1966) 89.
4.   Marquet, J. Acta Otolaryng. (Stockh.) 62 (1966) 459.
5.   Marquet, J. J. Laryng. Otology. 90 (196) 897.
6.   Kastenbauer, E., Hochstrasser, K. Arch. Ohr., Nas., Kehlk.
     Heilk. 203 (1973) 225.
7.   Veldman, J.E. Progress in Immunology III, 805, North Holland
     Publishing Company, Amsterdam (1977), eds. T.E. Mandel, C.
     Cheers, C.S. Hosking, I.F.C. McKenzie, G.J.V. Nossal.
8.   Veldman, J.E., Kuijpers, W., Overbosch, H.C. Clin. Otolaryngol.
     3 (1978) 119.

9.   Veldman, J.E., Kuijpers, W.   Clin. Otolaryngol. 3 (1978) in
      the press.
10.   Kuijpers, W., van den Broek, P.   Acta Otolaryng. (Stockh.) 80
      (1975) 283.
11.   Schoorl, T., Brutel de la Rivière, A., von dem Borne, A.E.G.Kr.,
      Feltkamp-Vroom, Th.M.   Am. J. Path. 84 (1976) 529.

SUMMING-UP - IMMUNOLOGICAL TOLERANCE (SUPPRESSION/DELETION)

J.R. Batchelor

Blond Laboratories, Queen Victoria Hospital

East Grinstead, London, England

This session which I have been asked to summarize has been to
a large extent concerned with questions about suppressor cells -
their characteristics such as sensitivity to irradiation, cyclophosphamide, or radiation leukaemia virus, their interactions with
other lymphoid cells, and their role in tolerance.

The orthodox story is that full differentiated T suppressors
are a subpopulation with the following characteristics. They are
still found after thymectomy and therefore long lived, but sensitive
to ALS. They carry Lyt 2, 3, and I-J region alloantigens, but not
Lyt 1 or I-A region alloantigens. The evidence of Drs. Zan-Bar and
Strober, and others made the important point that these fully
differentiated T suppressors are relatively resistant to radiation
i.e. long-lived but their precursors are radiation sensitive, i.e.
short-lived and they carry Lyt 1, 2 and 3. These precursors are
presumably the same population which was reported on recently by
Eardley et al. and Cantor et al. (1,2). These authors showed that
T helpers appear to activate the Lyt 1^+, 2^+, 3^+ population which
then in turn exert suppressive activity on the T helpers. It is not
at present clear whether the Lyt 1^+, 2^+, 3^+ population themselves
modulate the T helpers, or whether they first differentiate, possibly
into typical Lyt 1^-, 2^+, 3^+ suppressor cells.

In any case it is evident that experiments on suppressor cell
activity have to be very carefully designed and cautiously interpreted.
The possibility that more than one population may mediate suppression
has to be borne in mind, as Dr. Droege pointed out.

The role of suppressor cells in tolerance was another preoc-
cupation of this session. A number of participants reported the

363

finding of auto-reactive cells. Drs. Roder, Bell & Singhal described
auto-reactive B cell precursors in several mouse strains, and Drs.
Steele and Cunningham - autoreactive plaque forming cells reacting
with bromelain treated rbcs. These and other experiments suggest,
fairly strongly in my opinion, that self-reactive clones occur not
infrequently. Are then suppressor cells the normal physiological
mechanism responsible for preventing the expansion of these clones?

Dr. Kolsch and his colleagues discussed how suppressor cells
might act in low zone tolerance. Their suggestion was that the
activation threshold of suppressors was lower than that of helpers.
This might be taken to mean that suppressors have higher affinity
for antigen than helpers. Such an idea should be open to direct
experimental test now, perhaps using labelled antigen and purified
Lyt 1^-, 2^+, 3^+ T cell populations. The fact that in many systems
generation of detectable numbers of suppressor cells appears to need
high doses of antigen is an argument against suppressor cells having
uniquely high affinity for antigen.

One important need is for simple, direct, in vitro assays for
suppressor cells. Drs. Eisenthal, Nachtigel and Feldman described
such a system in which putative suppressor cells are added to a
mixed lymphocyte culture. Inhibition of the responder cells proliferation is measured. If it can be confirmed that fully differentiated,
Lyt 1^-, 2^+, 3^+, I - J+ cells mediate this effect specifically, it will
be a powerful tool for investigating the physiological and pathological
functions of suppressor cells.

But suppressor cells were not the only subject under consideration. Prof. Müller-Ruchholtz and Sir Gus Nossal have already referred
to clonal deletion or inactivation as another explanation of tolerance,
and the relative roles of these mechanisms in tolerance, or non-
responsive states continue to be hotly debated. It was perhaps disappointing that so little has been said today about mechanisms of
unresponsiveness to allografts. There was some interesting data from
Prof. Müller-Ruchholtz's group. They have raised antisera which react
predominantly with differentiated rat T cells and their immediate
precursors, and absorbed them with rat erythrocytes, foetal liver, and
lymphocyte-free peritoneal exudate cells. The absorbed sera were used
to treat CAP strain rat bone marrow which was then transplanted into
lethally irradiated Lewis rats or C3H mice. Graft versus host reactions could be virtually eliminated in this way and long lasting
chimaerism established. This approach to eliminating immunocompetent
T cells, but not harming other cells in the bone marrow looks to be
promising. If monoclonal antibodies can be produced with the appropriate specificity, preliminary absorptions ought to be required no
longer.

Lastly I have been asked to say something about immunologic
enhancement of allograft survival. Obviously a full discussion of

this topic would be out of place here. A recent review can be found
in (3). However in summary, current evidence supports the following
conclusions:

1.   Activation of helper T cells is crucial if MHC antigens are to
behave as "strong" immunogens.

2.   Platelets, purified lymphocyte membranes, liver membranes, ultra
violet light irradiated lymphocytes and long-surviving, enhanced
kidney allografts (minus passenger cells) fail to behave as strong
immunogens in vivo, despite carrying major histocompatibility system
(MHS) antigens. Probably this lack of immunogenicity is due to
failure to activate helper cells.

3.   Activation of helper T cells requires alloantigen plus another
signal. The nature of this "2nd signal" is not yet known.

4.   Continued presence of MHS antigen in the absence of helper cell
activation induces antigen specific unresponsiveness.

REFERENCES

1.   Eardley, D.D., Hugenberger, J., McVay-Boudreau L., Shen, F.W.,
     Gershon, R.K., Cantor, H. J. exp. Med. 147 (1978) 1106.
2.   Cantor, H., McVay-Boudreau, L., Hugenberger, J., Naidorf K.,
     Shen, F.W., Gershon, R.K. J. exp. Med. 147 (1978) 1116.
3.   Batchelor, J.R. The riddle of kidney graft enhancement.
     Transplantation 26: in press.

SESSION   A 4

IN VIVO RELEVANCE OF
NON-LYMPHOID CELLS IN THE IMMUNE REACTION

CHAIRPERSONS:

H. Dvorak

H. Fischer

INTRODUCTION - HETEROGENEITY OF THE CELLULAR IMMUNE RESPONSE

Harold F. Dvorak

Departments of Pathology, Massachusetts General Hospital

and Harvard Medical School, Boston, Massachusetts, U.S.A.

Our task this afternoon is to examine the relevance of non-lymphoid cells in immune reactions. Relevant non-lymphoid cells include at least the following: neutrophils, basophils, eosinophils, mast cells, monocytes/macrophages, reticular cells, and the endothelial cells of the microvasculature.

In introducing this session, I would like to report some data from our laboratory concerning mechanisms of syngeneic tumor and skin allograft rejection in experimental animals and man (1-3). The purpose of these remarks is 3-fold. First, I hope to convince you that basophils and the microvascular endothelium may be of great importance in biologically important reactions of cell-mediated immunity. Second, that an in vivo approach is not only useful but probably essential for an understanding of pathogenetic mechanisms of tumor and graft rejection. And third, I wish to convince you of the very great heterogeneity of cellular immune effector mechanisms.

Several lines of diethylnitrosamine-induced hepatocarcinomas may be grown in syngeneic strain 2 guinea pigs. Animals sensitized with these tumors develop delayed-type hypersensitivity, and tumor rejection, when it occurs, is effected by cellular mechanisms (4-14); antibody probably has no important role in this process in vivo.

The mechanisms by which the line 1 and 10 tumors are rejected depend to a large extent on the experimental conditions and the site of challenge. When sensitized animals were injected with line 1 tumor cells intraperitoneally, the principal finding 1-3 days later in the peritoneal cavity was variably sized aggregates or clumps of inflammatory and damaged or dying tumor cells (9). Cell clumps were composed largely of activated macrophages and lymphocytes but

basophils and rare eosinophils also participated. Very similar
results were reported by Snodgrass and Hanna (10) when line 10
tumor cells were injected intradermally in strain 2 animals along
with BCG. In these experiments macrophages formed numerous, complex
plasma membrane contacts and interdigitations with each other and
with tumor cells and contacts with macrophages seemed to be responsible in some way for tumor cytotoxicity. Macrophages did exhibit
evidence of phagocytosis but phagocytic mechanisms were probably
not a primary factor in tumor killing. These cellular aggregates
formed in vivo closely resembled those occurring in vitro among
peritoneal exudate cells whose migration from capillary tubes had
been inhibited by MIF (15), except that tumor cells and basophils
were also included in the former. In addition, both the peritoneal
cell aggregates and their counterparts in the in vitro migration
inhibition assay system had greatly reduced electron-dense cell
surface coat (15).

By contrast, injection of either line 1 or 10 tumor cells into
the skin of sensitized animals without BCG led to a quite different
result. Here, the delayed in time erythematous reactions that had
been thought to be typical of classic tuberculin hypersensitivity
were found instead to be manifestations of cutaneous basophil hypersensitivity, and, like reactions induced in sensitized animals with
non-cellular antigens, were comprised of extensive local infiltrations
of basophils which accounted for 12-23% of total inflammatory cells
(9). A striking feature of these reactions was the frequency of
intimate associations between infiltrating basophils and both viable
and necrotic tumor cells. Some of the granules of basophils disposed
about tumor cells lacked their usual affinity for Giemsa stain and
appeared pale, suggesting that portions of the granules' substance
responsible for normal staining had been lost. Most such basophils
had intact cell membranes and normal appearing nuclei but others
were disintegrating and could be recognized only by their characteristic granules. Degranulation of basophils was also observed and
basophil granules were occasionally found free in the tissues and
within the cytoplasm of macrophages. Galli et al. (16) have extended
these studies in vitro.

The preceding studies involved tumor cell suspensions that were
planted in the peritoneal cavity or in the skin of sensitized animals
and that were injected over relatively short periods of time (1-3
days); tumor cells remained as individual cells or as small clumps.
What happens in the case of solid tumor growth and rejection? Here
the mechanisms are substantially more complex (1). Within hours of
injecting 5×10^5 line 1 tumor cells into the subcutaneous space of
unsensitized syngeneic strain 2 guinea pigs these tumor cells formed
clumps and became invested in a semi-rigid, fibrin-gel cocoon. This
fibrin-gel comprised greater than 80% of the line 1 tumor mass and,
after day 3, became vascularized and was subsequently replaced by

fibrous connective tissue, giving the tumor the appearance of a
scirrhous carcinoma. Early injection sites appeared as largely
translucent, gelatinous papules containing one or more small, solid,
centrally placed, irregularly shaped, white to tan-pink colored areas.
Microscopically, only these central areas, occupying but a small
fraction of the overall mass, represented tumor cells. The bulk of
the mass perceived as tumor with the naked eye actually consisted of
an extensive, gelatinous, cocoon-like meshwork formed by separated
fibrin strands that were oriented in three dimensions and interspersed
in edema fluid. Fibrin was recognized by its characteristic fibrillar
appearance in 1μ Epon sections and its identity was confirmed by
immunofluorescence and by its characteristic banding pattern on
electron microscopy.

Beginning at about day 8 there was evidence of developing cellular immunity. Lymphocytes, basophils, and lesser numbers of monocytes
formed prominent cuffs about venules at the periphery of the tumor
mass, just outside the enveloping fibrous connective tissue. Many
lymphocytes in these cuffs appeared to be undergoing blast transformation. Nearly all macrophages remained at the periphery of the
tumor mass, separated from the tumor cells by the abundant fibrous
stroma. Macrophages were particularly prominent in peripheral zones
of microvascular hemorrhage where they were engaged in phagocytosing
extravasated erythrocytes and other debris. Unlike macrophages,
lymphocytes and basophils migrated into the granulation tissue
enveloping tumor, and occasional basophils entered the tumor clumps
where they were interspersed between individual tumor cells. Inflammatory cells were infrequent in the lumens of vessels that had penetrated the tumor and were not observed emigrating from these vessels.

Tumor cells developed progressive evidence of damage during this
period, culminating in widespread tumor death. The first sign of
injury consisted of cytoplasmic vacuolation of cells in the central
portions of tumor clumps. Within a few days these tumor cells became
necrotic and adjacent microfoci of dead tumor cells coalesced to form
larger zones of necrosis. A characteristic feature was the relatively
sudden and simultaneous destruction of large portions of the tumor
mass; i.e., the main tumor clumps were destroyed en masse, not by
the sequential, piece-meal death of individual tumor cells. Cellular
elements of the enveloping connective tissue were sometimes damaged
but generally to a lesser extent than tumor cells. Except for
scattered basophils, tumor necrosis was not preceded by, nor associated with, significant contacts between tumor cells and inflammatory
cells. Indeed, the tumor cells first affected, those at the center
of tumor clumps, were farthest removed from the mass of inflammatory
cells.

Tumor cell injury and necrosis were preceded by and correlated
with substantial and widespread microvascular compaction and damage
to endothelium of the small vessels supplying the tumor cells and the

surrounding connective tissue. Vessels remained patent, however, and thrombosis was not observed except as a late event, after extensive tumor destruction had already occurred, and then only irregularly. Occasionally, lymphocytes, basophils and other inflammatory cells were present within or adjacent to damaged vessels but contacts between inflammatory cells and necrotic endothelium were extremely rare.

What can be said about tumor regression under these circumstances? Literature review and the lymphocyte-and basophil-rich perivascular infiltrate argue that cellular immunity had indeed developed 8-10 days after a primary innoculation of line 1 hepatocarcinoma. However, the morphologic features associated with destruction of the main line 1 tumor mass differed significantly from previous descriptions of the cell-mediated rejection of line 1 and 10 tumor cell suspensions. Whether in the skin, peritoneal cavity, or in vitro, these last were characterized by intimate anatomic associations between individual tumor cells and inflammatory cells whether lymphocytes, basophils or macrophages. By contrast, regression of solid, vascularized line 1 tumors in the subcutaneous space could not be linked to anatomic contacts between tumor and either lymphocytes or macrophages. Basophils did infiltrate tumors but seemed too few to have initiated the extensive tumor damage observed on a cell contact basis.

Other possible mechanisms of tumor destruction must therefore be considered. The pattern of necrosis observed, beginning with focal tumor cell vacuolation and progressing over the course of a few days to generalized, nearly stimultaneous destruction of large groups of tumor cells, has many characteristics of ischemia progressing to infarction. Accompanying the first evidence of tumor cell necrosis, the vessels supplying the tumor and surrounding fibrous connective tissue exhibited dilatation and compaction, morphologic signs of static blood flow; widespread necrosis of vascular endothelial cells; and focal hemorrhages. What is the pathogenesis of these events and could they have an immunologic basis?

In support of an immunologic interpretation, microvascular alterations of the type described here have been observed in delayed hypersensitivity reactions of the skin following challenge with defined immunogens (2). More recently, studies of human skin allograft rejection have demonstrated extensive damage of the endothelial cells of the microvasculature supplying the graft and have pointed to the primacy of these changes in at least certain types of first set allograft destruction (3). The microvascular changes observed in the present study may, therefore, have an immunological basis. For example, microvascular damage could result from a primary toxic effect on blood vessel endothelium of a cytotoxic lymphokine. Alternatively, a mediator released by basophils or macrophages could have exerted

similar damage. Other possibilities may also be envisioned. Whatever
the mechanisms, endothelial necrosis would be expected to result in
greatly increased vascular permeability with consequences that
include local extravasation of plasma; retention within the vessels
of cellular elements, giving rise to locally increased viscosity;
stasis of blood flow; and tumor infarction.

Taken together, these data serve to illustrate the extreme
diversity and heterogeneity of the immune response. They indicate
that the response of the host to the same innoculum of tumor cells
varies enormously depending upon the immune status of the host and
the site of injection. Depending on the site of innoculation, tumor
may be rejected by mechanisms involving intimate anatomic contacts
with lymphocytes, macrophages, or basophils. On the other hand, the
host is also apparently able to reject solid tumors by another
mechanism involving compromise of the vascular supply.

The complexity and heterogeneity observed in this relatively
simple system is compounded when one looks to other species and other
tumors or grafts. For example, there is now solid morphologic and
functional evidence indicating that neutrophils play a crucial role
in allogeneic tumor rejection in the peritoneal cavity of the mouse
(17,18). In the case of renal allograft rejection in man, acute
episodes of rejection at early intervals after transplant are
associated with an infiltrate of basophils; by contrast, grafts
experiencing rejection at later intervals, months after transplant,
show a paucity of basophils but marked mast cell proliferation and
extensive vascular changes (19).

What are we to conclude from this confusing and paradoxical
heterogeneity? The answer, I think, is clear. We must recognize
that living organisms have developed multiple mechanisms for dealing
with foreign antigens, all of which may be effective at least under
certain conditions. Individual circumstances such as local factors
may indicate which of several possible pathways the immune system
may select in dealing with a particular antigenic challenge. We
must continue our in vitro investigations in order to elucidate the
potential functions of each of the cell types involved in the immune
response. This will require study not only of the currently
fashionable lymphocytes and macrophages but also of basophils,
neutrophils, and eosinophils. In addition, fixed tissue cells,
particularly mast cells and the microvascular endothelium, must not
be neglected because these very likely have important roles in most
inflammatory processes. We must not, however, in enthusiasm over
the beauty of our in vitro findings, then make the mistake of extra-
polating these literally and uncritically to the in vivo situation
without first subjecting our results to reality testing; that is,
the actual behaviour of the living organism.

REFERENCES

1. Dvorak, H.F., Dvorak, A.M., Manseau, E.J., Wiberg, L., Churchill, W.H. Growth patterns of line 1 and 10 solid tumors in unsensitized strain 2 guinea pigs. Relation to malignant behavior. Submitted for publication.
2. Dvorak, A.M., Mihm, M.C., Jr., Dvorak, H.F. Lab. Invest. 34 (1976) 179.
3. Dvorak, H.F., Mihm, M.C., Jr., Dvorak, A.M., Barnes, B.A. Fed. Proc. 36 (1977) 1071.
4. Rapp, H.J., Churchill, W.H., Jr., Kronman, B.S., Rolley, R.T., Hammond, W.G., Borsos, T. J. Natl. Cancer Inst. 41 (1968) 1.
5. Zbar, B., Tanaka, T. Science 172 (1971) 271.
6. Churchill, W.H., Jr., Rapp, H.J., Kronman, B.S., Boros, T. J. Natl. Cancer Inst. 41 (1968) 13.
7. Zbar, B., Bernstein, I.D., Rapp, H.J. J. Natl. Cancer Inst. 46 (1971) 831.
8. Meltzer, M.S., Oppenheim, J.J., Littman, B.H., Leonard, E.J., Rapp, H.J. J. Natl. Cancer Inst. 49 (1972) 727.
9. Dvorak, H.F., Dvorak, A.M., Churchill, W.J., Jr. J. Exp. Med. 137 (1973) 751.
10. Snodgrass, M.J., Hanno, M.G., Jr. Cancer Res. 33 (1973) 701.
11. Churchill, W.H., Jr., Zbar, B., Belli, J.A., David, J.R. J. Natl. Cancer Inst. 48 (1972) 541.
12. Osteen, R.R., Piessens, W.F., David, J.R., Churchill, W.J., Jr. J. Natl. Cancer Inst. 55 (1975) 873.
13. Piessens, W.F., Churchill, W.H., Jr., David, J.R. J. Immunol. 114 (1975) 293.
14. Churchill, W.H., Piessens, W.F., Sulis, C.A., David, J.R. J. Immunol. 115 (1975) 781.
15. Dvorak, A.M., Hammond, M.E., Dvorak, H.F., Karnovsky, M.J. Lab. Invest. 27 (1972) 561.
16. Galli, S.J., Dvorak, H.F., Churchill, W.F., Hammond, M.E., Connell, A.B., Galli, A.S., Dvorak, A.M. Fed. Proc. 36 (1977) 1324.
17. Dvorak, A.M., Connell, A.B., Proppe, K., Dvorak, H.F. J. Immunol. 120 (1978) 1240.
18. Nakayama, M., Sendo, F., Miyake, T., Fuyama, S., Arai, S., Kobayashi, H. J. Immunol. 120 (1978) 619.
19. Dvorak, H.F., Colvin, R.B. Lancet i. (1974) 212.

ACKNOWLEDGEMENT

This work was supported by U.S. Public Health Service Grant CA-16881.

MAST CELLS IN LOCAL ANTIBODY FORMATION AND ALLOGRAFT REJECTION

L. Jarosková[1], V. Viklicky[2], M. Holub[3], I. Trebichavsky[1],
R. Stepánková[1]

[1]Inst. Microbiol., [2]Inst. Mol. Genetics, [3]CSAV and IKEM,
Praha, CSSR

Besides various functions such as in blood clotting and fat
metabolism the mast cells (MC) and basophils participate in some
immunologic reactions and represent an integral part of connective
tissue metabolism. The quantity and quality of MCs reflect the
degree of maturation of the surrounding intercellular connective
tissues.

Two models are reported here in which an inverse relation exists
between the presence of MC and the extent or efficiency of the immune
response.

RESULTS

Rejection of skin allografts across a weak histocompatibility barrier in the mouse

In weak histocompatibility systems the transplantation of skin
allografts from newborn donors induces immunity early after transplantation in all cases although up to 50% of grafts survive permanently. The immune reaction is manifested by a round cell infiltration
in allografts, blastic reaction in regional lymph nodes and induction
of secondary response.

In the course of healing in of skin allografts there is a strong
overproduction of immature intercellular matrix, rich in glycosamino-
glycans (GAG). This is accompanied by appearance of immature forms
of MCs, at first close to the proliferating epidermis. Later the MCs

form continuous layers between epidermis and infiltrating cells and
reach a mature state. Such a great accumulation of MCs is always
associated with a permanent survival of the graft (Fig.1A). In a
situation in which the graft is being rejected and small necrosis
appear there is a complete disappearance of all types of MCs (Fig.1B).

Local antibody formation in omenta of germ-free (GF) and conventional (CV) rats

The omenta of GF and CV rats (Wistar strain, 2 months-old males)
differ markedly: in GF animals they have a lower content of lymphoid
cells and a larger number of immature forms of cells of various type,
including MCs. After immunization with horse radish peroxidase (HRP,
5 mg i.p.) there is an increase in the number of follicle-like dense
lymphatic areas (DLA) in perivascular structures in omenta of all
rats and only in CV rats a significant increase in DLA in free
omentum. Large and multilayer DLA, typical for CV rat omentum, are
nearly lacking in GF rats. In CV animals the numbers of MCs in
multilayer DLA in free omentum are low in comparison to the rich
content of lymphoid cells. In contrast, in GF rats there is a
striking accumulation of MCs in DLA in perivascular structures as
well as in DLA in free omentum (Tab.1, Fig.2A,B). Per individual DLA
there is an inverse relation between the numbers of lymphoid (and Ab-
containing cells) and MCs in all rats. The CV rats have in average
3-10 times more Ab-containing cells than GF rats.

DISCUSSION AND SUMMARY

During rejection of newborn skin grafts across a weak H-barrier
in mice as well as in local antibody formation to a soluble protein
antigen in GF rats a lower immune response was observed. In both
models a weak antigenic stimulus resulted in a weak response which is
more susceptible to regulatory factors. In the model of Wistar rats
using other antigens (SRBC, E.coli) the differences in plaque-forming
cells between the GF and CV state was not as pronounced (1) as in the
number of HRP-containing cells in omenta. With regard to antibody
formation studies in other GF models (pigs, rabbits) it was suggested
(1) that the differences in maturation pattern of the immunological
capacity in various species is not unified by the GF state and
signifies involvement of other physiological factors.

A significant common finding in the present results is the new
formation and reconstruction of young immature connective tissue
accompanied by an enormous accumulation of mast cells.

Recently the interest in the function of blood basophils and MC
in immune reactions has been intensified by the finding of receptors

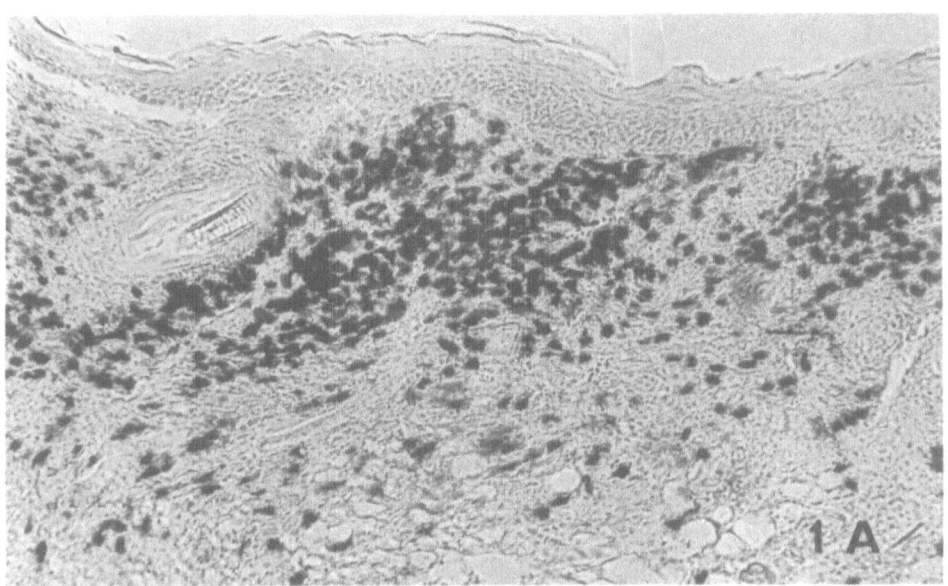

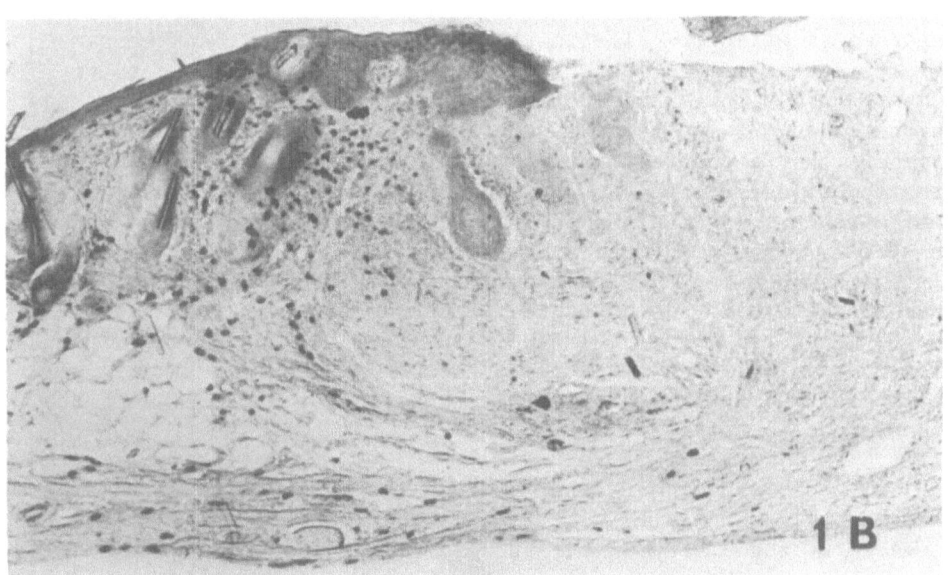

FIG. 1:   Newborn skin grafted across H-Y barrier in C57Bl/6 mice.
30 days after transfer. Toluidine blue, pH 2.

A - Graft without signs of rejection; continual layer of MCs
close to epidermis. Magn. 200x.

B - Part of the graft (right) is rejected. Abundance of MCs in
the other part. Magn. 120x.

TAB. 1:   Number of mast cells per 1 mm^2 of rat omentum.

Rats	DLA in perivascular structures[+]	DLA in free omentum[+]
GF control	513.0+ 68.2	poorly developed
GF HRP	1 629.8+236.4	524.0+94.6
GF saline	857.3+126.4	327.7+52.8
CV control	367.0+ 54.7	poorly developed
CV HRP	525.3+ 92.7	64.8+27.9
CV saline	667.8+ 84.3	123.5+31.5

Day 5 after i.p. administration of HRP (5 mg in saline or saline alone)

[+] Mean value $\pm$ S.E.   Counted in 6 animals in each group.

for IgE on MCs and the role of blood basophils in cutaneous basophil hypersensitivity (2). In both cases the basophils and MCs are regarded as effector cells in the immune reactions. At the same time using the same or other models an association of excessive numbers of basophils and MCs and inhibition of immune reaction was demonstrated (3,4). The effect of MC on the ongoing immune reaction may be either a suppressor one or the MCs may only signalize the presence of certain macromolecules in the environment in which the immune reaction is manifested. Those macromolecules have a marked regulatory effect on metabolic processes. It is histamine and GAG for which a regulatory effect on immune reactions of lymphoid cells has been repeatedly demonstrated. Such an effect may be exerted at the level of induction of immune reaction (5,6), at the level of re-distribution of lymphoid cells in the organism during immune reactions (7,8) or at the level of the effector phase of in vitro immune reactions (9,10).

Although one cannot fully exclude the possibility of masking the receptors which play role in the reactions, the basic mechanism seems to be the effect on the structures and functions of the membranes and thus on the processes which take place in the membranes of interacting cells.

The present paper shows a correlation of a high incidence of MCs with a lower rate of immune reactions.

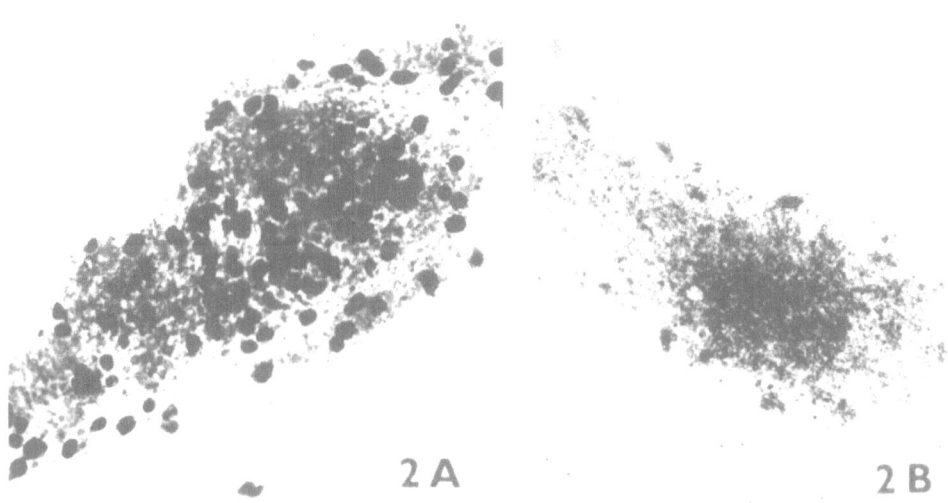

FIG. 2: DLA in free omentum of rats, immunized i.p. with 5 mg of HRP. Toluidine blue, pH 2.

A - GF rat. DLA with a massive amount of MCs. Magn. 300x.

B - CV rat. DLA with a few MCs. Magn. 100x.

REFERENCES

1. Tlaskalová, H., Sterzl, J., Stepánková, R., Abstracts 4th Europ. Immunol. Meeting (1978) Budapest, p.21.
2. Dvorak, H.F., Dvorak, A.M., Human Pathol. 3 (1972) 454.
3. Katz, S.I., Heatter, C.J., Paster, D., Turk, J.L., J. Immunol. 113 (1974) 1073.
4. Viklický, V., Poláckova, M., J. Immunogenetics 1 (1974) 131.
5. Darzynkiewicz, J., Balazs. E.A. Exp. Cell Res., 113 (1971) 123.
6. Dráber, P., Viklický, V., Lengerová, A., Folia Biol. 23 (1977) 81.
7. Bradfield, J.W.B., Born, G.V.R., Nature 222 (1969) 1183.
8. Viklický, V., Peknicová, J., Poláckova, M., Folia Biol. 22 (1976) 159.
9. Lippman, M., Nature 219 (1968) 33.
10. Brondz, B.D., Snegireva, A.E., Rassulin, Y.A., Shamborant, O.G., Immunochemistry 10 (1973) 175.

MARGINAL ZONE AND MARGINAL SINUS MACROPHAGES IN THE MOUSE ARE

DISTINCT POPULATIONS

John L. Humphrey

Department of Immunology, Royal Postgraduate Medical

School, Hammersmith Hospital, London W12 OHS, England

INTRODUCTION

The observations reported here arose from the finding that hapten-conjugated pneumococcal type 3 capsular polysaccharide (S3) is a potent specific inhibitor of anti-hapten antibody responses, especially secondary IgG responses (1). The mechanism involves inactivation of B lymphocytes with receptors for the hapten, and the relevant properties of the conjugate appear to be that suffi- cient hapten groups are attached to a high molecular weight polymeric carrier which does not itself elicit a thymus dependent response and which is only very slowly degradable in the body (e.g. 2). In a survey of other polysaccharide carriers which might be more readily available than S3 and equally effective after conjugation with haptens at suppressing anti-hapten antibody responses, a variety of neutral and negatively charged polysaccharides were examined. These were directly conjugated with DNP-lysine via CNBr (or via carbodi- imide in the case of pectin and alginic acid) and a small number of tryamine residues were introduced at the same time in order to make it possible to label the conjugates with ^{131}I or ^{125}I for metabolic and autoradiographic studies. The technique used for testing any immunosuppressive effects was to mix 15-25 million spleen cells from mice (C3H, CBA or CBA x C57 Bl Fl) primed with DNP-KLH with varying quantities of the substances to be tested and to transfer them i.v. into 850 r. irradiated syngeneic recipients. These were boosted next day with 20 µg fluid DNP-KLH, and the direct (IgM) and developed (IgG) anti-DNP plaque forming cells (PFC) were measured 6 to 8 days later (3). The findings will be reported fully elsewhere (4). Some examples are given in Tab.1, from which it is evident that conjugates with the acidic were much more effective than those with neutral

TAB. 1:   Inhibition of Secondary Anti-DNP Responses by Conjugates
7 Day Anti-DNP Responses (Total Spleen PFC) as % of Control.

		Dose of Conjugate (µg)			
		1	10	100	1000
DNP$_{2.7}$ S3*	Direct	12	18		
	Indirect	25	1		
DNP$_{4.6}$ S3	Direct	52	45	3	
	Indirect	90	1	1	
DNP$_{20}$alginate	Direct	18	18	11	
	Indirect	2	3	1	
DNP$_{16}$pectin	Direct	50	7	3	
	Indirect	21	0	0	
DNP$_4$Ficoll	Direct	95	135	62	33
	Indirect	112	69	45	15
DNP$_4$Levan	Direct	74	39	28	
	Indirect	49	18	11	
DNP$_5$Dextran	Direct	133	170	164	
2000	Indirect	103	138	144	

*   The degree of conjugation is given as mols DNP/50,000 daltons
irrespective of the molecular weight.

polysaccharides. In fact DNP conjugates of Ficoll, hydroxyethyl
starch (OEt starch) or levan injected in vivo in moderate doses
(50 - 200 µg) after an initial burst of IgM anti-DNP PFC gave a
lower but still substantial level of PFC lasting for many weeks.
(These represent a subpopulation of DNP responsive B cells different
from those responsive to DNP on a T-dependent carrier). The differences were not obviously correlated with the size of the carrier
moiety (which was usually heterogeneous and difficult to determine)
nor with the degree of conjugation provided that there were more
than 2 or 3 hapten groups/50,000 daltons.

METABOLISM AND FATE OF LABELLED POLYSACCHARIDES

The metabolic fate of conjugates labelled with radioiodine via
tyramine, injected i.p. or i.v. in doses from 10 - 100 µg, was
essentially similar. All were retained in the body for long periods,
elimination being exponential with half lives 20 - 60 or more days.
All were removed fairly rapidly from the blood stream, which contained only 0.5 - 5% of the injected dose after 2 days, but they
persisted at low levels (0.01 - 0.1%) up to 15 days, beyond which

TAB. 2:   Distribution of Different DNP-Polysaccarides (Average
between 1 and 12 Days), as Percentage of Dose Retained.

	Liver	Spleen	Skin*
DNP-S3	26	4	30
DNP alginate	22	6	20
DNP pectin	59	3	8
DNP levan	60	7	13
DNP dextran 2000	64	10	4
DNP Ficoll	49	16	12
DNP OEt Starch	13	26	7

*including underlying connective tissue

examination was not continued. However, despite the overall similarity in their overall metabolism, there were very marked differences
in their distribution in different tissues, examined between 1 and
12 days after injection. Although these distributions changed somewhat during this period, the general pattern remained the same, and
some mean values for the percentage of the retained label in liver,
spleen and skin are given in Tab.2. These are the tissues which
were also examined histologically.

The most relevant facts which emerge from the Table are the
relatively large proportions of neutral polysaccharides located in
the spleen, and of S3 and alginate in the skin. Except for OEt Starch
a substantial proportion of each polysaccharide was retained in the
liver.

Autoradiographic examination revealed some unexpected differences
in cellular distribution. Whereas the acidic polysaccharides were
exclusively detected in what are conventionally regarded as macrophages, the neutral polysaccharides were strikingly absent from liver
Kupffer cells (though in or on parenchymal cells) and strikingly
concentrated in macrophages of the marginal zone of the white pulp of
the spleen and in marginal sinus macrophages of peripheral lymph nodes.

Some extreme differences are illustrated in Figures 1 - 4.

Such observations could only be made because the labelled materials were indigestible and consequently retained within the cells which
had ingested them. Because differences in localization appeared to be
correlated with differences in the tolerogenic capacity of the conjugates, and presentation of antigens by marginal zone macrophages
might differ in important ways immunologically from presentation by
other macrophages to lymphoid tissues, it was decided to use fluorescent instead of radioactively labelled polysaccharides.

TAB. 3:   Cellular Distribution of Retained Polysaccharides in
Selected Tissues as Revealed by Autoradiography.

Conjugates of	Liver	Spleen	Lymph nodes	Skin
S3 Pectin Alginate	Kupffer cells++ (not in paren- chymal cells)	Red pulp MØ+ marginal zone MØ + or -	Medullary MØ+	Histio- cytes++
Ficoll OEt Starch Dextran 2000	Parenchymal cells (not in Kupffer cells)	Marginal zone MØ++ (not in red pulp)	Marginal sinus MØ++ Medullary MØ+	Histio- cytes+
Levan*	Parenchymal cells (Kupffer cells +)	Germinal centres++ (marginal zone MØ+)	not examined	

* Levan is exceptional in localizing rapidly in germinal centres
because it activates the alternative complement pathway (5).

DISTINCTIVE MACROPHAGES REVEALED BY
UPTAKE OF FLUORESCENT POLYSACCHARIDES

     S3, OEt starch and Ficoll were labelled with FITC or TRITC after
prior attachment of hexane 1, 6 diamine (via CNBr) to provide free
amino groups. Care was needed to avoid conjugating too many fluorescent residues, since conjugates of neutral polysaccharides with 5
or more residues/50,000 daltons tended to behave like acidic polysaccharides (e.g. to be taken up by Kupffer cells). However,
conjugates with 1 - 2 groups/50,000 daltons showed similar distributions to the radiolabelled conjugates. Fluorescence was examined
in frozen sections or dispersed cell preparations with a Leitz
Orthoplan microscope using epi-illumination, combined when required
with transmitted light. Cell viability was assessed by exclusion
of trypan blue or by uptake of fluorescein diacetate. Because the
fluorescent polysaccharides readily dissolved out of fixed or broken
cells into aqueous solutions, despite all conventional methods of
fixation, fixed preparations had to be mounted dry; it was also not
possible both to retain the fluorescence and to stain fixed specimens
by usual histological stains, and duplicate specimens had to be used
for this purpose.

     Fluorescent S3 was readily detected in frozen sections of spleen,

FIG. 1:   Liver ^{125}I S3 autoradiograph (Giemsa x 400).

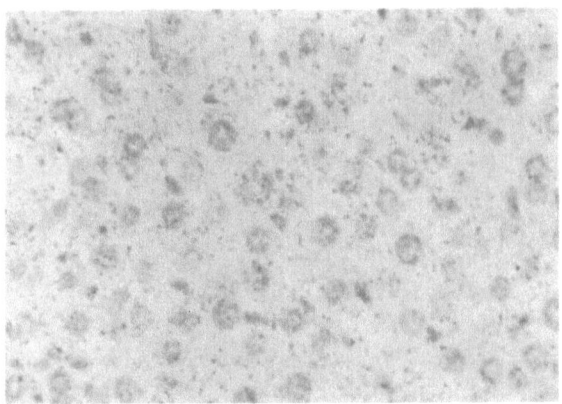

FIG. 2:   Liver ^{125}I - OEt Starch Autoradiograph (Giemsa x 400).

lymph nodes, liver, bone marrow, kidney and in connective tissue
spreads for at least 10 days after i.v. injection of 100 - 250 µg.
Little or none was seen in unstimulated free peritoneal macrophages.
Its localization was similar to that indicated in Tab.3; in
addition, it was present weakly in bone marrow macrophages, very
markedly in connective tissue histiocytes, and in mesangial cells of
the kidney. In mice killed more than 4 days after injection it was
also seen on dendritic cells in germinal centres, presumably because
rapidly formed antibody had formed complexes with the S3 still
circulating.

FIG. 3:   Spleen ^{125}I-S3 Autoradiograph (Giemsa x 140).

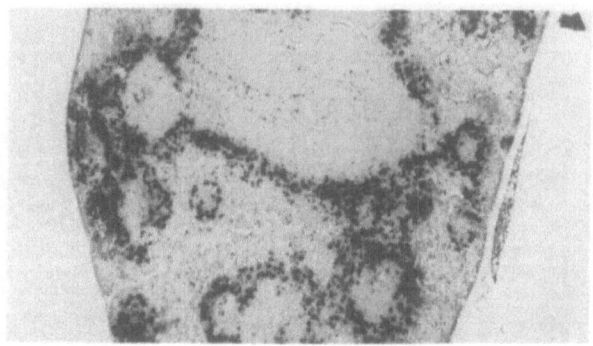

FIG. 4:   Spleen ^{125}I - Oet Starch Autoradiograph (Giemsa x 35).

Fluorescent OEt starch or Ficoll were very readily detectable after i.v. injection of 50 - 100 μg and persisted similarly to S3. They were confined to the marginal zones of the spleen white pulp, the marginal sinus of lymph nodes (though often with extension into the peripheral parts of the medulla), and to connective tissue histiocytes in which they appeared to be in somewhat lower concentration than S3. All the polysaccharides examined were present in small intracellular droplets, presumably phagolysosomes, which coalesced into larger droplets as time went on.

PROPERTIES OF SPLENIC MACROPHAGES

Mice were routinely injected i.v. with 100 μg TRITC OEt starch or Ficoll and 250 μg FITC S3 and examined 1 - 5 days later.   This colour combination was used because many liver, spleen and bone marrow macrophages, other than those of the marginal zone, had a dull red fluorescence, probably attributable to lipofuscin; although TRITC fluorescence was much brighter and could readily be recognized by eye it was less easily distinguishable by colour photography.

When spleens were teased to prepare dispersed cells in the usual way, green fluorescent red pulp macrophages were plentiful, but intact red fluorescent marginal zone macrophages were rarely present in single cell preparations. The 'debris' which had settled rapidly, and would normally be discarded, contained clumps of macrophages of both types. Marginal zone macrophages particularly seemed to be entangled with each other and with connective tissue, and readily broke if disentangled by force. Reasonably complete recovery of macrophages could be obtained by perfusing mice with collagenase (1 mg/ml), and then cutting the spleen into fragments which were incubated at $37^{o}C$ in medium (RPMI 1640 + 10% heat inactivated foetal calf serum) containing collagenase for 3/4 - 1 hour. The fragments readily broke up into single cell preparations, which were freed from collagenase by centrifugation twice through foetal calf serum gradients. Further separation from granulocytes or red cells could be achieved by centrifugation on ficoll - metrizamide gradients, the macrophages remaining with lymphocytes at the interface. Treatment with collagenase did not appear to affect viability of the cells, nor their capacity to ingest latex particles (0.8 nm diameter) compared with cells from spleens not so treated.

Since cells which contained fluorescent polysaccharides of either kind nearly all ingested latex particles, and cells which ingested latex were nearly all fluorescent, the doses of polysaccharides used presumably labelled virtually all the spleen macrophages. The total yield of labelled macrophages per spleen was variable, but in 4 - 6 month old C3H mice was around 1.5×10^{6}. Of these marginal zone macrophages (i.e. containing OEt starch or ficoll, often with some S3) made up approximately one tenth, but this proportion varied from mouse to mouse and was sometimes much less. This may have been due to incomplete dispersal despite collagenase treatment.

The marginal zone macrophages in suspension were generally larger than red pulp macrophages, and often had lymphocytes adhering to them. Unexpectedly, the majority of either kind failed to adhere to glass of plastic surfaces during 1 hour or overnight incubation - despite the fact that the non-adherent cells remained capable of ingesting latex. The proportion of marginal zone macrophages adhering was only about 10%. When examined for rosette formation with ox red cell EA and EAC (human) about 80% of the marginal zone macrophages and about 40% of the red pulp macrophages were positive for both.

Cyto-centrifuge preparations and glass adherent cells were
stained for acid phosphatase, nonspecific esterase and by Leishman
stain. The red pulp macrophages were strongly positive for both
enzymes, and had the typical morphology of mouse macrophages,
commonly with a ring shaped nucleus. The marginal zone macrophages
also stained strongly for both enzymes, but in Leishman stained
preparations were morphologically quite distinct, being larger with
round or oval open nuclei and pale blue-grey cutoplasm. Those
adherent to glass had long branching cytoplasmic processes, and
were usually surrounded by lymphocytes which appeared to adhere to
them.

If prelabelled mice were irradiated with 850r. whole body
γ -irradiation and killed 2 - 3 days later, when spleen and lymph
nodes were empty of lymphocytes, macrophages of both sorts remained
apparently intact and in their characteristic distribution - i.e.
they were radioresistant.

The origin, rate of turnover, immunological significance and
other properties of the marginal zone macrophages remains to be
determined. We are currently attempting to separate them in
sufficient numbers to permit further studies using the fluorescence
activated cell sorter and density gradients.

REFERENCES

1.   Mitchell, G.F., Humphrey, J.H., Williamson, A.R., Eur. J.
     Immunol. 2 (1972) 460.
2.   Klaus, G.G.B., Humphrey, J.H., Transplant. Rev., 23 (1975) 105.
3.   Klaus, G.G.B., Humphrey, J.H., Eur. J. Immunol. 4 (1974) 370.
4.   Humphrey, J.H., (in preparation).
5.   Klaus, G.G.B., Humphrey, J.H., Immunology 33 (1977) 31.

ACKNOWLEDGEMENTS

The skilled help of Ms. Deirdre Grennan is gratefully
acknowledged.

CELLS CONTAINING BIRBECK GRANULES IN THE LYMPH AND THE LYMPH NODE

E.C.M. Hoefsmit[1], B.M. Balfour[2], E.W.A. Kamperdijk[1] and
J. Cvetanov[2]
[1]Department of Electronmicroscopy, Medical Faculty, Free
University, Amsterdam, Holland
[2]National Institute for Medical Research, Mill Hill,
London, NW7 1AA, England

THE NORMAL LYMPH NODE

The lymph node is composed of functionally different compartments, each with a characteristic type of macrophage. In the
marginal zone the plasmacell reaction is induced, in the germinal
centre the memory B-cells are generated and in the paracortex recirculating T-cells are stimulated in thymus dependent humoral
responses and in cell mediated responses. In normal lymph nodes,
the reticulum and endothelial cells composing the stroma of these
areas, are clearly distinguished from the macrophages and the
lymphocytes (Hoefsmit 1975). Marginal zone macrophages, tingible
body macrophages (TBM) and interdigitating cells (IDC) seem to
differ in functional activity only.

The IDC resembles the epidermal Langerhans cell (Fig.1). These
cells form the same characteristic interdigitations with the
surrounding cells, having the electronlucent cytoplasm, the
irregularly formed nucleus and low phagocytic activity. However,
in non-stimulated lymph nodes Birbeck granules, which are the
characteristic organelles of the Langerhans cells, are not usually
present in IDC. In the concept of the mononuclear phagocyte system
(Langevoort et al 1970) all macrophages are bone-marrow derived and
should enter the node via the afferent lymph vessels or the blood
vascular system.

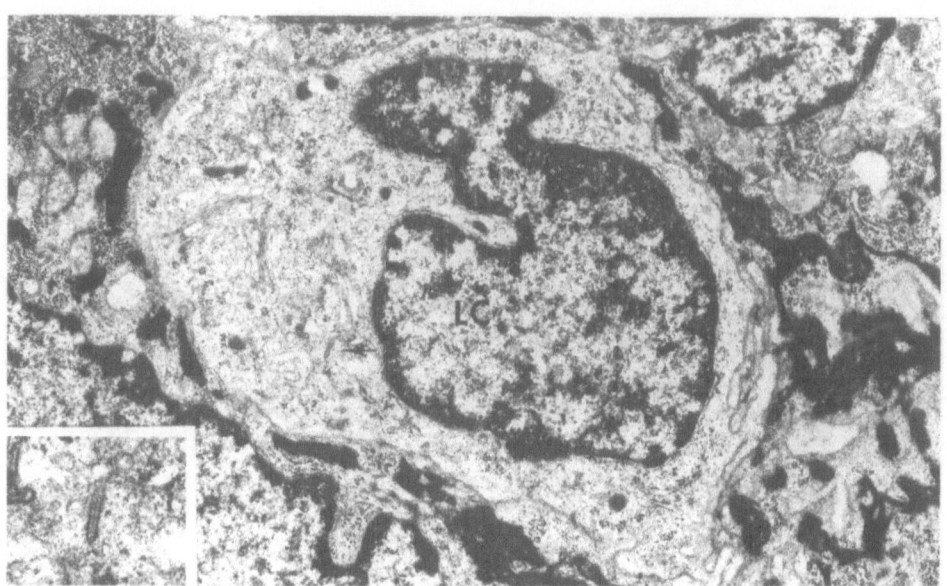

FIG. 1:   A Langerhans cell (LC) in the epidermis of a control rat
x 14.500.   Inset: a Birbeck granule.   (Reduced 40% for purposes of
reproduction.).

THE STIMULATED LYMPH NODE

Rats were given 0.1 ml parathyphoid vaccine, containing 5 x 10^9
formolkilled micro-organisms per ml, in one footpad.   The corresponding lymph node was studied at different intervals (Kamperdijk et
al. 1978).   This vaccine causes thymus dependent and thymus independent humoral immune responses. In the first 24 hours small, newly
arrived macrophages are present in the marginal sinus, the marginal
zone and in the paracortex.   At the same time the first immuno-blasts
are found in the marginal zone and the paracortex.   In the next days
transitional forms between the small macrophages and the IDC replace
the characteristic   IDC, which have largely disappeared from the
paracortex.   All these newly arrived macrophages, transitional forms
and IDC (Fig.2) may contain Birbeck granules and show more or less
phagocytic activity.   They often contain bundles of microfilaments.
When the blast reaction diminishes again the characteristic   IDC
gradually repopulate the paracortex.   However, Birbeck granules are
only seen in the macrophages during the first day of the response,
i.e. in the induction phase.   In IDC the presence of Birbeck granules
completes the resemblance with Langerhans cells.

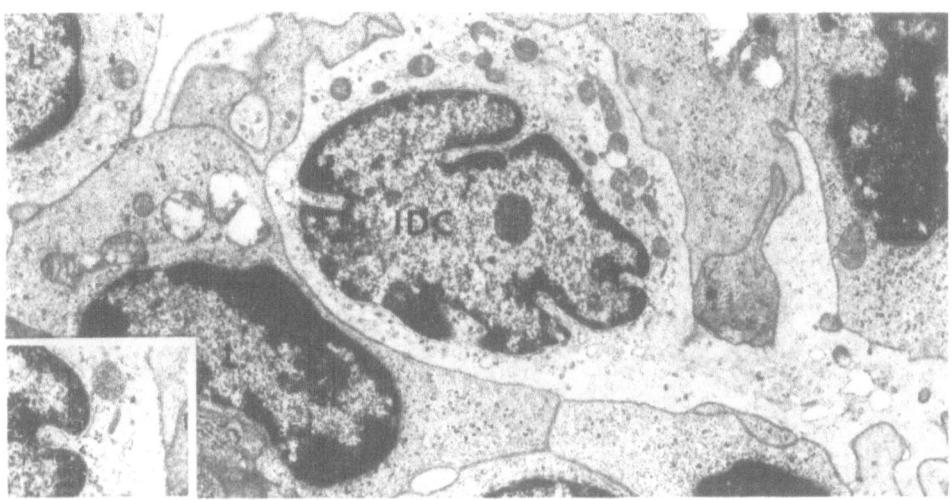

FIG. 2:   An IDC in the paracortex, 1 day after stimulation.   The
electronlucent cytoplasm shows Birbeck granules (arrows) x 13.000.
L = lymphocyte.   Inset: a detail of a Birbeck granule.   (Reduced
40% for purposes of reproduction.).

THE NORMAL LYMPH

Afferent vessels carrying lymph from the superficial tissues
of the hind foot to the popliteal lymph node of the rabbit were
canulated and the inflow examined (Kelly et al. 1978).   65% of the
mononuclear cells possess long actively moving cytoplasmic veils
which frequently made contact with other cells.   In the electron
microscope the veils could be identified as long, thin extensions.
Of the veiled cells 10 to 12% contained large phagolysomes, 4%
contained small lysosomes, 3% contained Birbeck granules (Fig.3) and
0.5% contained phagolysosomes and Birbeck granules.

THE LYMPH AFTER STIMULATION

Normal rabbits were injected in each footpad with diphtheria
toxoid containing 10 LF (flocculating units).   Lymph coming from the
site of the injection was examined.   The total number of veiled cells
varied from 0.6×10^5 cells per ml (day 0) to 1.8×10^5 cells per ml
(day 4).   On the first day after injection, half of the Birbeck
granule containing veiled cells also contained lysosomes and these
cells represented 8% of the total number of veiled cells.   These cells
were also present in small numbers on the third and fourth day after

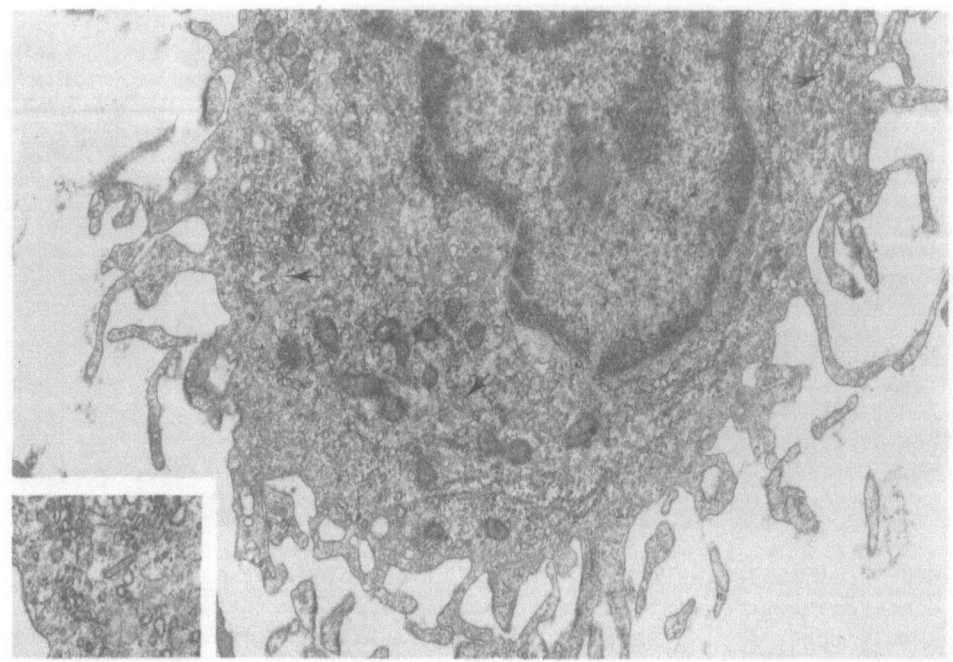

FIG. 3:   A veiled cell in the afferent lymph of a control rabbit
x 26.000.   Note Birbeck granules (arrows).   Inset: a Birbeck
granule (Reduced 40% for purposes of reproduction).

injection.   The absolute numbers of these cells are summarized in
Fig.4.   There was also an increase in the number of small smooth
surfaced mononuclear phagocytes in the first two days after antigen
injection being maximal on the second day.   In the corresponding
lymph nodes veiled cells are identified in the marginal sinus.   Also
macrophages containing Birbeck granules and large phagolysosomes
were seen penetrating the marginal zone in 3 and 6 hours after
stimulation.   However, we have not as yet found Birbeck granules
in the lymph node macrophages in later stages in the immune response.

     It is concluded that a proportion of the veiled cells present
in normal lymph have phagocytic abilities and a smaller number may
contain Birbeck granules.   Both these cell types were increased after
antigenic stimulation, the maximal increase occuring after the
induction of the immune response.   However, in the lymph node cells
containing Birbeck granules have so far only been found during the
induction phase.

All these observations taken together strongly suggest:

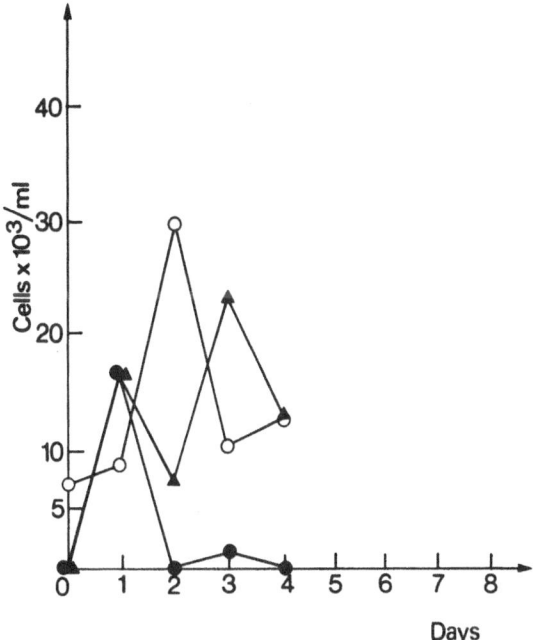

Days

FIG. 4:   The numbers of veiled cells in lymph at different intervals
after stimulation with diphtheria toxoid. Veiled cells with large
lysosomes (O) containing heterogeneous and/or recognizable cellular
material are counted separately from the veiled cells (●), which
only contain virginal and/or small secondary lysosomes. Veiled cells
containing Birbeck granules (▲) usually do not contain lysosomes.
If they contained lysosomes they were double counted.

1.   Veiled cells and IDC belong to the mononuclear phagocyte
      system.
2.   Veiled cells and other macrophages enter the node by way of the
      afferent lymphatics.
3.   These newly arrived macrophages may be identified by the
      presence of Birbeck granules and they probably play a role in
      the induction phase of the immune response in different
      compartments of the node.

REFERENCES

1.   Hoefsmit, E.Ch.M., Mononuclear phagocytes, reticulum cells and
      dendritic cells in lymphoid tissues. In: Mononuclear phagocytes in
      immunity, infection and pathology pp. 129-146 (R. van Furth, ed)
      Oxford-London-Edinburgh-Melbourne: Blackwell Scientific
      Publications (1975).
2.   Kamperdijk, E.W.A., Raaymakers, E.M., de Leeuw, J.H.S., Hoefsmit,
      E.Ch.M., Lymph node macrophages and reticulum cells in the

immune response: Cell and Tissue Research, in press.

3.   Kelly, R.H., Balfour, B.M., Armstrong, J.A., Griffiths, S.,
     Functional anatomy of lymph nodes. II Peripheral lymph-borne
     mononuclear cells.   The Anatomical Record 190 pp 5-22 (1978).

4.   Langevoort, H.L., Cohn, Z.A., Hirsch, J.G., Humphrey, J.H.,
     Spector, W.G., A proposal for a new classification. In: Mono-
     nuclear phagocytes pp. 1-6 (R. van Furth, ed) Oxford: Blackwell
     Scientific Publications (1970).

MACROPHAGE-LYMPHOCYTE INTERACTION FOLLOWING CONCANAVALIN A-STIMULATION AS MONITORED BY CHEMILUMINESCENCE

K. Wrogemann, M.J. Weidemann, B. Peskar, Hj. Staudinger and H. Fischer

Max-Planck-Institut für Immunbiologie
D-78 Freiburg, West Germany

INTRODUCTION

When phagocytic cells, like granulocytes or macrophages, are activated by phagocytosis of bacteria or zymosan particles they emit light (chemiluminescence, CL) which can be easily monitored in a scintillation counter (1-3). This CL is considered indicative for the generation of reactive species of oxygen (O_2^-, H_2O_2, $\cdot OH$) and singlet oxygen ($^1\Delta O_2$) which emit light in the presence of polysaturated fatty acids, polysaccharides or easily oxidizable substances like luminol (4). Recently we demonstrated that CL would also be generated if macrophages were activated by the calcium ionophore A23187 (3), although, luminol is required for this to occur (3). We were convinced of a great potential of this method if it could also be used to monitor early T-cell activation.

In this paper we show that CL can indeed be generated immediately after stimulation of thymocytes with concanavalin A, that it shares several properties with ConA stimulated thymidine in corporation which occurs many hours later, and that macrophages as well as soluble factor(s) enhance the CL response.

Thymocytes were prepared from 7-10 weeks old Lewis rats by teasing the organs with hypodermic needles (5). They were suspended in Dulbecco's modified Eagles medium without bicarbonate and indicator, buffered with 50 mM Hepes, pH 7.2. Rat macrophages were cultured from bone-marrow precursor cells as described elsewhere (5). CL was measured at 37°C in a Tricarb scintillation counter set in the off-coincidence mode. Thymocytes (10^8 cells) were placed in plastic vials with 5 ml Eagles-Hepes-Medium and the photons emitted after concana-

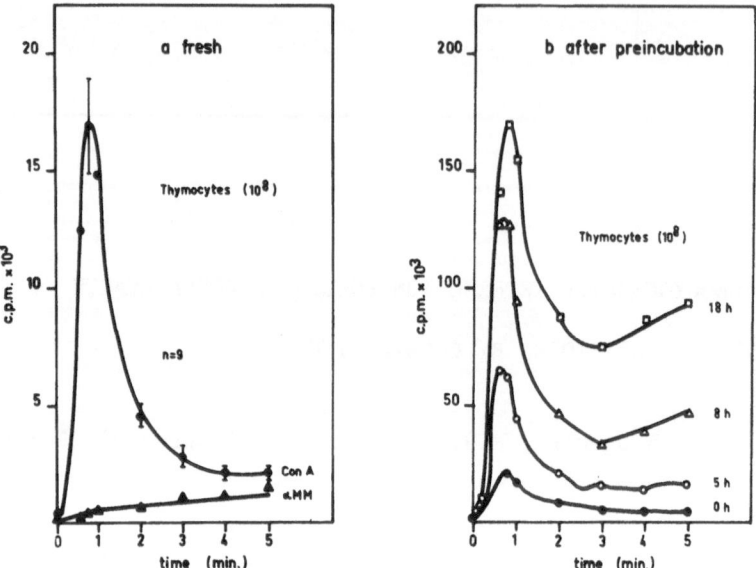

FIG. 1:   Time course of chemiluminescence of fresh (a) and (b)
preincubated rat thymocytes after 40 μg/ml ConA.

valin A addition (generally 40 μg/ml) monitored as counts/min. continuously for a period of 5 minutes. Details of the methods are
described elsewhere (3,5).

RESULTS AND DISCUSSION

Fig.1a shows the CL response from 9 different fresh thymocyte
preparations measured in 22 test runs. Characteristic is the quick
rise in CL immediately after ConA addition. It reaches very repro-
ducibly a peak after 50 seconds. The response is greatly enhanced
if the cells are preincubated at 37°C for extended periods (Fig.1b).
Under such conditions we have seen responses of up to 40 fold the
intensity observed in fresh cells. The degree of enhancement varies.

The optimal ConA concentration for eliciting a maximal CL
response is at 20-40 μg/ml. Higher concentrations become increasingly inhibitory (up to 160 μg/ml were tested). The response is
blocked by 50 mM   -methylmannoside (Fig.1a). It requires calcium,
and it is 50% inhibited by 0.6 μM prostaglandin E_1 (data not shown).
These characteristics are also observed in ConA stimulated thymidine
incorporation of thymocytes. But does the observed CL actually
originate on T-lymphocytes?

TAB. 1:   Effect of superoxide dismutase (S.O.D.) and catalase on
ConA-stimulated chemiluminescence.

Additions	Thymocytes	Macrophages
None	100%	100%
S.O.D.	80+6% (4)	85% (2)
Catalase	35+6% (4)	111% (2)

Thymocyte preparations are contaminated with macrophages (5,6)
and there is evidence that mitogen stimulation of T-lymphocytes
requires the presence of macrophages (6,7). Using the CL of zymosan
phagozytosing macrophages cultured from bone marrow precursor cells
(5) we have estimated the endogenous contamination of our thymocyte
preparation at 0.12% macrophages (5) on the assumption that the
macrophages in the thymus elicit an equal CL response to zymosan
phagocytosis as do the cultured cells. 100,000 macrophages, the
estimated contamination in 10^8 thymocytes, also emit light after
ConA addition (5). However, their contribution to the peak CL (Fig.1)
is insignificant, especially since the response to ConA evolves much
slower (5). It is possible though that a greater portion of the
"tail" response (Fig.1) between 2 and 5 minutes could originate on
macrophages.

What is the basis for CL in thymocytes? Some insight is obtained
from the action of enzymes that utilize reactive species of oxygen
(Tab.1). Thus, superoxide dismutase has little effect on the Cl
observed in either thymocytes or macrophages. However, catalase
suppresses the major portion of thymocytes CL, but does not inhibit
macrophage CL. We therefore have further support that the CL of
thymocytes is not generated on macrophages. Also H_2O_2 production
appears to be largely responsible for the observed CL.

Do macrophages play any role at all? When syngeneic bone marrow
derived macrophages are added (1 x 10^5 and 3 x 10^5) to 10^8 thymocytes
the CL response, after temperature equilibration, is more than the
sum of thymocytes and macrophages measured separately (Fig.2).
Furthermore, the enhancement of the CL response to ConA after preincubation at 37^0C (Fig.1b, Fig.2) is accelerated. An accelerated
response is also observed if the medium from 20h preincubated thymocytes is added to another, fresh preparation during preincubation.
During these preincubation periods cell aggregates are formed which,
on electronmicroscopic examination show cell contacts between lymphocytes and macrophages. These cell aggregates can easily be separated
by layering them over fetal calf serum and sedimenting them at 1xg
(Tab.2). Interestingly the fraction enriched with macrophages containing cell aggregates does not generate more CL after ConA stimu-

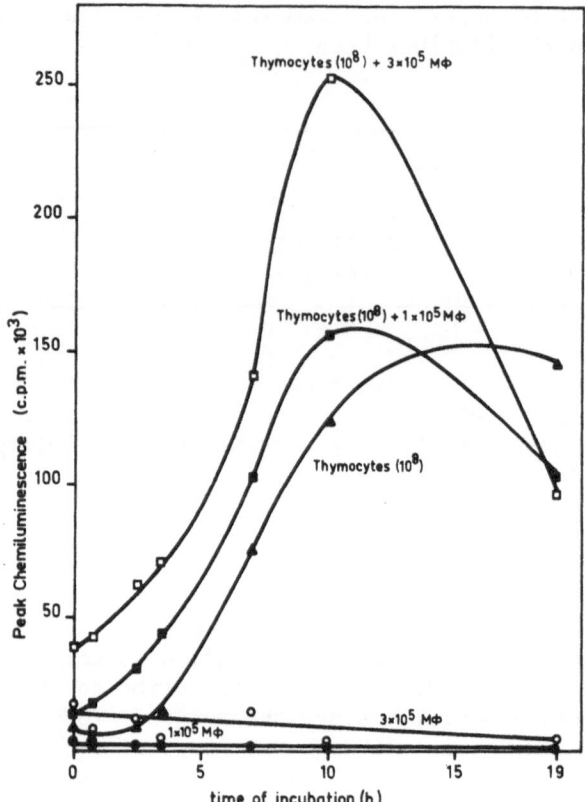

FIG. 2:   Peak chemiluminescence of thymocytes in the presence and absence of added macrophages after various times of preincubation.

lation. The fraction containing single cells only, which may have been in contact with macrophages before, appears to be devoid of macrophages but still emits at least an equally stong CL response. These results further support our finding that CL is generated on lymphocytes. They also show that after preincubation of thymocytes – containing endogenous macrophages – lymphocytes will give a CL response to ConA without macrophages being present at the time of ConA-addition.

CONCLUSIONS

    Chemilunimescence (CL) can be observed in thymocyte preparations immediately after ConA additon. The major portion of this CL originates on T-lymphocytes. It thus appears to be associated with (a) very early event(s) in T-lymphocyte activation. Macrophages as well as soluble factor(s) enhance the response. In spite of the

TAB. 2:   Chemiluminescence of single (macrophage-free) and aggregates (with macrophages) containing thymus cells after 20 hours preincubation.*

Expt. No.	1	2	3	4	$\bar{x}$
Single:	594	2238	368	711	100%
Aggregates:	208	1146	553	628	69%

*   Peak CL (cpm/10^6 cells).

long time span between this early CL response and the ConA stimulated thymidine incorporation the two processes have several characteristics in common. Chemiluminescence measurements alone and in combination with thymidine incorporation may therefore help to probe deeper into the events of mitogen stimulated T-cell activation. Furthermore, because of the immediate results by this method, chemiluminescence may become an effective approach to screen specificity and reactivity of T-lymphocyte populations, e.g. for tissue typing in organ transplantation.

REFERENCES

1.   Allen, R.C., Stjernholm, R.L., Steele, R.H. Biochem. Biophys. Res. Commun. 47 (1972) 679.
2.   Rosen, H., Klebanoff, S.J. J. Clin. Invest. 58 (1976) 50.
3.   Wiedemann, M.J., Peskar, B.A., Wrogemann, K., Rietschel, E.Th., Staudinger, Hj., Fischer, H. FEBS Letters 89 (1978) 136.
4.   White, E.H., Zafiriou, O., Kägi, H.H., Hill, J.H.M. J. Am. Chem. Soc. 86 (1964) 940.
5.   Weidemann, M.J., Wrogemann, K., Peskar, B.A., Staudinger, Hj., Rietschel, E.Th., Fischer, H. (submitted to Eur. J. Immunol.).
6.   Beller, D.I., Farr, A.G., Unanue, E.R. Fed. Proceed. 37 (1978) 91.
7.   Rosenstreich, D.L., Mizel, S.B. Immunol. Rev. 40 (1978) 102.

ACKNOWLEDGEMENTS

We thank Dr. H. Wekerle for helpful discussions, Dr. U. Ketelsen for performing the ultrastructural analyses and R. Marek for valuable technical assistance.

This work is supported by a grant from the Stiftung Volkswagenwerk.

CELL COOPERATIONS IN THE MITOGEN-INDUCED TRANSFORMATION OF HUMAN

BLOOD LYMPHOCYTES IN HEALTHY PERSONS AND IN HODGKIN'S DISEASE

M. Schlaak, P. Schröder and J.C. Wulff

1st Medical Clinic, University of Kiel

West Germany

Mitogen-induced lymphocyte transformation (LT) has been used extensively to describe proliferation abnormalities of lymphocytes in various diseases such as lymphoproliferative syndromes (1). Since LT results from the cooperation of different cell types (2) we further analyzed this phenomenon in order to define partial cellular defects underlying secondary immunodeficiency syndromes such as in Hodgkin's disease.

The experimental approach is based on the observation that there is a marked decrease in LT (expressed as ^{3}H-thymidine uptake) after the removal of adherent mononuclear cells (AMC) from mono- nuclear cell (MC) suspensions. Addition of AMC to column-separated purified lymphocytes results in the restoration of previous trans- formation rates. These AMC were isolated by glass surface adherence. According to dose response experiments only 1% of AMC are able to reestablish the LT capacity of purified lymphocytes. Therefore, the interpretation of abnormal LT data has to distinguish between lympho- cytic defects, deficient AMC helper effects or a combination of both.

In order to develop a test system in which cooperation defects can be analyzed in clinical situations comparative restitution experiments with syngeneic and allogeneic AMC have been performed; the results indicate that histocompatibility is not required in LT. The MLC-like lymphocyte activation occurring in allogeneic AMC restitu- ion experiments has no significant effect since the mitogeneic exceeds the allogeneic LT by usually about 15 times. Thus, allogenic AMC res- titution of purified lymphocytes can be used to further localize co- operation defects in LT.

In order to study the cellular requirements on the lymphocytic side in LT B- and T-cells were removed by SRBC rosetting technics

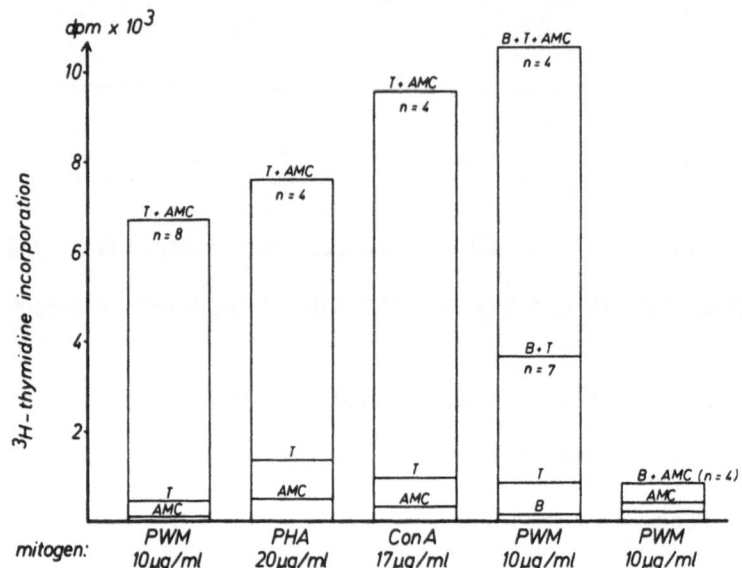

FIG. 1: Mitogenic stimulation capacity of human mononuclear blood cells after separation and recombination, T = T lymphocytes, B = B lymphocytes, AMC = adherent mononuclear cells; culture period 3d.

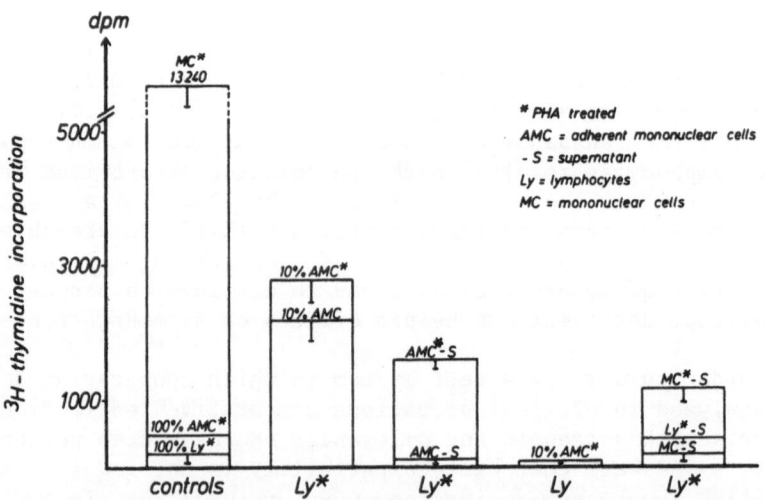

FIG. 2: Restitution of the stimulative capacity of purified human blood lymphocytes by AMC and the supernatants of various mononuclear cells cultured over 48 hrs.: culture period 3d.

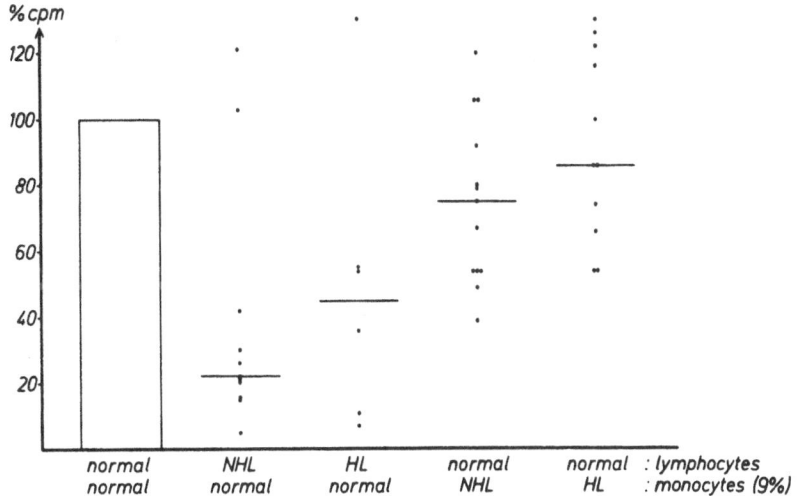

_3:   PHA(66 µg/ml) stimulation of purified lymphocytes from
homa patients and normal persons in various combinations;
ure period 3d.

centrifugation. As can be seen in Fig.1 neither T- nor B-cells
be stimulated by PHA, PWM and ConA in the absence of AMC.
tion of AMC leads to a complete restitution of LT in T- but not
-cells. On the other hand, there is some effect if B-cells are
d to T-cells in the absence of AMC (3).

The mechanism of the cooperation of lymphocytes and AMC has
  investigated by subjecting AMC to various pretreatments:
ruction of AMC by ultrasound abolished the helper effect,
ough pretreatment with mitomycin (25 µg/ml) or x-ray (2500 rad)
not. The AMC helper effect cannot be substituted by mercap-
hanol. Therefore, structurally intact AMC are required in LT.
s still controversial whether the lymphocyte-AMC cooperation in
s a result of direct cell-cell interactions or of soluble medi-
s. According to (4) lymphocyte agglutination is the consequence
er than the prerequisite of LT. Fig.2 shows the results of
riments investigating the helper activity of AMC supernatants.
an be seen there is a LT restitution only if the AMC supernatant
ves from mitogen treated AMC and is brought together with mitogen
ted lymphocytes, indicating a T-lymphocyte AMC cooperation
iring two mitogenic signals, the one derived from AMC and medi-
  by a soluble factor, recently named mitogenic protein (5), the
r enabling T-lymphocytes to respond to this factor.

The experiments so far presented in this paper have been designed
nable the clinician to identify partial cellular defects in

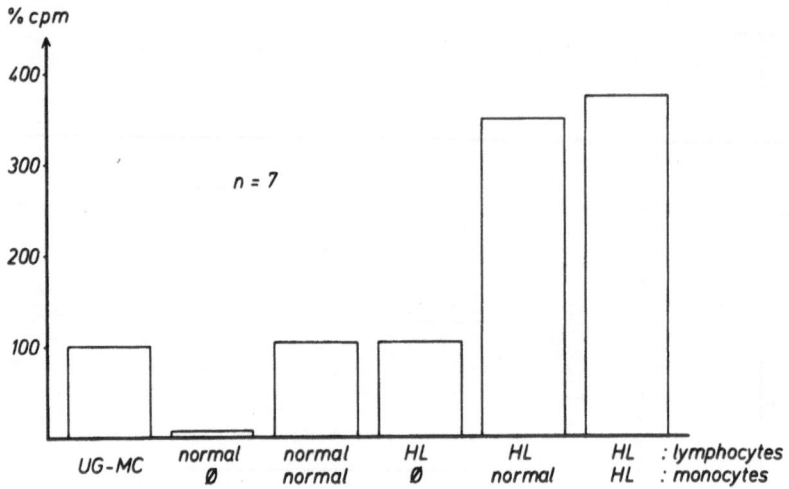

FIG. 4:   PHA (66 µg/ml) stimulation of purified and monocyte re-
combined Hodgkin lymphoma blood lymphocytes;   culture period 3d;
UG-MC = MC after whole blood centrifugation over a Urografin
gradient.

secondary immunodeficiencies.   In a first series 16 Hodgkin-(HL)
and 22 Non-Hodgkin lymphomas (NHL) stage III or IV have been tested
for isolated lymphocytic and/or AMC defects.   The LT of non-separated
mononuclear cells was reduced to 18% and 21% of normal in HL and NHL,
respectively, which is in accordance with (6).   HL-sera added to
cultures of normal MC depresses ConA-induced LT to 61% of normal;
this confirms data in (7).   When differentiating the cellular defects
in detail there is a major lymphocytic LT deficiency in both HL and
NHL, whereas the AMC defect is less pronounced (Fig.3).   Considering
the data depicted in Fig.2 this could reflect a disability of lymphocytes to respond to AMC mediator(s) or to the mitogenic signal that
usually enables them to react to this mediator.

    Apart from these data the test system revealed another effect
acting in HL LT: The separation of lymphocytes is not accompanied
by a reduction of the stimulative capacity (Fig.4) usually always
seen in controls and NHL.   The recombination of purified HL lymphocytes with control or HL AMC results in a substantial augmentation
of LT.   This can be explained by the existence of a subset of AMC
displaying suppressor activity in LT which is nylon wool but not
glass surface adherent and which possibly contributes further to the
depressed cell mediated immunity in HL.

REFERENCES

1. Willson, J.K.V., Zaremba, J.L., Pretlow, T.G. Blood 50 (1977) 783.
2. Rosenstreich, D.L., Farrar, J.J., Dougherty, S. J. Immunol. 116 (1976) 131.
3. Weksler, M.E., Kuntz, M.M. Immunol. 31 (1976) 273.
4. Dráber, P., Vicklický, V., Lengerová, A. J. Immunogenetics 5 (1978) 67.
5. Unnane, E.R., Kiely, J.-M. J. Immunol. 119 (1977) 925.
6. Case, D.C., Hansen, J.A., Corrales, E., Young, C.W., Dupont, B., Pinsky, C.M., Good, R.A. Blood 49 (1977) 771.
7. Amlot, P.L., Unger, A. Clin. exp. Med. 26 (1976) 520.

THE ANTIGEN BINDING DENDRITIC CELL OF THE LYMPHOID FOLLICLES:
EVIDENCE INDICATING ITS ROLE IN THE MAINTENANCE AND REGULATION
OF SERUM ANTIBODY LEVELS

[1]John G.Tew, Thomas Mandel, Antony Burgess and J. Douglas
Hicks

The Walter and Eliza Hall Institute of Medical Research,
Melbourne, Australia

INTRODUCTION

Antigen (Ag) is obligatory for the induction of immune responses.
It has been postulated that Ag continues to play a role in their
maintenance and regulation, however, the evidence for such a role is
largely circumstantial (1-5). In fact, the unequivocal demonstration
of a readily degradable Ag persisting in the presence of immune
clearance mechanisms has not been reported. The present investigation was undertaken to see how long a simple protein Ag could persist
in an immune animal and to see whether retained Ag might be implicated in the maintenance and regulation of antibody (Ab) production.

MATERIALS AND METHODS

Solubilization of the ^{125}I labeled antigen from lymph nodes.
The popliteal lymph nodes were removed, teased apart in phosphate
buffered saline (PBS) containing 5M guanidine hydrochloride and
100 μg/ml cold Human Serum Albumin (HSA). This mixture was incubated
in a 37° H_2O bath for 30 min and then dialized against PBS. After
centrifugation, 80 to 90% of the radiolabel originally present in the
lymph node was in the supernatant.

Coprecipitation. Sufficient rabbit anti-HSA was added to the
solubilized HSA to establish equivalence and the mixture was allowed

---

[1] This work was carried out while on leave from the Department of
Microbiology, Medical College of Virginia, P.O. Box 847, Richmond,
Virginia 23298, USA.

TAB. 1:   The Kinetics of Antigen Clearance from the Popliteal Lymph
Nodes of Immunized and Non-Immunized Mice.

Immune Status	Picograms ^{125}I-HSA per mg of tissue (mean $\pm$ SE (a)					
	day 0.2	day 1	day 3	day 6	day 11	day 28
Immunized	1,720+660	92+28	28+10	20+5	18+7	12.4+4
Non-Immunized	820+50	82+27	26+3	7+1	3+1	2.2+0.7

(a)   The popliteal lymph nodes from immune mice were much larger
than the nodes from non-immune mice. The data are therefore expressed
as picograms ^{125}I-HSA per mg of lymph node.

to incubate overnight at 4°C. The precipitate was collected by
centrifugation, washed twice, and the radioactivity was counted.

    Other methods.   Techniques for iodination of proteins, immuni-
zation of mice, autoradiography, cell culture, and the radioimmunno-
assay for mouse anti-HSA, have been described previously (6).

RESULTS

    The kinetics of clearance of ^{125}I labeled HSA from the popliteal
lymph nodes of immune and non-immune CBA/H WEHI mice was studied
(Tab.1). For the first 3 days radiolabel was cleared rapidly from
both groups of animals. However, by day 6 a difference between the
immune and non-immune groups was apparent. Less radioactivity was
present in the nodes from non-immune animals and this level was
declining rapidly. In contrast, radioactivity in the nodes from
immune animals declined slowly. In a separate experiment the half-
life of retained Ag was 2 mo (95% confidence interval between 1.3
and 5 mo) in the period between 10 and 45 days.

    Autoradiography revealed that 4 hours after injection, heavy
label was around germinal centers and over macrophages of the medulla
and superficial cortex. The same pattern was present at 24 hours
except there were very few grains left in macrophages. By the 3rd
day, long exposure times were required to detect radioactivity in
macrophages, but the labelling remained heavy in lymphoid follicles.
Electron microscopy in conjunction with autoradiography indicated
that retained radiolabel was associated with processes of dendritic
cells. To examine the rate of Ag catabolism in macrophages more
carefully, peritoneal macrophages were allowed to engulf radiolabelled

TAB. 2:   The Specific Coprecipitation of Radioactive Material
Released from Lymph Node Cells.

Time after injecting ^{125}I-HSA	Radioactivity coprecipitated with	
	HSA-anti-HSA	EA-anti-EA
(weeks)	(percentage)	(percentage)
2	90	2
4	96	2
12	89	3

Ag in the form of Ag-Ab complexes. Under these in vitro conditions
the half-life of Ag in macrophages was only 2 hours with a 95%
confidence interval between 1.5 and 3 hours.

The crucial question in these experiments was whether radioactivity is a reliable marker for Ag. If this is the case it
should be possible to specifically precipitate retained radiolabel
with anti-HSA. Solubilization of radiolabel was achieved by treatment with guanidine hydrochloride. The solubilized radiolabel was
then specifically coprecipitated with anti-HSA even after 12 weeks
in the animal (Tab.2). This solubilized radiolabel cochromatographed
with native HSA on Sepharacyl S 200 indicating the retained HSA was
still intact.

The retained Ag was localized in the draining lymph nodes (DLN)
of the immune mice. Cells taken from these nodes "spontaneously"
produced Ab when injected into irradiated recipients (Tab.3). However, exogenous Ag was required to stimulate cells from non-draining
lymph nodes (NDLN). The only apparent difference between the DLN
and NDLN appears to be the lack of Ag in the latter. Furthermore,
specific mouse anti-HSA blocked induction of Ab production in cells
from the DLN indicating that the inducer was specific and subject
to an Ab feedback mechanism.

DISCUSSION

These results imply that a major role of the Ag binding dendritic cells is to retain Ag which serves in conjunction with an Ab
feedback system to maintain and regulate serum Ab levels. This
concept is supported by the observation that: 1. Cells in the DLN
produce Ab at regular intervals or cycles (4). 2. The period between
intervals is related to the level of circulating Ab (3). 3. Cells
from DLN, which include dendritic cells with associated Ag, produce

TAB. 3:   Spontaneous Production of Anti-HSA in Recipients of Cells
from the Draining Lymph Nodes of HSA Immunized Mice.

Experiment No.	Source of cells	Serum or Antigen in Cell Culture Medium(a)	Mouse Anti-HSA (ng/ml serum ± SE)
I	DLN	15% FCS alone	150,000 ± 27,000
	NDLN	15% FCS alone	4,200 ± 1,100
	NDLN	15% FCS + 10 μg HSA/ml	90,000 ± 59,000
II	DLN	15% FCS alone	45,000 ± 6,000
	DLN	10% FCS + 5% mouse anti-HSA	10,000 ± 4,000
	DLN	10% FCS + 5% normal mouse serum	40,000 ± 14,000

(a) Cells were cultured for 5 hr at 37°C, transferred into irradiated recipients and 9 days later serum anti-HSA levels were determined by radioimmunoassay.

Ab spontaneously whereas cells from NDLN do not (present study). 4. Induction of Ab synthesis by DLN cells is subject to Ab feedback inhibition (present study). 5. Antigen retained on dendritic cells has a half-life of about 2 months which could explain maintenance of serum Ab for months or years (present study).

REFERENCES

1.   Graf, M.W., Uhr, J.W. J. Exp. Med. 130 (1969) 1175.
2.   Bystryn, J.C., Graf, M.W., Uhr, J.W. J. Exp. Med 132 (1970) 1279.
3.   Britain, S., Moller, G. J. Immunol. 100 (1968) 1326.
4.   Weigle, W.O. Adv. Immunol. 21 (1975) 87.
5.   Tew, J.G., Self, C.H., Harold, W.W., Stavitsky, A.B. J. Immunol. 111 (1973) 416.
6.   Tew, J.G., Mandel, T. J. Immunol. 120 (1978) 1063.

ACKNOWLEDGEMENTS

This study was supported by the National Health and Research Council of Australia, and Grants KAI00008A, Int-15635, and AI11101.

This is publication Number 2463 from the Walter and Eliza Hall Institute of Medical Research.

THE CONCEPT OF DRUG-CARRIERS IN THE TREATMENT OF PARASITIC DISEASES

P. Tulkens[1] and A. Trouet

Laboratoire de Chimie Physiologique, Université Catholique de Louvain and International Institute of Cellular and Molecular Pathology, avenue Hippocrate, 75, B-1200 Bruxelles, Belgium

In many parasitic diseases, the reticulo-endothelial system is the major site of infection. Linking antiparasitic drugs to macromolecular carriers may therefore extensively improve their therapeutical properties. The drug-carrier complex is no longer able to diffuse through the cell plasma membranes, and will be taken up preferentially by the cells which display high endocytic capacity. Complexed drugs will also be excreted at lower rate than free drugs, leading to increased plasma levels, for prolonged periods. Not the least, cells with low or no endocytic activity will be protected from adverse action of the drug, thus improving the overall therapeutic index of the complex with regard to the free drug.

Once endocytozed, complexed drugs will be conveyed to lysosomes and therein be exposed to a collection of acid hydrolases. Provided the link drug-carrier is sensitive to one of these enzymes, the drug will be released free and under an active form to act either within lysosomes, or even in the cytosol if it is able to diffuse out of lysosomes.

In this connection, the therapeutical effectiveness of Ethidium Bromide (EB) and EB complexed to DNA (EB-DNA) has been compared on mice infected with Trypanosoma Cruzi (1). EB forms stable intercalation complexes with DNA, DNA being itself easily endocytozed and

---

1   Chargé de Recherches of the Belgian F.N.R.S.

broken down in lysosomes by acid nucleases (2). Under its micro-
mastigote form, T. Cruzi invades and stays in lysosomal vacuoles,
where it resists to most available trypanocides. Animals receiving
EB alone fail to show definite remission, or display severe signs of
toxicity. In contrast, animals receiving EB-DNA showed up to 90%
long term cure, with no persistence of intracellular or extracellular
parasitosis, and no or little toxicity.

Linking drugs to more selective carriers is presently being
investigated; among these are antibodies directed against specific
surface antigens (3) or glycoproteins that are taken into a given
cell type, e.g. hepatocytes (4) or macrophages (5), by receptor-
mediated endocytosis.

REFERENCES

1.   Trouet, A., Jadin, J.M., Van Hoof, F. In: Biochemistry of
      parasites and host-parasite relationships. (H. Van den Bossche,
      ed.) Elsevier/North Holland Biomedical Press, Amsterdam, p. 519.
      (1977).
2.   Trouet, A., Deprez-de Campeneere, D., de Duve, C. Nature New
      Biology 239 (1972) 110.
3.   Tulkens, P., Schneider, Y.J., Trouet, A. Biochem. Soc. Trans.
      5 (1977) 1809.
4.   Ashwell, G., Morrell, A. Adv. Enzymol. 41 (1974) 99.
5.   Stahl, P.D., Rodman, J.S., Miller, M.J., Schlesinger, P.H.
      Proc. Natl. Acad. Sci. US 75 (1978) 1399.

RECYCLING (SHUTTLE) OF CELL SURFACE MEMBRANE DURING ENDOCYTOSIS

P. Tulkens[1], Y.J. Schneider and A. Trouet

Laboratoire de Chimie Physiologique, Université Catholique de Louvain and International Institute of Cellular and Molecular Pathology, avenue Hippocrate, 75, B-1200 Bruxelles, Belgium

The turn-over rate of plasma membrane constituents is much slower than expected from the endocytic activity of most cell types, i.e. the rate at which endocytic vesicles arise from cell surface and fuse with lysosomes (1,2). Two hypotheses have been put forward to account for this discrepancy : (a) only very discrete and small parts of plasma membrane are involved in endocytosis, and their fast turn-over has remained so far undetected (3); (b) after endocytosis, most of the plasma membrane constituents internalized are returned intact to the cell surface (4).

We present experimental evidence in favour of the 2d hypothesis. Fibroblasts were allowed to endocytose and to accumulate in lysosomes goat (antirabbit IgG) antibodies, which they retain therein and slowly digest under a subsequent wash-out. Coating the cells, during this wash-out, with rabbit antibodies directed specifically against plasma membrane antigens results in (i) unloading the goat (anti-rabbit IgG) antibodies (and not goat unspecific IgG, in control experiments) from lysosomes, and (ii) displaying part of these goat IgG on the cell surface. The necessary contact is believed to occur when the endocytic vacuole fuses with a lysosome, allowing the intra-lysosomal goat IgG to attach to the plasma membrane-bound rabbit IgG. Subsequent extrusion of the goat IgG indicates that the double-coated piece of plasma membrane shuttles back to the cell surface. At the same time, cells keep on endocytosing and accumulating in their lysosomes unrelated exogenous proteins, like horseradish peroxidase.

---

[1] Chargé de Recherches of the Belgian F.N.R.S.

Our findings indicate that during endocytosis, plasma membrane constituents are transiently, and perhaps repeatedly, exposed to the lysosomal hydrolases. If this applies to other cell types, we suggest this shuttle to play an important role in the modulation or alteration of the cell surface constituents and their ligands, e.g. in the handling of foreign antigens by macrophages (5).

REFERENCES

1. Doyle, D., Baumann, H., England, B., Frieman, E., Hou, E., Tweto, J. J. Biol. Chem. 253 (1978) 965.

2. Steinman, R.M., Brodie, S.E., Cohn, Z.A. J. Cell. Biol. 68 (1976) 665.

3. Berlin, R.D., Fera, J.P. Proc. Natl. Acad. Sci. US 74 (1977) 1072.

4. Tulkens, P., Schneider, Y.J., Trouet, A. In: Intracellular Protein Catabolism II (V. Turk, N. Marks, eds.) J. Stephan Institute, Ljubljana, and Plenum Press, New York, p. 73 (1977).

5. Rosenthal, A.S., Blake, J.T., Ellner, J.J., Greinder, D.K., Lipsky, P.E. In: Immunobiology of the Macrophage (D.S. Nelson, ed.) Academ. Press, New York, p. 131 (1976).

THE EFFECT OF VARIOUS PROSTAGLANDINS ON PLASMA MEMBRANE RECEPTORS AND FUNCTION OF MOUSE MACROPHAGES

E. Razin and A. Globerson

Department of Cell Biology, The Weizmann Institute of Science, 76100 Rehovot, Israel

INTRODUCTION

Mobility and redistribution of receptor molecules on the macrophage surface appear to be important for the interaction between macrophages and phagocytized particles and between macrophages and lymphocytes (1-3). It has been suggested that prostaglandins (PGs) may modulate the function of macrophages, since high doses (10^{-2}-10^{-3} mg/ml) inhibited phagocytosis of SRC, whereas lower doses (10^{-8}-10^{-4} mg/ml) enhanced phagocytosis (4). It was thus of interest to determine whether endogenous synthesis of PGs by the macrophage (5) is relevant in this process, and whether modulation by PGs is achieved by changing plasma membrane receptors. In this communication, we report that inhibition of PG synthesis in the macrophage interferes with phagocytosis and that PG treatment to macrophages leads to morphological changes in the membrane and to modulation of Con A and Fc cell membrane receptors.

MATERIALS AND METHODS

Animals: 2-4 month old (Balb/c x C57BL/6)F_1 male mice obtained from the Animal Breeding Center of the Weizmann Institute of Science were employed throughout this study.

Prostaglandins (PGs): PGE_2, $PGF_{1\alpha}$, $PGF_{2\alpha}$ and PGA_1 (kindly donated by Dr. J. Pike, Upjohn Company, Kalamazoo, Michigan) were dissolved in ethanol and then diluted in phosphate buffer saline (PBS) so that the final concentration of ethanol did not exceed 0.1% (v/v).

TAB. 1:   Effect of indomethacin with or without PGs on phagocytosis of IgG-coated SRC.

Series	Indo-metha-cin	mean cpm ± S.E.				
		PBS	PGE_2	$PGF_{2\alpha}$	$PGF_{1\alpha}$	PGA_1
A	+	1567±51[*]	3325± 78	3379±171	3403±99	3436±57
B	−	3349±29	4385±110	6137± 79	5690±76	5690±96

[*] Mean values of 3 replicates. Results represent one of 3 experiments. Total cpm added was 65 674.

Macrophage preparation and treatment: Adherent cells were separated from peritoneal exudate of thioglycollate injected mice or from spleens, as previously described (4). The cells were incubated in 10^{-6} mg/ml PG solutions for 20 min at 37°C then rinsed with PBS. Indomethacin (5 µg/ml) was applied for 1 hr at 37°C, followed by rinsing in PBS and reincubation for 45 min in the same solution. The cells were then washed in PBS. No change in viable cell numbers was found following treatment with PGs or indomethacin.

Phagocytosis assay: Phagocytosis was evaluated by incubating the macrophages with ^{51}Cr-opsonized sheep erythrocytes (SRC) (4).

Macrophage preparation for scanning electron microscopy (SEM): Specimens were fixed initially with 2.5% glutaraldehyde in PBS. Dehydration was performed with graded concentrations of ethanol. The fixed cells were flooded with acetone and dried by the critical point method (6). For surface conductivity specimens were coated with metallic gold alloy.

^{125}I-Con A binding to peritoneal macrophages: 1 ml of PBS containing 50 µg Con A, 10^{-1} M α-methyl-D-mannopyranoside (αMM) and 0.2% sodium azide (to prevent phagocytosis) were added to adherent cells. After 5 min incubation the cells were washed with PBS, exposed to 50 µg ^{125}I-Con A in 1 ml PBS and 0.2% sodium azide and washed. This last incubation was repeated 5 min before the final washing. All incubations were carried out at 37°C in an atmosphere of 5% CO_2/air. After addition of 2 ml of sodium dodecyl sulphate (2% SDS) to each plate, the cpm values of macrophage lysate were determined.

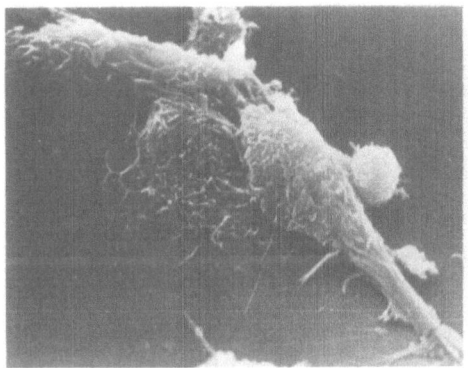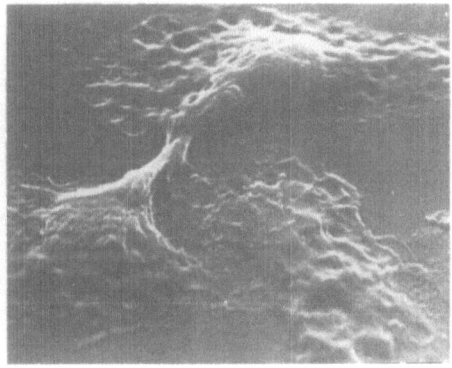

FIG. 1:   SEM preparations of peritoneal adherent cells treated
with PG (A) or PBS (B). (Mag. x3000)   (Reduced 10% for purposes
of reproduction.).

^{51}Cr-labelled IgG-sensitized sheep erythrocytes (SRC) binding
assay: Macrophages were incubated in 1 ml of PBS containing ^{51}Cr-
labelled SRC (4) and 0.2% sodium azide for 20 min at 4°C. The cells
were subsequently washed with PBS, lysed by 2% SDS, and cpm values
were determined.

RESULTS AND DISCUSSION

We first examined whether PG synthesis by macrophages plays any
role in phagocytosis. Splenic adherent cells were incubated with
indomethacin in PBS or together with PG (10^{-6} mg/ml) for 1 h (Tab.1,
series A). Control groups were incubated in PBS without indomethacin
(Series B). After rinsing with PBS, cells in Series A were treated
for 45 min with the same solutions as during the first hour and
series B were treated with PBS or PG, respectively. It was found
(Tab.1) that addition of indomethacin to the cultures led to a
decrease of about 50% in the phagocytosis of IgG-coated SRC. No
inhibition was observed when the various PGs were added to the
macrophages together with the indomethacin. PGs without indomethacin
enhances phagocytosis, as previously shown by us (4).

We then attempted to find out whether PG treatment to macrophages
manifests in any morphological change in the cell membrane. SEM
examination of adherent cells treated with PGs (10^{-6} mg/ml) indicated
dense population of microvillies, projections, and folds (Fig.1A) which
were not observed in the majority of PBS treated cells (Fig.1B). Hence,

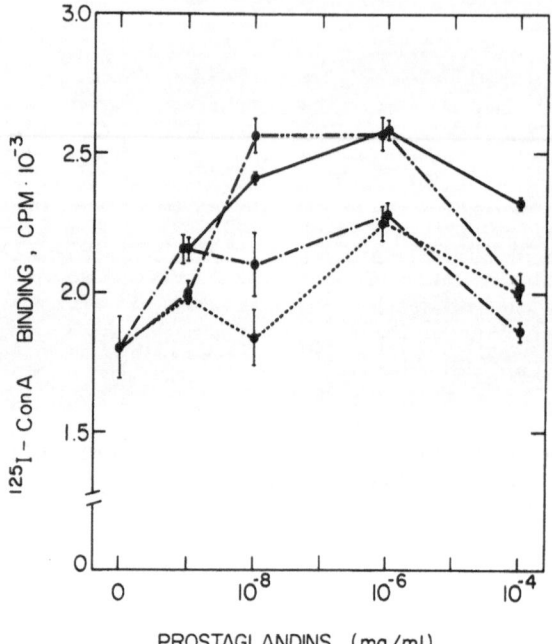

<u>FIG. 2</u>: ^{125}I-Con A binding to PG-treated macrophages.
$\overline{PGE_2}$ (●——●),   PGF$_{2\alpha}$ (●-·-·-●),   PGF$_{1\alpha}$ (●-··-··-●),   and PGA$_1$ (●---●).
Control cultures were treated in the same fashion in PG-free medium.
Total cpm initially added was 50,000.   Each point represents the
mean ± S.E. of 3 replicates.   The figure represents the results of
one out of 4 repeated experiments behaving in similar manner.

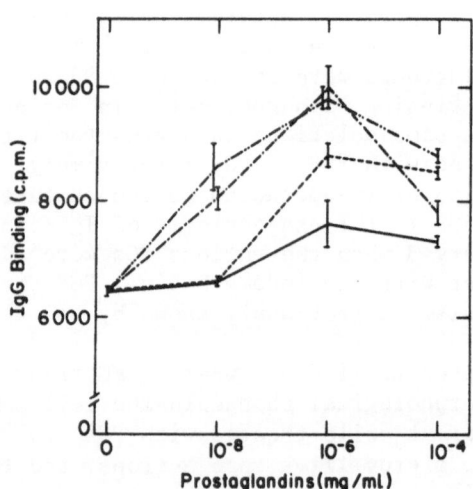

<u>FIG. 3</u>:   IgG binding to PG-treated macrophages.
Legend same as in Fig.2, but total cpm initially added was 54,000.

the PGs affect the macrophage cell membrane.

Further experiments were designed to test whether the effect on the cell membrane is expressed in change in activity of receptors. We thus investigated the function of Con A and Fc receptors in PGs as compared to PBS treated macrophages.

Dose-dependent enhancement of 50 μg/ml ^{125}I-Con A binding to peritoneal macrophages was obtained with various PGs (Fig.2). Maximal effect was noted at the concentration of 10^{-6} mg/ml.

In a similar manner, a marked enhancement in binding of IgG-sensitized ^{51}Cr-SRC was obtained with 10^{-6} mg/ml of PGs (Fig.3). These findings link the effect of the PGs on macrophages to a modification of cell membrane which influences the activity of plasma membrane receptors. The effect of PGs could be visualized as a possible rise in the accessibility and/or affinity of receptors to IgG and Con A. The observation that PGs enhance the binding capacity of surface proteins and receptors indicates that PGs may play an important role in modulating a variety of membrane-associated events. Whether the intrinsic PGs act by a similar mechanism as the PG applied externally remains to be determined.

REFERENCES

1. Oliver, J.M., Ukena, T.E., Berlin, R.D., Proc. Nat. Acad. Sci. US 71 (1974) 394.
2. Ptak, W., Naidorf, K.F., Gershon, R.K., J. Immunol. 119 (1977) 444.
3. Schmidt, M.E., Douglas, S.D., J. Immunol. 109 (1972) 914.
4. Razin, E., Bauminger, S., Globerson, A., J. Reticuloend. Soc. 23 (1978) 237.
5. Humes, J.L., Bonney, R.J., Pelus, L., Dahlge, M.E., Sadowski, S.J., Kuehl, F.A., Davies, P., Nature 269 (1977) 149.
6. Anderson, T.F., The American Naturalist 86 (No. 827) (1952) 91.

ACKNOWLEDGEMENTS

Partial support for these studies was provided by the Minerva Foundation.

MODULATION OF PHAGOCYTOSIS INDUCED PROSTAGLANDIN RELEASE FROM

MACROPHAGES

D. Gemsa, M. Seitz, J. Menzel, W. Grimm, W. Kramer and
G. Till
Institute of Immunology, University of Heidelberg,
Heidelberg, W. Germany

Prostaglandins of the E-class (PGE_1, PGE_2) are tissue hormones
which have been implicated to regulate inflammation and some
leukocyte interactions (1-4). Recently, we postulated (4,5) that
prostaglandins may play a role as modulators of immune reactions by:

1. a release in response to immune relevant stimuli,

2. a selective action towards leukocytes rendered particularly
    prostaglandin-sensitive.

A rapid enhancement of PGE_1 sensitivity of macrophages has already
been observed during alterations of the cell membrane such as
treatment with concanavalin A, colchicine, dextran sulfate and
phagocytosis (4,5). To gain more information about mechanisms
contributing to prostaglandin production, different classes of
leukocytes, their state of stimulation and the opsonization of
phagocytosable particles were examined in this study.

Leukocytes were obtained from guinea pigs. Eosinophils were
elicited by repeated intraperitoneal injections of Ascaris suis and
were purified by centrifugal elutriation (6). Neutrophils were
harvested 7 hours and macrophages 4 days after an intraperitoneal
injection of sodium caseinate (4). All leukocytes were more than
90% pure. A complement (C)-insensitive strain of E. coli was
opsonized with specific IgG and C as described (7). The degree of
phagocytosis was determined with ^{3}H-thymidine labelled E. coli (7).
PGE_1 and $PGF_{2\alpha}$ were measured in the incubation medium by radioimmunoassay (4). The incubation system consisted of glass tubes
with 5×10^6 leukocytes suspended in 2.5 ml Dulbecco's medium plus

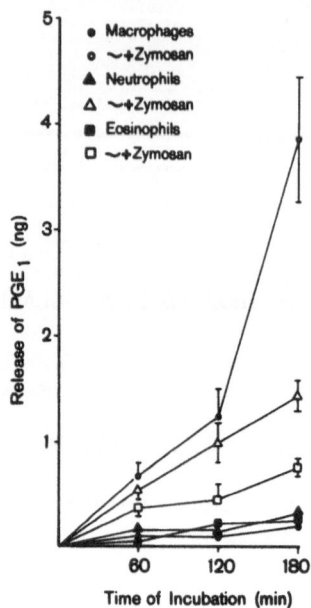

FIG. 1:   Phagocytosis-induced PGE$_1$ release from different phagocytes.
5x10^6 macrophages, neutrophils or eosinophils were incubated alone
or with added zymosan (1 mg).

5% heat-inactivated fetal calf serum with additions of bacteria or
zymosan particles as indicated.

When macrophages, neutrophils or eosinophils were incubated,
only little PGE$_1$ was released spontaneously (Fig.1). Addition of
zymosan particles, however, increased PGE$_1$ production from all
three cell types. A striking difference was observed in that
macrophages were by far the most potent producers of PGE$_1$ when
compared to neutrophils or eosinophils although the extent of
zymosan phagocytosis was similar. In macrophages, PGE$_1$ release
occurred at a lower rate during phagocytosis but at an accelerated
rate after phagocytosis had ceased. Indomethacin (10^{-5}M), an
inhibitor of prostaglandin synthesis, completely abolished
phagocytosis-induced PGE$_1$ formation. Latex particles, although
interiorized avidly by macrophages, completely failed to induce
PGE$_1$ release. To examine whether surface attributes of particles
may also affect PGE$_1$ production of macrophages, E. coli were
opsonized in different ways prior to incubation with macrophages.
Fig.2 shows that bacteria coated with specific IgG plus C were the
most efficient particles to induce PGE$_1$ release, although E. coli
coated only with IgG or C were phagocytosed to a comparable extent.
Since C activated on the surface of bacteria, either by IgG or via

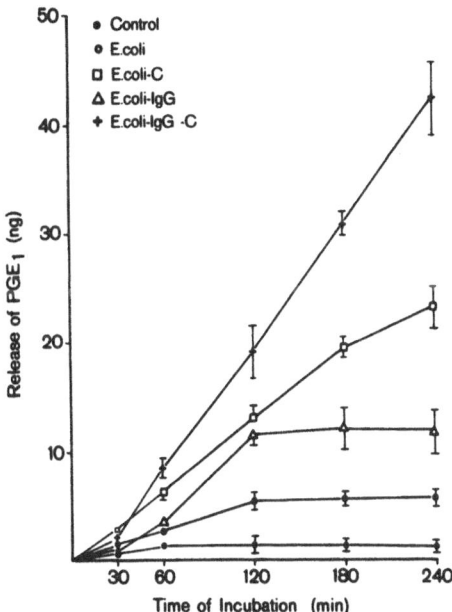

FIG. 2:   The effect of IgG and C on phagocytosis-induced PGE_1 release from macrophages. 5×10^6 macrophages were incubated with 2×10^7 E. coli which were opsonized as indicated.

the alternative pathway in the absence of IgG, apparently enhanced PGE_1 release from macrophages, it was of interest to study the effect of activated C fragments present in the fluid phase. When the chemotactically active fraction of zymosan-activated serum, mainly containing C5-derived leukotactic activity, was added to macrophages phagocytosing unopsonized E. coli, the PGE_1 release was completely abolished although the degree of phagocytosis was not affected (Tab.1). Similar results were obtained when bacteria were opsonized with IgG and C. Whether the state of macrophage stimulation would influence prostaglandin production was investigated with macrophages elicited with various agents. Macrophages obtained four days after an intraperitoneal injection of proteose peptone or casein exhibited features of stimulated cells whereas macrophages after injection of Corynebacterium parvum displayed properties of activated cells. Tab.2 demonstrates that all types of macrophages were phagocytically active to a rather similar degree. Their capacity to release prostaglandins, however, was markedly different. The highest spontaneous PGE_1 release was found in Corynebacterium parvum-induced macrophages, usually being 10 times higher than in other macrophages. On the basis of the low baseline PGE_1 production, phagocytosis-induced PGE_1 formation was very prominent in casein-

TAB. 1:   Effect of chemotactically active complement (C) on
phagocytosis-induced PGE_1 release

Macrophages $(5x10^6)$	Phagocytosis [a]	Migration (μm) [b]	$PGE_1 (ng)$ [c]
Resting	-	35	0.54 ± 0.03
Resting + activated C	-	92	0.35 ± 0.02
Phagocytosing	$0.47x10^6$	-	2.25 ± 0.30
Phagocytosing + activated C	$0.49x10^6$	-	0.29 ± 0.10

a.   Measured after 30 min. of incubation with $2x10^7$ unopsonized
     E. coli.
b.   Measured after 90 min. of incubation in a Boyden chemotaxis
     chamber.
c. PGE_1 release into the medium after 120 min. of incubation.

induced macrophages, although the highest absolute values were
obtained with macrophages 5 days after Corynebacterium parvum
stimulation. A different picture evolved when the release of $PGF_{2\alpha}$
was determined. Unstimulated and Corynebacterium parvum-induced
macrophages showed a notable spontaneous release, but in contrast
to PGE_1, phagocytosis clearly stimulated the highest $PGF_{2\alpha}$ release
from completely unstimulated macrophages.

Although the role of prostaglandins in the immune response is
far from clear, some observations indicate that particularly
macrophages are the main producers (4,8,9,10). Potent stimuli
appear to be all those agents which lead to a rapid perturbation
of the cell membrane such as phagocytosis and, under adverse
conditions, to a damage of the cell as described for silica or
carrageenan (4). The data presented here extend previous findings
in that the rate of prostaglandin generation may be influenced by
the composition of the phagocytosed particle. So far all available
evidence suggests that the phagocytosable particle should expose
opsonins, has to be degradable or should contain macrophage-
activating compounds such as ß (1-3) glucosidic linkages as in the
case of zymosan. Opsonization of bacteria with IgG and C clearly
enhanced PGE_1 production which may imply a role for both opsonins
in facilitating activation of phospholipases and mobilization of
precursor fatty acids. The preliminary findings described here,
showing that not cell-bound, biologically active C fragments
presumably C5a suppressed phagocytosis-induced PGE_1 synthesis

TAB. 2: Phagocytosis-induced prostaglandin release from differently stimulated macrophages

Macrophages (5x10^6)	Phagocytosis [a]	PGE$_1$ (ng) [b]		PGF$_2$α (ng) [b]	
		spontaneous	Phagocytosis	spontaneous	Phagocytosis
Unstimulated	6.87x10^6	0.12+0.10	1.70+0.40	1.06+0.35	5.90+1.27
Proteose Peptone	6.20x10^6	0.14+0.10	1.63+0.10	0.32+0.01	1.29+0.13
Casein	8.05x10^6	0.16+0.11	3.16+0.30	0.20+0.05	1.17+0.02
C. parvum (5d) [c]	6.70x10^6	1.97+0.14	6.52+0.42	1.10+0.01	2.13+0.18
C. parvum (14d) [c]	7.87x10^6	1.22+0.16	1.92+0.09	0.57+0.01	0.93+0.08

a. Measured after 30 min. of incubation with 2x10^7 opsonized (IgG+C) E. coli.

b. PGE$_1$ or PGF$_2$α release into the medium after 120 min. of incubation.

c. Macrophages were harvested 5 or 14 days after an intraperitoneal injection of Corynebacterium parvum (2mg).

remain to be further elucidated. Tentatively, it may indicate that various activated C products, depending on their localization, may act in an antagonistic manner on prostaglandin formation. PGE_1 synthesis of macrophages not only occurred under situations of rapid membrane alterations but also reflected spontaneous membrane activity typical of macrophages activated with Corynebacterium parvum. Thus, it may be conceivable that the previously described suppressive effects of highly activated macrophages on lymphocyte responses may be partially due to the immunosuppressive action of prostaglandins of the E-class. It remains to be seen whether prostaglandins of the F-class, which were produced to a higher degree by unstimulated macrophages, may assume a role different from PGE_1 and PGE_2. The data available suggest that macrophages, depending on their state of activation, may utilize prostaglandins as mediators to enhance or suppress an immune response.

REFERENCES

1. Kaley, G., Weiner, R., Ann. N.Y. Acad. Sci. 180 (1971) 338.
2. Braun, W., Lichtenstein, L.M., Parker, C.W., Cyclic AMP, Cell Growth and the Immune Response. Springer Verlag, Berlin, Heidelberg, New York, (1974).
3. Vane, J.R., In Advances in Prostaglandin and Thromboxane Research. Eds. S. Samuelsson, E. Paoletti. Raven Press, New York, Vol. 2 (1976) 791.
4. Gemsa, D., Seitz, M., Kramer, W., Till, G., Resch, K., J. Immunol. 120 (1978) 1187.
5. Gemsa, D., Steggemann, L., Till, G., Resch, K., J. Immunol. 119 (1977) 524.
6. Kownatzki, E., Till, G., Gagelmann, M., Terwort, G., Gemsa, D., Nature 270 (1977) 67.
7. Menzel, J., Junfer, H., Gemsa, D., Infect. Immun. 19 (1978) 659.
8. Seitz, M., Hirt, H.M., Gemsa, D., Kirchner, H., Z. Immun. Forsch. 153 (1977) 354.
9. Humes, J.L., Bonney, R.J., Pelus, L., Dahlgren, M.E., Sadowski, S.J., Kuehl, F.A., Davis, P., Nature 269 (1977) 149.
10. Kurland, J.I., Bockman, R., J. Exp. Med. 147 (1978) 952.

NEOFORMATION OF LYMPHATICS IN THE MOUSE OMENTUM

M. Holub[1], L. Jarosková[2], H. Fischer[3] and V. Viklicky[4]

[1]Institute for Clinical and Experimental Medicine
[2]Institute of Microbiology
[4]Institute for Molecular Genetics, CSAV, Praha, CSSR
[3]Max-Planck Inst. for Immunobiology, Freiburg, W. Germany

The omental immune response is connected with accumulation of phagocytic and lymphoid cells in follicle-like dense lymphatic areas (DLA) situated between the two mesothelial sheets (1,2). Concomitantly also lymphatics appear in the central part of the mouse omentum (3). Most of these lymphatics originate without connection with the vessels in the omental roots or occasional preexisting lymphatics in the central omentum; therefore the lining cells of the new lymphatics must differentiate from heterotypic precursors, not only by sprouting of other endothelia. The lymphatics disappear with the termination of the immune response (3).

Ip injection of 3.10^8 sheep red blood cells (SRBC) induces demonstrable neoformation of DLA and lymphatics; peak numbers were attained on days 3-4 and 8-10 and lowest scores on days 5 and 14-20 (Tab.1). Athymic nude (nu/nu) mice displayed higher numbers than euthymic mice. No difference was found between +/+ mice and nu/+ (panleucopenic) hybrids. Consequently the process is not thymus-dependent or T cell-controlled. The omentum is a B cell site in general (2,4). Since the macrophage system in nu/nu mice is known to be well equipped by precursor potential (5) and in an "activated" state (6), its involvement in the DLA and lymphatics formation was inferred from this experiment.

A seven times higher dose of SRBC after which virtually all omental macrophages appeared loaded with erythrocytes almost abolished the DLA and lymphatics formation (Fig.1). A booster dose of 3.10^8 SRBC provoked the highest reaction; here the bulk of the lymphatics counted is due to branching off of preexisting vessels,

TAB. 1:   Numbers of DLA and lymphatics per 100 mm^2 area of central omentum in mice of C57Bl/10Sn background after 2.10^8 SRBC ip (means from 5-8 mice ± S.E.M.)

Day	nu/+		nu/nu	
	DLA	lymphatics	DLA	lymphatics
0	7.29±2.06	0.51±0.38	10.04±1.87	0.99±0.29
3	19.10±1.75	8.26±4.27	24.67±0.62[1]	6.58±1.17
4	11.57±2.67[2]	6.53±3.31	32.63±9.09[1]	8.97±3.22
5	11.37±3.72[2]	2.11±1.32[2]	15.30±3.61[2]	3.05±0.52
8	15.34±3.24	3.24±0.75	34.68±8.33[1]	9.50±2.76[1]
10	28.60±8.27	5.34±1.50	14.65±1.12[2]	12.35±6.33

Only days with values significantly different (P < 0.01-0.05) from preimmunization (0 day) values given. No significant difference was found on days 1,2,6,7 and 14-20.

1.   Significant difference from nu/+ on the respective day.

2.   Value not significantly different from day 0.

but also new independent lymphatics were found in the 2nd peak. MIF provoked conspicuous accumulation of macrophages and lymphocytes and an intensive formation of specialized lymphatic bulbs (Fig.3). Activated complement induced only a prolonged granulocytic infiltration.

All substances tested produced biphasic reactions obviously due to two waves of PE cell immigration and emigration from the omentum and the resulting recruitment of cells lining the developing lymphatics.

The process starts with an alignment of some omental stromal cells in the prelymphatic pathways at the outskirts of a DLA. Long cytoplasmic projections of such cells appear on the omental surface and PE cells attach to them in high numbers (Fig.2). There is very little proliferation among the developing lining cells (3). Bulbs are formed on the tips of the lymphatics hanging from the omental surface. These bulbs as well as highly cellular DLA are the sites of the most intensive entry of fluid (patent blue tracing) or cells from the peritoneal cavity. Both intraomental and extraomental lymphatics are lined by cells which are acid phosphatase positive

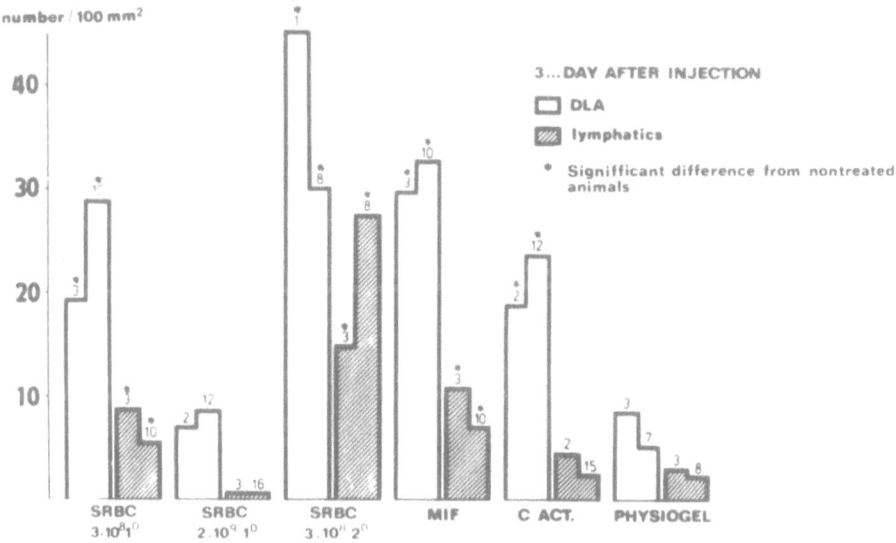

FIG. 1:   Peak numbers of DLA and lymphatics (as in Tab.1) after
different doses of SRBC, a second dose of SRBC given 3 weeks after
the first, MIF (supernatant from cultures of 3.10^7 mouse cells (3)),
zymosan-activated guinea pig complement and physiogel (non-immunogenic
modified gelatin). Inactivated complement, BSA, human sera and a
lymph node activating factor (7) yielded values in the range between
physiogel and act. complement.

and alkaline phosphatase negative, the cells of the tunics of the
large lymphatics are actively phagocytic (HRP tracing). Ultra-
structurally the cells found in the lumina of developing small
lymphatics correspond mostly to monocytes, the lining cells of the
differentiated lymphatics are typical endothelia attached by zonulae
adhaerentes to each other (Fig.5). Lymphatics are filled with
lymphocytes (Fig.5) and their persistence is strictly dependent on
the lymphocytic accumulation in the omentum (3).

    All this indicated again that PE macrophages play the essential
role in neoformation of lymphatics. An ip instillation of syngeneic
PE cells, activated in normal C57Bl/10Sn donors by proteose peptone
injection 3 days previously provoked the most intensive DLA and
lymphatics formation with only one peak on days 1 and 2, respectively
(Fig.6). Control animals received pooled lymph node cells from the
same donors and did not develop any conspicuous reaction. Lymphatics
were mostly intraomental and displayed very intensive branching (Fig.4).

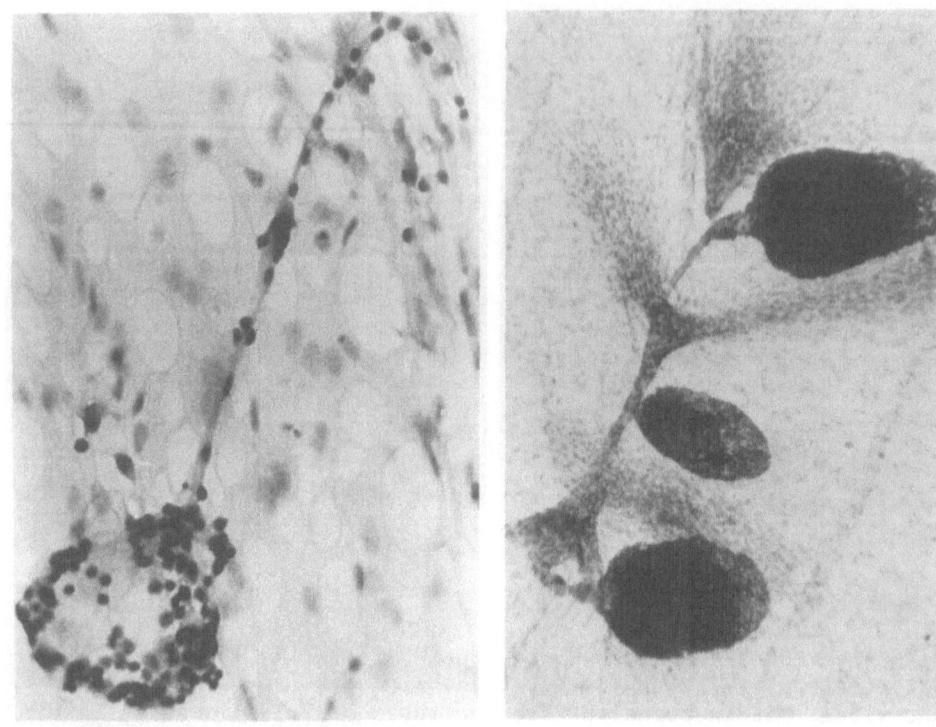

FIG. 2   FIG. 3

FIG. 2: 2° response to SRBC, day 8:   initial stage of a lymphatic.
HE, x 350 (Reduced 20% for purposes of reproduction.).

FIG. 3:   MIF, day 10:   lymphatic bulbs on the tips of lymphatics.
HE, x 56 (Reduced 20% for purposes of reproduction.).

The relatively low lymphocytic immigration may be responsible for
the short duration and persistence of the lymphatics.   Both
macrophages and conditioned media from 24 hours macrophage cultures
were found to provoke guinea pig corneal neovascularisation (8).   It
may be suggested that the angiopoietic stimulus in the omentum is a
humoral factor shed by the macrophages.   In addition some PE cells
may function as precursors of the lymphatics lining cells.   It is
likely that the vascular neoformation represents a general phenomenon
of the immune reaction occurring also in lymphatic organs (9).

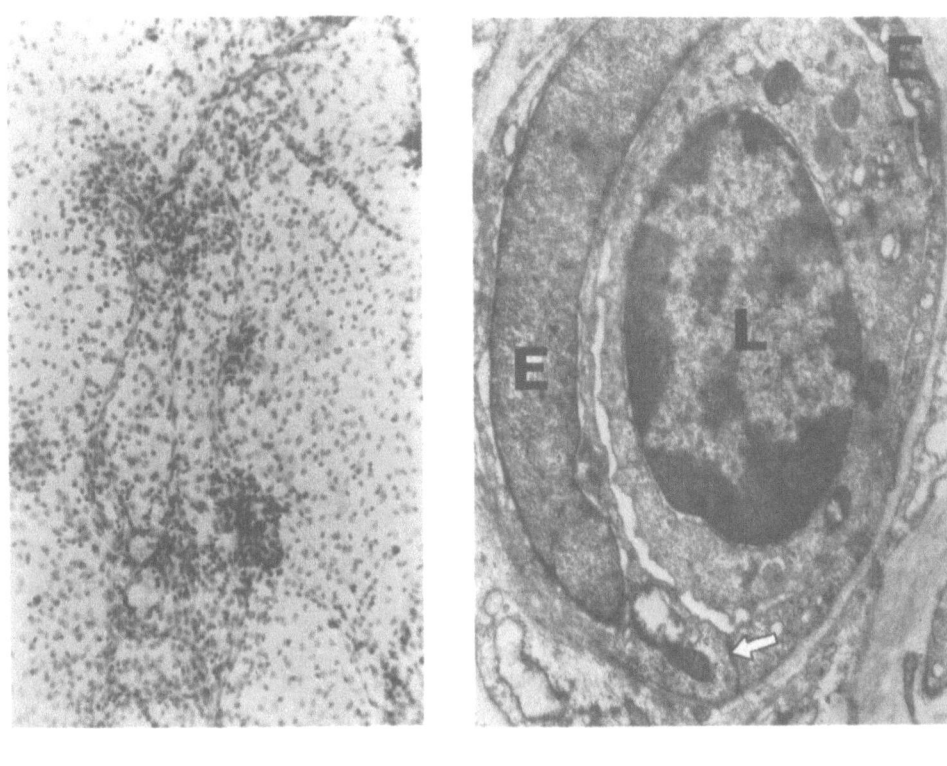

FIG. 4   FIG. 5

FIG. 4:   Act. macrophage transfer, day 2: branching off lymphatics.
HE, x 140.

FIG. 5:   1° response to SRBC, day 3: EM picture of a lymphatic;
L - lymphocyte in the lumen, E - endothelial cells, attached by a
z. adhaerens (arrow). x 12,000.

CONCLUSIONS

     Lymphatic neoformation occurs in the avascular central part of
the mouse omenta during the omental immune response. Inflammatory
agents (activated complement) or non-immunogenic material does not
provoke a demonstrable reaction. The development of lymphatics is
mediated by activated PE macrophages and their persistence is closely
related to the exudation and increased lymphocyte traffic in the
peritoneal cavity.

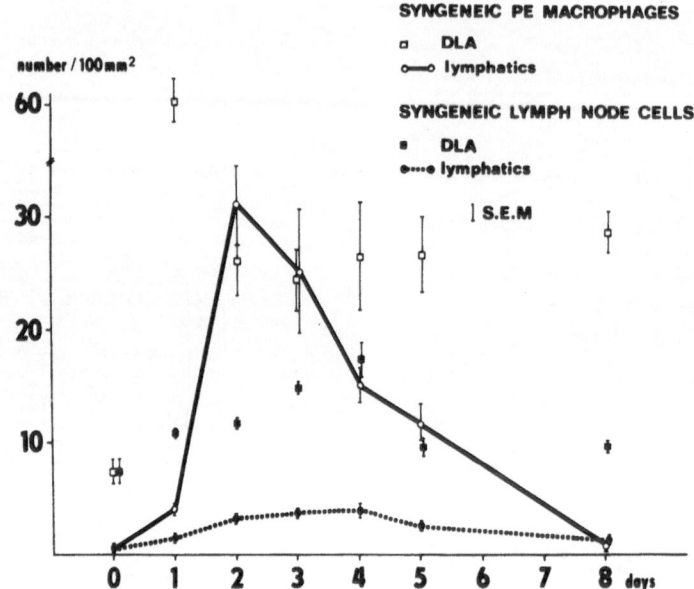

FIG. 6:   DLA and lymphatics formation after ip transfer of
syngeneic PE cells or lymph node cells (7-10.10^6 cells).

REFERENCES

1.   Kaboth, U., Ax, W., Fischer, H., Z. Naturforschung 21b (1966)
     789.
2.   Holub, M., Ax, W., Fischer, H., et al., Developmental Aspects
     of Antibody Formation and Structure, Academia, Prague (1970)
     p. 641.
3.   Holub, M., Polanová, E., in: Progress in Lymphology, Thieme
     Verlag, Stuttgart (1978) in press.
4.   Szaniawska, B., Arch. Immun. Ther. Exp. 23 (1975) 19.
5.   Wilson, F.D., Gershwin, M.E., Shifrine, M., Graham, R.,
     Developmental & Comp. Immunol. 1 (1977) 373.
6.   Rama Rao G., Rawls, W.E., Perey, D.Y.E., Tompkins, W.A.F.,
     J. Res. 21 (1977) 13.
7.   Korcáková, L., Holub, M., Allergie u. Immunol. 23 (1977) 287.
8.   Polverini, P.J., Cotran, R.S., Gimbrone, M.A. Jr., Unanue, E.R.,
     Nature 269 (1977) 804.
9.   Herman, P.G., Yamamoto, I., Mellins, H.Z., J. Exp. Med. 136
     (1972) 697.

PROPERTIES OF MONONUCLEAR PHAGOCYTES DERIVED FROM THE SMALL INTESTINAL WALL OF RATS

G.G. MacPherson[1] and H.W. Steer[2]

[1]Sir William Dunn School of Pathology, University of Oxford, Oxford, England

[2]Nuffield Department of Surgery, Radcliffe Infirmary Oxford, England

INTRODUCTION

A proportion of the mononuclear phagocytes (MNP) that enter tissue beds leave via afferent lymphatics. Under normal circumstances, these MNP are filtered out in the draining lymph nodes and do not appear in efferent lymph. However, following mesenteric lymphadenectomy in rats, macrophage-like cells appear in thoracic duct lymph (TDL) (G. Mayrhofer, personal communication). If these cells do derive from the small intestine, this model offers many advantages in the investigation of the properties of MNP derived from a tissue bed.

In this paper we present evidence that these cells are MNP and that they derive from the small intestine. In addition we have examined some of their functional properties.

MATERIALS AND METHODS

Specific-pathogen-free inbred rats were used. Mesenteric lymphadenectomy was carried out at least six weeks before thoracic duct cannulation. Thoracic duct cells were collected continuously and prepared for light and electron microscopy. Cytocentrifuge preparations were prepared for quantitation of MNP following non-specific esterase (NSE), staining using a α-napthyl butyrate as substrate. Lymph cells in suspension or adherent to glass coverslips were incubated with latex particles or sheep erythrocytes

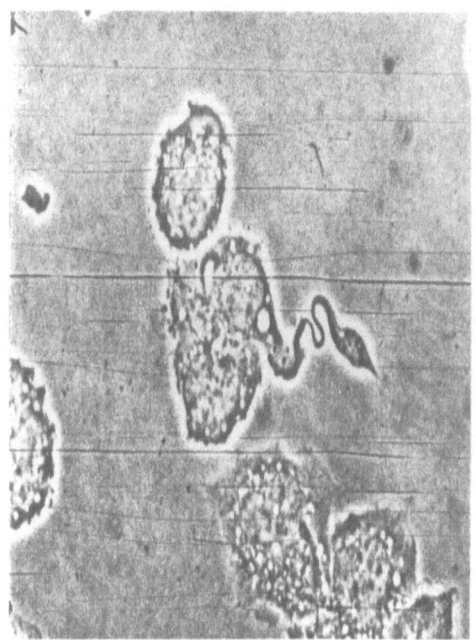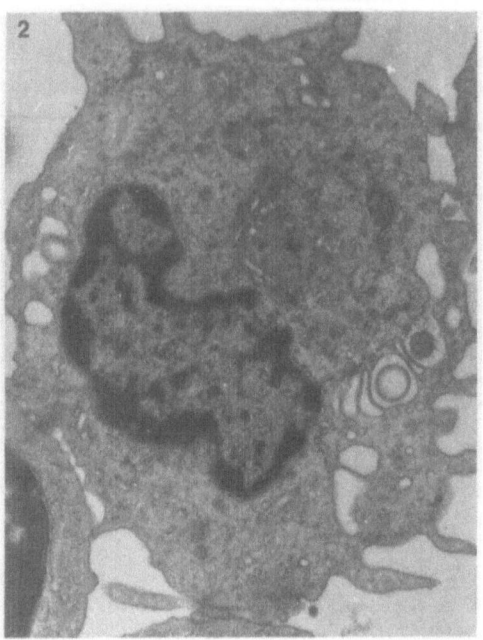

FIG. 1:   Fresh TDL mag. x 1,000. Nomanski interference. A large
MNP, four small and one large lymphocyte are present.

FIG. 2:   Electron micrograph of monocytoid cell in TDL.   mag. x
8,700. Pinocytotic vesicles and Golgi apparatus are conspicuous.

opsonized with whole antibody (EA) or the IgM fraction plus C'5-
deficient fresh mouse serum (EAC).

For the investigation of MNP kinetics, rats were injected intravenously with tritiated thymidine (^{3}HTdR) (1 μC/gm body weight) and
autoradiographs (ARG) made from washed TDL cells.

RESULTS

Morphology of MNP

Light microscopy revealed the presence of cells with features
of MNP (Fig.1). These cells, not found in normal TDL, ranged in
size from that of medium lymphocytes to cells larger than lymphoblasts. The nuclei were usually irregular and sometimes lobulated,
with nucleoli frequently present in the larger cells. Cytoplasm was

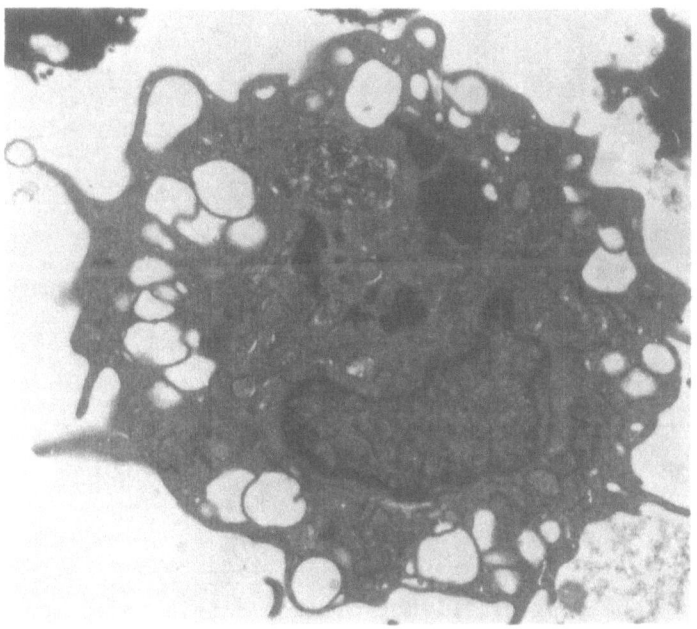

FIG. 3:   Macrophage-like cell in TDL. mag. x 7,100. Abundant
cytoplasm, residual bodies, pinocytotic vacuoles and cytoplasmic
veils.

sparse in smaller cells but abundant in large cells. Cytoplasmic
margins were irregular, especially so in large cells, where numerous
pseudopodia were usually present. Cytoplasmic inclusions were often
present in larger cells.

Electron microscopy confirmed these findings. NMP with monocytoid morphology were present (Fig.2) but these were often difficult
to distinguish from lymphocytes. Larger MNP were conspicuous in all
samples. These cells were often vacuolated (Fig.3) and many showed
extensive pseudopodia. In many of the larger cells, rough endoplasmic reticulum and Golgi apparatus were conspicuous, while some
large cells showed extensive smooth endoplasmic reticulum, often
extending into the pseudopodia and sometimes appearing to be surface
connected.

NSE staining of normal and experimental TDL was positive in a
proportion of small lymphocytes as one or two small dots. However,
in experimental TDL, cells with the morphological appearance of MNP
stained diffusely.The intensity of staining varied greatly, small

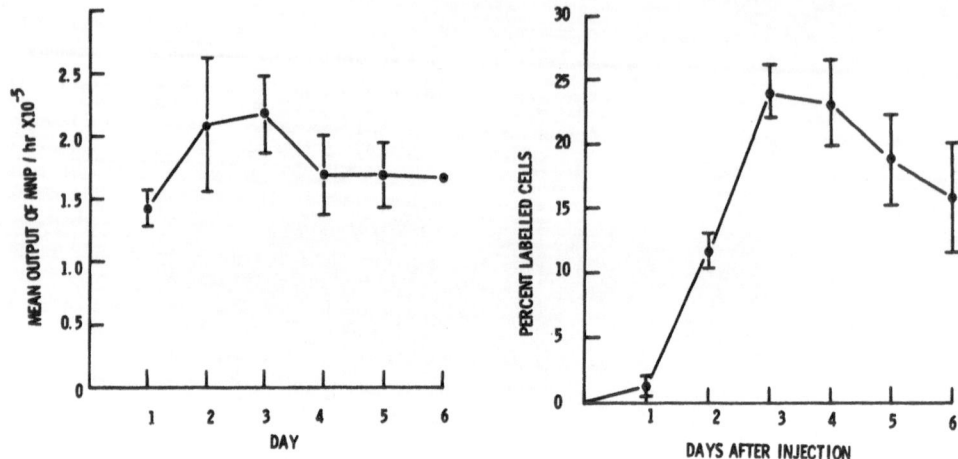

FIG. 4:   Hourly output of TDL MNP (Vertical bars = $^{+}_{-}$1 = S.E.M.)

FIG. 5:   % labelling of TDL MNP after a single injection of ^{3}HTdR (Vertical bars = $\pm$ 1 S.E.M.)

and medium sized cells usually giving a limited reaction confined to the nuclear 'hof', (+ - ++) whereas many large cells gave an extremely intense reaction, staining the whole cytoplasm and obscuring the nucleus (+++).

Quantitation of MNP

MNP were quantitated on NSE-stained cytocentrifuge preparations of fresh lymph. The proportion of MNP rose from about 1% of TDL cells at day 1 up to 5% by day 5-6. However, as the output of lymphocytes fell over this period, the actual hourly output of MNP remained relatively steady (Fig.4).

Glass Adherence

Lymph cells were incubated over glass coverslips. Adherent cells included all types identified as MNP by NSE staining and morphology. However, the smaller cells with less intense NSE staining were more strongly adherent.

TAB. 1

Particle	% phagocytic MNP			
	Total	NSE+	++	+++
Latex	73	91.2	75.6	36.0
EA	14	23	0	0

Phagocytosis

The results for phagocytosis of latex particles and EA are shown in Tab.1. 73% of cells with MNP characteristics ingested latex. The large, strongly NSE-positive cells were less phagocytic than the smaller cells. 5-10% of cells with ingested latex were not identifiable as MNP by morphology or NSE staining. Similarly, with EA, only occasional strongly NSE positive cells were phago- cytic, and 50% of the phagocytic cells did not possess MNP charac- teristics. A similar picture was seen with EAC.

Kinetics of MNP Production

ARG's of TDL labelled with ^{3}HTdR 'in vitro' and of NSE-stained sections of small intestine showed no labelled MNP. However, labelled MNP appeared in TDL by 24 hr post-injection and their frequency rose rapidly to reach 20-25% by day three, thereafter declining slowly (Fig.5) At day 1, only medium sized cells with weak NSE staining were labelled, but some of the most intensely stained cells were labelled by day 3.

Other Studies

Direct cannulation of intestinal afferent lymphatics has shown that cells with similar morphology and NSE staining are present in similar proportions to those in TDL.

DISCUSSION

Identity of MNP-like Cells

It is clear that there is a population of cells with MNP characteristics in TDL from lymphadenectomized rats. Cells which

are morphologically less mature and differentiated express typical
MNP properties of strong glass adherence and phagocytosis. However,
the more 'mature' cells are not strongly glass adherent or phagocytic, although cells of this type can be induced to phagocytose
latex. These large cells are similar to cells described in sheep
afferent lymph (Smith et al., 1970), rabbit afferent lymph (Kelly
et al., 1978), lymph draining pig skin (Balfour, personal communication) and to Langerhans cells seen in guinea pig epidermis, lymph
and lymph nodes (Silberberg-Sinakin et al., (1976). However,
despite an extensive search, no typical 'Langerhan granules' were
seen in TDL cells. Thus, as these cells are phagocytic, are glass-
adherent, and have the ultrastructural features of MNP, we see no
reason to classify them as a separate cell type. In addition, their
labelling kinetics with ^{3}HTdR closely parallel to those of blood
monocytes (Volkman and Gowans, 1965).

Original of TDL MNP

The finding of similar cells in TDL, afferent lymph and lamina
propria of the small intestine is conclusive evidence that at least
some TDL MNP are derived from the small intestine. However, it is
difficult to completely exclude the possibility that some may derive
from the peritoneal cavity. Roser (1976) has shown that after 5-6
days cannulation, MNP do appear in normal TDL and that they are
derived from the peritoneal cavity. However, injection of colloidal
carbon into the peritoneal cavity of cannulated lymphadenectomized
rats did not result in the appearance of labelled MNP in TDL until
6 days post cannulation.

CONCULUSIONS

Mesenteric lymphadenectomy allows the free passage of afferent
lymph cells into TDL. These cells include a population of MNP with
varying degrees of differentiation. The majority of these cells are
recently formed, probably from blood monocytes. This model allows
the opportunity for detailed investigation of MNP derived from a
tissue bed.

REFERENCES

1.   Kelly, R.H., Balfour, B.M., Armstrong, J.A., Griffiths, S.,
     Anat. Rec. 190 (1978) 5.
2.   Roser, B.J., Aust. J. Exp. Biol. Med. Sci. 54 (1976) 541.
3.   Silberberg-Sinakin, I., Thorbecke, G.J., Baer, R.L., Rosenthal,
     S.A., Berezowsky, V., Cell. Immunol. 25 (1976) 137.
4.   Smith, J.B., McIntosh, G.H., Morris, B., J. Anat. 107 (1970) 87.
5.   Volkman, A., Gowans, J.L., Brit. J. Exp. Path. 46 (1965) 50.

GRAFT-VERSUS-HOST INDUCED IMMUNOSUPPRESSION ASSOCIATED WITH AN

INCREASED THYMIC MITOGEN RESPONSE

W.S. Lapp and H. Kirchner

Institut für Virusforschung, Deutsches Krebsforschungs-

zentrum, 6900 Heidelberg, W. Germany

INTRODUCTION

The thymus gland is the site of production of T-lymphocytes
from pre thymic or stem cells. The gland is thus endowed with two
unique properties; firstly, it contains a large population of
immature T-cells, a small population of mature T-cells and virtually
no B-cells; secondly, the thymus gland selectively permits the
entry of stem cells while excluding mature T- and B-cells. Therefore, thymocytes normally respond poorly to the T-cell mitogen
phytohemagglutinin (PHA) and the B-cell mitogen lipopolysaccharide
(LPS) although there is usually a significant response to the T-
cell mitogen Concancavalin A (Con A) (1,2).

The graft-versus-host (GVH) reaction induces a state of permanent
immunosuppression (3-5). The later stage of immunosuppression is
associated with thymic dysplasia characterized by atrophy and the
abolition of Hassall's corpuscles and epithelial cells from the
medulla (6). The cause(s) of the destruction of epithelial cells,
which are considered to perform an important endocrine function in
T-cell ontogeny, is not known. One possibility is that sensitized
lymphocytes of donor origin gain entry into the thymus during the
GVH reaction and inflict the injury. We have, therefore, studied
the mitogenic response of thymus cells to PHA, Con A, and LPS
throughout the course of a GVH reaction since a significant increase
in the PHA and LPS responses would be strong evidence that mature
cells had entered the thymus.

TAB. 1:   Splenic PFC responses of $B_6D_2F_1$ mice to SRBC at different days post GVH induction.

Day post GVH[1]	Mean PFC response per spleen	
	Normal F_1	GVH
2	128,000	78,000
4	146,000	26,000
8	135,000	200
22	165,000	300

[1] Day post GVH when mice were immunized withSRBC.   PFC were determined four days later.

MATERIALS AND METHODS

Mice of the inbred strains DBA/2 (D_2), C57BL/6 (B6), and the $B_6D_2F_1$ hybrid were used.   GVH reactions were induced in adult $B_6D_2F_1$ mice by the intravenous injection of 50 - 70 x 10^6 B_6 or D_2 spleen and lymph node cells as described previously (3-6).   At different days post GVH induction animals were sacrificed and the mitogen responses of thymus cells to PHA, Con A and LPS were studied by the method described by Kirchner et al. (7).   It consisted essentially of cultering 6 x 10^5 cells with mitogens in RPMI 1640 supplemented with fetal calf serum for 48 hours in microtiter plates followed by 4-6 hours pulse with ^{3}H-thymidine.

The plaque forming cell (PFC) response to sheep erythrocytes (SRBC) was performed as described previously (3).   Mice were injected intravenously with 5 x 10^8 SRBC and the number of PFC was determined 4 days later.

RESULTS

The results shown in Tab.1 demonstrate that the PFC response to SRBC became severely suppressed by day 7 post GVH induction, thus confirming our earlier studies (3-6).

Tab.2 shows that thymus cells from normal mice displayed a negligible PHA and LPS mitogen response, but did produce a significant Con A response.   However, thymus cells from mice experiencing

TAB. 2:   Thymus cell response of $B_6D_2F_1$ mice to PHA, Con A and LPS at different days post GVH induction.

Day post GVH	Thymus Source[1]	Mitogen response $(\times 10^{-3})$[2]			
		No Mitogen	PHA[3]	Con A[3]	LPS[3]
2	NF$_1$	0.3	1.4	21.2	0.3
	GVH	0.4	2.3	37.2	1.6
6	NF$_1$	1.8+0.1	2.1+0.01	120.3+2.2	2.2+0.01
	GVH	3.8+0.01	7.2+0.7	144.3+0.01	14.3+0.6
7	NF$_1$	2.2+0.1	2.6+0.04	72.3+2.3	3.6+0.04
	GVH	6.5+0.2	9.3+0.1	120.8+1.5	20.2+0.4
11	NF$_1$	2.2+0.1	2.8+0.05	22.3+2.2	2.6+1.0
	GVH	2.6+1.9	6.8+0.7	51.5+2.1	8.8+0.3
19	NF$_1$	0.2	0.6	16.9+0.4	0.7
	GVH	0.3	1.9	2.7+0.09	0.7
49	NF$_1$	1.1	1.2	72.8+2.3	2.1
	GVH	0.2	0.2	4.2+0.2	0.1

[1] NF$_1$ = Normal $B_6D_2F_1$ mice, GVH = $B_6D_2F_1$ mice experiencing a GVH reaction.

[2] Mean of triplicate cultures. Standard errors are shown for days 6,7,11 and Con A responses for days 19 and 49.

[3] Optimum concentration of PHA, Con A and LPS were used which were 1.25 µg, 1.25 µg and 10 µg per ml respectively.

a GVH reaction developed a significant response to LPS by day 6 post GVH induction, which remained elevated until day 11 and returned to control values by day 19. The responses to both PHA and Con A were also elevated during the 6 to 11 day period post GVH induction. There was no significant thymic atrophy prior to day 12–15 in this combination. It can also be seen in Tab.2 that thymus cells from late GVH (days 19 and 49 post GVH induction) not only failed to respond to PHA and LPS but also displayed a markedly reduced Con A response when compared with normal F_1 mice.

Tab.3 shows that neither the injection of syngeneic cells $(B_6D_2F_1)$ nor treatment with hydrocortisone caused a significant increase in the LPS response although hydrocortisone did increase the PHA and Con A responses of normal thymus cells.

TAB. 3:   Thymus cell response of $B_6D_2F_1$ mice to PHA, Con A and LPS following treatment with syngeneic cells or hydrocortisone.

Treatment	Mitogen response $(x\ 10^{-3})$[1]			
	No Mitogen	PHA[2]	Con A[2]	LPS[2]
No treatment	1.4	1.7	31.7	1.6
Syngeneic cells	0.6	0.8	12.3	0.4
Hydrocortisone[3]	1.8	12.1	52.3	2.3

[1] Mean of triplicate cultures. Standard errors are not shown but were always less than 10%.

[2] As for Tab.2.

[3] 2mg of hydrocortisone as administered intraperitoneally two days before sacrificing the animals.

DISCUSSION

The results confirm our earlier studies in which we showed that the GVH reaction induced a state of permanent immunosuppression (3-6). The early suppression of the PFC response appeared to be due to macrophage suppression of helper T-cell function (4). It was postulated that the permanent or late suppression was possibly due to thymic dysplasia, characterized by destruction of medullary epithelial cells and Hassall's corpuscles (6). However, the cause of the thymic lesions is not known.

In the present study we demonstrate a significant increase in the PHA, Con A and most notably the LPS mitogen responses from days 6 to 11 post GVH induction. The increased thymic mitogen responses occur at a time when the splenic responses to all three mitogens are suppressed (Lapp and Kirchner in preparation). The increased responsiveness of thymic cells to both T and B cell mitogens suggests that mature lymphocytes have entered the thymus. It therefore appears that during the course of the GVH reaction there is some damage to the barrier, which normally excludes the entry of mature lymphocytes from the circulation, and therefore permits mature lymphoid cells to enter the intra thymic environment.

At present we do not know the genetic origin (donor or F_1) of the mitogen responding cells in the thymus, however, if they are of donor origin and sensitized to F_1 antigens it is conceivable that they could be responsible, at least in part, for the initial injury as well as the thymic dysplasia seen in the GVH mice.

The increased LPS response cannot be due to simply the increased number of cells or to stress related phenomenon, since neither the injection of syngeneic cells, nor hydrocortisone increased the LPS responsiveness (Tab.3), although hydrocortisone did increase the PHA and Con A responses. There have been reports that B cells have been detected in the thymuses of NZB/NZW mice (8) and 8JL/J mice (9). These two strains display a progressive age related decrease in immunoresponsiveness. It is of interest that B cells appear in the thymus of GVH mice at the time when they first become immunosuppressed. Thus, the present results argue quite strongly for the entry of mature lymphoid cells into the thymus during the early course of the GVH reaction.

The change in the Con A responsiveness is also of interest in the present study. Initially there was an increase in the Con A response, however, in the later stages of the GVH reaction it was severely depressed to rear background levels. The development of Con A responsive cells in the normal thymus is thought to be under the influence of thymic humoral factors released from the epithelial cells of the thymic medulla (1). The absence of Con A responsive cells in the late GVH thymus is suggestive evidence that T cell maturation is blocked. This lack of Con A responsive cells coincides with the GVH induced disappearance of medullary epithelial cells and Hassall's corpuscles (6). Therefore, it seems quite possible that a lesion in the thymic epithelial cells could lead to a state of permanent immunosuppression, to at last T cell dependent responses, since T cell maturation would be arrested. The lack of normal T cells and/or normal thymic function might also affect B cell ontogeny (10). Such a defect in the thymus would thus lead to a permanent immunodeficiency and may provide insight into the etiology of some types of immunodeficiencies seen in man.

REFERENCES

1. Bach, J.F., Carnaud, C., Prog. Altergy. 21 (1976) 342.
2. Shortman, K., Brunner, K.T., Cerottini, J.C., J. Exp. Med. 135 (1972) 1375.
3. Lapp, W.S., Wechster, A., Kongshavn, P.A.L., Cell. Immunol. 11 (1974) 419.
4. Elie, R., Lapp, W.S., Cell. Immunol. 34 (1977) 38.
5. Treiber, W., Lapp, W.S., Cell. Immunol. 37 (1978) 118.
6. Seemayer, T.A., Lapp, W.S., Bolande, R.P., Amer. J. Pathol. 88 (1977) 119.
7. Kirchner, H., Muchmore, A.V., Chused, T.M., Holden, H.T., Herberman, R.B., J. Immunol. 114 (1975) 206.

8.   Greenspan, J.S., Gutman, G.A., Talal, M., Weisman, I.L., Sugai,
      S., Clin. Immun. Immunopath. 3 (1974) 32.
9.   Ben-Yaakov, M., Haran-Ghera, N., Nature 255 (1975) 64.
10.   Sherr, D.H., Szewczuk, M.R., Siskind, G.W., J. Exp. Med. 147
      (1978) 196.

ACKNOWLEDGEMENTS

This work was supported in part by a grant from the MRC of
Canada to W.S. Lapp. We thank Ms. Anita Goldbach for her excellent
technical assistance and Ms. Maria Trautner for her excellent
secretarial assistance.

THYMIC MICROENVIRONMENT CHANGES ASSOCIATED WITH GRAFT-VERSUS-HOST

IMMUNOSUPPRESSION

E.F. Potworowski[1], T.A. Seemayer[2], R.P. Bolande[2] and
W.S. Lapp[3]

[1]Immunology Research Center, Institut Armand-Frappier;
[2]Department of Pathology, Montreal Children's Hospital and
[3]Department of Physiology,
McGill University, Montreal, Quebec, Canada

It is now well established that a graft-versus-host (GvH)
reaction suppresses both cell-mediated and humoral immune responses
(1-4). Restoration experiments have further shown that early
suppression of the humoral immune response was due to inhibition of
T helper function (4-6), presumably brought about by an excess of
adherent cells (7,8). Suppressor activity of GvH spleens has also
been demonstrated by their ability to inhibit antibody production
when added to normal spleen cells (5, 9-12). This suppression,
however, could not be demonstrated after day 21 (12) in spite of the
fact that animals, once suppressed, remained so indefinitely (4,12).
Earlier studies showed that when syngeneic thymuses were transplanted
into animals undergoing a GvH reaction, the intensity of the reaction
was significantly decreased, resulting in a rapid death of the
animals (13). This suggests that the GvH reaction had provoked a
functional deficiency in the autologous thymus which was corrected
by the transplant of a normal thymus.

Two antigenically distinct thymus stromal fractions described
previously (14) were monitored throughout the present study: a
soluble thymic factor (STF) and an insoluble thymic fraction (ITF).
STF (MW $\simeq$ 3000) was shown to participate in T cell maturation by
imparting Thy-1 antigens on T cell precursors, by confering cortico-
resistance on thymocytes and by stimulating helper T function. ITF,
on the other hand, was shown to stimulate the migration of myeloid
precursor cells into the thymus (15). STF was localized within
thymic reticuloepithelial cell cytoplasm while ITF was found in the
membranes surrounding medullary blood vessels (16).

TAB. 1:   Mean Number of PFC x 10^3 per spleen.

DAYS POST-GvH	7	35
NORMAL MICE	120.5	118.5
GvH MICE	1.73	0.3

MATERIALS AND METHODS

The method used to induce GvH reactions was described previously
(6). It consisted essentially of injecting adult CBA x AF_1 mice
intravenously with 75 x 10^6 A strain spleen and lymph node cells.
Since A and CBA share the K region of the H-2 complex, the GvH
reaction induced was of the chronic type.

Plaque forming cells (PFC's) were assayed using a modification
of the technique of Cunningham and Szenberg (17,18). Sheep red
blood cells were used as the antigen.

Rabbit anti-STF and goat anti-ITF antisera used for immunofluorescence were prepared and rendered specific as described
previously (14,19). A double sandwich technique was used throughout
with rhodamine conjugated guinea-pig anti-goat immunoglobulin and
fluorescein-conjugated goat anti-rabbit immunoglobulin. The
staining intensity was graded from - (negative) to ++++ (strongly
positive).

The animals inoculated on day 0, were divided into three groups
and studied at sequential intervals from day 7 to day 71. The first
group was used for splenic PFC response, the second for light and
electron microscopy and the third for immunofluorescence with antibodies to STF and ITF.

RESULTS

PFC response

Immunosuppression was demonstrable in experimental animals at
day 7 and 35 post GvH reaction induction (Tab.1). These results
confirm previous studies which revealed that once animals become
immunodepressed following a GvH reaction, they do not recover their
ability to form PFC's or antibody to thymus-dependent antigens (4).

TAB. 2:   Reticuloepithelial cell staining with anti-STF.

DAYS POST-GvH	7	14	16	28	36	42	56	71
IMMUNOFLUORESCENCE STAINING INTENSITY	++++	++++	++	-	-	-	-	-

Histological observation

The principal histological features of the thymuses of animals undergoing a GvH reaction included a complete effacement of cortico-medullary demarcation, a gradual reduction with ultimate total disappearance of Hassall's corpuscles, and marked progressive lymphoid depletion.

At the ultrastructural level, the epithelial cells displayed some chromatin homogenization as well as areas of irregular chroma-tolysis. Emperiopolesis of epithelial cells by intact lymphocytes was also observed, although not commonly. Intact and injured epithelial cells contained degenerating, necrotic and/or partially lysed lymphocytes. Cytolysosomes, replete with lipid and electron dense membranous and granular debris were abundant. The progressive accumulation of intraepithelial cytoplasmic cellular fragments was a most striking and consistent observation. Mitochondria, struc-turally intact in the control animals, were rarified in appearance due to swelling, fragmentation, and partial loss of cristae.

Changes in STF and ITF

STF within reticuloepithelial cells of experimental mice stained as intensely as in controls on days 7 (Tab.2) and 14, although some disorganization in the staining pattern was evident on that day. On day 16, the staining intensity of the majority of reticuloepithelial cells was markedly reduced. On day 28, although rare identifiable cells displayed some fluorescence, the reaction was generally negative. From day 36 until the conclusion of the experiment, no reticuloepithelial cells were stained with anti-STF serum.

The staining by anti-ITF of perivascular medullary membranes remained generally strong throughout the experiment. The appearance of marked pericapillary fluorescence seemed to coincide with the light microscopic changes of thickening of perivascular medullary membranes. With the thickening of the perivascular membranes, it became progressively evident that these were often double, separated by a clearly definable space.

DISCUSSION

The principal changes in the thymus following the induction of GvH reaction are thymocyte depletion, perivascular membrane thickening and reticuloepithelial cell injury.

The changes observed in the perivascular basement membranes of the medulla cannot easily be interpreted. However, previous work has suggested that lymphoid traffic out of (and possibly into) the thymus occurs through the medullary blood vessels and that ITF injections in mice increase the influx into the thymus of prothymocytes of myeloid origin (14,15). It is therefore conceivable that modifications in the thymus cell traffic occur during the GvH reaction and that thickening of the perivascular membranes of medullary vessels affect this transit.

The marked decrease of STF-containing cells probably reflects a loss of thymic hormone which could be responsible for the permanent immunosuppression observed in animals undergoing chronic GvH, as postulated by Grushka and Lapp (13).

Since the thymic lesion produced by a GvH reaction mimics that seen in some human immunodeficiency conditions, it is possible that a GvH reaction might be responsible for the development of certain T-cell congenital deficiency states (20). If the reaction and deficiency are initiated in a fetus or infant, either by transplacental or postnatal transfusion of immunocompetent lymphocytes, thymic transplants in such a patient might have an adverse effect, by intensifying the pre-existing GvH reaction.

REFERENCES

1. Howard, J.G., Woodruff, M.F.A., Proc. Roy. Soc. 154 (1961) 532.
2. Lapp, W.S., Möller, G., Immunology 17 (1969) 339.
3. Möller, G., Immunology 20 (1971) 597.
4. Lapp, W.S., Wechsler, A., Kongshavn, P.A.L., Cell. Immunol. 11 (1974) 419.
5. Parthenais, E., Elie, R., Lapp, W.S., Cell. Immunol. 13 (1974) 164.
6. Elie, R., Lapp, W.S., Cell. Immunol. 21 (1976) 31.
7. Elie, R., Lapp, W.S., In: Immune recognition (A.S. Rosenthal, Ed.) p. 563, Academic Press, New York, (1975).
8. Lapp, W.S., Treiber, W., Elie, R., Transplant. Proc. 7 (1975) 393.
9. Sjoberg, O., Clin. Exp. Immunol. 12 (1972) 365.

10. Byfield, P., Christie, G.H., Howard, J.G., J. Immunol. 111 (1973) 72.
11. Lapp, W.S., Elie, R., Parthenais, E., In: Suppressor Cells in Immunity (S.K. Singhal, N.R. St. C. Sinclair, Eds.) p. 127, University of western Ontario, London, Ontario (1975).
12. Shand, F.L., Immunology 29 (1975) 953.
13. Grushka, M., Lapp, W.S., Transplantation 14 (1974) 157.
14. Potworowski, E.F., Fournier, M., Zollinger, L., Teodorczyk, J.A., Ann. Immunol. (Institut Pasteur) 128C (1977) 407.
15. Zollinger, L., Fournier, M., Potworowski, E.F., Rev. Can. Biol. 36 (1977) 245.
16. Potworowski, E.F., Clin. Exp. Immunol. 30 (1977) 305.
17. Cunningham, A.J., Szenberg, A., Immunology 14 (1968) 599.
18. Kongshavn, P.A.L., Lapp, W.S., Immunology 22 (1972) 227.
19. Potworowski, E.F., Borduas, A.G., Lussier, G., J. Immunol. 111 (1973) 1292.
20. Seemayer, T.A., Lapp, W.S., Bolande, R.P., Amer. J. Pathol. 88 (1977) 119.

ACKNOWLEDGEMENTS

This work was supported by the MRC and the National Cancer Institute of Canada.

LOCAL CELLULAR REACTIONS FOLLOWING INTRACUTANEOUS INJECTIONS OF

VARIOUS ADJUVANTS IN RATS AND GUINEA-PIGS

E.D. Wachsmuth

Research Department, Pharmaceuticals Division,

CIBA-GEIGY Limited, CH 4002 Basel, Switzerland

INTRODUCTION

Complete Freund's adjuvant (cFA), one of the most commonly used immunological adjuvants, consists of a water-in-oil emulsion containing mycobacteria and antigen (1,2). Replacement of the mycobacterial component of cFA with bacterial endotoxin (3,1), lipopolysaccharide (4) and muramyldipeptides (5) for instance, has been shown to enhance the immune response. Cell-mediated immune responses were only stimulated when the antigens were incorporated in the adjuvant mixtures (6). The question thus arises in what way reactions at the injection site contribute towards the immune response. One approach to this problem is to analyse the cells involved in the inflammatory reactions to different adjuvants. For this purpose it is preferable to inject the antigen intracutaneously, since this minimizes its diffusion and spread and permits the study of the inflammatory reaction in vivo.

METHODS

Male rats ($\sim$150 g) and guinea-pigs ($\sim$270 g) were given two single intracutaneous injections (0.05 ml) into two different sites of the back of one of the following adjuvant mixtures: 5 mg muramyldipeptide (N-acetyl-nor-muramyl-L-alanyl-D-isoglutamine) (MDP) in phosphate-buffered saline (PBS); complete Freund's adjuvant (cFA); incomplete Freund's adjuvant (iCF); iCF with 5 mg MDP (iCF + MDP); adjuvant 65 (A65); A65 with 5 mg MDP (A65 + MDP). A65 was prepared from 2 g monostearate, 10 g aracel 80 and 106 g peanut oil (7). Three weeks later, the injections were repeated at two different sites.

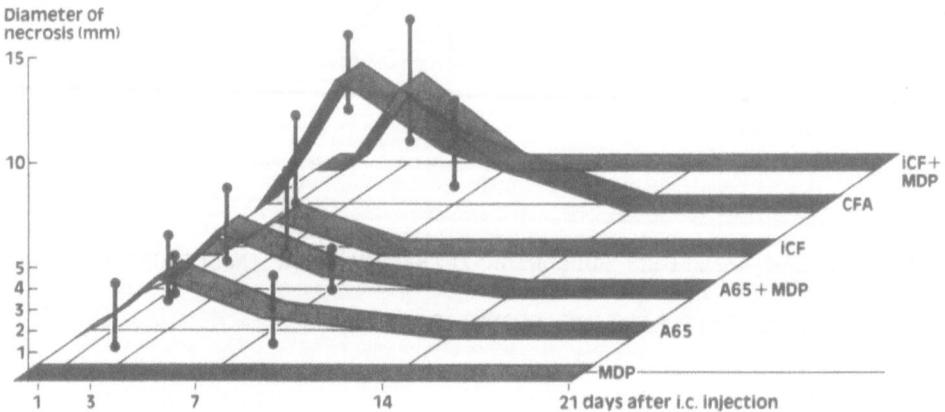

FIG. 1:   Development of necrosis in rat skin. The diameter of
necrosis after i.c. injection of different adjuvants was measured.
Mean values of at least 16 injection sites and their standard
deviations are given. Note the rather homogenous, fast and short-
lasting reaction compared with that seen in the guinea-pig (Fig.2).

The injection sites were observed over periods of up to six weeks
and examined grossly for changes in the diameter of erythema and
necrosis and microscopically for changes in cell composition and
tissue organization.

INFLAMMATORY RESPONSE IN RATS

Erythema developed rapidly after injection of the different
adjuvant preparations, with the exception of MDP + PBS, which gave
rise to necrosis (Fig.1) reaching its maximum after three days.
These effects vanished within two weeks in all cases. Three weeks
after the first injection, the animals were reinjected at a different
site on the back with the same adjuvant preparations as before. The
gross manifestations of the inflammatory reaction at the new site
followed the same course as had been observed after the first
injection. The first site remained unaffected.

The microscopical findings of granulocytic invasion and ulceration correlated with the macroscopic signs of necrosis (Fig.3). All
the adjuvants additionally provoked lymphocyte and monocyte infiltration, which was followed by the formation of epithelioid cells,
giant cells and granulomata in the corium and subcutis from the third
day onwards. The granulocyte infiltration observed after the injection of MDP, A65 and iCF was less marked and more transient than

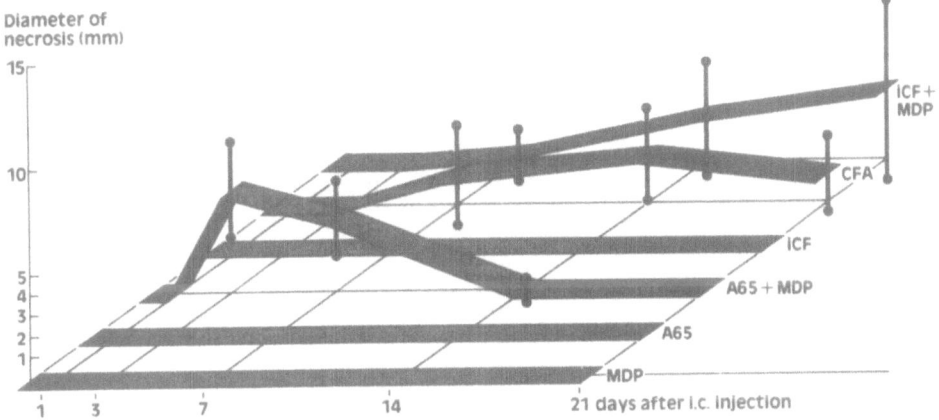

FIG. 2: Development of necrosis in guinea-pig skin. Treatment and
evaluation as in Fig.1. Note the large standard deviations for
values obtained with cFA and iCF + MDP due to some non-reactive
animals and the slow, delayed reaction compared with that of the rat
(Fig.1).

that induced by the other adjuvants. No epithelioid-cell development
was seen after MDP, but oedema was visible in the corium at the site
of injection, which was surrounded by some mononuclear cells and
granulocytes. In the epidermis at the site of the injection this
caused the development of subcorneal vesicles filled with granulocytes (Fig.3). As the reaction subsided, acanthosis was seen in all
cases. No signs of inflammation were observed 14 days after injection.
Nevertheless, the initial inflammatory reaction in the rat was extensive, and accordingly adjuvant deposits (oil droplets) were eliminated
rapidly.

INFLAMMATORY RESPONSE IN GUINEA-PIGS

In contrast to the findings in rats, the inflammatory responses
in guinea-pigs were slower and more persistent. Erythema developed
rapidly after the injection of all the adjuvant mixtures with the
exception of MDP in PBS. Subsequent necrosis only occurred after
A65 + MDP, iCF + MDP and cFA (Fig.2). The rate of development of
necrosis after the injection of A65 + MDP was fast, similar to that
seen in rats, whereas after cFA or iCF + MDP it was slow and persisted
three to five times longer than in rat. Upon challenge at another
site, the rate and extent of the reaction were similar to those
observed after the initial injection.

Microscopically, granulocytic invasion was seen in all cases.

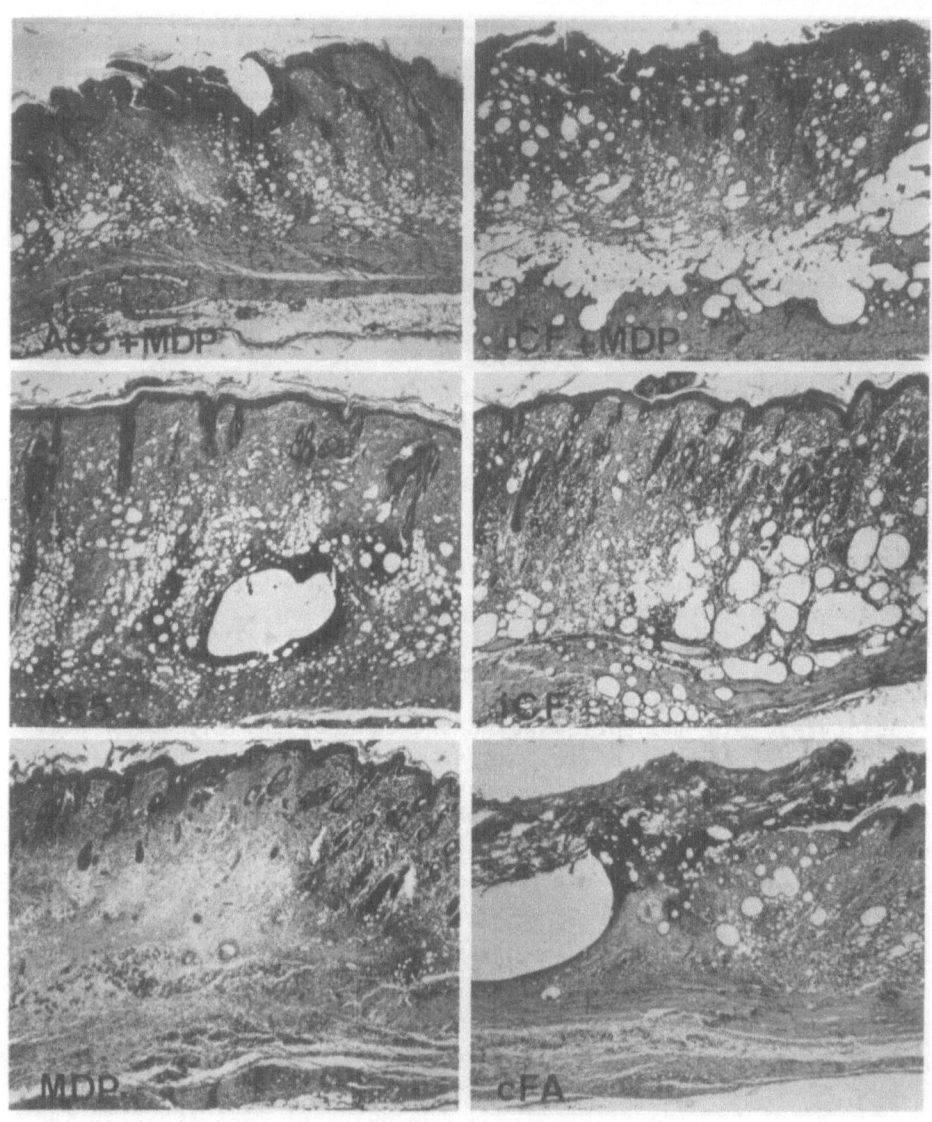

FIG. 3:   Acute inflammation in rat skin 3 days after i.c. injection
of different adjuvants. Note superficial subcorneal vesicles filled
with neutrophil granulocytes after MDP, extensive ulceration after
A65 + MDP, iCF + MDP and cFA. Mag. 21 x.

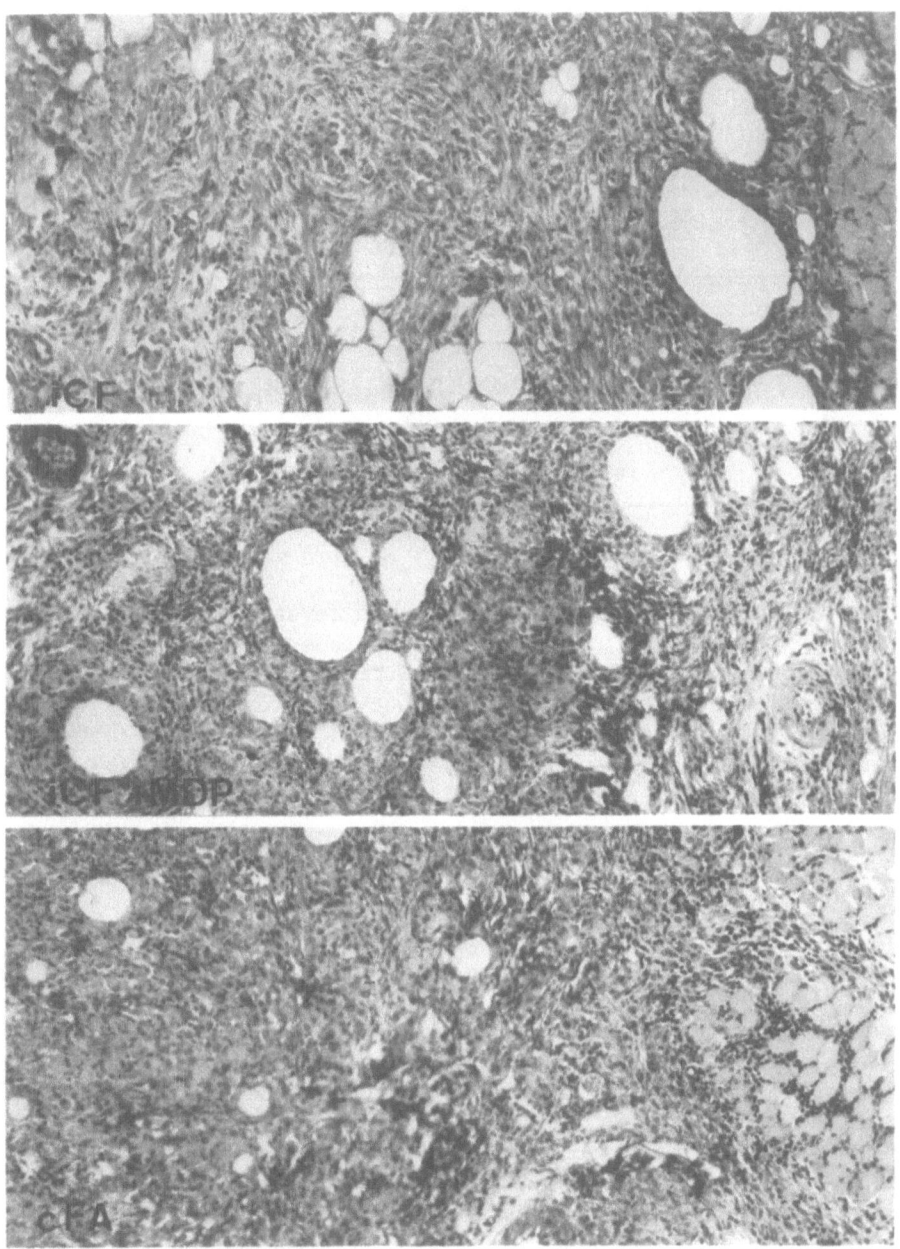

FIG. 4: Inflammatory reaction in guinea-pig skin 3 weeks after i.c. injection. On the right muscularis, on the left corium. Note epithelioid and giant cells and granuloma in all 3 samples. Granulocytes in the two bottom samples only surrounding granulomata and in muscularis. Mag. 120 x.

TAB. 1:   Effect of MDP on the cellular events of the local inflammatory reaction after intracutaneous injection in rats (R) and
guinea-pigs (G). Sections from animals injected with MDP in different media were compared with those injected with corresponding
media without MDP. Differences as observed over a period of 3
weeks after injection are given semiquantitatively.

		Granulocyte infiltration	Epithelioid-cell development	Granuloma formation	Ulceration
PBS	R	(+)	0	0	0
	G	+	+	(+)	0
A65	R	+	0	0	0
	G	+	0	0	+++
iCF	R	++	0	0	+
	G	+++	0	0	++

Infiltration persisted for not more than seven days after the injection of MDP in PBS or of A65 and for an even shorter time after
the injection of iCF (Fig.4). In addition, there was a more
persistent mononuclear cell and lymphocyte invasion, which was
followed by the development of epithelioid cells, giant cells and
granulomata, to increasingly greater extents after MDP, A65, A65 +
MDP, iCF, iCF + MDP and cFA, in that order.

                            EFFECT OF MDP

     The injection of MDP in PBS did not cause lasting erythema,
either in the rat or in the guinea-pig. However, granulocytes and
mononuclear cells were attracted to the injection site. This
resulted in an accumulation of granulocytes around the growing
oedema in the corium at the injection site and the development of
granulocyte filled (impetigo-like) subcorneal vesicles. In addition,
there was a moderate invasion by lymphocytes and monocytes which, in
guinea-pigs, was followed by some epithelioid-cell development.
Eventually fibroblast substitution took place. No ulceration
occurred. The reaction was more extensive and lasted longer in
guinea-pigs than in rats.

     Addition of MDP to either A65 or iCF augmented the extent of
the inflammatory reaction (Figs.1,2) elicited by the two oil bases
alone and provoked ulceration, mainly due to increased granulocyte
infiltration. However, the granulocyte-stimulating effect of MDP

was much more marked with iCF than with A65. Furthermore, in guinea-pigs it lasted longer with iCF than with A65. The results are summarized semiquantitatively in Table 1. As judged by cytological criteria, MDP substituted for mycobacteria in complete Freund's adjuvant in guinea-pigs and to a lesser extent in rats.

CONCLUSION

MDP has been successfully used as a substitute for mycobacteria in complete Freund's adjuvant for the stimulation of immune responses (7). In the local inflammatory reaction to intracutaneously injected incomplete Freund's adjuvant, the addition of MDP to the adjuvant base augumented granulocyte infiltration and led to a prolonged reaction similar to that elicited by complete Freund's adjuvant. On the other hand, MDP in adjuvant 65 or MDP in incomplete Freund's adjuvant augmented the extent of the local inflammatory reaction in guinea-pigs, but did not prolong the reaction time. While complete Freund's adjuvant or MDP in incomplete Freund's adjuvant effectively stimulate both cell-mediated and humoral immunity, MDP in adjuvant 65 increases only the humoral antibody response (8). If the generation of an immune response were dependent on an initial inflammatory reaction, then our observations would indicate that granulocytes play a more important role during the induction of immunity than has hitherto been believed. Moreover, persisting local inflammatory reactions and granulocyte infiltration might be prerequisites to the development of cell-mediated immunity.

REFERENCES

1.   Freund, J. Am. J. Clin. Pathol. 21 (1951) 645.
2.   Freund, J. Adv. Tubercul. Res. VII (1956) 130.
3.   Johnson, A.G., Gaines, S., Landy, M. J. Exp. Med. 103 (1956) 225.
4.   White, R.G. Ann. Rev. Microbiol. 30 (1976) 579.
5.   Ellouz, F., Adam, A., Ciorbaru, R., Lederer, E. Biochem. Biophys. Res. Comm. 59 (1974) 1317.
6.   Chase, M.S. J. Invest. Dermatol. 67 (1976) 136.
7.   Hilleman, M.R. Progr. Med. Virol. 8 (1966) 131.
8.   Dietrich, F.M., Gisler, R.H., personal communication.

ACKNOWLEDGEMENTS

The excellent technical assistance of Mr. H.P. Baum and M. Talmon-Gros is gratefully acknowledged.

SUMMING-UP

H. Fischer

Stübeweg 51

78 Freiburg-Zähringer, West Germany

As Dr. Dvorak has made it very clear in his introductory
remarks, a multitude of non-immune cells participate in immune
reactions in vivo. Although the complexity of their interaction
with immune cells is far from being understood, one is not permitted
to disregard their importance. Future attempts of comparative studies
must therefore try to close the gap between the simplified - and often
misleading - in vitro systems and the complex events in vivo.

Dvorak has added to the panel of well-known non-immune reactants
(granulocytes, easinophils, basophils, mast cells) the vascular lining
endothelial cells which are important in the later stages of immune
graft rejections, in tumor necrosis and in Shwartzman-like phenomena.
In other sessions of our Conference Dr. Lennert has repeatedly called
our attention to epithelioid cells,which due to their high metabolic
and secretory power might play a key role in a number of chronic
immune diseases. So, one of the messages and take home lessons of
this Congress is - at least for myself - to learn more about the
morphogenesis, the biochemistry and the regulatory role of these cells.

I will, however, from now on carefully avoid running into the
jungle of those cellular changes and reactions which accompany and
specify the later stages of immune responses. Instead, I will try
to focus on the question: What news have we heard about the importance
of non-immune cells during the initiation of immune responses.

Here of course, a few words have to be said first on the status
of the macrophage. While until recently the answer to the Gretchen-
question "Wie hältst Du's mit dem Macrophagen" made a clear distinction
between the scholars of intellectual and applied immunology, new data

have had a reconciliating effect: Since it has been discovered that macrophages carry on their membranes those products of the HLA-complex which decide whether antigen is recognized or not, tremendous efforts are being directed to the further clarification of this phenomonon. Macrophage receptors, maturation, and subpopulations have become a fascinating new branch of immunological research. A number of excellent monographs on these topics have recently been published (1,2).

We have heard today about the distinct morphology and function of marginal and dendritic macrophages in contributions by John Humphrey and J.G. Tew and collaborators. G.G. MacPherson and H.W. Steer have reported on the direct cannulation of lymphatics and appearance of macrophages which obviously have traversed the intestinal wall and are on their way to mesenteric lymph nodes. M. Schlaak and his colleagues from Kiel have demonstrated that vital human blood monocytes are needed for the mitogen-induced transformation of T and B lymphocytes and have opened the discussion on the sort of signals provided by the macrophage that are important for cell co-operation.

Now that the pendulum has swung and the immune aspects of macrophage function have been widely accepted, we should keep in mind that macrophages do not respond only to immunogens and therefore are not exclusively immune cells. They can be activated via numerous stimuli, some including phagocytosis, some not. Their potentiality of making use of different metabolic pathways, of secreting enzymes, complement components and a number of "monokines", not to forget the rapid synthesis and release of prostaglandins and endoperoxides, are expressions of their non-immune function and of their immune function as well.

It is obvious that both, immune and non-immune functions mutually influence each other when they are elicited in a local environment together. The macrophage really is the "Treffpunkt" where specific and non-specific events meet, and where they can be optimally studied!

We have heard about some promising new approaches towards this goal. So, as P. Tulkens pointed out, the flow and recycling of membranes in activated and non-activated cells may be entirely different; refined determinations of prostaglandins and endoperoxides have already provided us with new aspects of macrophage funtion and their regulatory role. I refer here to the interesting contribution of D. Gemsa, of E. Razin, and I. Wrogemann. And last, but not least, measurements of chemiluminescence might become a powerful tool to evaluate the role of free radicals in the co-operation between macrophages and lymphocytes during immune stimulation!

Now, with all these new aspects and techniques in mind let me come back to the original problem: the in vivo relevance of non-immune cells for immune stimulation. The classical observation of Ramon (3), which led to the discovery of the adjuvant effect, to my mind still represents the key for a more refined analysis. Ramon found that antigen injected into sites of inflammation elicits a much higher antibody response compared to injections into non-inflamed areas. Wachsmuth today has shown us how such an analysis can be initiated using morphometry and time sequence of cellular events. A close relationship between the course of local cell infiltration and the extent of cell mediated immunity as caused by various adjuvants could indeed be verified.

What is the molecular explanation for this correlation? At present one can vaguely assume that nutrients and factors from activated or degraded non-immune cells gain access to the draining lymphatics of lymph nodes. The report of Lydia Jarosková on de novo formation or hypertrophy of lymphatics, following immune stimulation (of the mouse omentum) is absolutely on line with this assumption. So, as a result of adjuvant application, a stream of nutrients and mediators will reach the lymph nodes together with the antigen.

In lymph nodes T and B lymphocytes are normally kept "silent", in a resting state. Their situation may be compared to the one of learned poor monks in a trappist cloister. They live under strict commandments (suppression?), their compartments are narrow and food supply is limited. The response to foreign messages will be poor and restricted, so long as the condition of a vita minima does not change. This change does, however, occur, when foreign messages, together with a stream of nutrients remove the environmental restriction, permit encounters, collaboration, "body building" and in later stages prolif- eration of lymphocytes. Perhaps germinal centers are privileged areas for the turning on of otherwise suppressed cells.

So, let me conclude: without non-specific material the lympho- cytes cannot respond to specific signals! This speculation, vague as it seems at first, is able to be tested: In recent publications an increasing number of observations report on in vitro maturation of lymphocytes (4,5) or acceleration of their response towards mitogen, following preincubation. Dr. Wrogemann's findings of accelerated chemiluminescence in preincubated thymocytes certainly are in accordance with this line of thought.

May I finish in saying that the facts presented in our session have given a true picture about our improved knowledge of the inter- action between non-immune and immune cells; they are to my mind most stimulating for the planning of future in vivo and in vitro experi- ments.

REFERENCES

1.   Role of Macrophages in the Immune Response. Immunol. Rev. 40 (1978).

2.   Symposion "Macrophage Functions in Immunity. Fed. Proc. 37
     (1978).
3.   Ramon, M.G. Compt. Rend. Acad. Sci. 181 (1925) 157.
4.   McCombs, C.C., Michalski, J.P., Talal, N. J. Immunol. 120
     (1978) 532.
5.   Wrogemann, K. et al.: this volume.

SESSION   A 5

SOLUBLE MEDIATORS OF IMMUNITY

CHAIRPERSONS:

J. David

A. de Weck

STUDIES ON MIF AND THE ROLE OF MACROPHAGE ASSOCIATED ESTERASES IN THE RESPONSE OF THE MACROPHAGE TO MIF

Heinz G. Remold, Alma D. Mednis and Philip L. McCarthy

Harvard Medical School and Robert B. Brigham Hospital

Boston, Massachusetts 02115, USA

It has been known for some time that "activated" macrophages obtained from immune animals have altered morphology and metabolism, and that they show enhanced capacities to deal with a number of microorganisms (1,2). A number of these studies have shown that the lymphocyte is involved in these activation processes (3,4). Their action can be partially explained by the production of soluble mediators such as macrophage activating factor (MAF) which increases the capacity of macrophages to kill bacteria and tumor cells (5,6). This factor cannot be distinguished from migration inhibitory factor (MIF) (7,8,9).

In the following, we will report new biochemical data on guinea pig MIF, and we will then turn to the problem of the interaction of MIF with the macrophage involving macrophage associated esterases.

These studies were carried out using casein- and oil-induced guinea pig peritoneal exudate cells. The mediators used were produced by incubating lymphocytes from sensitized guinea pigs with concanavalin A (Con A). The MIF-containing and control lymph node cell supernatants were prepurified on Sephadex G-100 columns and were then subjected to sucrose density gradient electrophoresis in a 0.2 M Tris acetate buffer, pH 8.6. The active fractions from this step were subjected to isoelectrofocussing in a sucrose density gradient from 0 to 47% sucrose and a pH gradient ranging from pH 2 to 6.2. The MIF-containing and control fractions from the isoelectro-focussing column were then filtered over a Sephadex G-75 column in the presence of bovine serum albumin (10). MIF was assayed in a capillary tube macrophage migration assay (11).

<u>Fractionation of Guinea Pig MIF into Two Different Species</u>:
MIF-containing and control lymph node cell supernatants were
partially purified by the methods described. The active fractions
from the sucrose density gradient electrophoresis were then
subjected to isoelectrofocussing. Two MIF fractions were recovered.
We called the one with an isoelectric point of 3.0-4.5 pH3-MIF, and
the one with an isoelectric point of 5.0-5.5 pH5-MIF (10).

In order to show whether pH3-MIF and pH5-MIF have also different
characteristics on Sephadex gel chromatography,both species were
filtered over Sephadex G-75. It could be shown that pH3-MIF elutes
with albumin (molecular weight 65,000), whereas pH5-MIF elutes
between chymotrypsinogen and ovalbumin (molecular weight of 25,000-
40,000) (10).

Thus, the two MIF species can be clearly separated on the basis
of their different isolectric points and their chromatographic
behavior on Sephadex G-75 columns.

In an attempt to correlate MIF activity with a specific protein
band, we incubated Con A stimulated lymph node cells in the presence
of ^{3}H-leucine, a method introduced by Sorg and Bloom (12). The
supernatants were then purified as described above. The purified
fractions were then tested for MIF activity, and another aliquot of
each fraction was subjected to SDS polyacrylamide slab gel electrophoresis (13) and was then autoradiographed (14). Under these
conditions, control lymphocytes did not produce any of the proteins
of interest. Autoradiography of the radiolabelled fractions from
the isoelectrofocussing columns revealed a number of radioactively
marked proteins. However, in the pH3-MIF region, only one band
having a molecular weight of 39,000 was common to the active
fractions. In the pH5-MIF regions, about 9 different proteins
could be discerned. We therefore fractionated the pH5-MIF fraction
with the highest amount of the activity on Sephadex G-75 columns.
When these fractions were electrophoresed and autoradiographed, it
was found that the fractions with MIF activity contained only one
band with a molecular weight of 39,000, whereas the other labelled
proteins lacked MIF activity. We do not know yet whether the
protein bands which correlate with the MIF activity are indeed MIF.

We reported earlier that crude MIF is a glycoprotein which is
neuraminidase sensitive and fractionates on cesium chloride density
gradients in fractions containing molecules denser than and with
the same density as albumin, a pure protein (15). These results
and the different isoelectric points of pH3-MIF and pH5-MIF indicate
that they might differ in their carbohydrate content. To investigate
this, we subjected pH3-MIF and pH5-MIF to cesium chloride density
centrifugation. In these experiments, pH3-MIF activity was found
exclusively in the dense part of the gradient, whereas pH5-MIF had

the density of albumin. The results suggest that pH3-MIF is a glycoprotein, whereas pH5-MIF has a density of a pure protein.

Modulation of the MIF by Pretreatment of the Macrophages with Esterase Inhibitors: Sometime ago, we showed that the effect of MIF on the macrophage can be enhanced if these cells are preincubated with diisopropylfluorophosphate (DEP) or other serine esterase inhibitors (16,17). A possible explanation for the enhancement would be the following hypothesis: Normally, a proteinase inactivates a certain amount of mediator reaching the cell. Blockage of this enzyme by an esterase inhibitor leads to an accumulation of MIF which manifests itself in an increased response of the macrophage to the mediator. This hypothesis could be tested when we found that guinea pig MIF can be fractionated into pH3-MIF and pH5-MIF. When we incubated pH3-MIF and pH5-MIF with macrophages and measured the remaining MIF activity, pH5-MIF was inactivated by incubation with macrophages and pretreatment with DFP of the macrophages prior to incubation with pH5-MIF abolished their ability to inactivate pH5-MIF (18). This finding is consistent with the action of a serine esterase(s) on the macrophage (pH5-MIF inactivator). When, on the other hand, pH3-MIF was incubated with macrophages, the activity was not abolished, indicating that pH3-MIF is resistant to treatment with macrophages. We then compared the specificity of the pH5-MIF inactivator on pH3-MIF and pH5-MIF with a number of proteinolytic enzymes such as trypsin, plasmin, thrombin, and chymotrypsin. Incubation of pH5-MIF with trypsin abolishes the activity of pH5-MIF, whereas pH3-MIF activity is unaltered. Trypsin thus resembles the pH5-inactivator in its specificity to MIF species. Thrombin and plasmin are proteinases with a narrower specificity and do not alter the activity of both MIF's. On the other hand, chymotrypsin inactivates both MIF's due to its broad specificity.

Our studies demonstrate a new regulatory component of the guinea pig macrophage, a serine esterase which activates pH5-MIF but not pH3-MIF. The macrophage, the target cell for MIF, participates in the regulation of the MIF concentration at the cell. Cell associated esterases have been involved in the control of several other biological processes, including the chemotaxis of polymorphonuclear leukocytes, the histamine release of mast cells and erythrophagocytosis (19,20, 21). It would be of interest to investigate whether the mechanism described here is a common regulatory step in hormone-effector cell interaction of other systems.

REFERENCES

1.   Lurie, M.B., In "Resistance to Tuberculosis: Experimental Studies in Native and Acquired Defensive Mechanisms", Harvard Univ. Press, Cambridge (1964).

2.   Mackaness, G.B., J. Exp. Med., 120 (1964) 105.
3.   Mackaness, G.B., J. Exp. Med., 135 (1972) 1104.
4.   Lane, F.C., Unanue, E.R., J. Exp. Med. 135 (1972) 1104.
5.   Piessens, W.F., Churchill, W.H., David, J.R., J. Immunol. 114 (1975) 293.
6.   Fowles, R.S., Fajardo, I.M., Leibowitch, J.L., David, J.R., J. Exp. Med. 138 (1973) 952.
7.   Bloom, B.R., Bennett, B., Science 153 (1966) 80.
8.   David, J.R., Proc. Natl. Acad. Sci., 56 (1966) 72.
9.   Nathan, C.F., Remold, H.G., David, J.R., J. Exp. Med. 137 (1973) 275.
10. Remold, H.G., Mednis, A.D., J. Immunol. 118 (1977) 2015.
11. Remold, H.G., Katz, A.B., Haber, E., David, J.R., Cell. Immunol., 1 (1970) 133.
12. Sorg, C., Bloom, B.R., J. Exp. Med. 137 (1973) 148.
13. Laemmli, U.K., Nature 227 (1970) 680.
14. Bonner, W.M., Laskey, R.A., Eur. J. Biochem. 46 (1974) 83.
15. Remold, H.G., David, J.R., J. Immunol. 107 (1971) 1090.
16. Remold, H.G., J. Immunol. 112 (1974) 1571.
17. Remold, H.G., Rosenberg, R.D., J. Biol. Chem. 250 (1975) 6608.
18. Remold, H.G., Mednis, A.D., Fed. Proc. Abs. 37 (1978) 1590.
19. Ward, P.A., Becker, E.L., J. Exp. Med. 127 (1968) 693.
20. Becker, E.L., Austin, K.F., J. Exp. Med. 120 (1964) 491.
21. Pearlmann, D.S., Ward, P.A., Becker, E.L., J. Exp. Med. 130 (1969) 745.

ACKNOWLEDGEMENTS

Supported in part by USPHS Grant AI12110 and a Grant-in-Aid from the American Heart Association. Dr. Remold is the recipient of an Established Investigatorship from the American Heart Association.

CHEMICAL CHARACTERIZATION OF RADIOLABELED LYMPHOCYTE ACTIVATION PRODUCTS OF GUINEA PIG ASSOCIATED WITH MACROPHAGE MIGRATION INHIBITORY ACTIVITY (MIF)

W. Klinkert and C. Sorg

Department of Experimental Dermatology

University of Münster, West Germany

Lymphokines are products of activated lymphocytes which in minute quantities produce profound biological effects. Due to the small quantities their chemical characterization is tedious and usually has to rely on time consuming and poorly reproducible biological assay systems. In order to circumvent some of these problems Sorg and Bloom (1) developed a radioactive double labeling technique which allowed to detect those products of activated lymphocytes which were produced either de novo or in increased amounts. Among the many products three more prominent ones could be identified with a Mw 60.000 (a), 45.000 (b) and 30.000 (c) which had a very similar isoelectric point of 5.2. The molecule of Mw 45.000 designated as b could be associated with the biological activity of MIF. While these studies were in progress, Geczy et al. (2) succeeded in raising an antiserum in the rabbit against highly purified fractions containing MIF. The antiserum obtained displayed some striking biological effects in vivo and in vitro (3, 4,5). If injected locally or systemically the serum suppressed totally delayed type hypersensitive reactions in the guinea pig and the antibody if conjugated to a solid matrix specifically removed MIF activity from active supernatants. An analysis of the serological specificity (6) revealed that the serum reacted preferentially with three lymphocyte activation products of the Mw 60.000, 45.000 and 30.000 which all had the same isoelectric point of around 5.2.

In the following we will describe the purification and some further biochemical characteristics of these products of activated lymphocytes reacting with the anti-lymphokine serum. Supernatants from Concanavalin A (Con A) stimulated guinea pig lymph node cells

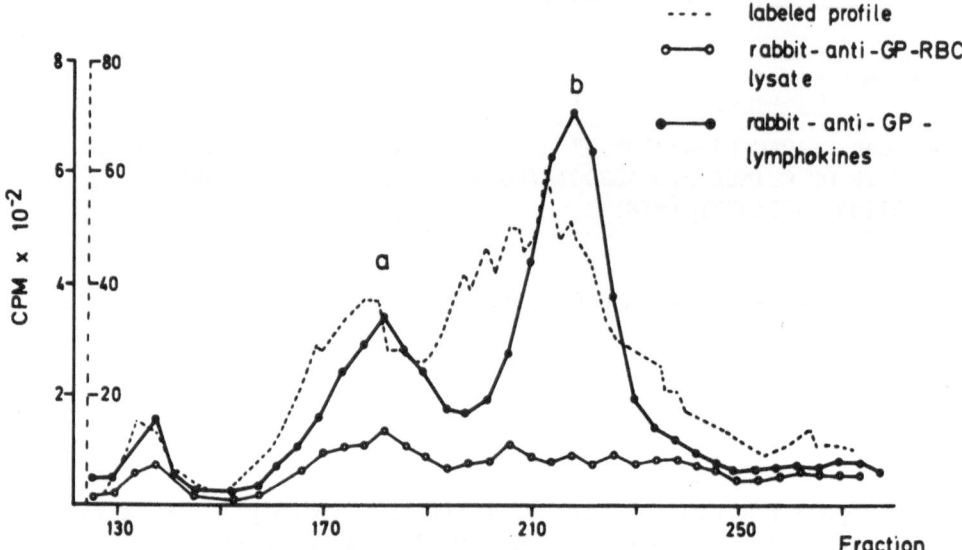

FIG. 1:   Rechromatography on Sephadex G 100 of pooled fractions from Sephadex G 75 chromatography (Mw-range 30.000 -70.000). Aliquots were reacted with anti-lymphokine serum or anti-guinea pig red blood cell lysate serum and immune precipitated.

were labeled with ^{3}H-leucine and chromatographed first on Sephadex G 75.   Pooled fractions of a Mw range from 70.000 - 30.000 were rechromatographed on Sephadex G 100.   Individual fractions were then assayed for binding material with the anti-lymphokine serum and an anti-guinea pig red blood cell lysate serum.   The anti-lymphokine serum specifically reacted with two distinct molecular entities with a molecular weight of 60.000 and 45.000 (Fig.1).   In this preparation molecules c had been cut off after the first chromatography on Sephadex G 75.

Material of G 100 fractions in the molecular weight range of a, b and c were subjected to isoelectric focusing in polyacrylamide gels containing a pH gradient of 3.5 - 10 (Fig.2).   Most material of a, b and c focused at pH 5.2.   This material was also found to

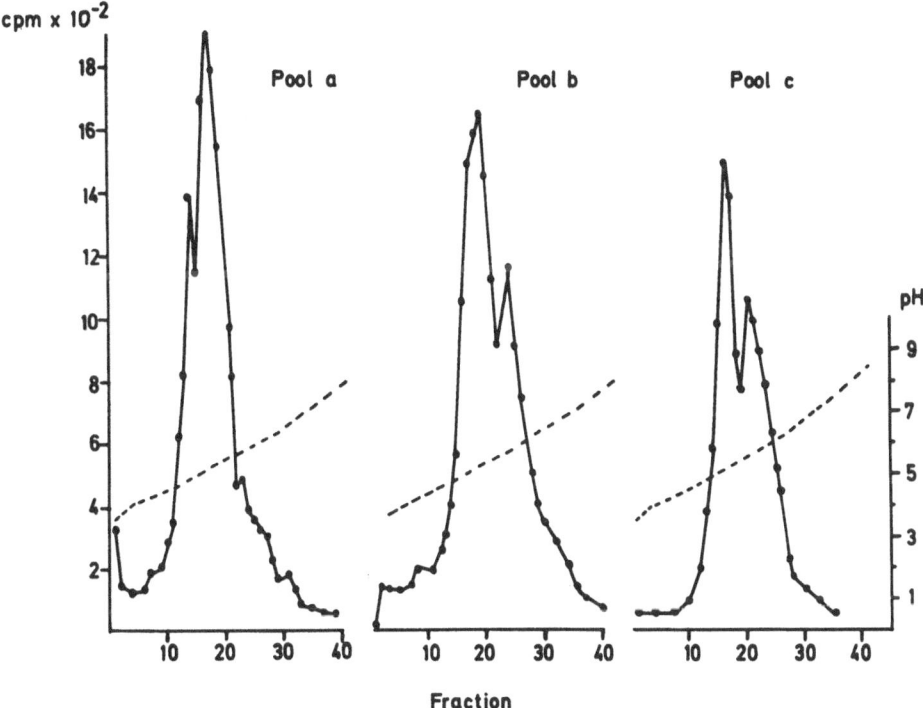

FIG. 2: Isoelectric focusing of pools of radiolabeled material after rechromatography on Sephadex G 100 (Mw a=60.000; b = 45.000; c = 30.000).

react specifically with the anti-lymphokine serum. When peak fractions at pH 5.2 were collected and assayed in the macrophage migration test, a, b and c contained significant inhibitory activity compared to identical fractions from non-stimulated lymphocyte culture supernatants which had been reconstituted with Con A before fractionation.

With the preparations a, b and c some further characterizations were performed. Since it has been suggested earlier that the migration inhibitory factor of guinea pig was a glycoprotein (7) radiolabeled a, b and c were subjected to isopycnic centrifugation in caesiumchloride gradients. It was found that all material concentrated at a density of 1.278 which was very similar to the density of radiolabeled albumine run in parallel. Since it had been reported that migration inhibitory activity was sensitive to neuraminidase treatment (7) a, b and c was also treated with neuraminidase from vibrio comma (cholerae). If focused before and after treatment no shift to an isoelectric point greater than 5.2 could be observed.

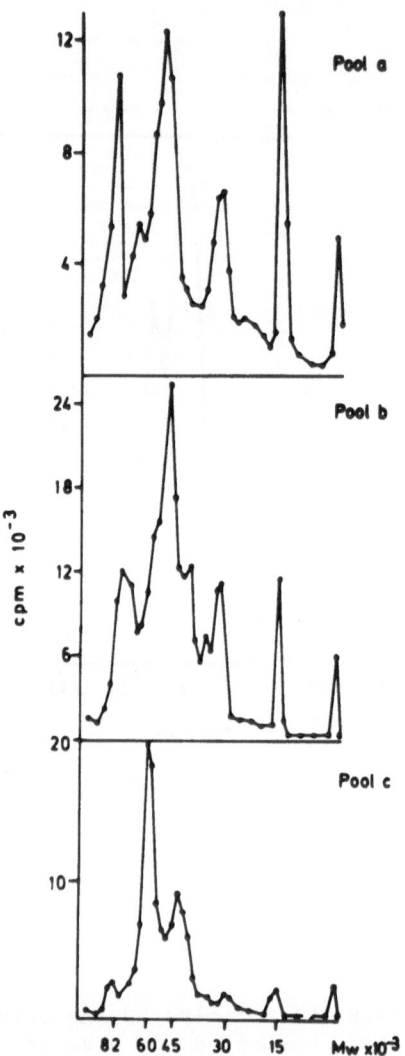

FIG. 3: SDS – PAGE (12.5%) of radiolabeled material of a, b and c
after rechromatography on Sephadex G 100 and isoelectric focusing
in presence of 8 molar urea.

However, in some preparations material with identical molecular
weight but a pI of 3.5 – 4.5 was found which after neuraminidase
treatment focused at pH 5.2 (Sorg and Geczy, submitted).

Since the three molecules were similar with respect to some
functional and biochemical properties, we thought about the possibility that they were composed of the same subunit structure. In
order to test this possibility the purified materials were treated
with 8 molar urea and fractionated on Disc-polyacrylamide gels

without SDS. All three preparations contained only high molecular
weight material. If aliquots from the same preparations were
treated with 8 molar urea, SDS and 2 - mercaptoethanol and then
analyzed in presence of these agents the profile did not change
either indicating that the molecules are not composed of non
convalently or disulfide linked subunits. The profiles in both
systems are very similar even though Disc-polyacrylamide gel electrophoresis separates for size and charge whereas SDS - polyacrylamide gel electrophoresis separates for size only. Pool c shows
high molecular weight material which is similar in charge and size
to that of pool a and b. The resistance to urea, SDS and 2 -
mercaptoethanol shows that these materials are not simply aggregates.
It rather appears that the material of pool c has the tendency to
polymerize. In Fig.3 this phenomenon is shown more clearly.
Different preparations of a, b and c were run on polyacrylamide gels
in presence of SDS and 8 molar urea. Compared to marker proteins
run in parallel gels the molecular weight of peaks in preparation
a, b and c were determined at 15.000, 30.000, 45.000, 60.000 and
82.000. It is remarkable that the preparation of pool c contained
a 60.000 molecule as the major component even though molecules of
this size had been removed before by repeated Sephadex chromatography. It is also remarkable that after purification steps

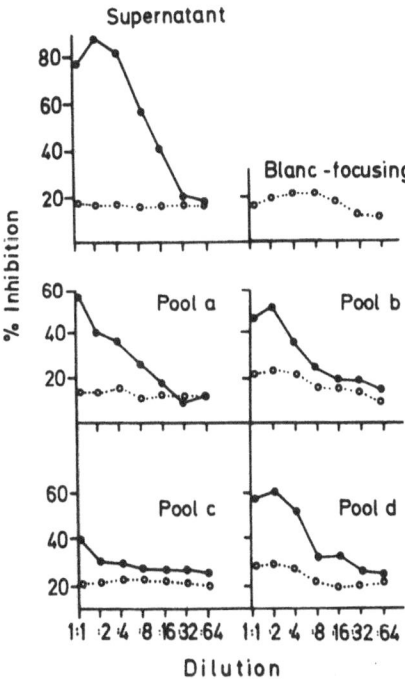

FIG. 4:   Migration inhibitory activity of MIF containing supernatant, purified a, b, c and d, analogue preparations from non-
stimulated control supernatants and a blank isoelectric focusing.

according to size and charge all preparations contained material
with the molecular weight of 15.000. In a systematic search it
was possible to detect the 15.000 molecular weight material in cell
lysates and in very low amounts in stimulated culture supernatants.
The isoelectric point of this molecule was determined at 5.2 which
is identical with the pI of a, b and c. The 15.000 Mw molecule
also reacts with the anti-lymphokine serum.

As can be seen from Fig.4 all four products of activated
lymphocytes show significant migration inhibitory activity compared
to identical preparations from control non-stimulated supernatants
and a blank isoelectric focusing. The analysis of the highly
purified a, b and c shows that each preparation contained material
with characteristics of the other preparations which should have
been removed by preceeding fractionation procedures. In order to
explain this phenomenon the best fit hypothesis would be that the
different molecules are oligomers of a common subunit of Mw 15.000
which has a pI 5.2. The generation of covalently linked oligomers
could be brought about either by an autocatalytic mechanism
suggesting that MIF itself is an enzyme or by contaminating enzymes.
While there are known examples for enzymes which can polymerize
proteins degradation to smaller oligomers could be explained by a
contaminating proteolytic enzyme. However, no such activity could
be detected in any of the three preparations. Even though a
possible structural relationship of the various molecular entities
needs further experimental proof, at this stage the conclusion
might be justified that migration inhibitory activity is not
associated with a single molecular entity but rather with a group
of molecules.

REFERENCES

1.   Sorg, C., Bloom, B., J. Exp. Med. 137 (1973) 148.
2.   Geczy, C.L., Friedrich, W., de Weck, A.L., Cell Immunol. 19
     (1975) 65.
3.   Geczy, C.L., Geczy, A.F., de Weck, A.L., J. Immunol. 117 (1976)
     1824.
4.   Geczy, C.L., Geczy, A.F., de Weck, A.L., J. Immunol. 117 (1976)
     66.
5.   Hentges, F., Geczy, C.L., Geczy, A.F., de Weck, A.L., Immunology
     32 (1977) 905.
6.   Sorg, C., Geczy, C.L., Eur. J. Immunol. 6 (1976) 688.
7.   Remold, H.G., David, J.R., J. Immunol. 107 (1971) 1090.

MURINE MIF DOES NOT CONTAIN Ia DETERMINANTS

Alice L. Kühner and John R. David

Harvard Medical School and Robert B. Brigham Hospital

Boston, MA., USA

In recent years, a number of soluble lymphocyte factors have been found to contain determinants encoded by genes within the I-region of the major histocompatibility complex (MHC) of the mouse. These factors, such as those described by Taussig (1), Tada (2), Kapp (3), and co-workers either enhance, support, or suppress various immune responses. Furthermore, they can generally be categorized as being antigen-specific in nature and also as displaying certain MHC restrictions in their action on cells of the immune system. In the studies reported here, the lymphokine murine MIF, (migration inhibitory factor), also a soluble lymphocyte mediator, has been investigated for the presence of I-region gene products, using anti-Ia immunoadsorbants. Murine MIF, in contrast to the above-mentioned factors, is not antigen-specific and does not display MHC restrictions in its action on cells of the immune system.

METHODS

Production of Murine MIF

MIF for these studies was produced by antigen-stimulation of lymph node (LN) cells. Briefly, B10.A mice were infected with 2 x 10^6 BCG organisms via footpad injection. Four to five weeks later, the axillary and inguinal LN were collected from these mice and single cell suspensions made. Lymphocyte cultures containing 24 x 10^6 cells/ml were incubated in enriched MEM containing 2% fetal calf serum, according to a method previously described (4). PPD, 20 µg/ml, was added to half of the cultures, while the other half served as the unstimulated control culture. After incubation for 72 hr at 37C the

supernatant fluids were collected and PPD was added to the unstimulated control supernate. The supernates were then dialyzed and
lyophilized in preparation for fractionation on Sephadex G-100
columns.

Murine MIF Assay System

MIF activity was measured using a capillary tube MIF assay, as
previously described (4). Peritoneal exudate cells from normal B10.A
mice, which had been induced by injection of 3.0 ml of Marcol oil I.P.
4 days before collection, were used as the indicator cells in the MIF
assay. A total of 6 capillaries was tested in each media, and the
percentage of inhibition was calculated by comparing the mean area of
migration of macrophages incubated in MIF-containing fractions, with
the mean area of migration of macrophages incubated in control
fractions.

Molecular Weight Determination

Lyophilized supernates from PPD-stimulated and control cultures
were re-dissolved in 0.01 M sodium phosphate-buffered saline, pH 7.4,
and chromatographed on Sephadex G-100 columns, according to a method
previously described. Following chromatography, the various fractions
were tested for MIF activity.

Polyacrylamide Gel Electrophoresis

MIF-containing and control Sephadex G-100 fractions were
subjected to discontinuous acrylamide gel electrophoresis at pH 8.9
for 2-3 hr according to the method previously described (4).

Immunoadsorption Procedure

MIF-containing and control Sephadex G-100 fractions equivalent
to 50 ml of original supernate were brought up to 2.0 ml in 0.2 M
NaKPO$_4$ buffer, pH 7.2, divided in half, and each portion incubated
in parallel with an excess of the appropriate immunoadsorbant for 1
hr at 4C with constant stirring. The following glutaraldehyde-
insolubilized antisera were used in this study: A.TH anti-A.TL which
contains antibodies directed against the products of the $\underline{I}^k$ region
(and reacts with the Ia molecules of B10.A mice), and (B10.D2n X AQR)-
F$_1$ anti-B10.T(6R) which is the control anti-Ia serum and contains
specificity for products of the $\underline{I}^q$ region. Normal mouse serum (NMS)
was used as the serum toxicity control throughout this study. These
sera were kindly donated by Drs. M. Dorf and B. Benacerraf. After
the incubation period, the insolubilized antisera were removed by

centrifugation, and the supernatant fluids dialyzed overnight, and tested in an MIF assay.

RESULTS AND DISCUSSION

MIF was produced by PPD-stimulation of lymphocytes obtained from BCG-sensitized mice. Following Sephadex G-100 column chromatography, MIF activity eluted in a broad band in Sephadex fractions II, III, and IV, corresponding to molecules having the molecular weight (MW) 134,000-48,000. Peak activity was found in fraction III, containing molecules with the MW 87,000-67,000. This MW distribution was found to be somewhat different than that previously reported for MIF produced by Con A-stimulation of spleen cells (4). While MIF produced both by spleen and LN cells elutes in the MW range 87,000-48,000, MIF activity in LN supernates was found in addition in fraction II, containing a higher MW range, 134,000-87,000. Since such a high MW MIF had not been found before, and since it had been shown that other things such as antigen-antibody complexes can also cause inhibition of migration (5), it was necessary to characterize this activity further.

All MIF-containing and control fractions were then subjected to discontinuous electrophoresis in polyacrylamide gels. The migratory behavior of MIF activity in Sephadex fraction II was compared with that found in the other MIF-containing fractions. It was found that the MIF activity in all of the fractions migrated to the same region, which was cathodal to albumin. This finding was in agreement with the electrophoretic mobility of MIF produced by spleen cells, which has been previously described (4). These findings indicate therefore, that the inhibition of migration seen in the high molecular weight fraction II was due to MIF activity.

Partially purified Sephadex fractions II, III, and IV containing MIF and their corresponding control fractions were then incubated with anti-Ia immunoadsorbants or with the control adsorbants. In 4 experiments, MIF activity remaining after incubation with the anti-Ia^k immunoadsorbant was compared with the activity found after incubation with the NMS control. In 1 experiment, MIF activity remaining after incubation with the anti-Ia^k immunoadsorbant was compared with the activity found after incubation with the anti-Ia^q control. No significant decrease in MIF activity was seen. The mean inhibition of migration following adsorption with the anti-Ia^k immunoadsorbant was 31%, while the mean inhibition of migration remaining in the controls was 34% (6).

At the present, no anti-murine MIF sera exists which could be prepared in the same manner as the immunoadsorbants and thus used as a positive control. There is indirect evidence, however, which strengthens our findings: these antisera had previously been shown to have a very strong specific cytotoxic activity before insolubilization, and the same antisera had also been used as immunoadsorbants to specifically adsorb 2 other soluble lymphocyte factors-allogeneic effect factor (7) and the antigen-specific suppressor factor of Tada (2). Considering this evidence, and the fact that MIF activity was not removed by this immunoadsorption procedure, these results suggest that MIF does not contain Ia determinants.

It appears then that perhaps MIF belongs to a different category of soluble lymphocyte factors than those that contain Ia determinants. Indeed, those factors that are Ia positive, generally have one or more of the following characteristics: (1) they display antigen-specificity in their action on cells of the immune system; (2) their activity shows certain H-2 restrictions; and (3) they are not easily obtained in soluble form, and extraction procedures are sometimes required. Whereas, using MIF as an example, it may be found later that Ia negative factors will show one or more of the following characteristics: (1) they do not display antigen-specificity in their action on cells of the immune system; (2) their activity is not H-2 restricted; and (3) they are easily obtained in soluble form from supernatant fluids of mitogen or antigen-stimulated lymphocytes. It will be interesting to see if, in the future, other lymphokines, which also share some of the same characteristics as MIF, are also Ia negative.

REFERENCES

1.   Taussig, M.J., Munro, A.J. In: Immune Recognition. A.S. Rosenthal (ed). Academic Press, New York (1975) p. 791.
2.   Taniguchi, M., Hayakawa, K., Tada, T. J. Immunol. 116 (1976) 542.
3.   Thèze, J., Kapp, J.A., Benacerraf, B. J. Exp. Med. 145 (1977) 839.
4.   Kühner, A.L., David, J.R. J. Immunol. 116 (1976) 140.
5.   David, J.R., David, R.A. In: Progress in Allergy, Vol. 16. P. Kallos, B.H. Waksman, A. de Weck (eds). Karger, Basel (1972) p.300.
6.   Kühner, A.L., Pisani, N., David, J.R. Manuscript in preparation (1978).
7.   Armerding, D., Sachs, D.H., Katz, D.H. J. Exp. Med. 140 (1974) 1717.

DIFFERENT CELLULAR SITE FOR THE PRODUCTION OF MURINE MACROPHAGE

MIGRATION INHIBITORY FACTOR AND IMMUNE INTERFERON (TYPE II)

Christine Neumann and C. Sorg

Department of Experimental Dermatology

University of Münster, W. Germany

Macrophage migration inhibitory factor (MIF) and interferon (IF) belong to the biological activities found in lymphocyte cultures upon stimulation with antigen or mitogen (1,2). Further, both mediators were found to appear simultaneously in the serum of mice which had been immunized with BCG (3,4). As they could not be separated on a molecular weight basis, it was concluded that both activities might be two different functions of the same molecule.

Interferons are defined by their potent anti-viral activity which renders cells unresponsive to virus replication. The IF which is produced by cells of the immune system is called "immune interferon" or "Type II interferon". Recently IF has evoked considerable interest because of a possible role in immune regulation.

In a previous report we gave evidence that macrophages stimulated in vitro by T cell products can produce IF which shares some properties with the immune – IF found in lymphocyte cultures (5). It was concluded that macrophages are a prime source for IF in an immunological situation. On the other hand, the role of T cells in MIF production is well established (6). It, therefore, was hypothesized that immune IF and MIF are derived from different cellular sources. Here, we present evidence that both activities can be dissociated by dissecting the cellular requirements for their in vitro production.

Thymus, lymph node and spleen cells were stimulated with Concanavalin A (Con A) by a pulse exposure method washing the lymphocytes several times after stimulation (7). After further

TAB. 1:   Production of mediators by Con-A stimulated lymphocytes of different compartments.

		unfractionated	
	spleen	lymph node	thymus
migration inhib. (percent)	78	75	56
interferon (units)	500	8	0
proliferation (stim. index)	5	28	265
macrophages (percent)	10	2	1

incubating 25 - 65 hr the supernatants were collected and tested for MIF and IF. The removal of Con A was an absolute prerequisite because Con A interferes with the macrophage migration inhibition assay. Monitoring for Con A was done by incubating stimulated cultures at $4^{o}C$ which does not allow MIF production to occur (7). In several experiments highly enriched T cells were prepared from spleen and lymph node by passage over adherence columns (5). Percentage of T cells, B cells and macrophages in the cell preparations were monitored by anti-theta serum, fluorescent anti-mouse globulin and unspecific esterase staining using α-naphthylacetate and α-napthylbutyrate as a substrate.

Results of mediator production by the different lymphocyte types were as follows (Tab.1). Spleen cells produced IF and MIF. Lymph node cells produced considerable amounts of MIF but only low or no IF. Thymus cells when cultured at high cell density (1 x 10^{7}/ ml) produced considerable MIF activity but no IF. The interferon activity produced by the different types of lymphocyte cultures correlated positively with the number of esterase positive cells.

Spleen cells which produced MIF and IF were depleted of macrophages and enriched for T cells by passage over adherence columns. The purified T cells had lost the capacity to produce IF while MIF production and blast transformation were retained (Tab.2). These results show that the cellular requirements for the production of IF and MIF upon mitogen stimulation are different. It also suggests that MIF is produced by highly purified T cells, while for the production of IF other than T cells play a crucial role. Together with our previous finding that the interferon response can be restored when bone marrow or spleen macrophages are added to unresponsive T cells it can be stated that there is absolute requirement for macrophages in the production of interferon by mitogen stimulated lymphocytes.

TAB. 2:   Production of mediators by Con-A stimulated T-lymphocytes.

	spleen – T	lymph node – T
migration inhib. (percent)	79	54
interferon (units)	8	0
proliferation (stim. index)	15	141
macrophages (percent)	1	1

The results shown in Fig.1 would allow the interpretation that macrophages can produce interferon upon immunologic stimulation. Macrophages grown from bone marrow or spleen could be activated to produce IF when exposed to supernatants from Con A stimulated spleen T lymphocytes which themselves did not contain IF. The peak production in macrophage cultures occurred at about 45 h. Macrophages could also be activated by pulse exposure to lymphocyte supernatant. The supernatants were removed after 6 or 15 h. The macrophages were washed and IF was found to be released after another 25 - 40 h culture. Presence of Con A in the supernatants had no marked effect nor had supernatants from unstimulated lymphocytes (not shown).

While in the above situation MIF but no IF was produced by T cells, in the following experiments a situation is described where IF but no MIF was produced by macrophages. IF containing supernatants from lymphokine activated bone marrow macrophages were tested for MIF activity and were usually found to be negative (Tab. 3A). Macrophages treated with conventional interferon inducers such as poly rI : rC and corynebacterium parvum (Tab.3B) secreted IF but no MIF into the culture medium.

Finally, the interferon activity in supernatants from stimulated lymphocytes containing IF and MIF was neutralized by an anti-interferon serum (kindly provided by Dr. I. Gresser). MIF activity however, was not reduced. It seemed unlikely that immune complexes were responsible for the persisting migration inhibitory activity, becuase no migration inhibition occurred when a fibroblast interferon was neutralized with the antiserum.

MIF and IF were produced by different cell types under the conditions described. Con A stimulated T cells had the capacity to produce high MIF activity whereas macrophages could be induced to release IF upon stimulation with T cell supernatants. Thus macrophages can be considered as candidates for the production of IF in the course of an immune response. MIF and IF seem to exert different

TAB. 3:

A.   Bone marrow macrophages induced with lymphocyte supernatants
      produce IF but no MIF

IF : 23 - 125 IU/ml	MIF : < 25% migration inhib.
7 of 8 experiments positive	7 of 8 experiments negative

B.   Bone marrow macrophages induced with conventional interferon
      inducers also produce IF but no MIF

IF : 47 - 188 IU/ml	MIF : < 25% migration inhib.
6 of 6 experiments positive	6 of 6 experiments negative

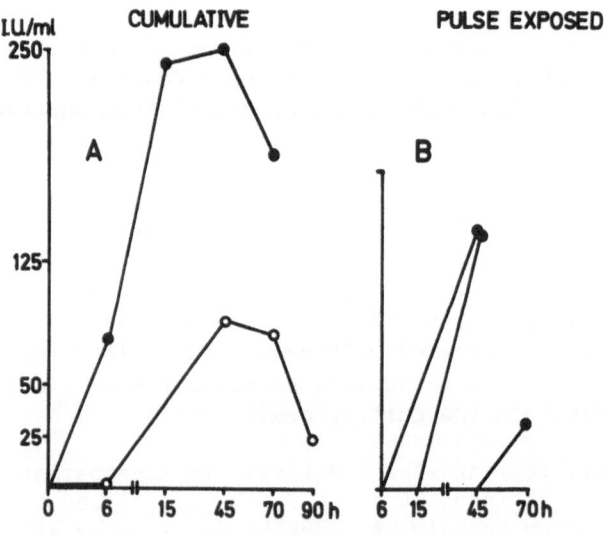

FIG. 1:   Interferon production in macrophage cultures induced by
lymphocyte supernatant.

Macrophages were cultured from bone marrow. Lymphocyte supernatants
derived from spleen T cells which had been stimulated with Con A for
25 h. Different symbols represent different experiments.

functions in an immune reaction. IF is thought to possess immunoregulatory functions mainly in the sense of mediating immune
suppressive effects (8,9). MIF on the other hand could not be
distinguished from macrophage activating factor sofar (10). Thus
it is conceivable that MIF primarily produced by T cells activates
macrophages to produce IF. Interferon in turn would counteract the
immune response in a regulatory suppressive way.

REFERENCES

1. Bloom, B.R., Adv. Immunol. 13 (1971) 101.
2. Wheelock, E.F., Science 149 (1965) 310.
3. Salvin, S.B., Younger, J.S., Lederer, W.H., Infect. Immun. 7 (1973) 68.
4. Younger, J.S., Salvin, S.B., J. Immunol. 111 (1973) 1914.
5. Neumann, Ch., Sorg, C., Eur. J. Immunol. 7 (1977) 719.
6. Morita, C., Soekawa, M., Poult. Sci. 51 (1972) 433.
7. Manheimer, S., Pick, E., Immunol. 24 (1973) 1027.
8. Brodeur, B.R., Merigan, T.C., J. Immunol. 114 (1975) 1323.
9. De Maeyer, E., De Maeyer – Guignard, J., Vandeputte, M., Proc. Nat. Acad. Sci. 72 (1975) 1753.
10. David, J.R., Fed. Proc. 34 (1975) 1730.

BIOCHEMICAL CHARACTERIZATION OF THE HUMAN LYMPHOKINE LEUKOCYTE
MIGRATION INHIBITORY FACTOR (LIF):   ROLE OF cGMP AS A SPECIFIC
INHIBITOR OF THE LIF ESTERASE ACTIVITY

K. Bendtzen

Laboratory of Clinical Immunology, Department of
Medicine TA, Rigshospitalet University Hospital,
Copenhagen, Denmark

Many phenomena associated with cell-mediated immunity are
believed to involve soluble lymphocyte products termed lymphokines
(7). These mediators are released by antigen- or mitogen-stimulated
T- and B-lymphocytes;   like hormones, they bind to membrane components
of inflammatory cells and induce a series of largely unknown intracellular reactions, which result in an altered state of reactivity
of the responder cells. Since lymphokines are produced in very small
amounts, they usually escape detection by conventional biochemical
techniques, and their characterization in molecular terms is as yet
quite incomplete (7).

One of the best characterized lymphokines is the human leukocyte
migration inhibitory factor (LIF), which is capable of reducing the
migration of polymorphonuclear leukocytes under agarose or out of
capillary tubes (7). LIF is relatively heat stable but highly
unstable when stored even at -20°C. It is a protein of MW 60,000,
and it is susceptible to the blocking effect of the irreversible
serine esterase and protease inhibitors phenylmethylsulfonyl fluoride
(PMSF) and diisopropylfluorophosphate (DFP) (1,3,12). The PMSF-
induced inactivation of LIF is dose-,time- and temperature-dependent
and hydrolyzed PMSF is ineffective in blocking the lymphokine.
Furthermore, the ability of arginine esters and amides to selectively
protect LIF against PMSF inactivation, and the fact that PMSF-
inactivated LIF regains full biological activity after treatment with
the nucleophilic agent, pralidoxime methansulfonate, confirm that LIF
belongs to a group of hydrolytic enzymes characterized by a reactive
serine in their catalytic centres (3-5).

Using a sensitive radioenzymatic assay, Rocklin & Rosenthal
recently demonstrated arginine-specific esterase activity in rather

crude LIF-rich supernatants (12). Unfortunately, this finding is of
doubtful significance in demonstrating esterolytic activity of LIF,
since supernatants of cultured lymphocytes, whether stimulated or
not, contain several other arginine-specific esterases (8).

We have pursued the characterization of LIF along two lines, an
indirect and a more direct one, to clarify the molecular biology of
LIF and, in particular, the putative role of cGMP as a modulator of
LIF.

COMPETITION EXPERIMENTS USING PMSF

The use of highly purified LIF preparations does not appear to
be necessary for competition experiments using the irreversible
serine esterase inhibitor, PMSF (4,5). In these types of experiments
various reagents are allowed to compete with PMSF for the reactive
site(s) on the LIF molecule. After a limited reaction period, the
agents are removed by dialysis, and residual LIF activity is tested
by bioassay. As already mentioned, arginine esters and amides
selectively counteract PMSF-induced blockade of LIF activity,
probably by preventing the inhibitor in gaining access to the
catalytic site of the lymphokine (4,5).

When testing a variety of synthetic esters for a similar effect,
we discovered that the phosphodiester, bis-p-nitrophenyl phosphate
but not various phosphomonoesters preserved LIF activity in the
presence of PMSF (4). Since this unexpected finding suggested a
selective affinity of LIF also for phosphodiesters, we proceeded by
testing the natural phosphodiesters, cGMP, cAMP, and a range of
other purine and pyrimidine derivatives. The results of some of
these experiments are summarized in Table 1. Only cGMP and, to a
lesser extent, 2',3'-cCMP were able to reduce the ability of PMSF
to inactivate LIF. The effect of cGMP was highly specific, since
minor differences in the position of the diester bond (2',3'-cGMP),
in the sugar residue (2'-deoxy-cGMP), or in the purine base (cAMP)
rendered the molecules ineffective. The ester also had to be a
cyclic phosphodiester, since the monoesters, 5'-GMP and GTP, and
the noncyclic phosphodiesters, guanylyl (3'-5') cytidine and cyti-
dylyl (3'-5') guanosine, were ineffective (Tab.1 and ref.9). The
protection afforded by 2',3'-cCMP was also specific, since the
cytidine monophosphates, 2'-CMP and 3'-CMP, and the parent nucleoside,
cytidine, were all inactive, as were esters of the pyrimidine base,
uracil (9).

As shown in Table 2, the relative rather than the absolute concentrations of cGMP and PMSF determined the degree of protection
afforded by cGMP. This response would be expected, if the nucleotide
competes with the inhibitor for the catalytic site of LIF, or if cGMP

TAB. 1:   Protective effect of cGMP and 2',3'-cCMP and PMSF-induced inactivation of LIF.

| Nucleotide | % loss of LIF activity after pulse treatment with | | |
	10^{-3}M PMSF	Nucleotide +10^{-3}M PMSF	P
10^{-3}M cGMP	58 + 17	3 + 8	<0.05
10^{-4}M cGMP	52 + 11	14 + 20	<0.05
10^{-5}M cGMP	50 + 11	33 + 21	ns
10^{-3}M 2',3'-cGMP	51 + 15	39 + 15	ns
10^{-3}M 2'-deoxy-cGMP	55 + 16	49 + 22	ns
10^{-3}M GTP	50 + 16	41 + 10	ns
10^{-3}M 5'-GMP	50 + 13	47 + 17	ns
10^{-3}M cAMP	52 + 15	49 + 18	ns
10^{-3}M 2',3'-cCMP	56 + 13	16 + 8	<0.05
10^{-4}M 2',3'-cCMP	49 + 13	42 + 16	ns

LIF activity was determined by bioassay using a leuckoyte migration agarose technique (6,9). The results are means ± 1 SD of four different experiments. P >0.05 was considered not significant (ns) (Mann-Whitney rank sum test).

TAB. 2:   Competitive nature of protection afforded by cGMP.

| (M) | % loss of LIF activity | |
	10^{-3}M PMSF	3 x 10^{-3}M PMSF
0	48 (43 to 53)	78 (69 to 89)
10^{-5}	21 (16 to 25)	
10^{-4}	3 (-4 to 14)	67 (42 to 79)
10^{-3}	8 (-2 to 14)	40 (29 to 50)
10^{-2}		12 (-14 to 32)

LIF activity was determined by bioassay. The results are means of three different experiments. Ranges in parentheses.

TAB. 3:   Inhibitory effect of cGMP and 2',3'-cCMP on LIF—mediated
esterolysis.

cGMP (M)	% loss of esterolytic activity [+]		2',3'-cCMP (M)	% loss of esterolytic activity [+]	
			10^{-3}	18 ± 7	(P $\angle 0.05$)
10^{-4}	34 ± 13	(P $\angle 0.05$)	10^{-4}	7 ± 11	(ns)
10^{-5}	23 ± 12	(P $\angle 0.05$)	10^{-5}	3 ± 9	(ns)
10^{-6}	18 ± 6	(P $\angle 0.05$)			
10^{-7}	15 ± 8	(P $\angle 0.05$)			
10^{-8}	7 ± 6	(ns)			

[+] Determined by radioenzymatic assay using tritiated tosyl arginine
methylester as substrate (8). The results are means of five different
experiments. P $\searrow$0.05 was considered not significant (ns) (Mann-
Whitney rank sum test).

binds to a subsite distinct from the catalytic centre, provided that
the attachment of cGMP induces an allosteric change in the LIF
molecule resulting in a decreased affinity for PMSF (11).

EFFECT OF cGMP ON THE
ESTEROLYTIC ACTIVITY OF PURIFIED LIF

To gain further insight into the putative regulatory role of
cGMP, we have recently attempted to purify LIF and to test directly
the LIF-mediated esterolysis, using a slight modification of a highly
sensitive radioenzymatic assay originally described by Roffman et al.
(13). To follow the effects of the purification procedures, the
supernatant serine esterases were specifically labeled with the active
site-directed inhibitor, ^{3}H-DFP. Most enzymes were removed by a
gentle three-step procedure, allowing more than 50% of the initial
LIF activity to be recovered. The steps were: 1) irreversible
blockade of contaminating histidine esterases by means of tosyl lysine
chloromethyl ketone (8), 2) Sephadex G-100 chromatography for removal
of unreacted inhibitor, and for fractionation of the proteins, and
3) immunosorption of the eluted LIF-rich fractions with Sepharose-
immobilized antibodies against protein contaminants of LIF-rich supernatants (2,8). The resulting esterase concentration was approximately
10^{-11}M, and the esterolytic activity corresponded to that of 0.3 ng
human thrombin per ml (both calculated on the basis of unconcentrated
supernatants) (8).

When radioenzymatic assay of purified LIF was carried out in
the presence of cGMP at concentrations down to 10^{-7}M, the rate of

TAB. 4:   Selective effect of cGMP on LIF-mediated esterolysis.

Nucleotide (10^{-4}M)	% loss of esterolytic activity [+]
cGMP	38 (32 to 45)
GTP	4 (0 to 10)
5'-GMP	-8 (-12 to -2)
cAMP	1 (-2 to 5)

[+] Determined by radioenzymatic assay. The results are means of three different experiments. Ranges in parentheses.

esterolysis was repeatedly reduced (Tab.3). Again, the inhibitory effect of cGMP was highly specific, since several related cyclic and noncyclic nucleotides were ineffective; an exception was 2',3'-cCMP that was slightly inhibitory but only at concentrations of 10^{-3}M (Tabs. 3 and 4).

Throughout these experiments supernatants of nonstimulated lymphocytes, devoid of LIF activity, were always processed and tested in parallel, and inhibitory effects of cGMP, 2',3'-cCMP, or any of the other nucleotides, were never encountered (data not shown).

The natural substrate(s) for LIF is unknown as is the biological significance of the cGMP-mediated modulation of LIF activity. Indeed, the exact biological role of LIF is uncertain, since the lymphokine may have effects on the leukocytes other than those involved strictly in cell migration. A likely intracellular mediator of such a variety of effects could be cGMP. Thus, LIF might initiate a series of consecutive biosynthetic reactions leading to an increase in cellular cGMP levels. This would provide an attractive mechanism by which LIF activity could be regulated. Many similar examples of end-product regulatory systems are known in biology (14).

Finally, since cGMP is thought to play a role in lymphocyte activation and proliferation (10), the possibility should be considered that LIF, a lymphocyte product whose biological activity is regulated by cGMP, might exercise important biological functions also in processes governing lymphocyte activation and gene expression.

REFERENCES

1.   Bendtzen, K.   Acta path. microbiol. scand. Sect. C. 84 (1976) 471.
2.   Bendtzen, K.   J. Immunol. Methods 13 (1976) 321.

3.   Bendtzen, K.   Scand. J. Immunol. 6 (1977) 125.
4.   Bendtzen, K.   Scand. J. Immunol. 6 (1977) 133.
5.   Bendtzen, K.   Scand. J. Immunol. 6 (1977) 1055.
6.   Bendtzen, K.   Scand. J. Immunol. 6 (1977) 1357.
7.   Bendtzen, K.   Allergy (1978) In the press.
8.   Bendtzen, K.   J. Clin. lab. Immunol. (1978) In the press.
9.   Bendtzen, K.   Scand. J. Immunol. (1978) In the press.
10.   Hadden, J.W., Johnson, E.M., Coffey, R.G., Johnson, L.D., in
      Rosenthal, A. (ed) Proc. IXth Leuk. Culture Conf., New York,
      Academic Press (1975) p. 359.
11.   Koshland, D.E.   The Enzymes 1 (1970) 341.
12.   Rocklin, R.E., Rosenthal, A.S.   J. Immunol. 119 (1977) 249.
13.   Roffman, S., Sanocka, U., Troll, W.   Anal. Biochem. 36 (1970)
      11.
14.   Stadtman, E.R.   The Enzymes 1 (1970) 397.

SOME CHARACTERISTICS OF THE ANTIGEN - DEPENDENT MIGRATION

INHIBITION FACTOR

J. Pekárek, J. Krejcí, L. Rozprimová and J. Svejcar

Institute of Sera and Vaccines, Praha, Czechoslovakia

INTRODUCTION

From the very first studies of the mediators of cellular hyper-sensitivity it has been known that in the interaction of hypersensi-tive lymphocytes with a specific antigen, in addition to mediators of pharmacological nature, also such mediators are released which possess an immunological activity, i.e. they are able to react specifically with the antigen. Apart from the transfer factor it was the so called antigen-dependent migration inhibition factor (MIF) first described in 1967 (1,2). Supernatant of lymphocytes cultured with a minute dose of specific antigen which had no migration inhibitory activity by itself became inhibitory, however, after further addition of specific antigen into the testing system. This activity was gradually proved in a whole number of antigen and different species. Later it was shown that the respective factor is able to influence macrophage behavior in such a way that these originally pharmacologically active but immuno-logically incompetent cells suddenly become able to react like immuno-logically competent ones. In contrast to lymphocytes of which only a restricted number can react with one antigen the macrophages when influenced by this antigen-dependent factor can react specifically both with more antigens and as the whole macrophage population. Instead of a few hypersensitive lymphocytes the organism can dispatch into the fight almost the whole population of pharmacologically active macro-phages which apart from their own digestive function acquire with the assistance of factors of lymphocyte origin the ability to react specifically with antigen.

In our previous papers (3,4) we have described some chemical pro-perties of the antigen dependent migration inhibiting factor (MIF). In this paper we are going to show the affinity of the substance to speci-fic antigen (to which it was produced) and the possibility to raise antibodies against it.

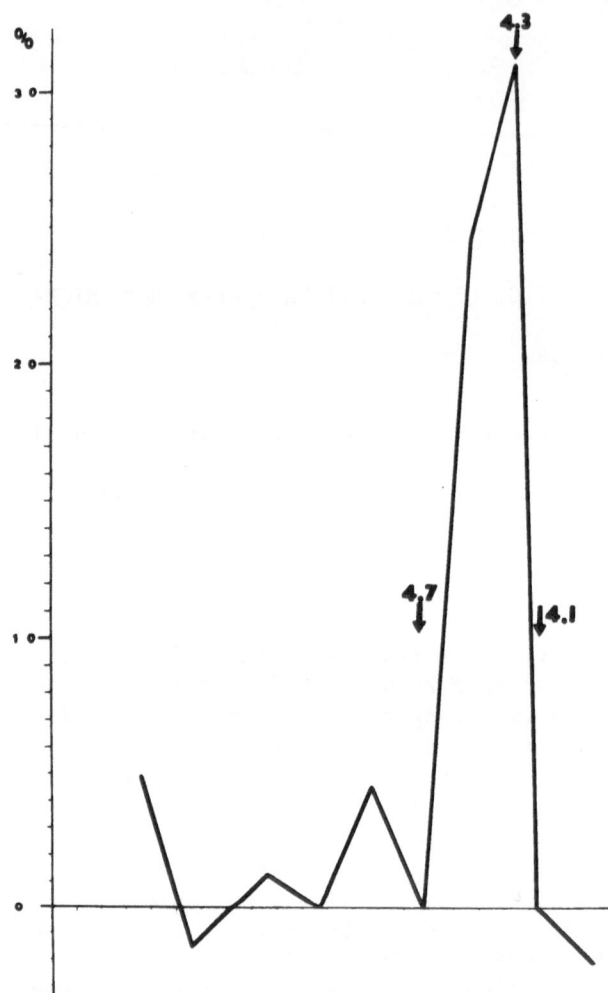

FIG. 1:   Migration inhibiting activity of the fractions eluted at
various pH from PPD - Sepharose column. Note: The arrows mark the
pH changes.

MATERIALS AND METHODS

Animals: C57Bl/6 mice were used as source of lymphocytes.
Chinchilla rabbits were used as donors of spleens for testing.
Pigs of 70 kg b.w. were used for immunization.

Preparation of the antigen-dependent MIF as well as the partial
purification on Amicon membranes were described in the previous
papers (3,4). Original supernatants and the respective fractions
were tested for migration inhibition of rabbit spleen explants by
the method described previously (4). Fifty μg PPD/ml of tested

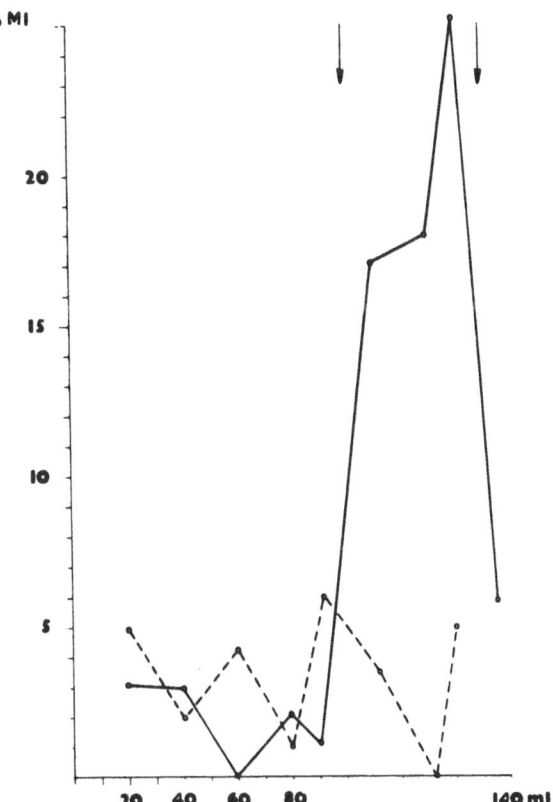

FIG. 2:   Migration inhibiting activity of the fractions eluted at
various pH from PPD - Biogel column. Note: the arrows mark the pH
changes.

sample was added to visualize antigen dependent migration inhibition
activity. Each fraction was reconstituted before testing by dialysis
against distilled water followed by dialysis against medium.

    Raising of antiserum: Two pigs were injected with 1.0 ml of
active Amicon fraction mixed with 1 : 6 ratio of Al-span-oil adjuvant.
Four of such injections were repeated in 14 days interval. Seven
days after the last booster the pigs were bled out and the antiserum
prepared. Gamma globulin fraction was prepared by the method using
caproic acid at pH 4.5 (5). Each antiserum was tested for its antibody content by IEP against whole mouse serum, whole active supernatant and active Amicon fraction.

    Preparation of immobilized PPD: PPD as antigen was bound both
to Sepharose 4 B and to Biogel P 100. Immobilization of PPD by means
of Sepharose was done according to the directions of the producer. The
immobilization by Biogel P 100 was performed by the method of Avrameas
(6).

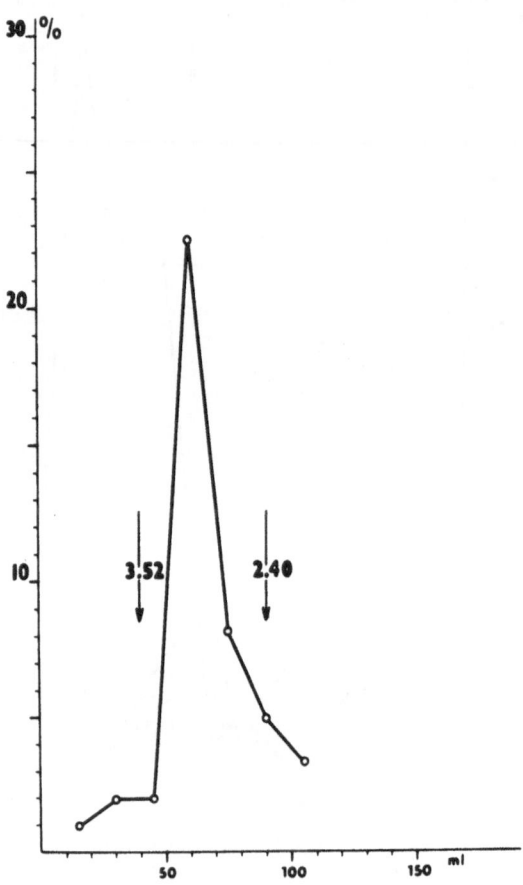

FIG. 3:   Migration inhibiting activity of the fractions eluted
from antiserum - Sepharose column at various pH values.   Note:
The arrows mark pH changes.

Chemicals and media: Powdered RPMI 1640 with glutamine
(Gibco, USA) fetal calf serum lyophilized (Gibco, USA), PPD tuberculin, powdered and liquid (mammalian PPD - Central Veterinary Labs.,
Weybridge, England).   Before use the PPD was dialysed for 24 hours
in the cold against saline to remove the preservative.   CNBr
activated Sepharose 4B (Pharmacia Uppsala, Sweden), Biogel P 100
(BIO-RAD LABS, USA),   ethanolamine (Lachema, Czechoslovakia),
rabbit anti mouse polyvalent serum (Boehringwerke, Marburg/Lahn,
BRD), Al-span-oil adjuvant (SEVAC, Czechoslovakia).

RESULTS

Supernatants containing antigen-dependent migration inhibitory activity were allowed to react with PPD immobilized on Sepharose 4B illustrated in Figure 1. The activity was completely retained on the column. Subsequently it was possible to elute the activity with acetate buffer pH 4.7. Further lowering of pH did not bring any additional activity. In view of the fact that Sepharose showed a certain degree of nonspecific adsorption, in further experiments Biogel P 100 was used which did not react nonspecifically. In this column with PPD, the activity could be bound and later released at pH 4.7, too (Fig. 2).

In further experiments the production of specific antisera was checked. The sample of results from affinity chromatography experiment using antiserum immunosorbent column is depicted in Figure 3. The activity was completely removed from the supernatant after the passage through the immunosorbent column and was recovered by elution with acetate buffer pH 3.5.

The active fractions of the immunosorbent column were analysed by means of IEP. Proteins contained in the eluate from the immunosorbent developed precipitation lines when reacted with the antiserum. The "in situ" absorption of the antiserum with fetal calf serum caused disappearance of those lines.

DISCUSSION

Previous experiments described elsewhere (3,4) have shown that antigen-dependent MIF is a relatively low molecular weight T cell product. This activity when bound to cell surface has specific affinity to antigen thus rendering the macrophages to slow their movement (7) and to phagocyte specifically the corpuscular antigen (8). In this paper we were able to demonstrate such affinity also to insoluble antigen and to show the immunogenicity of the factor by its ability to bind selectively to antibody. It remains to be found to what degree this factor is related to or even identical with the other antigen dependent factors. At the present time we know a lot of similar antigen dependent factors, e.g. macrophage arming factor (9), specific T and B cooperation factor (10), transfer factor (11), specific suppressor factor (12), receptors for antigen on lymphocytes, etc. Due to their ability to influence the reactivity of effector cells (macrophages) to the specific antigen they are believed to play a role in some important biological processes as e.g. in antitumor immunity, defense against various infections, induction of the immune response (cell cooperation) and its regulation (suppressor function). Some of them transfer passively the cellular hypersensitivity.

We have stated that some of these factors can be proved by a relatively simple migration inhibition test due to their ability to bound onto macrophages. Because of its simple nature this test also enables us a relatively simple control of various fractionation and isolation procedures. We are aware of the fact, however, that the biological significance of these factors is certainly broader than its mere ability to influence the migration ability of macrophages and that is why we have concentrated on it lately.

REFERENCES

1.   Bennett, B., Bloom, B.R.   Transplantation 5 (1967) 996.
2.   Svejcar, J., Johanovský, J., Pekárek, J.   Z. Immun. Forsch. 133 (1967) 259.
3.   Hochová, B., Krejcí, J., Pekárek, J., Svejcar, J., Johanovský, J.   Immunology 29 (1975) 321.
4.   Krejcí, J., Pekárek, J., Rozprimová, L., Svejcar, J., Johanovský, J.   Immunology 31 (1976) 283.
5.   Steinbach, M., Adran, R.   Arch Biochem. & Biophys.   134 (1969) 279.
6.   Weston, P.D., Avrameas, S.   Biochem. & Biophys. Res. Comm. 45 (1971) 1574.
7.   Svejcar, J., Pekárek, J., Johanovský, J.   Z. Immun. Forsch. 138 (1969) 342.
8.   Svejcar, J., Pekárek, J., Johanovský, J.   Experientia 28 (1972) 467.
9.   Evans, R., Grant, C.K., Cox, H., Steele, K., Alexander, P.   J. exp. Med. 136 (1972) 1318.
10. Munro, A.J., Taussig, M.J., Cambell, R., Williams, H., Lawson, Y.   J. exp. Med. 140 (1974) 1579.
11. Lawrence, H.S.   Adv. Immunol. 11 (1969) 195.
12. Zembala, M., Asherson, G.L., Mayhew, B., Krejcí, J.   Nature 253 (1975) 72.

A MEDIATOR ACTING AS A COSTIMULATOR FOR THE DEVELOPMENT OF

CYTOTOXIC RESPONSES IN VITRO

K.J. Lafferty, Hilary S. Warren and J.A. Woolnough

Department of Immunology, John Curtin School of Medical
Research, Australian National University, P.O. Box 334
Canberra City, A.C.T., Australia

INTRODUCTION

There is now evidence that alloantigen alone does not provide
a sufficient stimulus for lymphocyte activation (1,2). Cells killed
by any of a variety of means do not stimulate although they can be
shown to express antigen. Furthermore, not all viable cells can
stimulate. Antigen bearing non-lymphoid cells such as cultured
fibroblasts or erythrocytes will not stimulate allogeneic lymphocytes. We earlier proposed a model for allogeneic lymphocyte interactions in which the cell stimulating lymphocyte activation not only
provided a source of foreign antigen but also provided an inductive
signal for the responding cell. We summarize the evidence here that
this inductive signal which we call the lymphocyte costimulator can
be provided by the supernatant from Con A-activated spleen cells
(CS) and provide data on the species specificity of the costimulator
and the cellular requirements for the production of costimulator.

MATERIALS AND METHODS

Preparation of Con A-activated cell supernatant (CS): 10^8
CBA/H (H-2^k) spleen cells or cells as indicated were plated out in
10 mls of serum-free Eagles medium containing 0.1mM 2-mercaptoethanol
and 5 µg/ml Con A in 25 cm^2 surface area plastic culture flasks.
After 2 hrs at 37°, the cell monolayer which had formed was washed
to remove Con A, culture medium was re-added, and the cells incubated
for a further 16-18 hrs at 37° (3). The supernatant was concentrated
10-fold over a PM-10 Diaflo membrane, sterile filtered and stored at
-20°. Unless otherwise stated CS was used as a 5% addition in the
culture system.

497

TAB. 1:   The role of CS in T cell activation.

cell cultures	CS	cytotoxic activity $\log_{10}$ CU/culture
C57B1/6 LNC + γ-P815	–	5.4
C57B1/6 LNC + UV-P815	–	<2.5
C57B1/6 LNC + UV-P815	+	6.0
C57B1/6 LNC	+	<3.7

Cell cultures and cytotoxic assays: Cytotoxic responses were
generated in 1 ml cutures containing 10^6 C57B1/6 lymph node cells
(LNC) and 1.6 x 10^5 P815 which were either γ-irradiated (5000 r)
or UV-irradiated.   P815 was UV-irradiated in a suspension 1 mm deep
for 4 min with a 30-W germicidal lamp at an intensity of 960 uW/cm^2
in the 230 to 270 nm range.   Cytotoyic activity was measured after
5 days as described previously (4,5) and is expressed as cytotoxic
units (CU)/culture.

RESULTS AND DISCUSSION

Alloantigen alone does not induce cytotoxic T cell activation:
Tab.1 shows data obtained in an experiment designed to determine
the requirements for cytotoxic T cell activation in vitro.   Activation of C57B1/6 (H-2^b) lymph node cells to P815 (H-2^d) antigens
occurs when γ-irradiated P815 is used as the stimulating cell
population.   UV irradiation of the P815 tumour inactivates its
metabolic activity and renders the cell non-stimulating.   The
addition of CS to the cultures restores the response to antigens
carried by the UV-irradiated cell.   No detectable cytotoxicity for
the P815 tumour was generated when CS was added to cultures of
C57B1/6 lymph node cells alone.   From this data we can conclude that
transplantation antigen presented on the surface of the UV-irradiated
tumour is not a sufficient requirement for allogeneic lymphocyte
activation.   The results support our contention that specific T cell
activation is a two signal process requiring both antigen presentation to the lymphocyte and a second inductive stimulus (the lymphocyte costimulator) (1).   The inactivation of the stimulator capacity
of P815 cells by UV-irradiation can be attributed to the inactivation
of the metabolic function required for the production and or release
of the costimulator.

Requirement for CS during development of the allogeneic response:
Costimulator provided by the CS preparations must be present early

TAB. 2:   The requirement for CS during activation of C57B1/6 LNC
to UV-P815.

Period in days during which CS was present	0-5	1-5	2-5	3-5	0-3	not present
cytotoxic activity after 5 days $\log_{10}$ CU/culture	5.7	5.6	<3.7	<3.7	3.9	<3.7

TAB. 3:   Phylogenetic specificity of CS preparations.

Source of Responding Lymphocytes	Treatment of P815	$\log_{10}$C.U./culture with various CS Preparations					
		None	Mouse	Rat	G.Pig	Bovine	Human
Mouse L.N.	U.V.	<3.9	5.8	6.2	<3.9	<3.9	<3.9
Guinea Pig L.N.	γ-ray	<3.9	<3.7	NT	5.3	NT	NT
Bovine L.N.	γ-ray	<3.9	<3.9	NT	NT	4.7	NT
Human P.B.	γ-ray	<3.9	<3.9	NT	NT	NT	4.7
Mouse L.N.	γ-ray	5.5	NT	NT	NT	NT	NT
Rat L.N.	γ-ray	5.2	NT	NT	NT	NT	NT

NT = not tested   L.N.= lymph node   P.B. = peripheral blood

in the interaction between antigen and responsive T cells for a full
response to develop (Tab.2). Furthermore, CS must remain for the
entire culture period. If the cells were washed on day 3 and reconstituted in fresh medium the response was aborted. These findings
can be interpreted in two ways. There may be two activities in CS
preparations - an early acting costimulator and a late acting
maintenance or amplifier factor. Another possibility is that the
costimulator acts by interfering with an intrinsic 'switch off'
system that is operative in the lymphocyte. In such a case, removal
of the costimulator at any stage during the culture period would
abort the response.

Phylogenetic specificity of the costimulator: CS shows no
strain specificity for cytotoxic responses generated in the mouse
system. CS does however show phylogenetic specificty (Tab.3). Only
CS preparations from mouse and rat allowed the development of

TAB. 4:   Production of costimulator activity by spleen cells from normal and athymic (nude) mice.

Source of CS	cell equivalents of CS in 1 ml cultures	cytotoxic activity from cultures of C57Bl/6 LNC, UV-P815 and CS $\log_{10}$ CU/culture
CBA/H spleen	5×10^6 5×10^6	6.2 5.6
Nude spleen (mixed CBA/H, BALB/c background)	8×10^6 12×10^6 10×10^6	5.7 4.4 <3.7

TAB. 5:   Cellular requirements for costimulator production.

Nude spleen (BALB/c background)	nylon wool filtered T cells from BALB/c LNC	Cytotoxic activity generated in cultures of C57Bl/6 LNC, UV-P815 and 10% CS $\log_{10}$ CU/culture
10^8	0	<3.7
0	2×10^7	<3.7
10^8	1×10^6	<3.7
10^8	5×10^6	5.4
10^8	1×10^7	5.7
10^8	2×10^7	6.1

cytotoxic responses of mouse lymphocytes to the UV-irradiated mouse tumour. This phylogenetic restriction shown with CS preparations reflects that found with xenogeneic responses to the γ-irradiated mouse tumour. Only mouse and rat lymphocytes responded to the mouse tumour while lymphocytes from other species did not. In our model we postulated that the species specificity of lymphocyte activation was likely to reside in the species specificity of the costimulator (1). The above results support this postulate since xenogeneic responses do occur provided that the CS preparation is obtained from the same species as the responding lymphocytes (Tab.3).

Cellular requirements for costimulator production: Costimulator activity is present in CS preparations from normal spleen.
The amount of costimulator activity can vary between different
preparations and in Tab.4 is listed an upper and lower value from
the many preparations tested. Spleen cells from nude mice can also
produce costimulator activity but the amount produced in different
preparations is variable and in about one third of the preparations
was not detectable. When T cells purified by twice filtering over
nylon wool were added to nude spleen cells the amount of costimulator activity produced increased with increasing numbers of T cells
(Tab.5). The T cells alone did not produce detectable costimulator
activity. The data indicate that cells of the nude spleen can
produce low levels of costimulator following Con A-stimulation.
The level of costimulator production is greatly amplified by the
addition of syngeneic T cells to the nude spleen population
indicating that either T cells in the presence of nude spleen cells
are induced to produce a high level of costimulator or that these
cells modulate the level of costimulator production by a cell from
the nude spleen population.

REFERENCES

1. Lafferty, K.J., Cunningham, A.J., Aust. J. Exp. Biol. Med. Sci.
    53 (1975) 27.
2. Batchelor, J.R., Welsh, K.I., Burgos, H., Nature 273 (1978) 54.
3. Talmage, D.W., Woolnough, J.A., Hemmingsen, H., Lopez, L.,
    Lafferty, K.J., Proc. Natl. Acad. Sci. USA 74 (1977) 4610.
4. Lafferty, K.J., Bootes, A., Dart, G., Talmage, D.W., Trans-
    plantation 22 (1976) 138.
5. Warren, H.S., Woolnough, J.A., Denaro, C.P., Lafferty, K.J.,
    (1978) This volume.

COLONY STIMULATING ACTIVITY OF HUMAN SPLEEN CELL CULTURE SUPERNATANTS

H. Laukel, W.D. Gassel and K. Havemann

Department of Medicine, University of Marburg

Marburg, W. Germany

INTRODUCTION

It has been demonstrated by semisolid agar or methylcellulose culture systems (1,2) that proliferation and differentiation of myelopoietic progenitor cells (CFU_c) into mature granulocytes and monocytes depend on the continuous presence of specific humoral regulators of glycoprotein nature, given the operational term "colony stimulating factors" (CSF) or "colony stimulating activity" (CSA).

Mouse CFU_c inducing activities (CSA_m) are obtained from a variety of mouse and human tissues such as lung, liver, spleen, kidney and brain (3), from conditioned media of peripheral leucocytes (4) but also from human urine (5). Active material stimulating human CFU_c (CSA_h), however, has only been detected in human tissues and conditioned media (2,4,6-13), but not in human urine.

The CSA producing cells in human leucocyte cultures have been identified as monocytes (14) however, CSA may also be produced by stimulated lymphocytes (15). Great heterogeneity of CSA from human sources showing molecular weight from less than 1300 to 150,000 and stimulating either mouse and human or only human CFU_c has been reported (4,8,11,12,16). Our study had three aims: first, to find out a suitable way for mass production of CSA, which would more easily allow final characterization and purification of the factor(s), second, to compare CSA_h from different sources by molecular weight, and third, to check some purification procedures for their availability to separate the biological activities from the main protein impurities.

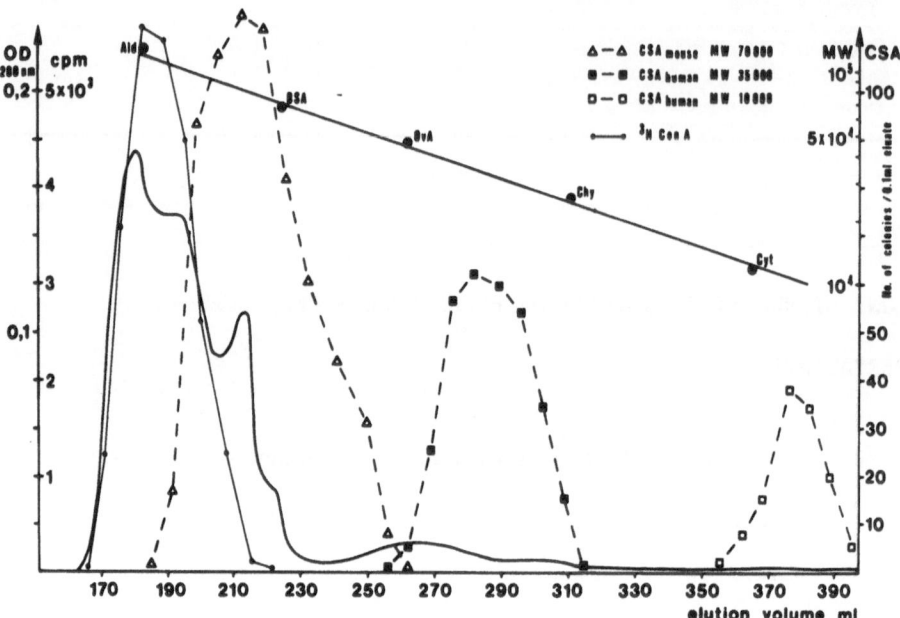

FIG. 1:   Protein-, activity- and Con A-elution profile of concentrated (100 ml to 2 ml) human spleen cell supernatant on Sephadex
G 100. Experimental data: bovine serum albumin (BSA), ovalbumin
(OvA), chymotrypsinogen (Chy) and cytochrome C (Cyt) served as
proteinmarkers, column 2.6 x 100 cm, buffer Earles's salts, flow
rate 17.5 ml/h.

MATERIALS AND METHODS

Assay Systems

Mouse bone marrow cultures in semisolid agar were done according
to Bradley and Metcalf (1), human bone marrow cultures were performed
according to Pike and Robinson (2).

Isolation of Cells and Preparation of Culture Supernatants

Pieces of human spleen were prepared to single cell suspensions.
Erythrocytes were removed by hypotonic shock, the remaining cells
were washed serumfree in Medium 199. Cultures (100 ml in Roux
bottles) containing 1×10^7 cells/ml in Medium 199 were stimulated
with 5-10 μg Concanavalin A (Con A)/ml and incubated for a period of
40-48 h at 37°C, in a humidified atmosphere containing 7.5% CO_2 in
air. Controls and experiments varying in doses of mitogen, number
of cells and time of incubation were done in 10 ml cultures. Cell
free supernatants were obtained by centrifugation at 3000 rpm for 20
minutes.

Ficoll mononuclear leucocytes (monu Le) and acute monocytic
leukaemia (AMoL) cells were used for Con A- and MLC-stimulated
cultures (monu Le only). Con A-stimulated culture conditions were
the same as those of spleen cell cultures. To carry out MLC-
stimulated cultures monu Le were adjusted to 3 x 10^6/ml/donor in
those cultures containing 2% AB serum and to 1 x 10^7 cells/ml/donor
in the serumfree cultures. Two-way MLC's (2 ml in plastic culture
vessels) in Medium 199 were incubated for a period of 72 h.

Chromatographic Techniques

All chromatographic procedures were performed as standard
techniques and have been described elsewhere (17,18).

RESULTS AND DISCUSSION

Yield of CSA_h from Different Human Sources

Cultures of Con A-stimulated spleen cells, Con A- and MLC-
stimulated monu Le and Con A-stimulated AMoL cells as well as the
appropriate unstimulated controls (conditioned media) were studied
for release of CSA_h. Except AMoL cells which already showed high
spontaneous production without further augmentation after stimulation,
all stimulated cultures revealed a marked increase of CSA generation
over control cultures. Under identical conditions stimulated spleen
cell cultures showed a significant higher yield (about 3 fold) than
stimulated cultures of monu Le. As the number of cells obtained
from one spleen was about 30 times higher than the yield of monu Le
from one blood pack, total amount of CSA produced by one spleen was
approximately 100 fold. The considerably higher yield from AMoL
cultures containing less than 5% lymphocytes compared with stimulated
monu Le and the accordance in molecular weight between the CSA from
different sources including AMoL (as below) suggests a monocyte
origin of CSA. The production of CSA in Con A- or MLC-stimulated
cultures of mononuclear cells might therefore be the result of
induction of lymphokines which then stimulate monocytes to release
CSA.

Optimal Conditions of Spleen Cell Cultures

In order to define the optimal conditions for spleen cell
cultures, incubation time, cell concentration and Con A doses were
varied. Using a constant cell concentration of 1 x 10^7/ml unstimulated cultures and cultures stimulated with Con A doses up to 1 μg/ml

FIGS. 2 - 4:   Protein- and activity-elution profile of concentrated (100 ml to 2 ml) human spleen cell supernatant on:

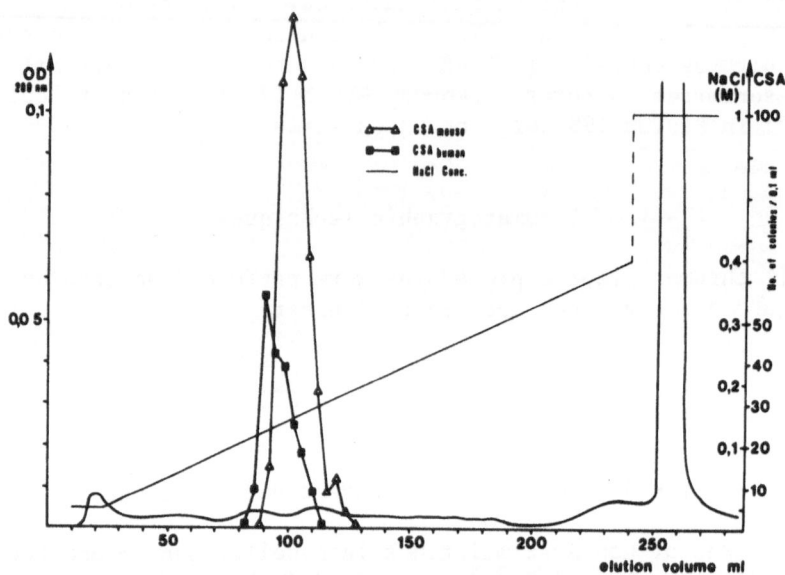

FIG. 2:   DEAE-cellulose. Experimental data: column 1.6 x 10 cm, gradient 0-0.4 M NaCl in Earle's salts followed by batch elution at 1 M NaCl, flow rate 20 ml/h.

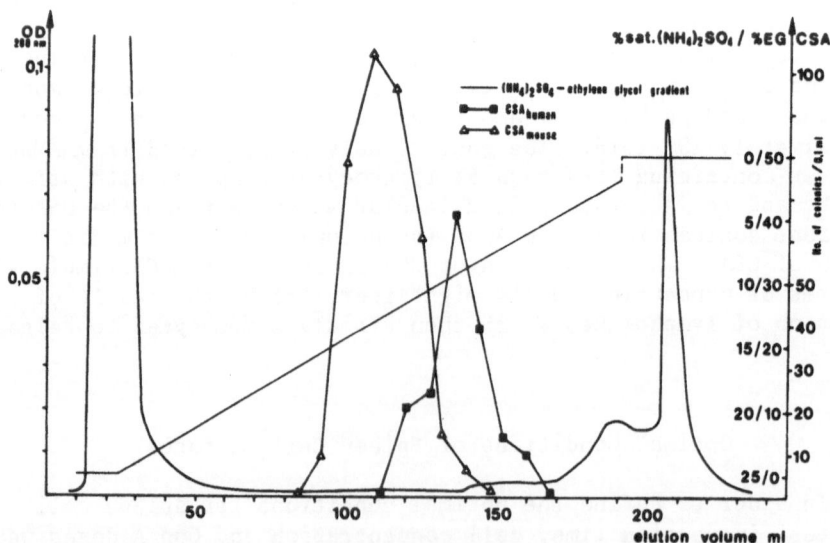

FIG. 3:   Phenylsepharose. Experimental data: column 1.6 x 10 cm, gradient decreasing ammonium sulphate (25% sat.-0) and increasing ethylene glycol (0-50%) in 0.01 M Na-phosphate buffer pH 7.0, flow rate 20 ml/h.

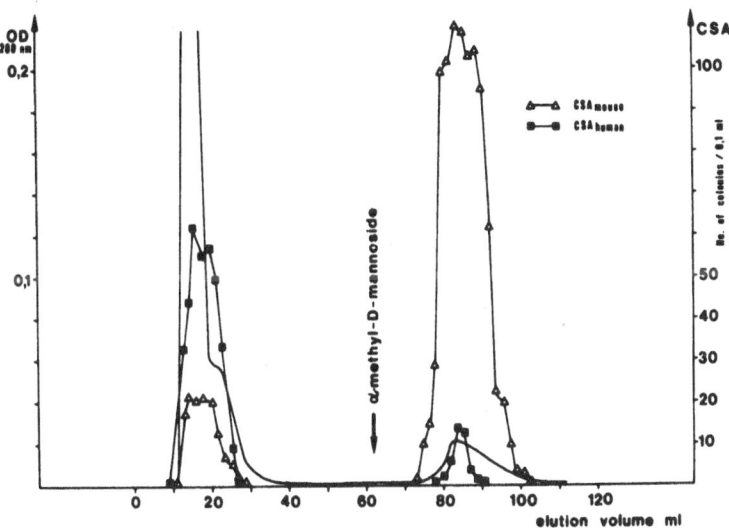

FIG. 4:   Con A-sepharose. Experimental data: column 1.6 x 10 cm,
elution buffer 0.15 M alpha-methyl-D-mannoside in Earle's salts,
flow rate 20 ml/h.

demonstrated only a slight increase of activity. Cultures stimulated with Con A doses between 5 and 50 μg, however, showed a marked
increase of CSA reaching a maximum between 40 and 48 h.   Cultures
containing only 5×10^6 or less cells/ml exhibited significantly
lower CSA levels.   Therefore cultures containing 1×10^7 cells and
5 μg Con A/ml incubated for 48 h were used for the following experiments.   Average yield of a culture from one spleen under these
conditions was about 3×10^{10} cells/spleen, 3000 ml supernatant and
$2.5-3 \times 10^6$ over-all induced colonies.

Characterization of Human Spleen Cell Derived CSA

Gelfiltration of concentrated spleen cell culture supernatants
(Fig.1) revealed three regions of activity with molecular weights
of 70,000, 35,000 and 10,000 daltons. Whereas the fraction with
MW 70,000 stimulated only mouse CFU_c, both other fractions were
active only on human bone marrow. These CSA, especially the human
activities, were separated from the main protein impurities by this
technique. In further experiments concentrated supernatants were
extensively dialyzed which resulted in an almost complete loss of
the MW 10,000 CSA_h. The dialyzed supernatants were then subjected
to different chromatographic procedures and tested for mouse and
human CSA. Both activities were eluted from DEAE cellulose at
0.12-0.19 M NaCl overlapping each other (Fig.2). A similar elution
profile was obtained applying hydrophobic interaction chromatography

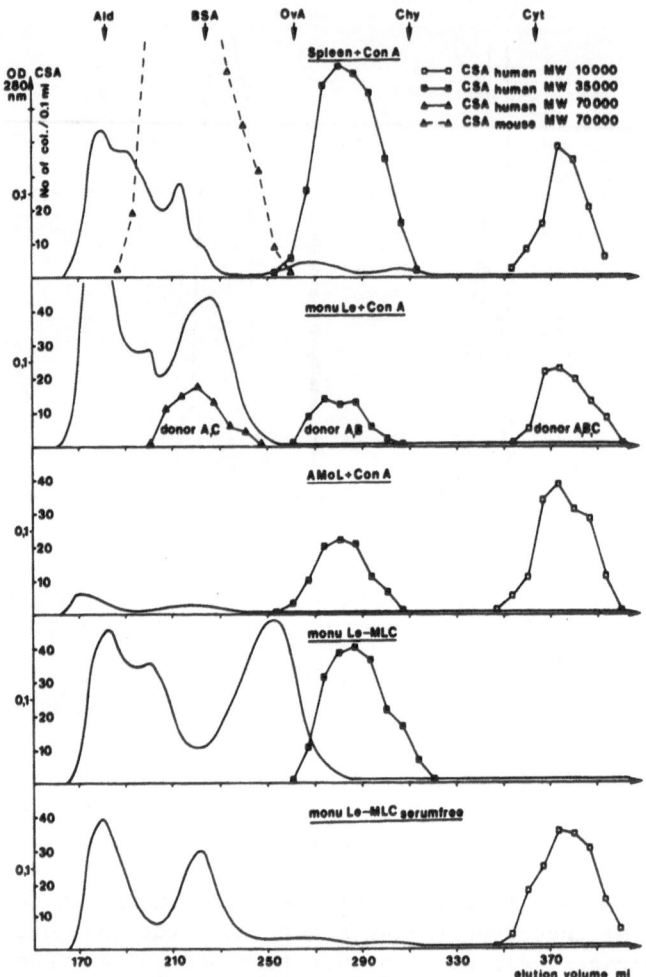

FIG. 5: Protein- and activity-elution profile of concentrated
(100 ml to 2 ml). Spleen cell supernatant (Spleen + Con A), Con A-
stimulated supernatants of mononuclear leucocytes (monu Le + Con A)
and acute monocytic leukaemia cells (AMoL + Con A) and MLC-stimulated
supernatants of mononuclear leucocytes incubated with (monu Le-MLC)
and without 2% AB serum (monu Le-MLC serumfree) on Sephadex G 100.
Experimental data: see Fig.1. In monu Le + Con A the individual
CSAs were only detectable in cultures from donor A, B or C.

on Phenylsepharose with a decreasing ammonium sulphate and an
increasing ethylene glycol gradient (Fig.3). Although both techniques
were not sufficient for separating mouse and human activities, they
were quite useful to remove more than 95% of accompanying proteins.
Con A Sepharose chromatography showed almost complete binding of
CSA_m, whereas the bulk of CSA_h passed the column (Fig.4).

Gelfiltration of Human CSA from Various Leucocyte Cultures

Concentrated culture supernatants of Con A-stimulated spleen cells, monu Le, AMoL-cells and MLC-stimulated monu Le (with and without serum) were subjected to Sephadex G 100 chromatography; the fractions were tested on mouse and human bone marrow (Fig.5). CSA_m could only be detected in Con A-stimulated spleen cell cultures. Although the presence of human activities varied in the different supernatants, they always eluted at 35,000 and/or 10,000 daltons; only the Con A-stimulated supernatants of monu Le showed an additional CSA_h with MW 70,000. The corresponding MW suggest identity between CSAs from different sources. The heterogeneity of CSA_h leads to the possibility that the different activities are monomeres (11,500) trimeres (35,000) and hexameres (70,000) of one active subunit.

Identity of Human Urinary CSA_m and CSA_m from Spleen Cell Cultures

Comparing spleen CSA_m and human urinary CSA_m by means of elution profiles in different chromatographic methods, including gelfiltration (G 100: MW 70,000), ionexchange chromatography (DEAE: eluted at 0.15 M NaCl) affinity chromatography (Con A-Seph.: 90% bound), hydrophobic interaction chromatography (Phenyl-Seph.: eluted at 13.5% saturated ammonium sulphate and 23% ethylene glycol) and isoelectric focussing (PH 4), complete identity was detected (17,18). In addition a monospecific antiserum against human urinary CSA completely inactivates human spleen cell derived CSA_m. This suggests that both activities are identical.

REFERENCES

1. Bradley, T.R., Metcalf, D., Aust. J. Exp. Biol. Med. Sci. 44 (1966) 287.
2. Pike, B.L., Robinson, W.A., J. Cell. Physiol. 76 (1970) 77.
3. Sheridan, J.W., Metcalf, D., J. Cell. Physiol. 81 (1973) 11.
4. Shah, R.G., Caporale, L.H., Moore, M.A.S., Blood 50 (1977) 811.
5. Robinson, W.A., Stanley, E.R., Metcalf, D., Blood 33 (1969) 396.
6. Chervenick, P.A., Boggs, D.R., Science 169 (1970) 691.
7. Iscove, N.N., Senn, J.S., Till, J.E., McCulloch, E.A., Blood 37 (1971) 1.
8. Price, G.B., Senn, J.S., McCulloch, E.A., Till, J.E., Biochem. J. 148 (1975) 209.
9. Paran, M., Sachs, L., Barak, Y, Resnitzky, P., Proc. Nat. Acad. Sci. US 67 (1970) 1542.
10. Brown, C.H. III., Carbone, P.P., J. Nat. Cancer Inst. 46 (1971) 989.

11. Burgess, A.W., Wilson, E.M.A., Metcalf, D., Blood 49 (1977) 573.
12. Fojo, S.S., Wu, M.C., Gross, M.A., Yunis, A.A., BBA 494 (1977) 92.
13. Gassel, W.D., Havemann, K., v. Manteuffel, G.E., Laukel, H., Exp. Hemat. 6 (1978) 391.
14. Chervenick, P.A., Lo Buglio, A.F., Science 178 (1972) 164.
15. Cline, M.J., Golde, D.W., Nature 248 (1974) 703.
16. Price, G.B., McCulloch, E.A., Till, J.E., Blood 42 (1973) 341.
17. Laukel,H., Gassel, W.D., Dosch, H.M., Schmidt, W., Havemann, K., J. Cell. Physiol 94 (1978) 21.
18. Laukel, H., Gassel, W.D., Havemann, K., in preparation.

DETECTION OF THYMOSIN IN THYMIC EPITHELIAL CELLS BY AN IMMUNOPER-OXIDASE METHOD

[1]J.G. van den Tweel, [1]C.R. Taylor, [2]J. McClure and [2]A.L. Goldstein

[1]Department of Pathology, Hematopathology Section, University of Southern California School of Medicin, Los Angeles, California 90033, USA

[2]Department of Biochemistry, University of Texas Medical Branch, Galveston, Texas, USA

INTRODUCTION

For some decades scientists have maintained the view that the thymus plays a crucial role in the development of the lymphocyte and the functioning of the immune system.

The classical thymic extirpation experiments pioneered by Comsa 1938 (1) and extended and reviewed by others provided confirmation of the importance of the thymus in the development of cell mediated immunity. Subsequent reconstitution experiments, particularly those utilizing thymic implants in millipore chambers for the prevention of post-thymectomy syndrome (2) led to the hypothesis that the thymus might exert its effect by the secretion of one or more hormone-like substances.

Several attempts have been made to isolate and define an active thymic hormone, and currently four main 'factors' have been defined by different groups of investigators :

1. Thymosin (3), 2. Thymic Humoral Factor (4), 3. Thymic Factor (5), and 4. Thymopoietin (6). Although the possible interrelation of these factors has still to be defined, they do appear to have biological activities in common (7).

The cellular origin of thymosin remains a matter of conjecture. The reticuloepithelial cells of the thymus have long been under

suspicion as the site of synthesis, for they do show electron microscopic features consistent with active protein synthesis (8), and an
active thymic factor can be demonstrated in the supernatant of
thymic epithelial cell cultures (9,10). Immunofluorescence methods
have provided some evidence in support of this contention, but the
interpretations of results have been confused by the poor morphology
and cellular resolution in immunofluorescence preparations, and by
uncertainty concerning the specificity of the antisera (11).

The present report describes the application of an immunoperoxidase technique in an attempt to determine the precise intracellular localization of thymosin within bovine thymus. The method
adopted has been used extensively by the authors for the demonstration
of a wide variety of intracellular antigens (12,13) in fixed embedded
tissues. The antisera used in this study were those prepared (J.M.
and A.G.) using thymosin extracted from bovine thymus.

MATERIALS AND METHODS

Fresh calf thymus was fixed either in buffered formalin or in
B-5 fixative and embedded in paraffin. Serial 5μ sections were cut,
deparaffinized, and examined for the presence of thymosin by the PAP
immunoperoxidase method (12,14) using anti-thymosin sera. This
method is a sensitive multistep procedure and depends upon the
addition of an excess of swine antiserum against rabbit immunoglobulin in order to link the primary anti-thymosin serum (raised in
rabbit) with the PAP reagent (an immune complex of horseradish
peroxidase and rabbit antibody to peroxidase) added subsequently.

Diaminobenzidine was employed as the chromogenic substrate for
the horseradish peroxidase label. This produces a permanent brown
color clearly visible by light microscopy in contrast to the blue
of the hematoxylin counterstain.

Six anti-thymosin antibodies were tested in this system. For
each antibody a checkerboard study was set up using increasing
serial dilutions (1/50 to 1/10,000) of antiserum applied to serial
sections of formalin and B-5 fixed bovine thymus. Bovine kidney
was used as a negative tissue control; in addition, the presence
of contrasting staining reactions of the different cell types
present within the thymus served as an intrinsic control in each
section.

Parallel sections of thymus and kidney were also treated with
normal rabbit serum and with rabbit antisera of irrelevant specificity (rabbit anti-human IgG, rabbit anti-human lysozyme) at dilutions
from 1/5 to 1/1,000 to control for the presence of naturally occurring
'anti-bovine epithelial cell' activity in any of the antisera used in
the immunoperoxidase system.

TAB. 1:

Antiserum	Thymic Eipthelial Cells[1]		Kidney Epithelial Cells[2]	
	Non-absorded	Absorbed	Non-absorbed	Absorbed
Anti-F_5				
1/50	++++	++++	+++	+
1/500	++++	++++	++	+
1/1000	++++	++++	+	±
1/5000	+++	++	−	−
Anti-F_6				
1/50	++++	+++	+	+
1/100	++++	++	+	±
1/500	+++	±	−	±

[1]   Similar staining was observed in epithelial cells of cortex and medulla, except that anti-F_6 (adsorbed) showed significantly less staining of cortical epithelial cells.

[2]   Scores represent patterns of staining in epithelial cells of collecting tubules and distal tubules. Glomeruli were always totally negative. In higher concentrations some staining of proximal tubular epithelial cells was observed, possibly reflecting re-absorption of thymosin from the glomerular filtrate.

RESULTS

The results of staining with each antiserum were assessed by two observers independently (CRT, JGvdT) and were scored on a semi-quantitative scale according to the intensity of staining of positive cells (Tab.1). In general the results obtained in B-5 fixed tissue were superior to those obtained following formalin fixation. Unabsorbed antisera against both fraction-5 and fraction-6 showed localized staining of thymic reticulo-epithelial cells, both in the cortex and in the medulla, at dilutions of antisera from 1/100 to 1/5,000. There was no staining of thymic lymphocytes, but a small number of mononuclear cells of uncertain type showed variable staining in all cases.

In the bovine kidney (negative tissue control) these antisera also showed positive reactivity against proximal and distal tubular epithelium at dilutions from 1/100 to 1/500 (anti F6) and 1/100 to 1/1500 (anti F5) beyond which the staining of the kidney cells disappeared, while the staining of thymic epithelial cells persisted to a dilution of 1/3000 (anti F6) and 1/5000 (anti F5). Using absorbed antisera to anti F5 and anti F6 (previously absorbed with

bovine kidney) a dramatic reduction in the staining in renal epithelium was observed. Staining was abolished in the distal   tubules
and greatly reduced in the proximal tubular cells, while staining
of thymic epithelial cells and Hassal's corpuscles persisted at
dilutions of 1/100 to 1/1000. The substitution of normal rabbit
anti-lysosome or anti-immunoglobulin anti-serum for the rabbit anti-
thymosin antibody (negative antibody control) showed no evidence of
staining of thymic epithelial cells (positive granulocytes were seen
with anti-lysosome, and occasional plasma cells were seen with anti-
immunoglobulin antibody).

DISCUSSION

These findings should be interpreted in relation of our assessment of the specificity of the antisera employed and the immunoperoxidase procedure used. Regarding the antisera, their specificity for
thymosin has been demonstrated in radioimmunoassay and in biological
systems and the immunizing antigens used in the preparation of these
antisera clearly appears to be thymosin. In the peroxidase procedures,
significant activity against bovine epithelial cells was detected with
all antisera, and resulted in labelling of epithelial cells of thymus
and kidney. Any specific staining for thymosin appeared to be masked
by this anti-epithelial cell antibody at least at the high concentrations of the antisera. Following absorptions of the antisera with
bovine kidney, the activity of the anti-epithelial cell antibody was
almost abolished as evidenced by the failure to stain distal tubules
of the kidney. Strong staining persisted in a proportion of thymic
epithelial cells, and in Hassall's corpuscles, and this is interpreted
as being indicative of the presence of thymosin within these cells.
This does not constitute the presence of in situ sythesis, but taken
with the knowledge of the ultrastructure of these cells, and the
evidence from thymic eipithelial cell cultures does suggest that the
thymic epithelial cells do constitute an endocrine organ with the
function of synthesizing thymosin. The presence of some residual
staining of renal proximal tubular cells following absorption of
bovine kidney might be indicative of a high concentration of "epithelial antigen" on these cells (compared to distal tubular cells which
were negative) or most likely might reflect the reabsorption of
thymosin form the glomerular filtrate by the proximal tubular cells.

Further studies are being undertaken to elucidate these findings
and to examine the possibility of applying this methodology to the
study of the human thymus.

REFERENCES

1.   Comsa, J. C.R. Soc. Biol. 127 (1938) 903.
2.   Osoba, D., Miller, J.F.A.P. J. Exp. Med. 119 (1964) 177.

3. Goldstein, A.L. et al in: Biological Activity of Thymic Hormones.
    (ed. D.W. van Bekkum) p. 173, Kooyker Scientific Publications,
    Rotterdam (1975).
4. Trainin, N. et al, ibidem p. 117.
5. Bach, J.F. et al, ibidem p. 145.
6. Goldstein, G. in Progr. im Immunology III, p. 891, Austr.
    Acad. of Science (1977).
7. Kruisbeek, A.M. in: Biological Activity of Thymic Hormones
    (ed. D.W. van Bekkum) p. 209, Kooyker Scientific Publications,
    Rotterdam (1975).
8. Clark, S.L. Am. J. Anat. 112 (1963) 1.
9. Pike, K.W., Gelfand, E.W. Nature 251 (1974) 421.
10. Hensen, E.J. et al. Clin. Exp. Immunol. in press.
11. Teodorczyk, J.A. et al. Nature 258 (1975) 617.
12. Taylor, C.R. Eur. J. Cancer 12 (1976) 61.
13. Taylor, C.R., Skinner, J. Blood 47 (1976) 305.
14. Taylor, C.R. Lancet 2 (1974) 802.

During this study Dr. van den Tweel was a fellow of The
Netherlands Organization for the Advancement of Pure Research (ZWO).

CHARACTERIZATION OF THYMUS EXTRACTS WHICH STIMULATE INCORPORATION

OF GALACTOSE INTO GLYCOCONJUGATES OF RAT BONE MARROW CELLS

D.A. Monner and P.F. Mühlradt

Gesellschaft für Biotechnologische Forschung mbH

Mascheroder Weg 1, D-3300 Braunschweig, W. Germany

INTRODUCTION

Many stages of lymphocyte differentiation are recognized by antigenic specificities at the cell surface, most of which reside in the glycoconjugates of the cell membrane (1). It is known that mitogen-induced changes in lymphocyte glycoconjugates can be detected by the increased incorporation of radioactive galactose into their acid insoluble material (2,3).

We reasoned that an assay based on this principle could be used to search non-specifically for putative factors involved in immune maturation. Calf thymus extracts, which are reported to contain a number of factors active at different stages of T-cell maturation (for review see 4), were tested for their in vitro effect on galactose incorporation into immature lymphocytes.

MATERIALS AND METHODS

Calf thymus extracts were prepared after the method of G. Goldstein (5) through the ultrafiltration steps. The concentrate was then chromatographed on a Bio-Gel P-2 column, and the void volume fraction used as a crude extract.

Animals. Female Lewis rats, 80-120 grams, and male CBA-mice, 4-6 weeks old, were from the Zentralinstitut für Versuchstierzucht, Hannover. C3H/HeJ nonresponder mice were a gift from F. Hoffmann – La Roche & Co., Basel/Switzerland.

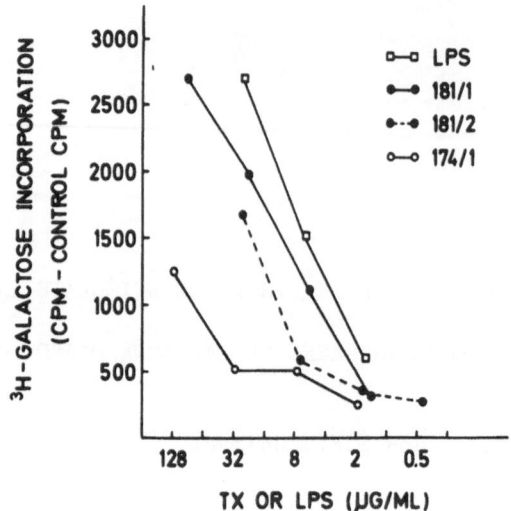

FIG. 1:   Stimulation of ^{3}H-Galactose Incorporation in C3H/HeJ
Mouse Bone Marrow Cultures: Dependence on Concentration of
Lipopolysaccharide and Thymus Extract.

Cell preparation.   Culture medium was RPMI 1640 with 20 mM
NaHCO$_3$, 10 mM Hepes, 100 ug/ml streptomycin, 65 μg/ml penicillin,
2 mM glutamine and 5% heat inactivated fetal calf serum. Cells in
medium were gently pressed through a 40 micron mesh nylon sieve,
washed once, counted with Türks solution, and adjusted to the
desired concentration.

Assay for galactose incorporation.   To microtiter plates with
flat bottomed wells was added 1.5 x 10^6 cells in 0.2 ml medium per
well. Other additions were included in this final volume. Incubation was at 37°C in 5% CO$_2$ in air. At the desired time ^{3}H-galactose,
0.5 μCi in 10 μl of 400 μM galactose, was added per well. Incorporated radioactivity was precipitated using a Skatron cell harvester.
All assays were in triplicate.

RESULTS AND DISCUSSION

Initial experiments showed that thymus extracts would stimulate
incorporation of galactose into acid insoluble material in rat bone
marrow cell cultures. The effect was generally two- to three-fold.
Kinetic studies revealed that, when extract was added at the
beginning of the culture time, maximal stimulation of galactose
incorporation occurred from 8 to 24 hours of incubation. Thus cells

TAB. 1:   Effects of Thymus Extract on Concanavalin A Response of
Density Gradient Separated Mouse Spleen Cell Fractions.

Cell Fraction (Density Cut)	^{3}H-Thymidine Incorporated in Cells (CPM+SEM[1])			
	Control	TX[2]	Con A[3]	TX[2] + Con A[3]
Unseparated	1,150+ 72	1,555+17	30,742+1,092	41,398+1,016
1.07 - 1.08	733+ 60	635+40	57,504+1,831	44,417+1,975
1.08 - 1.09	1,928+147	2,357+28	18,751+ 355	29,146+ 975
1.09 + 1.10	1,061+ 73	907+43	18,977+1,180	22,779+1,831

1)   All cultivations lasted 72 hours. ^{3}H-Thymidine, 1 µCi/culture,
was added the last 24 hours.

2)   Thymus extract, 125 µg/ml, was added at the beginning of
cultivation.

3)   Concanavalin A, 1 µg/ml, was added after 24 hours of cultivation.

were routinely labelled from 4-20 hours.   Thymidine incorporation
experiments showed no mitogenic activity in the extracts.   The
effects of the extracts were the same when fetal calf serum was
withheld from the medium.

The specificity of this effect of thymus extracts was investigated using different lymphocyte sources from rat and mouse.
Significant stimulation of galactose incorporation was found in bone
marrow and spleen cells of both rat and mouse.   In thymus there was
no effect, which may indicate that the extract, if it acts on T-cell
maturation, only affects pre-thymic cells.

Some stages of T-cell maturation can be induced by cyclic AMP,
either directly or via the ß-adrenergic receptor (6,7).   We
therefore tested the effect of cyclic nucleotides and ß-adrenergic
agents on galactose incorporation in rat bone marrow cell cultures.
Neither cAMP or cGMP at 10^{-4}M, nor agents which increase cyclic
nucleotide concentrations in vivo (theophylline and isoproterenol),
stimulated galactose incorporation.   The ß-adrenergic stimulator
isoproterenol at 10^{-5}M appeared to inhibit the basal level of
galactose incorporation, an effect which has not been further
investigated.   Propranolol (5×10^{-5}M), which blocks the ß-adrenergic
receptor, did not affect the action of thymus extract.   From these
experiments we concluded that our extract-stimulated galactose
incorporation was not mediated via cyclic nucleotides.

Lipopolysaccharide (LPS) was found to be active in nanogram

amounts in the galactose incorporation assay. It was conjectured that LPS contamination in the extracts could be the sole source of activity. Therefore, C3H/HeJ LPS nonresponder mouse bone marrow was used for a comparative titration of the activities of several extracts and LPS in a standard assay (Fig.1). LPS was still active in the microgram range, but it was clear that LPS contamination, unless it were over 50%, could not account for the extract activity.

The effect of preincubating splenocyte fractions with thymus extract on their response to the T-cell mitogen concanavalin A was measured by thymidine incorporation (Tab.1). The extract alone had no effect. In combination with concanavalin A it caused increased mitogenic activity in unseparated cells (35%) and cells of density 1.08-1.09 (55%). A suppression of mitogenic activity was seen in extract-treated cells of density 1.07-1.08 (23%). These opposing effects on Thymidine incorporation could be interpreted as extract-induced maturation of two (or more) precursor cell subsets having different potentialities.

Our findings support the use of this assay as a convenient method to screen for factors involved in the differentiation of lymphoid cells.

REFERENCES

1. Vitetta, E.S., Uhr, J.W., Biochim. Biophys. Acta. 415 (1975) 253.
2. van Eijk, R.V.W., Mühlradt, P.F., Eur. J. Biochem. 78 (1977) 41.
3. Rosenfelder, G., van Eijk, R.V.W., Monner, D.A., Mühlradt, P.F., Eur. J. Biochem. 83 (1978) 571.
4. Friedman, H., ed., Ann. N.Y. Acad. Sci. 249 (1975).
5. Goldstein, G., Nature 247 (1974) 11.
6. Bach, M.-A., Fournier, C., Bach, J.-F., Ann. N.Y. Acad. Sci. 249 (1975) 316.
7. Scheid, M.P., Goldstein, G., Hämmerling, U., Boyse, E.A., Ann. N.Y. Acad. Sci. 249 (1975) 531.

GENERATION OF AN EOSINOPHILOTACTIC FACTOR FROM HUMAN PMNs BY VARIOUS MECHANISMS OF CELL ACTIVATION

W. König[1], N. Frickhofen and H. Tesch

Institute of Medical Microbiology, Johannes Gutenberg-Universität, Mainz, W. Germany

[1]Correspondence to : Institut für Med. Mikrobiologie, Hochhaus am Augustusplatz, D-6500 Mainz, W. Germany

INTRODUCTION

It is well established that an increase in the number of eosinophils both in tissue and in the circulation is a feature of many clinical conditions based on delayed (1,2) and immediate type hypersensitivity reactions (3,4). Since eosinophils have been recognised to exert specific killer function on parasites (5) and to be prominent participants at sites of inflammation, the mechanisms of their chemo-attraction are of major importance. In immediate type hypersensitivity reactions, eosinophils have been demonstrated to counteract the mediators of inflammation such as histamine (6), the SRS-A (7) and the platelet aggregating factor (8).

Recently, several eosinophilotactic factors have been described which are lymphocyte- (1,2), mast cell- (9,10,11), and serum-derived products (12). The mast cell derived factor ECF-A has been studied best with regard to structure and eosinophilotactic properties. ECF-A is preformed within mast cells and consists of two tetra-peptides which have been recently analysed (9). In addition, oligo-peptides with eosinophilotactic properties have been shown to be released from mast cells during the allergic reaction (11). Furthermore, lipid factors such as HHT and HETE which were obtained by incubation of arachidonic acid with the microsomal fraction of platelets were able to attract eosinophils and neutrophils by chemo-kinesis and chemotaxis (13).

While intensive research on eosinophilotactic factors primarily has been focussed on mast cells, recent discoveries emphasized the

521

role of neutrophils in the secretion of mediators on inflammation.
It has been demonstrated that neutrophils can release the spasmo-
genic substance "SRS" which is similar to the SRS-A derived from
mast cells during the allergic reaction (14). Furthermore, a non-
preformed, low molecular weight eosinophilotactic factor which
with regard to its molecular weight is indistinguishable from the
ECF-A of mast cells could be released from human PMNs with the Ca-
ionophore (15), phagocytosis (16) and with arachidonic acid (17).

These results clearly underline the interdependence of allergic
and inflammatory processes. The purpose of this paper is to clarify
by careful analysis and enzyme studies the generation of ECF induced
by various stimuli and its inactivation. These studies will help to
understand the molecular basis and the mechanisms of mediator
secretion from human PMNs.

MATERIALS AND METHODS

The preparation of human PMNs, the assay systems for eosinophil
and neutrophil chemotaxis, buffers used for the release process of
ECF, the methods of subcellular breakage, the fractionation and
equilibrium density gradient centrifugations have been described in
detail (15-18).

RESULTS

Human PMNs were incubated with the calcium ionophore. At
different time intervals the samples were centrifuged and the
supernatants were assayed for eosinophilotactic activity and enzyme
release. As was shown by us previously, ECF activity rapidly
appears in the supernatant and decreases markedly at later times
of secretion. Since ECF was shown to represent a rather stable
biological activity, we suggested that a cell derived inactivator
might induce the decrease in activity. As to the enzyme release,
it is apparent that the calcium ionophore represents a non cytotoxic
stimulus as was determined by the enzyme lactate dehydrogenase.
Among the granular markers, lysozyme which is present in specific
granules was released up to 40%, ß-glucuronidase up to 20% and
peroxidase which is present in the azurophilic granules up to 15%
after 60 min of incubation. Only negligible amounts of microsomal
activity appeared in the supernatant on stimulation. As is apparent
from our data, ECF activity appears prior to the maximum of enzyme
release. Its release pattern is clearly different from that of a
granular mediator such as histamine, which parallels the lysosomal
enzyme release.

A more biological system of ECF generation occurs during phago-

TAB. 1:   Release pattern of ECF and enzymes from human PMNs on
stimulation with the calcium ionophore (5×10^{-6}(14)), opsonized
zymosan (mg/ml) and arachidonic acid (0.35 mM).

time (minutes)	ECF (Eos/5HPF)	Lyso-zyme %	ß-glucu-ronidase %	peroxidase %
		Ionophore		
4	490	14	5	2
8	420	25	6	3
20	110	38	8	3
		phagocytosis		
4	80	20	10	4
8	250	28	15	8
20	150	48	18	15
		arachidonic acid		
4	250	8	2	0.5
8	180	9	3	1
20	70	15	4	3

cytosis (16). It has been demonstrated that plain zymosan and
opsonized zymosan particles are potent stimuli for ECF generation
and release. With opsonized zymosan particles, a more rapid ECF
release occurs as compared to experiments in which plain zymosan
particles have been used. The pattern of ECF release resembles
that induced by the ionophore and occurs prior to the maximum of
enzyme release. Again, after a rise in ECF activity a donor
dependent decline in ECF activity occurred. As to the lysosomal
enzymes, activities present within the specific granules are
released to a better degree as compared to the azurophilic enzyme
marker peroxidase. A similar release pattern for ECF can be obtained
on stimulation of human PMNs with arachidonic acid. It is well
established that arachidonic acid serves as an important precursor
molecule for the generation of biologically active substances (19-
21): A cyclooxigenase can convert arachidonic acid into PGG2 and a
lipoxygenase is responsible for the production of HETE, as has been
shown with platelets. Factors such as HETE and HHT have been recently
shown to stimulate human eosinophils and PMNs by chemotaxis and random
migration. In contrast, the PMN derived AA induced ECF is highly
specific for eosinophils and does not attract human or guinea pig

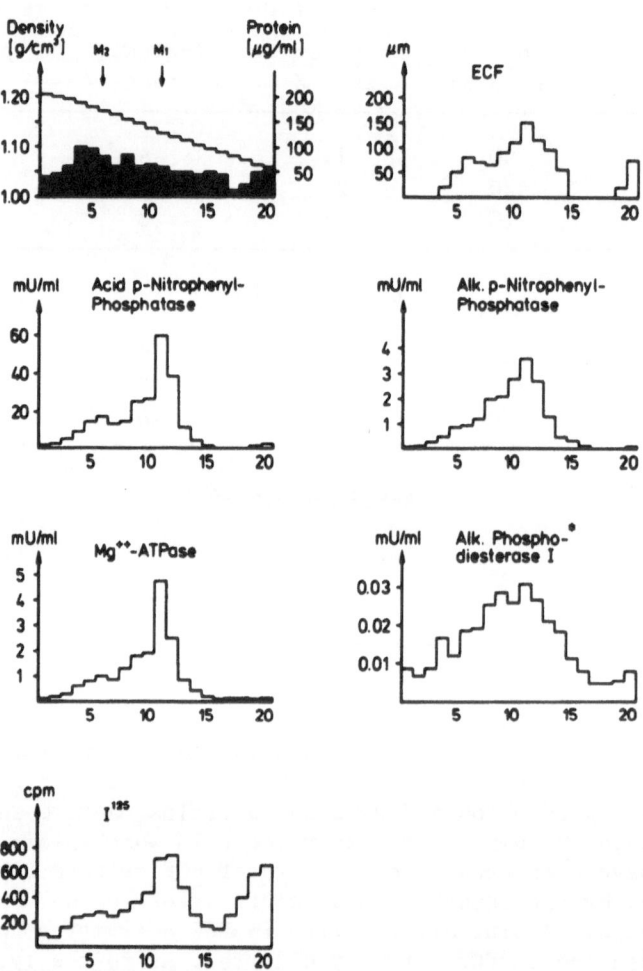

FIG. 1:   Localization of structurally bound ECF after ultracentrifugation of the 200 000 xg precipitate of stimulated PMNs on a
linear sucrose gradient; 1,2 = separation of microsomal components;
μm = distance of migration into the filter.

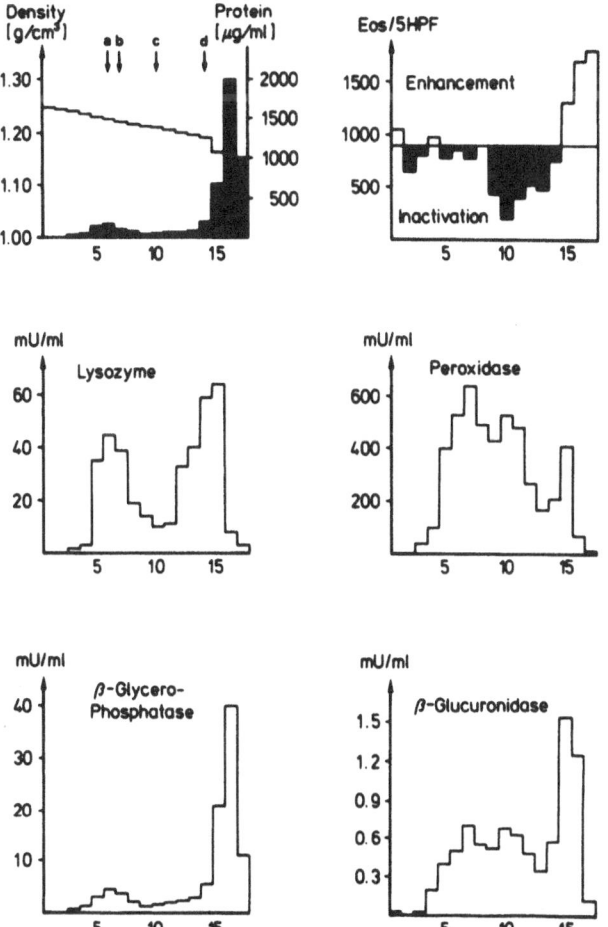

FIG. 2: Separation of PMN granules and localization of the inactivator for ECF. A - C represent the position of the granules. Inactivator is measured as decrease in activity of a standard ECF
after incubation with the fraction.

PMNs (17). Furthermore, it has been shown that incubation of AA
with guinea pig PMNs leads to products other than HETE and HHT with
unknown biological activity (22). The AA induced ECF release can
occur in cytotoxic and non-cytotoxic dose range. In the kinetics
demonstrated here a non-cytotoxic concentration for ECF release was
chosen. The ECF release pattern is similar to those induced by
other stimuli.

The data reported so far indicate that ECF activity can be
released from human PMNs on stimulation with quite different stimuli.
Since it is known that the calcium ionophore increases the calcium
flux across the membrane and since the phagocytic stimuli lead to
membrane pertubation, the question arises as to the mechanism of ECF
generation from PMNs on stimulation with arachidonic acid. Apparently,
these three totally different stimuli initiate a common pathway of
cell membrane activation resulting in the generation and release of
ECF. One may speculate from our data that the common molecular basis
for ECF generation might be due to the activation of the membrane
phospholipids leading to the turnover of arachidonic acid. According
to this hypothesis ECF represents either a biological activity
distinct from AA and its split products or represents a known or
unknown conversion product of AA with potent effects on eosinophils
at minimal concentrations.

Subcellular fractionation studies and equilibrium density
gradient experiments were performed to localize ECF synthesis and
its inactivator. Stimulated human PMNs were disrupted and various
fractions were obtained by differential centrifugation at 400, 3000,
20 000, 200 000 g with a final 200 000 g supernatant. The 200 000g
fraction containing ECF activity was placed on a sucrose gradient.
After centrifugation, enzyme and ECF activities were assayed for
each fraction. It is apparent that ECF activity coelutes with the
microsomal enzyme markers (Fig.1). Since our previous experiments
favoured the hypothesis that a PMN derived inactivator might be
responsible for the decline of ECF activity, experiments were carried
out to localize the inactivator for ECF. Unstimulated human PMNs
were disrupted in hypotonic sucrose; fractions at 3000 and 20 000 g
were obtained and separated on a shallow sucrose gradient. It is
apparent that inactivator activity coelutes with the peroxidase
positive subpopulation of the azurophilic granules (Fig.2).

In view of our data that ECF activity peaks prior to the enzyme
release and that by subcellular fractionation technique, ECF coelutes
with the microsomal enzymes, we favour the following hypothesis: On
stimulation with the ionophore, during phagocytosis or by arachidonic
acid, ECF is generated by an unknown mechanism within the cell
membrane and released as a low molecular weight mediator from the
plasma membrane. During stimulation, azurophilic granules containing
ECF inactivator are mobilized and fuse with the plasma membrane.
Inactivation of ECF could be due to the interaction of ECF with the
secreted inactivator in:

1.   fluid phase,

2.   inside the azurophilic granules by interaction with a structurally bound inactivator or

3.   the inactivator could modulate ECF release from the cell
membrane.

These data indicate that one cell is able to generate, secrete
and modulate the biologically active mediator which specifically
attracts eosinophils. Since eosinophils have been recognized as
prominent participants at sites of delayed and immediate type
hypersensitivity, the mechanisms of their chemoattraction appear to
be of major importance in order to understand the biological role
of eosinophils.

REFERENCES

1.   Colley, D.G., Eosinophils and immune mechanisms. 1. Eosinophil
      stimulation promoter (ESP): A lymphokine induced by specific
      antigen or phytohemagglutinin. J. Immunol. 110 (1973) 1419.
2.   Cohen, S., Ward, P.A., In vitro and in vivo activity of a
      lymphocyte and immune complex-dependent chemotactic factor for
      eosinophils. J. Exp. Med. 133 (1971) 133.
3.   Kay, A.B., Stechschulte, D.J., Austen, K.F., An eosinophil
      leukocyte chemotactic factor of anaphylaxis. J. Exp. Med. 133
      (1971) 602.
4.   Goetzl, E.J., Modulation of human eosinophil polymorphonuclear
      leukocyte migration and function. Am. J. Path. 85 (1976) 419.
5.   Mahmond, A.A.F., Warren, K.S., Peters, P.A., A role for the
      eosinophil in acquired resistance to schistosoma mansoni
      infection as determined by anti eosinophil serum. J. Exp. Med.
      142 (1975) 805.
6.   Zeiger, R.S., Twang, F.J., Colten, H.R., Histamine release from
      human granulocytes. J. Exp. Med. 144 (1976) 1049.
7.   Wasserman, S.I., Goetzl, E.J., Austen, K.F., Inactivation of
      slow reacting substance of anaphylaxis by human eosinophil
      arylsulfatase. J. Immunol. 114 (1975) 645.
8.   Kater, L.A., Goetzl, E.J., Austen, K.F., Isolation of human
      eosinophil phospholipase D. J. Clin. Invest. 57 (1976) 1173.
9.   Goetzl, E.J., Austen, K.F., Purification and synthesis of
      eosinophilotactic tetrapeptides of human lung tissue: Identifi-
      cation as eosinophil chemotactic factor of anaphylaxis. Proc.
      Nat. Acad. Sci. 72 (1975) 4123.
10.   Clark, R.A.F., Gallin, J.I., Kaplan, A.P., The selective eosino-
      phil chemotactic activity of histamine. J. Exp. Med. 142 (1975)
      1462.
11.   Boswell, R.N., Austen, K.F., Goetzl, E.J., Immunologic release
      of eosinophil chemotactic factors (ECF) from purified rat
      peritoneal mast cells. Fed. Proc. 36 (1977) 1328.

12. Ward, P.A., Cochrane, C.G., Müller-Eberhard, H.J., The role of serum complement in chemotaxis of leukocytes in vitro. J. Exp. Med. 142 (1976) 1462.

13. Goetzl, E.J., Woods, J.M., Forman, R.R., Stimulation of human eosinophil and neutrophil polymorphonuclear leukocyte chemotaxis and random migration by 12L-hydroxy-5,8,10,14-eicosatetraenoic acid. J. Clin. Invest. 59 (1977) 179.

14. Jakshik, B.A., Falkenhein, S., Parker, C.W., Precursor role of arachidonic acid in release of slow reacting substance from rat basophilic leukemia cells. Proc. Natl. Acad. Sci. 74 (1977) 4577.

15. Czarnetzki, B.M., König, W., Lichtenstein, L.M., Eosinophil chemotactic factor(ECF). I. Release from polymorphonuclear leukocytes by the calcium ionophore A 23187. J. Immunol. 117 (1976) 229.

16. König, W., Czarnetzki, B.M., Lichtenstein, L.M., Eosinophil chemotactic factor (ECF). II. Release during phagocytosis of human polymorphonuclear leukocytes. J. Immunol. 117 (1976) 235.

17. König, W., Tesch, H., Frickhofen, N., Generation and release of eosinophil chemotactic factor from human polymorphnuclear neutrophils by arachidonic acid. Europ. J. Immunol., in press.

18. Frickhofen, N., König, W., Subcellular localization of the eosinophil chemotactic factor (ECF) and its inactivator in human PMNs. Manuscript submitted.

19. Granström, E., In: Prostaglandins and Thromboxanes. Edited by F. Berti, B. Samuelsson, G.P. Velo. Published by Plenum Press, New York, London p.1 (1977).

20. Vane, J.R., In: Inflammation, Mechanisms and Controls. Eds. I.H. Lepow, P. Ward. Academic Press, Inc. New York, p. 261 (1972).

21. Hamberg, M. Samuelsson, B., Prostaglandin endoperoxides. Novel transformation of arachidonic acid in human platelets. Proc. Nat. Acad. Sci. 71 (1974) 3400.

22. Borgeat, P., Hamberg, M., Samuelsson, B., Transformation of arachidonic acid and homo-linolenic acid by rabbit polymorpho-nuclear leukocytes. J. Biol. Chem. 251 (1976) 7816.

ACKNOWLEDGEMENTS

This work was supported by the Deutsche Forschungsgemeinschaft, SFB 107, A 6 at Mainz.

THE EFFECT OF HISTAMINE ON LYMPHOCYTES :   RELEASE OF AN INHIBITOR

OF EOSINOPHIL CHEMOTACTIC MIGRATION

E. Kownatzki, G. Till and D. Gemsa

Institut für Immunologie und Serologie,

Universität Heidelberg, Heidelberg, W. Germany

Mast cells and basophil granulocytes have been shown to accumu-late in certain local immune reactions (1,2). Their secretory product histamine has been reported to suppress the destruction of target cells by cytotoxic T lymphocytes (3), the number of plaque forming cells in vitro (4,5), the production of lymphokines (6) and the incorporation of ^{3}H-thymidine after stimulation by phytohemag-glutinin (6). We recently described a stimulatory action of histamine on mononuclear cells, leading to the release of a small molecular weight inhibitor of eosinophil chemotactic migration (7). The present study indicates that the histamine sensitive and inhibitor producing cells are lymphocytes stimulated by antigen or mitogen.

Outbred guinea pigs received a crude aqueous extract of Ascaris suis, 4 mg of which were injected intraperitoneally twice weekly for at least 2 weeks. Four days after a last injection peritoneal exudate cells were collected by lavage with Hanks' balanced salt solution (HBSS) containing heparin 10 U/ml. The cells were fraction-ated by centrifugal elutriation to yield an eosinophil rich fraction containing 75 - 95% eosinophils, and an eosinophil poor fraction containing 93 - 98% mononuclear cells and a few mast cells. Eosinophils were tested for their chemotactic migration in a modified Boyden chamber. Micropore filters of 8 μm pore size were used and the leading front of migrating cells into the filter was measured. Normal human serum, which was treated with baker's yeast to activate complement, was used as chemotactic attractant.

Mononuclear cells to be tested for their ability to generate the inhibitor of eosinophil migration were incubated in HBSS con-

TAB. 1:   Centrifugal elutriation of guinea pig peritoneal exudate cells.

Fraction	RPM	Counter current (ml/min)	Cells ($\times 10^6$)	Eosino-phils (%)	Residual cells	Inhibitor
0 [a)]	–	–	180	29	MN [b)]	+
I	2770	15	11	2	small MN	–
II	"	20	51	75		
III	"	25	30	24		
IV	0 [c)]	40	32	2	large MN	+

[a)]   Cells before fractionation.

[b)]   Mononuclear cells.

[c)]   Fraction collected with centrifuge stopped.

taining histamine at 10^{-8} mol/l for 45 minutes. The cells were centrifuged and eosinophils of more than 75% purity were suspended in the supernatant, incubated for 10 minutes at 37°C and then added to the upper compartment of a Boyden chamber. Controls included eosinophils suspended in HBSS only and in HBSS containing histamine 10^{-8} mol/l.

Inhibitor producing cells were originally discovered in the exudate cells from animals injected with Ascaris extract. They were also detected in a suspension of mesenteric lymph node cells from these animals. However, no activity was recovered from histamine treated nuchal lymph node cells, spleen cells and peripheral blood lymphocytes. Cells from untreated animals could not be induced at all to release the inhibitor. Inhibitor generation did not depend on the injection of Ascaris extract, since peritoneal exudate cells and mesenteric lymph node cells from animals injected with bovine serum albumin were also capable of releasing the inhibitor.

Mononuclear cells from the peritoneal cavity of injected animals were fractionated by adherence on Petri dishes into an adherent and a nonadherent fraction. After incubation with histamine the chemotaxis inhibitor was only released from the nonadherent fraction and none was detected in the supernatant of adherent cells. This finding taken together with the production of inhibitor from lymph node cells, which contain very few macrophages, strongly favors lymphocytic cells as the source of the inhibitor.

Centrifugal elutriation allows the fractionation of cells mainly

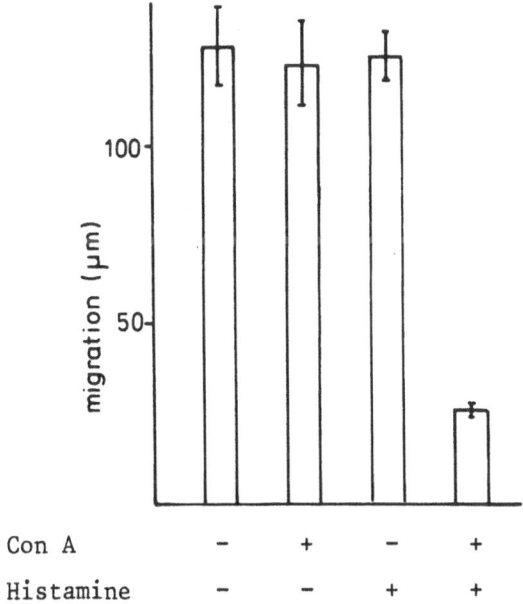

<u>FIG. 1</u>:   Generation of inhibitor producing cells by 24 hr culture
with Con A.   Cells were incubated for 24 hr with (+) or without (-)
Con A and subsequently for 45 min with (+) or without (-) histamine.

on the basis of size (8).   A typical separation is shown in Tab.1.
In addition to providing the eosinohpil rich fraction II, mononuclear
cells of different size were obtained.   Fraction I contained small,
fraction IV large mononuclear cells.   Inhibitor was liberated from
the large mononuclear cells only.

    Since inhibitor was released by lymphocytic cells from animals
repeatedly injected with antigen, it was of interest to examine
whether mitogen was capable of converting non-producing to inhibitor
producing cells.   Spleen cells from an untreated guinea pig were
cultured in RPMI containing 5% fetal calf serum with concanavalin
A 2.5 µg/ml added to some cultures and omitted from others.   After
24 hr the cells were harvested, washed twice with HBSS, divided into
two parts, one of which was treated with histamine for 45 min at 37°C,
the other was incubated without histamine.   As shown in Fig.1, no
inhibitor was released by cells which were treated with only one
stimulant, either Con A or histamine.   Inhibitor release was only
observed with those cells which had undergone a dual stimulation,
first by Con A for 24 hr and then by histamine for 45 min.

    The results suggest that the ability to release the inhibitor

of chemotactic migration upon treatment with histamine is restricted
to a limited population of lymphocytes. Only cells stimulated by
Con A or antigen were capable of releasing inhibitor and it is well
possible that only a small fraction of these were active. Inhibitor
generating cells were detected at or near the site of antigen
administration, i.e. in the peritoneal cavity and the regional lymph
nodes. Extraregional lymph nodes, the spleen or the blood did not
contain these cells in quantities which could be detected by the
assay procedure. This suggests that the cells are involved in the
local handling of antigen.

Inhibition of chemotactic migration of eosinophils was the
method by which the factor was detected and analyzed. There is
evidence that the factor also inhibits the chemotactic migration of
polymorphonuclear leukocytes (9). The previously observed inhibition
of chemotactic migration of basophil granulocytes (10) may well be
caused by the mechanism described here. An understanding of the
biological role of this histamine-induced process in local immune
reactions has to await further elucidation of the inhibitor effects
on its target cells.

REFERENCES

1. Ogilvie, B.M., Love, R.J., Transpl. Rev. 19 (1974) 147.
2. Dvorak, H.F., Dvorak, A.M., Progress in Immunol. II, Vol. 3,
    p. 171 (1974).
3. Plaut, M., Lichtenstein, L.M., Gillespie, E., Henney, C.S.,
    J. Immunol. 111 (1973) 389.
4. Melmon, K.L., Bourne, H.R., Weinstein, Y., Shearer, G.M., Kram,
    J., Bauminger, S., J. Clin. Invest. 53 (1974) 13.
5. Fallah, H.A., Maillard, J.L., Voisin, G.A., Ann. Immunol. 126
    (1975) 669.
6. Rocklin, R.E., J. Clin. Invest. 57 (1976) 1051.
7. Kownatzki, E., Till, G., Gagelmann, M., Terwort, G., Gemsa, D.,
    Nature 270 (1977) 67.
8. Glick, D., v. Redlich, D., Juhos, E.T., McEwen, C.R., Exp. Cell
    Res. 65 (1971) 23.
9. Till, G., Kownatzki, E., Gemsa, D., Fed. Proc. 37 (1978) 1656.
10. Lett-Brown, M.A., Leonard, E.J., J. Immunol. 118 (1977) 815.

SUMMING UP: SOLUBLE MEDIATORS OF IMMUNITY

A.L. de Weck

Institute for Clinical Immunology, University of Bern

Bern, Switzerland

I do not believe that this audience really expects a summing
up of all what has been said this morning and even less of what has
not been said about soluble mediators of immunity. What I would
rather do is to stress on the basis of some experiments and of
results obtained in our laboratory some of the pitfalls and
difficulties encountered by people dealing with lymphokines and
monokines. At the same time I shall emphasize some of the new
perspectives and possibilities which, in my opinion, will give a
great impulse to cell mediator research during the next years.

The first point which I would like to tackle briefly is that
of specific antibodies against lymphokines or monokines. In the
past years, several groups including our own, have reported the
production of antibodies against guinea pig or human lymphokines
(Table 1). Some of these antibodies have been shown in the guinea
pig to inhibit biological functions in vivo such as delayed-type
hypersensitivity reactions (1,2) and to bind in vitro to newly
sensitized proteins which have been internally radiolabelled in
culture (3). These antibodies react with molecules which are
secreted by the cells and not with constituents of the cell membrane.
Anti-lymphokine antibodies are therefore quite distinct from anti-
lymphocyte immunoglobulins obtained by immunisation with whole
lymphoid cells. Recently we have also been able to obtain an antiserum which appears to react with human macrophage inhibition
factor (MIF).

It is certainly by no means easy to produce antibodies against
lymphokines, for the following reasons:

TAB. 1:   Antibodies against some human and guinea pig lymphokines.

Antibodies directed against:	Author:	Reference:
Guinea pig macrophage migration Inhibiting factor (MIF)	Yoshida T. et.al. Geczy C.L. et.al.	J.Immunol. 114(1975)688 Cell.Immunol.19(1975)65
Guinea pig lymphotoxin (LT)	Gately M. et.al.	J.Immunol. 115(1975)817
Guinea pig allogeneic mitogenic factor (MLC-MF)	Geczy C.L.	J.Immunol.119(1977)2107
Human Lymphotoxin (LT)	Boulos G.N.et.al. Lewis J.E. et.al.	J.Immunol.112(1974)1347 J.Immunol. Methods 14 (1977)163
	Walker S.M. and Lukas Z.J.	J.Immunol. 113(1974)813
Human macrophage migration inhibiting factor (MIF)	Geczy C.L. McLeod T.F.et.al.	Cell.Immunol.27(1976)332 Cell.Immunol.32(1977)370
Human leukocyte migration inhibiting factor (LIF)	Bendtzen K.	Cell.Immunol.29(1977)382

1.   The amounts of lymphokines produced in terms of protein are very small. According to some estimate (4) it is for LIF (leucocyte migration inhibiting factor) of the order of 200 picograms/10^6 cells. This means that the handling of about 5 liters of culture supernatant at a concentration of 10 x 10^6 cells/ml is required to isolate at most 10 µg of material.

2.   It is rather striking that up to now the antibodies produced against lymphokines of a given species have been very specific; e.g. the antibodies against guinea pig lymphokines do not react with human, rat or mouse lymphokines. Vice versa, the anti-human lympo- kine antibody did not react with guinea pig or mouse lymphokines. On the other hand, there is a relatively broad cross-reactivity of lymphokines among species in terms of biological activity. A first but still speculative conclusion is that there are provably extensive molecular identities among the mammalian lymphokines. In order to produce antibodoes against a common portion of the mammalian lympho- kines, it will therefore probably be advantageous to immunize phylogenetically distant species.

TAB. 2:   Properties of guinea pig mitogenic factors.

		PPD - MF	MLC - MF
Molecular weight	a)	22 - 25000	18000
	b)	45000	
pI	a)	7.5	6.5
	b)	5.4	
Heat stability (1 hr, 56°)		stable	stable
Activity inhibited by 0.1 M fucose		no	yes
Absorbed by:			
anti-MIF serum*		no	yes
anti-MLC-MF serum		no	yes

*   serum containing anti-MIF and anti-MLC-MF antibodies or anti-MIF antibodies cross-reacting with MLC-MF.

Another point to which I would like to call attention is the choice of target-cells to assess lymphokine activity. These do not appear to be indifferent and may be the cause of much variability in the results. Caroline Geczy in our laboratory (5) identified two different types of mitogenic factors, produced by either antigen or mitogen stimulation on one hand or mixed lymphocyte reaction (MLC) on the other hand (Table 2). It was clearly demonstrated that the mitogenic factor produced by MLC (MLC-MF) does not act on any third party target-cells but that all target-cells possessing the B_2 antigen of the guinea pig major histocompatibility system (GPLA system) are not or very poorly responding. This is the case even if the cells used for generating the MLC-MF do not possess the B_2 antigen (6). In other words, variability in the target cells used for assessing lymphokine activities may be a frequent cause of erratic results in this field.

Another important point to assess lymphokine activities are the conditions in which lymphokine or monokine-producing cells are grown. We have observed that the addition of 2-mercaptoethanol (2-ME) to cultures of human mononuclear cells has both quantitative and qualitative effects on the lymphokines produced. For example, the addition of 2-ME to one-way or two-ways MLC cultures considerably increases the mitogenic activity of supernatants on third party cells. Appropriate controls demonstrate that more activity is really generated and that the increased activity does not merely reflect increased sensitivity of the test system. A similar effect has been observed on the production of human lymphocyte activating factor (LAF) as tested on mouse thymocytes (Fig.1). Qualitative effects

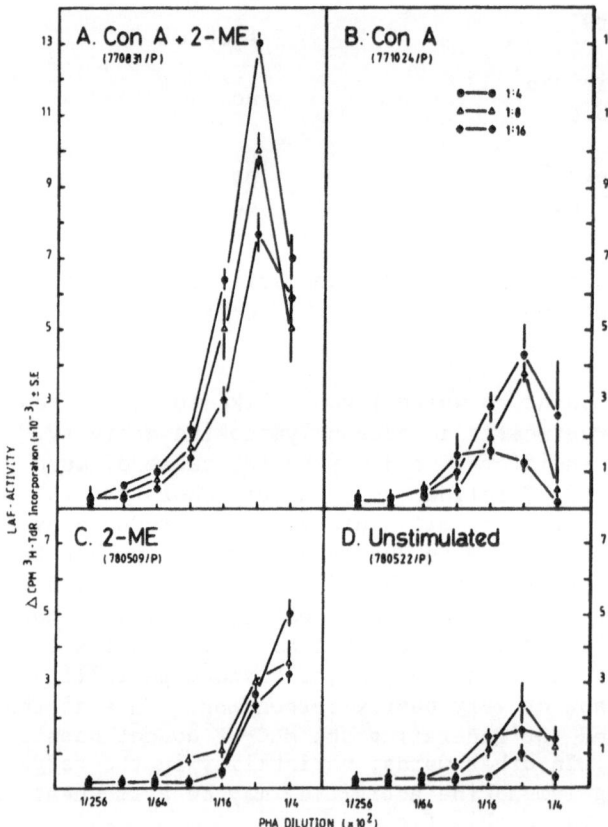

FIG. 1: Influence of 2-mercaptoethanol (2-ME) on the production of human lymphocyte activating factor (LAF) by peripheral blood mononuclear cell populations.

also appear in cultures from Con A-stimulated human lymphocytes.
Normally, MIF activity appears to be restricted to one major molecular moiety of approximately 25 000 daltons. By contrast, in
cultures performed in the presence of 2-ME a second peak of activity
at approximately 12 500 daltons regularly appears. Since the 25 000
daltons peak cannot be reduced to smaller active molecules in the
presence of 2-ME in vitro, these results suggest that a basic unit
of 12 500 daltons is secreted by the producing cells only in the
presence of 2-ME.

Another problem of great actuality is the cellular origin of
the various biological activities encountered in culture supernatants
from mononuclear cell populations. Such studies on mixed populations
of cells are difficult because stimulating factors may act on several
cell types causing cascade reactions among various types of cells.
This is certainly an argument for suggesting cell lines, cell subpopulations and possibly hybridomas as new and more selective sources
for the production of lymphokines, monokines and similar biologically
active factors.

As exemplified by several communications in this meeting, provided logistical problems are solved and a combination of immunochemical and biological methods used, it has become possible to
attack the lymphokine and monokine problem at the molecular level.
The time is not far away, where these molecules will become amenable
to radioimmunological and enzymatic assays. In view of their role
as effector and/or regulatory molecules, it is a whole new biological
world opening up. It is also to be hoped that some links will be
developed between this type of molecular and biochemical approach
and classical immunopathological and morphological studies, permitting
thereby to follow the presence and activity of lymphokines in tissues.

REFERENCES

1.   Geczy, C.L., Geczy, A.F., de Weck, A.L. J. Immunol. 117 (1976)
     66.
2.   Yoshida T., Bigazzi, P.E., Cohen, S. J. Immunol. 114 (1975)
     688.
3.   Sorg, C., Geczy, C.L. Eur. J. Immunol. 6 (1976) 688.
4.   Bendtzen, K. Cell. Immunol. 29 (1977) 382.
5.   Geczy, C.L. J. Immunol. 119 (1977) 2107.
6.   Geczy, C.L., Geczy, A.F. Eur. J. Immunol. 8 (1978) 236.

ACKNOWLEDGEMENTS

Personal work supported in part by the Swiss National Research
Foundation (grants No. 3.468.75 and 3.850.077).

SESSION   B 1

FUNCTIONAL AND MORPHOLOGICAL
ASPECTS OF MALIGNANT LYMPHOMAS

CHAIRPERSONS:

M. Seligmann

K. Lennert

INTRODUCTION - FUNCTIONAL AND MORPHOLOGICAL ASPECTS OF MALIGNANT

LYMPHOMAS

Karl Lennert

Institute of Pathology, University of Kiel,

2300 Kiel, W. Germany

The inclusion of our session in the program has two intentions:

1.   to demonstrate some of the progress made by the investigation
of malignant tumors of immunocompetent cells by means of immunological methods, and

2.   to stimulate thinking about the function of normal cells on the
basis of new facts about neoplastic cells, since malignant lymphomas,
being masses of usually monoclonal cell populations, offer a special
opportunity to be studied with immunological and biochemical methods.
In this context, we should not forget that the first biochemically
analyzed and characterized immunoglobulin was a myeloma protein.

Morphological feedback phenomena can also be expected from
immunological studies and have indeed been found. For instance, it
has been shown that lymphocytes with azurophilic granules are T-
lymphocytes, probably T-suppressor cells. So the immunological
approach to malignant lymphomas is a good example of give-and-take
between morphology and function.

The prerequisite for lymphoma studies is a subtle histological,
cytological, cytochemical, and, in some cases, electron microscopical
study of the tumor. There are two reasons for this:

1.   In lymphatic tissue we can distinguish some morphologically
distinct forms of lymphoid cells and their derivatives that can be
found with a corresponding morphology in tumors derived from the same
cells.

2.   The normal and the neoplastic cells can also be characterized
by immunological markers.

    An immunological characterization is no longer necessary for
some common cell types, however, because morphology can stand for
function: we can recognize cells of germinal centers and the plasma
cell series as B-cells quite well. Therefore, tumors consisting of
cells of germinal centers and the plasma cell series are clearly B-
cell lymphomas. That is not true, however, for all lymphoid cells.
Many cells, especially small lymphocytes, cannot be recognized as B-
or T-cell derivatives by their morphology alone. Thus we need other
aids. One is provided by cytochemistry and another by the histological features of a lymphoma.

    Acid phosphatase and, perhaps more efficiently, acid nonspecific
esterase can be used as good markers of T-cells, if we use strict
criteria. That was shown for lymphoblastic lymphomas of the T-cell
type, which show marked paranuclear acid phosphatase reactivity.
Unfortunately, however, the reaction may be negative in exceptional
cases, even those of isomorphic tumors. Dr. Poppema will present a
special B-cell lymphoma that is positive for alkaline phosphatase.
The neutral and acid nonspecific esterase reactions are good methods
for recognizing histiocytic neoplasms.

    Amongst the histological criteria, nodularity is highly estimated
by pathologists, because, if cytology corresponds, it reflects B-cell
lymphomas of a high frequency. Another histological criterion is the
site of primary infiltration in the lymph node, i.e. whether the
lymphoma infiltrates the B- or the T-cell area first. That may be of
help, for instance, in the differential diagnosis of chronic lymphocytic leukemia (CLL) and Sézary's syndrome. The third histological
criterion might be the demonstration of B- or T-specific structural
components, namely, dendritic reticulum cells in neoplasms of germinal
centers, and interdigitating reticulum cells and epithelioid venules
in T-cell neoplasms. We have to be careful with the content of
venules, however, because there are also occasional cases of B-cell
lymphomas that contain increased numbers of venules.

    Since 1974, we have another method for studying malignant
lymphomas in histological sections, viz.: the immunoperoxidase
technique of Taylor. It provides a way of identifying intracytoplasmic immunoglobulins and other substances in routine material.
That allows us to identify Ig-secreting tumor cells. Dr. Burkert
and Dr. van den Tweel will report on such investigations. It also
allows us to define monoclonality as an important criterion for
malignancy in unclear cases; for instance, one can distinguish CLL
with reactive plasma cells from immunocytoma, or reactive follicular
hyperplasia from follicular lymphoma.

If we apply all the morphological techniques I have mentioned, then we can recognize a given lymphoma as B- or T-cell-derived in about 85% of the cases. In the remaining cases immunological techniques applied to fresh tissue or cell suspensions are necessary for a clear diagnosis. Immunological analyses will show that a number of lymphomas are neither B- nor T-cell-derived and, in many cases, are probably tumors of stem cells. Even after exclusion of these non-B/non-T lymphomas, however, there will be a small number of tumors in which an immunological diagnosis cannot be given.

In our session, we shall get a lot of information about special new data on the correlation between structure and function of lymphoma cells. In addition, there will be some presentations covering special approaches to the immunological and biochemical characterization of neoplastic B- and T-cells. Finally, there will be two contributions dealing with the pathogenesis of malignant lymphomas.

All that I have said so far concerns the so-called non-Hodgkin's lymphomas, which are presently in the focus of attention. That is also reflected by our program: only one presentation deals with Hodgkin's disease. One of the reasons for that is the complexity of interacting cells in Hodgkin's lymphomas. I expect, however, that there will be many more contributions on Hodgkin's lymphomas at the next germinal center conference.

MULTIDISCIPLINARY STUDY OF NON-HODGKIN LYMPHOMAS:

ELECTRON MICROSCOPY, IMMUNE- AND ENZYME-HISTOCHEMISTRY[+]

C.A. Feltkamp[1], Th.M. Feltkamp-Vroom[2], J. Koudstaal[2],
P.v. Heerds[1], H. Spiele[1], C.B. de Graaff-Reitsma[2]
[1]Antoni van Leeuwenhoekhuis, The Netherlands Cancer Inst.
[2]Slotervaart Ziekenhuis, Amsterdam, The Netherlands

In order to characterize in greater detail the cells of 39 malignant non-Hodgkin lymphomas, the tissues were studied simultaneously.

Immediately after removal of the lymph node, the tissue sample was processed as follows: One part was fixed for light microscopy after preparations of imprint smears for cytology. For EM a 1 mm thick cross section was fixed and cut into wedge-shaped blocks with known orientation. Selection of parts to be studied was made on 1 μ sections, covering the entire depth of the biopsy. The remaining part was frozen in liquid nitrogen and used for immunefluorescence with antisera against human lymphocytes (ALS), T cells, heavy and light immunoglobulin chains (M, D, G, A, E, κ and λ) and for enzyme histochemistry demonstrating activities of a.o. 5'nucleotidase, ATPase, alkaline phosphatase, acid phosphatase and α -naphthyl acetate esterase (short and long fixation).

For comparison of the data the lymphomas were grouped according to the commonly used classification of Rappaport.

FOLLICULAR LYMPHOCYTIC LYMPHOMAS (9 cases)

All tumors consisted of monoclonal B cells with bright fluorescence of the outer rim, presumably the cell membrane, positive for M+D or G together with κ in nearly all cases. In

[+]Studies of cell suspensions of the same lymphomas will be published separately (A.A. Bom-van Noorloos e.a., Cancer, in the press).

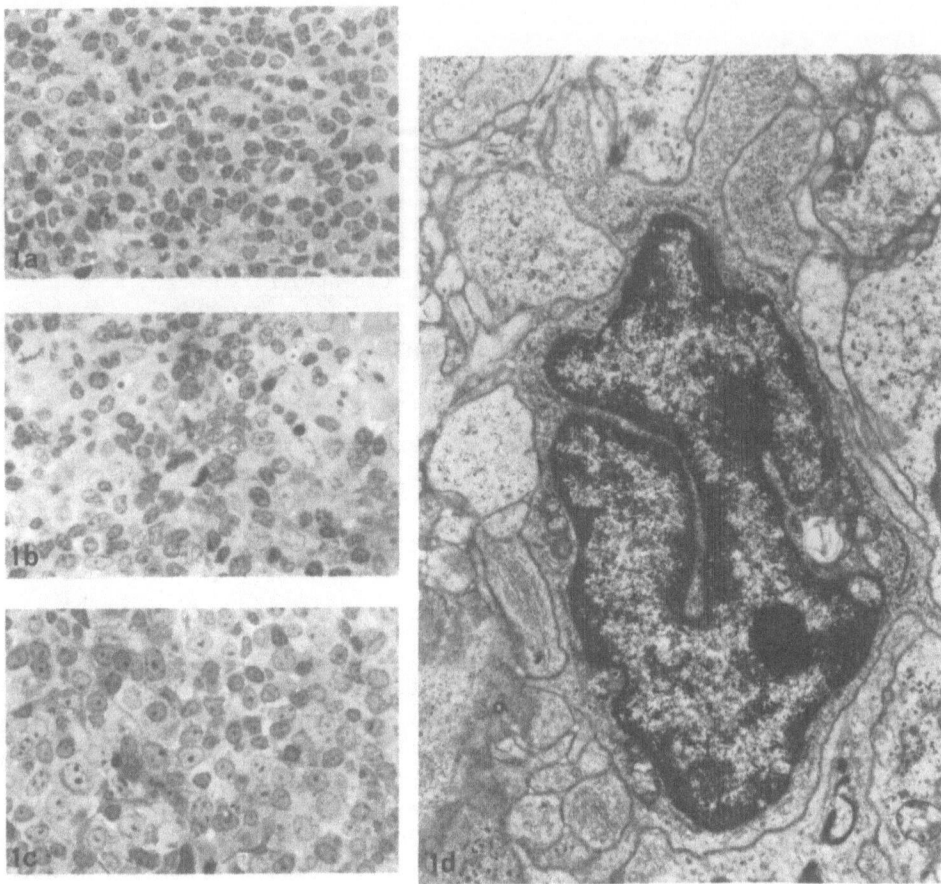

FIG. 1 a, b, c: Follicular lymphomas respectively consisting of small cells, small+blast-like cells, blast-like cells.   x 300.

FIG. 1 d: Small cell with irregular nucleus, surrounded by an elaborate network of cell protrusions.   x 10,000.

every tumor a part of the tumor cells showed a low to moderate activity of 5'nucleotidase, while three of nine tumors possessed a number of cells with clear ATPase activity. Four of the follicular lymphomas had tumor cells with alkaline phosphatase activity. The tumor cells were either small and moderately differentiated (ovoid/irregular nucleus, moderately condensed chromatin, free ribosomes), or larger and more blast-like (regular nucleus, dispers chromatin, multiple marginal nucleoli, free polysomes). The ratio between

TAB. 1:   Diffuse "Histiocytic" Lymphomas

light microscopy, immunology, enzyme histochemistry

pat. nr	sex, age	predom. cell type	s Ig	5'nucleot.	ATPase	Alk.ph	Ac.ph.
69	m 35	IB	-)'	-	>75 ++	-	>75 ±
122	f 62	IB	-	-	>75 +++	-	-
134	m 27	IB	-)"	-	<50 ±	-	<25 ±
153	f 74	IB	-	-	<25	-	-
70	m 68	CC	A κ	>75 +	>50 ++	-	-
119	m 64	CC	- λ	-	-	-	-
139	m 50	CC	-	-	>75 +++	-	>50 +
77	m 65	CB	M λ	-	>75 ++	-	-
79	f 65	CB	-	-	-	-	-
120	m 67	CB	M κ	-	>75 +++	-	-
152	f 55	CB	-	<50 ++	>75 +	<25 ±	-
157	m 24	CB	-	-	<25 +	-	-
165	f 72	CB	M κ	-	<25 ±	-	-
174	f 78	CB	-)"'	-	>75 ++	-	-

)' cytoplasmic A κ;)" cytoplasmic M λ;)"' cytoplasmic M κ

- = no activity; ± = trace activity; + = low activity; ++ = moderate
activity; +++ = high activity; > resp. < means more resp. less percent of the total tumor cells that had enzyme activity

both was variable (Fig.1 a-c). One case consisted almost exclusively of blasts on which no heavy Ig chains, but only κ light
chain was detected. The most intense ATPase activity was found in
two cases that contained mainly moderately differentiated cells.

The surface of the cells had many protrusions that often formed,
together with dendritic reticulum cells an elaborate network (Fig.1d).

Between and often closely against the border of the follicles
many T cells were present. The intrafollicular areas contained also
normal B cells, some tumor cells and cells of other types. Within
the follicles few, generally inactive histiocytic cells were seen.

DIFFUSE LYMPHOCYTIC LYMPHOMAS (7 cases)

The predominant cells in all cases were monoclonal B cells.

Two cases consisted of well differentiated cells (round nucleus, condensed chromatin, free ribosomes). They showed weak rim-like fluorescence, positive for M+D and κ ; they had low 5' nucleotidase but high ATPase activities. Only very few, rather inactive histiocytic cells were seen.

The other five cases contained less differentiated cells, similar to those in follicular lymphomas. They showed moderate rim-like fluorescence of M or M+D, and κ or λ . The activity of ATPase was rather high, that of 5'nucleotidase low or absent. The cell surface was more irregular than that of well differentiated cells, but did not form an elaborate network. The number of histiocytic cells was higher than in the well differentiated subgroup.

DIFFUSE "HISTIOCYTIC" LYMPHOMAS (14 cases)

In contrast to the former groups, this group showed much variety in morphology, immunology and enzyme histochemistry (Tab.1).

Eight lymphomas consisted of monoclonal B cells with immuno-globulin either at the cell surface (rim-like) or intracellular. In one case of the latter subgroup (69), most cells showed strong cytoplasmic fluorescence of A κ , and contained many swollen cisternae of rough ER (Fig.2a). The acid phosphatase activity in nearly all cells was caused by a relatively high number of lysosomes in the Golgi area of the tumor cells. In both other cases the cytoplasmic fluorescence could not convincingly be correlated with plasmacytoid morphology (Fig.2b). The five cases with surface Ig consisted of cells that resembled enlarged forms of both cell types in follicular lymphomas (Fig.3a,b).

The remaining six lymphomas were negative with anti immunoglob-ulin and anti T cell sera, but positive with ALS. The pattern of enzyme activities varied from completely negative (79) to high activity of ATPase (122, 139). The morphology of the tumor cells also showed much diversity. Some cases (139, 152) showed similarity with follicular lymphoma cells, others (79, 134) consisted of very large cells that were more conform EM descriptions of "immunoblasts" (e.g. very large nucleoli, high amount of free polysomes, variable number of ER profiles). However, no clearcut correlation between the data obtained with different disciplines was found.

Most lymphomas of the diffuse "histiocytic" group contained many, often very actively phagocyting histiocytes.

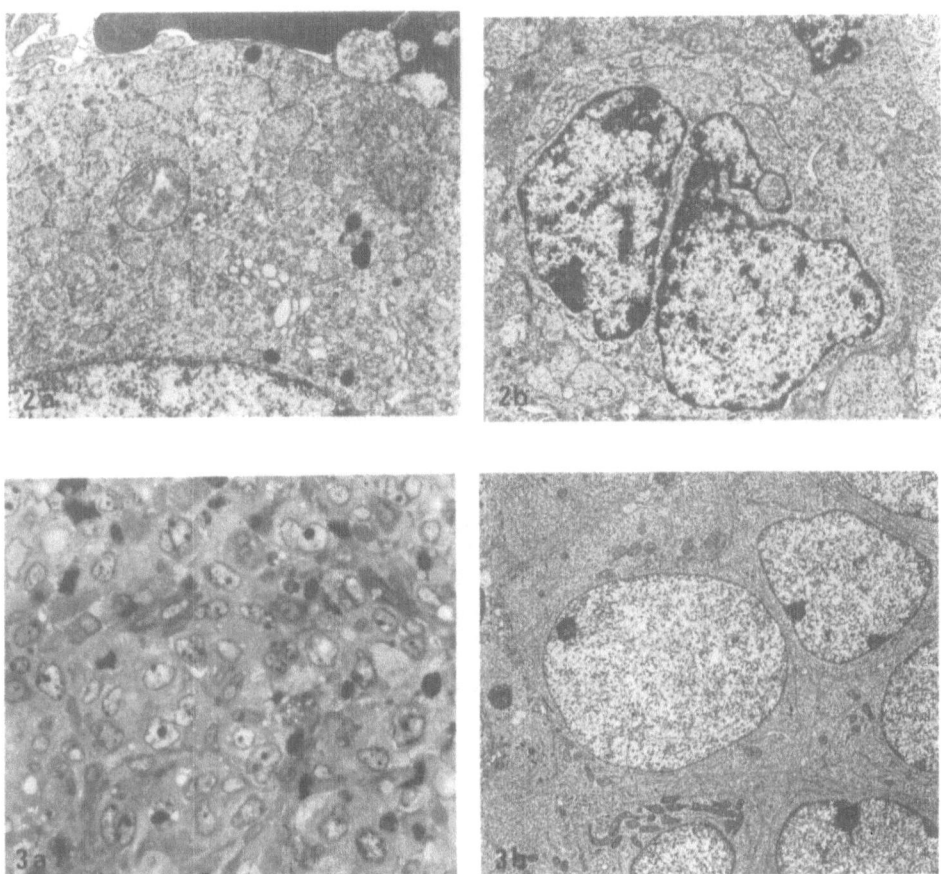

FIG. 2a: Well developed rough ER cisternae (case 69).   x 9,000.

FIG. 2b: Tumor cell with few ER profiles (case 175).   x 4,000.

FIG. 3a, b: Tumor cells resemble enlarged forms of cells found in follicular lymphomas (cases 70 and 165).   x 300(a);   x 3,000(b).

"UNDIFFERENTIATED" LYMPHOMAS (6 cases)

The age of patients in this group was considerably lower than in other groups. Two cases did not show sIg or T cell fluorescence, but were positive with ALS. They had low or no enzyme activities. The cells had ovoid/irregular nuclei, rough dispers chromatin, free ribosomes and polysomes.

The tumor cells of the four other cases (all males) reacted with anti human T cell serum, and showed focal acid phosphatase activity, but no α-naphthyl acetate esterase activity, even not

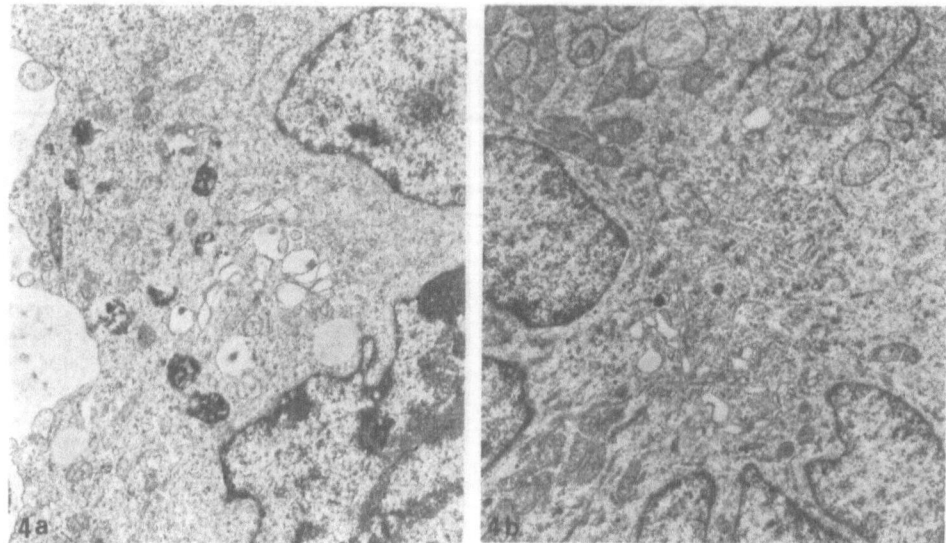

FIG. 4a: Malignant histiocytic cell with swollen Golgi cisternae and secondary lysosomes. x 7,000.

FIG. 4b: Malignant histiocytic cell with tubulo-vesicular Golgi apparatus. x 7,000.

after long fixation. Most nuclei contained very homogenous, densely dispers chromatin, and were broadly indented at one side.

MALIGNANT HISTIOCYTIC TUMORS (3 cases)

The cells of three lymph node tumors did not react with ALS, anti-Ig or anti T cell sera. The cells were large and had a very well developed Golgi apparatus. However, differences were found between the fine morphology of the three cases and between the enzyme patterns of two cases tested. One showed high acid phosphatase and α-naphthyl acetate esterase activities and no activities of other enzymes; the other had high ATPase, but no acid phophatase or α-naphthyl acetate esterase activities. The Golgi apparatus of the first consisted of swollen cisternae with many lysosomes (Fig.4a), while that of the latter was formed by a fine tubulo-vesicular system without lysosomes (Fig.4b). We suppose that these differenes are reflections of differences between subtypes of histiocytic cells from which the tumors originate.

CONCLUSIONS

Follicular and diffuse lymphocytic lymphomas consist of mono-clonal B cells with moderate or weak sIg fluorescence, respectively. Most tumors with 5'nucleotidase activity are found in the group of follicular lymphomas.

Generally the ATPase activity of tumor cells of B-type lymphomas is more intense than the activity of lymphoid cells in the cuff of normal lymph follicles.

"Histiocytic" lymphomas are not a homogeneous group. They consist either of B cells or of non B non T cells. The latter are possibly in part derived from B cells that have lost certain characteristics.

"Undifferentiated" lymphomas are either non B non T cells, or T cells.

Malignant histiocytic tumors have variable morphology and enzyme patterns, that possibly reflect differences between subtypes of the original histiocytic cells.

REFERENCES

1. Brouet, J.C. et al., J. Natl. Cancer Inst. 56 (1976) 631.
2. Jaffe, E.S. et al., Cancer Treat. Rep. 61 (1977) 953.
3. Kaiserling, E., Non-Hodgkin Lymphome, Stuttgart, G. Fischer Verlag (1977).
4. Leech, J.H. et al., J. Natl. Cancer Inst. 54 (1975) 11.

CORRELATION OF BIOCHEMICAL AND IMMUNOLOGICAL MARKERS WITH
CONVENTIONAL MORPHOLOGY AND CLINICAL FEATURES IN 120 PATIENTS
WITH MALIGNANT LYMPHOMAS

R. Mertelsmann, D.A. Filippa, B. Koziner, E. Grossbard,
J. Beck, M.A.S. Moore, P.H. Lieberman, B.D. Clarkson,
S. Gupta and R.A. Good
Memorial Sloan-Kettering Cancer Center
New York, N.Y. 10021, U. S. A.

INTRODUCTION

The striking heterogeneity of clinical features, morphological
characteristics and prognosis in patients with neoplastic lymphoproliferative disorders has stimulated attempts to reclassify these
diseases according to the phenotypic characteristics of the predominating cell type (1-6). This approach is based on the following
hypotheses: 1) the neoplastic cell type is the most important determinant of biological behavior, 2) the different neoplastic cell types
represent proliferations, "frozen" at distinct stages of the normal
development sequence of a specific cell lineage, and 3) all cells
with proliferative capacity can give rise to neoplasia. Various
approaches have been successfully employed for the phenotypic
characterization of hematopoietic tumors utilizing immunological,
functional, biochemical, cytogenetic and in vitro culture techniques.
In this study, we have attempted to assess the significance of a
comprehensive methodology employing cell surface marker characterization, assay for terminal deoxynucleotidyl transferase activity,
and conventional morphology in the clinical evaluation of 122 patients
with known or suspected lymphoid neoplasias.

MATERIALS AND METHODS

Peripheral blood, bone marrow and biopsy specimens from different
lymphoid tissues were obtained from 122 adult patients as part of
their diagnostic evaluation at Memorial Sloan-Kettering Cancer Center.
Techniques for characterization of cell surface markers (1,2), and
determination of terminal deoxynucleodityl transferase activity (4)

TAB. 1:   Distribution of TdT in Normal Human Tissues

Tissue	Cases Studied	TdT activity (mean $U/10^8$ cells)
Thymus	1	132.0
Bone Marrow		
- mononuclear cells	19	0.12
- sed. veloc. 3.5mm/h	3	16.5
Tonsil	2	0.05
Peripheral Blood, Spleen, Lymph Node		
- mononuclear cells	28	<0.01
- B cells	4	<0.01
- T cells	4	<0.01
- null cells	4	<0.01

were as described previously. Fc receptors for IgG and IgM on T
lymphocytes were assayed according to Gupta et al. (7). Colony
formation in soft agar by myeloid committed stem cells was assayed
in all patients with bone marrow involvement according to Moore (8).
Histopathological classification of lymph node biopsies was performed
according to Rappaport (9).

RESULTS AND DISCUSSION

Distribution of Terminal Deoxynucleotidyl
Transferase in Normal Tissues

Analysis of normal human tissues for terminal deoxynucleotidyl
transferase (TdT) activity has confirmed the restricted distribution
of this enzyme to thymocytes and to a subpopulation of human bone
marrow cells under physiological conditions (Tab.1). The TdT positive
bone marrow cells could be enriched approximately 100-fold by cell
separation according to sedimentation velocity. These cells could
then be induced to express the HTLA marker, an early T-cell antigen,
following in vitro incubation in the presence of thymopoietin,
strongly suggesting that an immature cell of T-cell lineage is the
TdT positive cell in normal human marrow (5). In contrast, human
bone marrow myeloid progenitor cells (CFU-c), highly enriched T, B
and null (non-T, non-B) cells from peripheral blood, lymph node,
spleen and tonsil specimen, as well as a mouse pluripotent stem cell
fraction (N. Williams, unpublished) revealed low or undetectable TdT

TAB. 2:   TdT and Cell Surface Markers in Malignant Lymphomas.

Phenotype	Histological Diagnosis	Cases studied	Specific PB	Activity BM	LN/Biop.
		n	mean(units/10^8 cells)		
null, TdT$^+$	LBL	21	3.57	6.59	.43
	DHL	2	–	10.6	–
	CML, LB	1	–	–	7.08
null, TdT$^-$	Ca. anaplastic	3	–	–	< .02
	AML	2	–	–	< .01
	CML, MB	1	–	–	< .05
T, TdT$^+$	LBL	5	11.4	–	–
T, TdT$^-$	DPDL, LBL, DHL	3	–	–	< .01
	Sezary's S., MF	2	–	–	< .01
B, TdT$^{(+)}$	Burkitt's L.	3	.14	–	< .01
B, TdT$^-$	Burkitt's L.	1	<.01	–	–
	DPDL, NPDL	27	<.05	<.05	< .05
	DHL, DML, NHL	17	<.05	<.05	< .05
	IBLA	1	–	–	< .07
	DWDL, CLL	14	<.01	<.05	<.03
	Plasmacytoma	2		<.01	<.01
'Mono', TdT$^-$	DHL	1	<.01	<.01	–
'H', TdT$^-$	Hairy Cell L.	8	<.01	<.02	<.02
?, TdT$^-$	Hodgkin's d.	6	<.01	<.10	<.05

activity (Tab.1). These observations demonstrate the highly
selective expression of the TdT genome in apparently T-cell related
bone marrow progenitor cell and in thymocytes with the subsequent
disappearance of this enzyme during maturation to a peripheral blood
T cell. While the presence of TdT in a common progenitor cell for T
and B cells cannot be ruled out, it is clearly neither present in
normal mouse pluripotent stem cells, human myeloid stem cells,
chicken bursa cells (10), nor in mature cells of any cell lineage.

TdT and Cell Surface Markers
in Malignant Lymphomas

Cell marker phenotypes, histopathological diagnoses, and TdT activities of tissue samples from 122 patients presenting with a tentative diagnosis of malignant lymphoma, are summarized in Table 2. The non-B, non-T ("null") phenotype could be further subdivided according to the presence or absence of high levels of TdT activity (specific activity >0.5 U/10^8 cells). The phenotype "null, TdT$^+$" carried morphological diagnoses of lymphoblastic lymphoma (LBL), diffuse histiocytic lymphoma (DHL) or chronic myeloid leukemia (CML) in lymphoblastic acute phase (LB), while "null TdT$^-$" was the predominant cell type in lymph nodes from patients with metastasizing carcinoma (Ca), acute myeloid leukemia (AML) and CML in myeloblastic acute phase (MB). The phenotype "T, TdT$^+$" was only observed in LBL. One case of LBL was "T, TdT$^-$", suggesting a more mature T-cell related neoplasia, as was observed in one case each of diffuse poorly differentiated lymphocytic lymphoma (DPDL) and diffuse histiocytic lymphoma (DHL). A similar phenotype was observed in Sezary's syndrome, Mycosis Fungoides, and occasionally in patients with T-cell ALL (5). We have previously shown that lymphoblastic lymphomas showed similar cell markers as seen in ALL and also exhibited a very similar clinical course (11). The 2 cases of "null TdT$^+$" DHL with peripheral blood and bone marrow involvement (Tab.2), were clinically very similar emphasizing the strong correlation between cell phenotype and clinical features, independent of the histopathological classification. Based on the available literature and on our own studies, the basic phenotypes of the various neoplasias of T-cell lineage have been tentatively classified in Table 3. However, a more detailed analysis of 18 cases of T-cell LBL and acute lymphoblastic leukemia (ALL) employing SRBC rosetting at 4° (E^4) and 37° (E^{37}), EAC-rosetting (EAC$^+$) and demonstration of receptors for IgG (Tγ) and IgM (Tμ) revealed even further heterogeneity of the "T3" phenotype (Tab.3). The following cell marker patterns were observed (in order of decreasing TdT activity): a) E^4, TdT$^+$, EAC$^+$; b) E^4, TdT$^+$, EAC$^+$, Tμ, Tγ; c) E^{37}, TdT$^+$, EAC$^+$, Tγ; d) E^{37}, TdT$^+$, Tγ; e) E^4, EAC$^+$, TdT$^-$; f) E^4, Tγ, TdT$^-$. It still remains unsettled whether these cell marker patterns are associated with particular clinical features, e.g. attributable to specific homing properties of certain surface marker constellations, since the numbers of patients in each subgroup are still small. Further studies of T cell related neoplasias employing these and additional markers are continued at present and should help to elucidate the clinical and biological significance of specific cell characteristics and the ontogeny of normal and neoplastic T cells. The majority of malignant lymphomas of adults were found to be of "B, TdT$^-$" type including diffuse and nodular poorly differentiated lymphocytic lymphoma (DPDL, NPDL), diffuse and nodular histiocytic (DHL, NHL), diffuse mixed lymphoma (DML), immunoblastic lymphadenopathy (IBLY), diffuse well differentiated lymphoma (DWDL),

TAB. 3: Cell Marker Findings in Neoplasias of T-Cell Lineage.

Type	Cytology	a-ALL a)	AcP b)	Hex.I c)	E-Rosette 4°	E-Rosette 37°	TdT	Diagnoses
T1 "null" (pre-thymic)	lymphoblast	-	-	-	-	-	+++	ALL, LBL,
T2 "common" (pre-thymic)	lymphoblast	+	-	+	-	-	+++	CML-LB, MPS-LB d) rare: DHL
T3 (thymic)	lymphoblast +/- conv. nucleus	-	+/- (Golgi)	-	+	+	+++	ALL, LBL
T4 (post-thymic)	lymphocyte variable size azurophilic granules	-	+	-(?)	+	-	-	T cell CLL rare: DPDL, ALL, LBL
T5 (post-thymic)	lymphocyte cerebriform nucleus (EM)	-	+ (gran)	-(?)	+	-	-	Mycosis F. Sezary's S.

a) a-ALL = anti-ALL serum (17).
b) AcP = acid phosphatase, cytochemical reaction (11).
c) Hex.I = Hexosaminidase I, biochemical assay (17).
d) MPS-LB - myeloproliferative syndrome in lymphoblastic acute phase (5,18); for other abbreviations, see text.

TAB. 4:   Cell Marker Phenotypes in Malignant Lymphomas.

Cell Phenotype		"null" TdT$^+$	T TdT$^+$	T TdT$^-$	monocytoid TdT$^-$	B TdT$^-$
Diagnosis	n			incidence (%)		
Lymphoblastic	27	77	19	4	0	0
Histiocytic	21	10	0	5	5	80
poorly differen- tiated lymph.	28	0	0	4	0	96
well differen- tiated lymph.	14	0	0	0	0	100

chronic lymphocytic leukemia (CLL) as well as plasmocytoma (Tabs.2,4).
Detailed descriptions of the various B-cell related neoplasms have
been reported previously (1,2). One case of DHL revealed monocytoid
features with phagocytosis of latex particles and a CFU-c growth
pattern as seen in acute myeloid leukemias, suggesting the myelo-
monocytic lineage of this patient's neoplasia ("true histiocytic
lymphoma"). All other patients studied for CFU-c formation, revealed
a low normal or no growth in soft agar culture as seen in lymphoid
leukemias or in lymphomas with bone marrow involvement (8). While
the cell lineage has not been definitely established for the "Hairy
Cell" of leukemic reticuloendotheliosis (hairy cell leukemia) and
for the malignant cell in Hodgkin's disease, neither of these two
diseases reveals any TdT activity in involved tissues.

We have observed slightly elevated levels of TdT activity in
peripheral blood cells (Tab.2) from 2/4 patients with Burkitt's
lymphoma in leukemic phase. Whether this reflects the presence of
low levels of this enzyme in other than pre-T cells, e.g. a common
progenitor cell for T and B lymphocytes, or the admixture of a small
number of pre-T cells to the predominating Burkitt's cells, is unknown
at this point. It has been shown that in some cases of ALL (12) and
of CML-LB (M. Greaves, personal communication) cells with intracytoplasmic IgM ("pre-B cells") can exhibit elevated TdT activity.

CONCLUSIONS

The majority of adult malignant lymphomas are related to the B-
cell lineage (1-3,6,13,14). However, phenotypic characterization of
the predominating cell type by multiple cell markers reveals some
heterogeneity with respect to cell lineage within the various histopathological diagnoses (Tab.4). These observations might explain

part of the clinical heterogeneity observed in these patients. Because clinical features, response to therapy and prognosis, and cell phenotype appear to correlate closely (11,15,16), it is suggested that chemotherapeutic protocols should be selected according to cell phenotype whenever possible. The phenotypes "null, TdT$^+$" and "T, TdT$^+$" probably require intensive chemotherapy as used for ALL in order to prevent leukemic progression (11), the "monocytoid, TdT$^-$" phenotype as used for AML. The phenotypic subgroups of the B cell related neoplasms appear to be associated with characteristic clinical features (1,2). Further comprehensive analysis of this group of malignant lymphomas is required, however, to assess the contribution of phenotypic analysis to clinical management in these patients.

REFERENCES

1. Koziner, B., Filippa, D.A., Mertelsmann, R., Gupta, S., Clarkson, B.D., Good, R.A., Siegal, F.P. Am. J. Med. 63 (1977) 556.
2. Filippa, D.A., Lieberman, P.H., Erlandson, R.A., Koziner, B., Siegal, F.P., Turnbull, A., Zwiring, A., Good, R.A. Am. J. Med. 64 (1978) 259.
3. Lukes, R.J., Collins, R.D. Cancer Treat. Rep. 61 (1977) 971.
4. Mertelsmann, R., Mertelsmann, I., Koziner, B., Moore, M.A.S., Clarkson, B.D. Leukemia Research 2 (1978) 57.
5. Mertelsmann, R., Koziner, B., Filippa, F., Grossbard, E., Incefy, G., Moore, M.A.S., Clarkson, B.D. in: Modern Trends in Human Leukemia III, Springer-Verlag (1978) in press.
6. Preud'Homme, J-L., Seligman, M. Blood 40 (1972) 777.
7. Gupta, S., Good, R.A. Clin. Exp. Immunol. 30 (1977) 222.
8. Moore, M.A.S. Blood Cells 2 (1976) 109.
9. Rappaport, H. Atlas of Tumor Pathology, Section 3, Fasc. 8, Washington, D.C., Armed Forces Institute of Pathology (1966).
10. Modak, M.J., Bhatt, H., Seidner, S., Hahn, E.C., Gupta, S., Good, R.A. Biochem. Biophys. Res. Commun. 83 (1978) 266.
11. Koziner, B., Mertelsmann, R., Filippa, D.A. in: Differentiation of normal neoplastic hematopoietic cells, Cold Spring Harbor (1978) in press.
12. Vogler, L.B., Crist, W.M., Bockman, D.E., Pearl, E.R., Lawton, A.R., Cooper, M.D. N. Engl. J. Med. 298 (1978) 872.
13. Kung, P.C., Long, J.C., McCaffrey, R.P., Ratliff, R.L., Harrison, T.A., Baltimore, D. Am. J. Med. 64 (1978) 788.
14. Donlon, J.A., Jaffee, E.S., Braylan, R.C. N. Engl. J. Med. 297 (1977) 461.
15. Marks, S.M., Baltimore, D., McCaffrey, R. N. Engl. J. Med. 298 (1978) 812.
16. Bloomfield, C.D., Kersey, J.H., Brunning, R.D., Gajl-Peczalska, K.J. Cancer Treat. Rep. 61 (1977) 963.
17. Ellis, R.B., Rapson, N.T., Patrick, A.D., Greaves, M.F. N. Engl. J. Med. 298 (1978) 476.

18. Hoffman, R., Esteen, S., Kopel, S., Marks, S.M., McCaffrey,
     R.P. Ann. Int. Med. 89 (1978) 71.

ACKNOWLEDGEMENTS

This work was supported in part by ACS Grant PDT-95, NCI grants
CA-08748, CA-17353, CA-17085, the Gar Reichman Foundation and a
grant from the "Eosinophilic Granuloma Task Force, Merlin Foundation".

BIOLOGY OF LYMPHOMA TRANSFORMATION

[1]C.R. Taylor, [1]R.J. Lukes and [1,2]J.G. van den Tweel

[1]Sections of Immunopathology and Hematopathology,
University of Southern California Medical School,
Los Angeles, California, U.S.A.

[2]Department of Pathology, University of Leiden,
Leiden, The Netherlands

INTRODUCTION

The question of the exact nature of Hodgkin's disease, and its relationship to other tumors of the lymphoid organs, has long excited the imagination of pathologists. For many years the reticulum cell was, by popular consensus, considered to be the primordial cell not only of Hodgkin's disease but also of the other lymphomas: "A group of diseases of the reticulum exists in which proliferation is possible into one or several of the possible cell progeny" (Pullinger, 1932) (7). Thus the relationship of Hodgkin's disease with other lymphomas has at times been considered close ("I join Warthin, Ginsberg, Herbut et al and others who regard all tumors of lymphoid tissue as related variants of one disease" (Willis, 1948))or distant. In recent years the general adoption of the term 'non-Hodgkin lymphoma' reflects the current consensus of opinion that Hodgkin's disease is distinct from other lymphomas, at least in terms of cellular origin.

Nevertheless Hodgkin's disease sometimes occurs in intimate association with a variety of 'non-Hodgkin lymphomas'. Such cases fall into the general diagnostic category of composite lymphomas (1). This paper seeks to re-examine the occurrence of Hodgkin's-non-Hodgkin's composite tumors in the light of current concepts relating the different forms of lymphoma to the process of lymphocyte transformation.

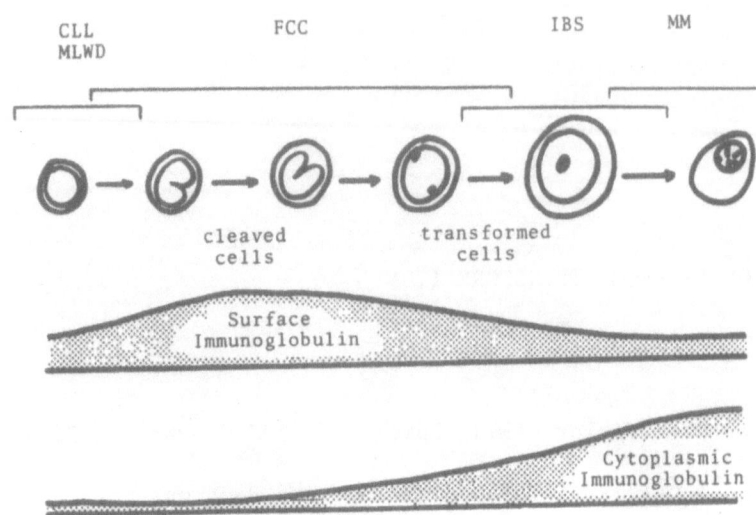

FIG. 1:   Postulated relationship of B cell neoplasms to B lymphocyte transformation and maturation to the plasma cells.   There are
radical changes in morphology and staining for surface and cytoplasmic immunoglobulin.

PATIENTS AND METHODS

     Ten cases falling into the general diagnostic category of
composite lymphoma (1) were selected from the files of the University
of Southern California-Los Angeles County Medical Center.   Cases
were classified according to Rappaport (8) and Lukes and Collins (5)
(Tab.1).   In every case formalin paraffin sections were stained by
immunoperoxidase technique described elsewhere (9) to determine the
immunoglobulin content of the neoplastic cells.   Morphological and
immunological findings were interpreted in accordance with the
postulate that the morphology and behavior of malignant lymphomas
can be related to the corresponding normal progenitor lymphocytes
(Fig.1).

DISCUSSION

     The occurence of Hodgkin's disease with a 'non-Hodgkin'
lymphoma, or the occurrence of two different histological types of
'non-Hodgkin' lymphoma, together in one tissue biopsy, has long been
recognized.   Custer proposed the term composite lymphoma for this
phenomenon (1).   This intimate association of neoplastic cell types
was thought by some to indicate a close developmental relationship
between the co-existing tumors (2).   With the passing of the reticulum cell concept, and the emergence of new classifications, this

TAB. 1: Composite Lymphoma, Immunohistological Features and Clonal Origin[1].

Histology of the Composite Tumors According to Lukes-Collins[5]	Rappaport[8]	Immunoperoxidase Staining for Cytoplasmic Ig	Interpretation of Diverse Morphologic Appearances within a Single Neo-plastic Clone
1 S cl/L n-cl FCC	PDLN/DH	Both components negative	Variable morphol-ogy of lymphocyte in FCC stage
2 S cl/L cl FCC	PDLN/DH	Both components negative	As for case 1
3 L cl FCC/MM	DH/MM	Matching mono-clonal Ig	As for case 1; in addition a small proportion mature to plasma cells
4 IBS/L cl FCC	PCPD/DH	Monoclonal Ig in PC/IBS only	As for case 3; with a high proportion of dividing cells (immunoblasts)
5 PC/IBS	PC/DH	Monoclonal Ig in both; heavy chains differ	Clone matures to plasma cells; many dividing cells (immunoblasts in 2nd biopsy)
6 IBS/MM	DH/MM	Matching mono-clonal Ig	As for case 5
7 PC/IBS	PC/DH	Monoclonal Ig in PC only	As for case 5
8 PC/IBS/HDNS	PC/DH/HDNS	Matching mono-clonal Ig inclu-ding Reed-Stern-berg cells	As for case 5; in addition Hodgkin/Reed-Sternberg cell component may be lymphocyte derived
9 L cl FCC/HDMC	DH/HDMC	Matching Ig not clearly mono-clonal	As for case 1; in addition Reed-Sternberg cells may be lymphocyte derived
10 IBS/HDNS	DH/HDNS	Both components negative	Clone shows a high proportion of lymphocytes in dividing phase (im-munoblasts); in addition Hodgkin/Reed-Sternberg cells may be lymphocyte derived

[1]   See figure 1 for diagramatic representation of variations in morphologic expression of the lymphocyte.

LN = lymph node;   BM = bone marrow;   Ig = immunoglobulin;   FCC = follicular center cell lymphoma;   S cl = small cleaved;   L cl = large cleaved;   L n-cl = large non-cleaved;   MM = multiple myeloma;   IBS = immunoblastic sarcoma;   PDLN = malignant lymphoma poorly differentiated lymphocytic nodular;   DH = malignant lymphoma diffuse histiocytic;   HDNS, HDMC = Hodgkin's disease, nodular sclerosis and mixed cellularity;   PC = plasmacytoma, extramedullary plasmacytic neoplasm occurring in absence of myeloma.

---

idea soon fell into disrepute. For example, most of the reported cases of composite lymphoma consist of two types of 'non-Hodgkin' lymphoma (usually malignant lymphoma lymphocytic poorly differentiated and malignant lymphoma histiocytic) (4). According to the Rappaport scheme (8) these two tumor types are considered to be of separate lineage (lymphocytic and histiocytic).

More recently the development of an increased understanding of lymphocyte morphology and function has produced yet a further reappraisal of the nature of the cells comprising some of the lymphomas. It now seems probable that at least some so-called composite lymphomas are composed of closely related neoplasms with a common cellular origin (10,12). Thus the various histological subtypes of follicular center cell lymphomas (5) are now considered to represent extreme morphologic variation of a single neoplastic cell type, the lymphocyte, rather than entirely distinct neoplasms, each of separate origin. This belief is central to the concept summarized in Figure 1, that the various histological types of lymphoma can be related to the different functional and morphological expressions of the lymphocyte during transformation. The essence of this scheme has been confirmed by immunologic studies from several laboratories (6, 10). Immunohistological studies have also established a common clonal origin for some plasma cell neoplasms (cases of multiple myeloma and plasmacytoma) and immunoblastic sarcomas of B cell type, occurring in the same patient (11). Similarly chronic lymphocytic leukemia and follicular center cell lymphoma may evolve to malignant large cell lymphoma, formerly classified as reticulum cell sarcoma or malignant lymphoma histiocytic (10), but here designated as immunoblastic sarcoma, emphasizing a common developmental relationship of these cell types (Fig.1).

The occurrence of any two of the above B cell neoplasms (Fig.1) in a single patient might then be considered to represent the morphologic extremes of a single neoplasm, rather than a true composite

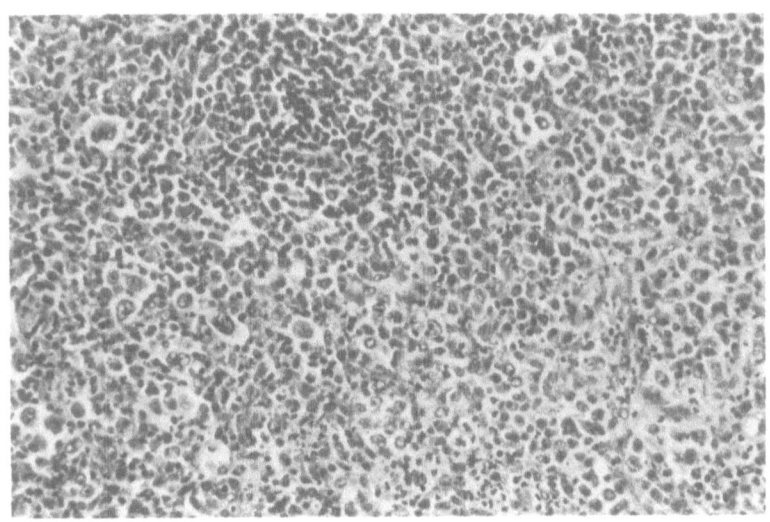

FIG. 2:   Case 8, 'composite lymphoma', Hodgkin's disease (left),
immunoblastic sarcoma (center), plasmacytoma (right). Patient had
several recurrences of classical nodular sclerosing Hodgkin's
disease, plus a Coombs positive hemolytic anemia and a monoclonal
IgG κ serum protein.

lymphoma composed of two or more neoplasms of separate cellular
origin. The immunohistological studies performed on the seven 'non-
Hodgkin composite lymphomas' reported here support this contention,
for the observed patterns of immunoglobulin staining in the diverse
histologic components were in accordance with those anticipated
(Fig.1) in five of the seven cases. In a sixth case the heavy chain
components differed (plasmacytoma κγ, IBS α only), but again this
finding is not without precedent in the normal B cell series (3).

Thus the original concept of Custer (2) that the intimate
association of two lymphomas in a composite lymphoma might be indicative of a common cellular origin appears to be valid for many so-
called composite lymphomas composed of diverse histological types of
B cell lymphoma.

The question remains as to whether the concurrence of Hodgkin's
disease and B cell lymphomas carries a similar implication. The
origin of the neoplastic cell of Hodgkin's disease, the Hodgkin or
Reed-Sternberg cell, remains uncertain, and indeed controversial (10).
Immunoperoxidase studies of the pattern of immunoglobulin staining
in the three Hodgkin-non-Hodgkin composite lymphomas reported here
are thus of interest. In case 10 neither the immunoblastic nor the

Hodgkin-Reed-Sternberg cell components contained detectable immunoglobulin, which of course proves nothing. In case 9 both the large
cleaved and the Hodgkin-Reed-Sternberg cell components contained
cytoplasmic immunoglobulin, but this was not clearly monoclonal,
and the interpretation was thus uncertain. In case 8 (Fig.2), however, the pattern of immunoglobulin staining was quite remarkable
in that all three morphologic components (plasmacytoma, immunoblastic sarcoma, and Hodgkin-Reed-Sternberg cells) showed identical
monoclonal immunoglobulin staining. By current concept this is
indicative of a common cellular origin for these three neoplastic
cell types, and suggests that at least some cases of Hodgkin's
disease might be B cell derived, thus having a closer relationship
to the non-Hodgkin lymphomas than currently envisioned.

REFERENCES

1.   Custer, R.P. Proc. 2nd National Cancer Conference. Vol. I.
     Amer. Cancer Soc.p.556 (1954).
2.   Custer, R.P., Bernhard, W.G. Am. J. Med. Sci. 216 (1948) 625.
3.   Gearhardt, P.J., Sigal, N.H., Klinman, N.R. Proc. Natl. Acad.
     Sci. 72 (1975) 1707.
4.   Kim, H., Dorman, R.F. Cancer 33 (1974) 657.
5.   Lukes, R.J., Collins, R.D. Br. J. Cancer 31 Suppl.2 (1975) 1.
6.   Lukes, R.J., Taylor, C.R., Parker, J.W., Lincoln, T.L., Patten-
     gale, P.K., Tindle, B.H. Am. J. Path. 90 (1978) 461.
7.   Pullinger, B.D. Histology and Histogenesis. Rose Research in
     Lymphadenoma. Bristol, John Wright, p. 117 (1932).
8.   Rappaport, H. Atlas of Tumor Pathology. Sect. 3, Fasc. 8.
     A.F.I.P., Washington (1966).
9.   Taylor, C.R. Arch. Pathol. Lab. Med. 102 (1978) 113.
10. Taylor, C.R. Hodgkin's Disease and the Lymphomas. Annual
     Research Reviews, Vol. I & II. Montreal, Eden Press; Edinburgh/
     London, Churchill, Longman, Livingstone (1977) Vol. I, (1978)
     Vol. II.
11. Taylor, C.R., Mason, D.Y. Clin. Exp. Immunol. 18 (1974) 417.
12. van den Tweel, J.G., Lukes, R.J., Taylor, C.R. Pathophysiology
     of lymphocyte transformation (submitted for publication).
13. Willis, R.A. Pathology of Tumors. London, Butterworths (1948).

DEMONSTRATION OF INTRACYTOPLASMIC IMMUNOGLOBULIN, LYSOZYME, AND ALBUMIN AND ISOELECTRIC FOCUSING PATTERN OF TISSUE IMMUNOGLOBULIN IN SO-CALLED RETICULUM CELL SARCOMA (IMMUNOBLASTIC OR LARGE CELL LYMPHOMA)

M. Burkert, H. Stein, H. Bouman and K. Lennert

Institute of Pathology and Institute of Biochemistry
University of Kiel, 2300 Kiel, W. Germany

INTRODUCTION

In 1930, Roulet (14) separated a tumor of large cell type from other lymphomas and believed it was derived from reticulum cells. This concept was generally accepted. Accordingly, the tumor was called retothelsarcoma, or more often reticulum cell sarcoma. Rappaport (13) also agreed to Roulet's concept in principle and introduced the term "malignant lymphoma, histiocytic". That was before it was discovered that lymphocytes can transform into blast cells.

The detection of lymphocyte markers in recent years has made it possible to examine the concept of histiocytic or reticulocytic origin of large cell malignant lymphomas. Nevertheless, immunologic studies (1,3,4,6,7,12,16,17,20,21) have so far not led to general agreement on the incidence of so-called reticulum cell sarcomas that are actually derived from macrophages and of those derived from lymphoid cells. A comparison of the various histologic descriptions given in the literature reveals a large number of discrepancies. Some of these are probably due to the inclusion of different types of tumors in different workers' studies. One morphologic feature shared by all descriptions is the large size of the tumor cells. Tab. 1 is a list of large cell neoplasms that are often confused with each other, especially when only hematoxylin-eosin-stained sections are examined. Like our earlier studies (15,16), the present investigation deals only with the large cell neoplasms whose cells resemble reactive immunoblasts in Giemsa-stained sections.

TAB.1:   Large cell tumors that resemble malignant lymphoma,
immunoblastic.

Malignant lymphoma, centroblastic
True reticulosarcoma (malignant lymphoma, histiocytic)
Malignant reticulosis
Hodgkin's sarcoma (Hodgkin's disease, lymphocyte
        depleted type)
Myelosarcoma (granulocytic sarcoma)
Metastasis of anaplastic carcinoma, especially naso-
        pharyngeal carcinoma (lymphoepithelioma)

The aim of this study was to determine how many of the immunoblast-like large cell lymphomas in our series can be identified as
B-cell-derived and how many as histiocyte-derived neoplasms by
examining a relatively large number of cases and using cytoplasmic
immunoglobulin (cIg) as a marker of B cells and lysozyme as a
marker of histiocytes.

MATERIALS AND METHODS

Fifty routinely formalin-fixed and paraffin-embedded lymph node
biopsies were examined. All were histologically classified in
Giemsa-stained sections as large cell lymphoma or malignant lymphoma,
immunoblastic according to the criteria previously described in
detail (8,9). For the detection of cytoplasmic immunoglobulin (cIg),
lysozyme, and albumin we applied the triple-layer antibody enzyme
bridge method, i.e., the so-called PAP or immunoperoxidase technique
developed by Sternberger et al. (18) and modified by Taylor and
Burns (21). In five cases saline extracts of biopsy tissue and the
corresponding sera were subjected to isoelectric focusing (IEF).
The plates were developed with radioiodine-labeled antibodies
directed against one light chain type or against mu chains (2).

RESULTS

The data obtained with the immunoperoxidase technique are
summarized in Tab. 2. We were not able to detect either cytoplasmic
lysozyme or cytoplasmic albumin in any of the 50 large cell lymphomas.
In 26 out of the 50 cases, or 52%, however, we found cIg in the tumor
cells. Nineteen out of the 50 cases showed a monotypic pattern, with
restriction to one light chain. Kappa light chains could be demon-

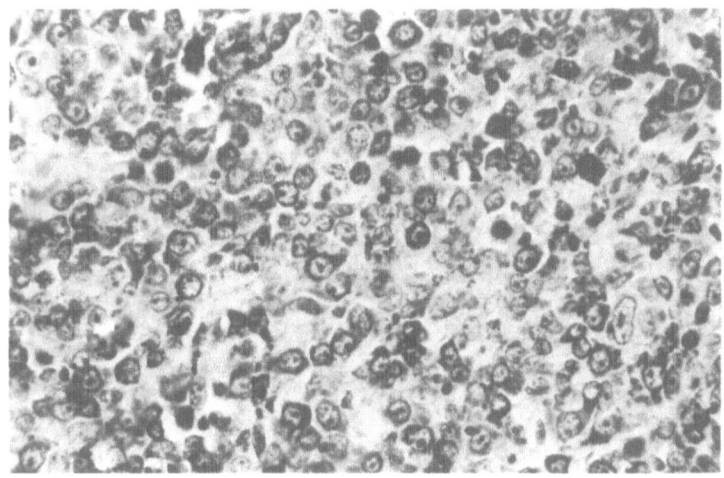

FIG. 1:   Large cell lymphoma (malignant lymphoma, immunoblastic) immunostained for cytoplasmic kappa chains.   Numerous tumor cells are positive.   Counterstaining with hemalum. X 300.

strated about twice as often as lambda chains. Heavy chains were not stainable in the tumor cells from all cases except for one. In the exceptional case we found cytoplasmic IgM/kappa.

In five of the monotypic cases we subjected saline tumor tissue extracts and corresponding sera to IEF.   In contrast to the diffuse, polyclonal IEF pattern of the patients' sera, the tumor tissue extracts revealed a monoclonal IEF pattern showing two to ten bands (2).

In seven out of 50 cases both kappa and lambda chain-positive tumor cells were present. In three of these bitypic cases there were no heavy chains. In the four other bitypic cases the tumor cells stained for gamma chains.

By studying serial sections and by double labeling by means of the method of Nakane (10), we determined that at least some of the tumor cells contained kappa and lambda chains simultaneously.

DISCUSSION

In 19 out of 50 cases, i.e. 38% of the large cell malignant lymphomas whose cells resembled reactive immunoblasts in morphology with Giemsa staining, the tumor cells stained for only one light chain. The Ig chains extracted from biopsy tissue from five of these cases revealed a monoclonal IEF pattern. These findings are

TAB. 2:   Intracytoplasmic immunoglobulin, lysozyme, and albumin in
50 cases of so-called reticulosarcoma (large cell lymphoma) demonstrated by the immunoperoxidase technique

	Incidence	(%)
Immunoglobulin	26/50	52
Monotypic (restriction to		
one light chain)	19/50	38
kappa	13/50	26
lambda	6/50	12
Bitypic (presence of both		
light chains)	7/50	14
without heavy chains	3/50	6
with one heavy chain (IgG)	4/50	8
Lysozyme	0/50	0
Albumin	0/9	0

strong evidence of synthesis of the Ig chains by the tumor cells
and thus of a B-cell origin.

In seven out of 50, or 14% of the cases both light chains were
detected in the tumor cells. It is difficult to explain this
bitypic staining, however, since the presence of kappa and lambda
chain-positive tumor cells in the same section conflicts with the
concept of monoclonality and the simultaneous presence of kappa
and lambda chains in the same tumor cells conflicts with the concept
of allelic exclusion (5). Therefore, one might assume that the
simultaneous prescence of kappa and lambda chains reflects phagocytosis rather than synthesis of Ig by the tumor cells. To check
this alternative, sections from all 50 cases were subjected to
immunostaining for lysozyme. We always found lysozyme in neutrophils,
monocytes, and histiocytes, but never in tumor cells. This finding
makes the histiocytic origin of the bitypic cases at least unlikely.

Another possible explanation for the presence of both kappa
and lambda chains in the tumor cells is passive absorption of the
chains from the serum. If this were the case, then the cells of
the bitypic cIg-positive tumors should have also absorbed other
proteins, such as albumin, which are present in large amounts in
the serum. It has been shown that Hodgkin and Sternberg-Reed cells
of some cases of Hodgkin's lymphoma contain easily detectable amounts
of albumin in their cytoplasm (11). In contrast, the tumor cells of

the present tumor group were consistently negative when anti-albumin serum reabsorbed with purified Ig chains was used. The serum in blood vessels on the sections, on the other hand, showed a strongly positive staining for albumin, indicating the specific activity of the antisera and the preserved antigenicity of albumin on the sections.

The data presented here may be summarized as follows: (a) 38% of all immunoblast-like large cell lymphomas we studied were Ig producers and thus of B-cell origin. (b) In 14% of the cases the tumor cells showed a bitypic staining pattern, as do most Hodgkin and Sternberg-Reed cells. The significance of this finding could not be clarified. (c) In none of the 50 cases we studied did we obtain evidence of a histiocytic nature of the tumor cells, which suggests that true histiocytic lymphomas usually do not occur among large cell lymphomas whose cells resemble reactive immunoblasts in morphology.

REFERENCES

1. Aisenberg, A.C., Long, J.C., Amer. J. Med. 58 (1975) 300.
2. Bouman, H., Lüsebrink, W.D., Havsteen, B., Stein, H., FEBS Lett 64 (1976) 201.
3. Braylan, R.C., Jaffe, E.S., Mann, R.B., Frank, M.M., Berard, C.W.,in:Haematology and Blood Transfusion, Vol. 20, pp. 47-52. Thierfelder, S., Rodt, H., Thiel, E., Eds., Berlin-Heidelberg-New York: Springer (1977).
4. Brouet, J.C., Preud'Homme, J.L., Flandrin, G., Chelloul, N., Seligmann, M., J. nat. Cancer Inst. 56 (1976) 631.
5. Fröland, S.S., Natvig, J.B., J. exp. Med. 136 (1972) 409.
6. Garvin, A.J., Spicer, S.S., McKeever, P.E., Amer. J. Path. 82 (1976) 457.
7. Krüger, G., Uhlmann, C., Hellriegel, K.P., Sesterhenn, K., Samii, H., Fischer, R., Wustrow, F., Gross, R., in: Hämatologie und Bluttransfusion, Vol. 18, pp. 17-31. Löffler, H., Ed., München:Lehmanns (1976).
8. Lennert, K., Mohri, N., Stein, H., Kaiserling, E., Brit. J. Haemat. 31 (Suppl.) (1975) 193.
9. Lennert, K., Stein, H., Kaiserling, E., Brit. J. Cancer 31 Suppl.II (1975) 29.
10. Nakane, P.K., J. Histochem. Cytochem. 16 (1968) 557.
11. Papadimitriou, C.S., Stein, H., Lennert, K., Int. J. Cancer 21 (1978) 531.

12. Ralph, P., Moore, M.A.S., Nilsson, K., J. Exp. Med. 143 (1976) 1528.
13. Rappaport, H., Atlas of Tumor Pathology, Sect.3, Fasc.8, Washington, D.C., Armed Forces Inst. of Pathology (1966).
14. Roulet, F., Virchows Arch. path. Anat. 277 (1930) 15.
15. Stein, H., Bouman, H., Lennert, K., Fuchs, J., Havsteen, B.,in: Haematology and Blood Transfusion, Vol. 20, pp. 315-327. Thierfelder, S., Rodt, H., Thiel, E., Eds., Berlin-Heidelberg-New York: Springer (1977).
16. Stein, H., Kaiserling, E., Lennert, K., Virchows Arch. A 364 (1974) 51.
17. Stein, H., Lennert, K., Parwaresch, M.R., Lancet (1972) II, pp.855-857.
18. Sternberger, L.A., Hardy, Jr., P.H., Cuculis, J.J., Meyer, H.G., J. Histochem. Cytochem. 18 (1970) 315.
19. Taylor, C.R., Lancet (1974) II, pp. 802-807.
20. Taylor, C.R., Hodgkin's disease and the lymphomas. Montreal: Eden Press (1976).
21. Taylor, C.R., Burns, J., J. clin.Path. 27 (1974) 14.

ACKNOWLEDGEMENTS

This work was supported by the Deutsche Forschungsgemeinschaft, SFB111/C7, C3 and D2.

ALKALINE PHOSPHATASE POSITIVE LYMPHOMAS AND LYMPHOCYTES

S. Poppema[1], J.D. Elema[1] and M.R. Halie[2]

From the departments of Pathology[1] and Medicine[2]
(Division of Haematology), University of Groningen
The Netherlands

During an enzymehistochemical and immunological study of 50
cases of non-Hodgkin lymphoma 5 appeared to have alkaline phosphatase
staining of the neoplastic cell membranes (Fig.1). According to
Rappaport these should be classified as lymphocytic, poorly differentiated. Some had a mixed character with small, intermediate and
large lymphocytes (Fig.2) and a vaguely nodular structure. Others
were diffuse and consisted nearly entirely of large lymphocytes with
many mitoses and a starry sky pattern (Fig.3). These lymphomas are
not prepresented in the classification of Lukes and in the Kiel
classification. Probably they should be classified as large cleaved
cells or as lymphoblastic "unclassified".

All 5 patients had marked splenomegaly and leukemic dissemination,
although in 3 cases less than 10.000 leukocytes/mm^3 were counted. 4
patients had lymphadenopathy. In all cases strong membrane immunofluorescence was found for IgM with monoclonal kappa or lambda light
chains on the lymphocytes in the tumor cell suspensions as well as in
peripheral blood. Furthermore C3 receptors could be identified by
means of EAC rosettes on frozen sections. EA, E sheep and E mouse
rosettes were not formed by these lymphoma cells (Tab.1). The only
other cases with alkaline phosphatase positive membranes were 2 out
of 4 Burkitt type lymphomas. However, in contrast to the group of
lymphomas presented here, these did not have demonstrable C3 receptors
in frozen sections.

Alkaline phosphatase positive lymphomas were described by Lennert
(1961) and by Nanba (1977). The 7 cases described by Nanba seem to
have the same morphological and immunological characteristics as our
5 cases. From these results it is quite clear that the alkaline

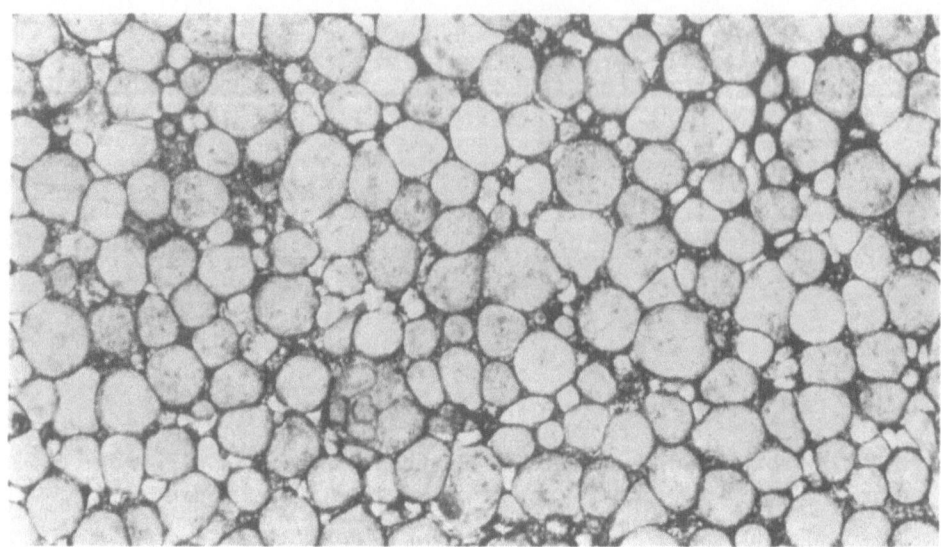

FIG. 1:   Imprint of lymph node stained for alkaline phosphatase.
Note that all tumor cells are stained positive (x 500).

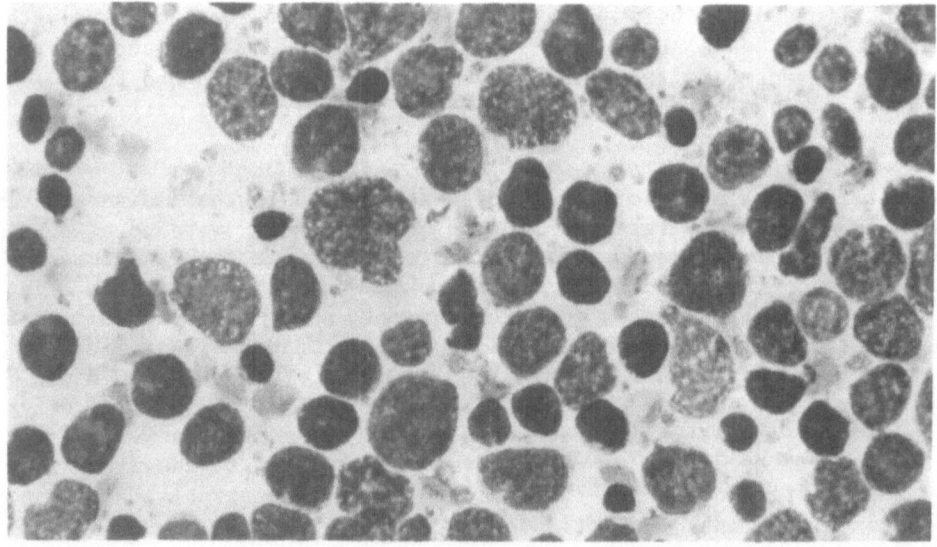

FIG. 2:   Imprint of lymph node showing small, intermediate and large
lymphocytes with sometimes irregular nuclei (x 800, M.G.G.).

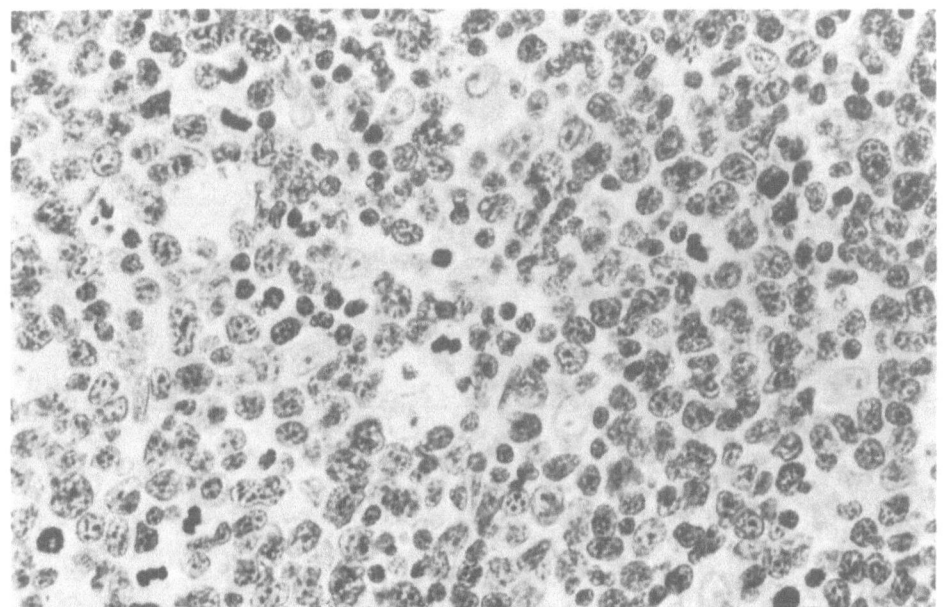

FIG. 3:   Diffuse proliferation of large lymphocytes with irregular
nuclei, many mitoses and several histiocytes (x 500, H&E).

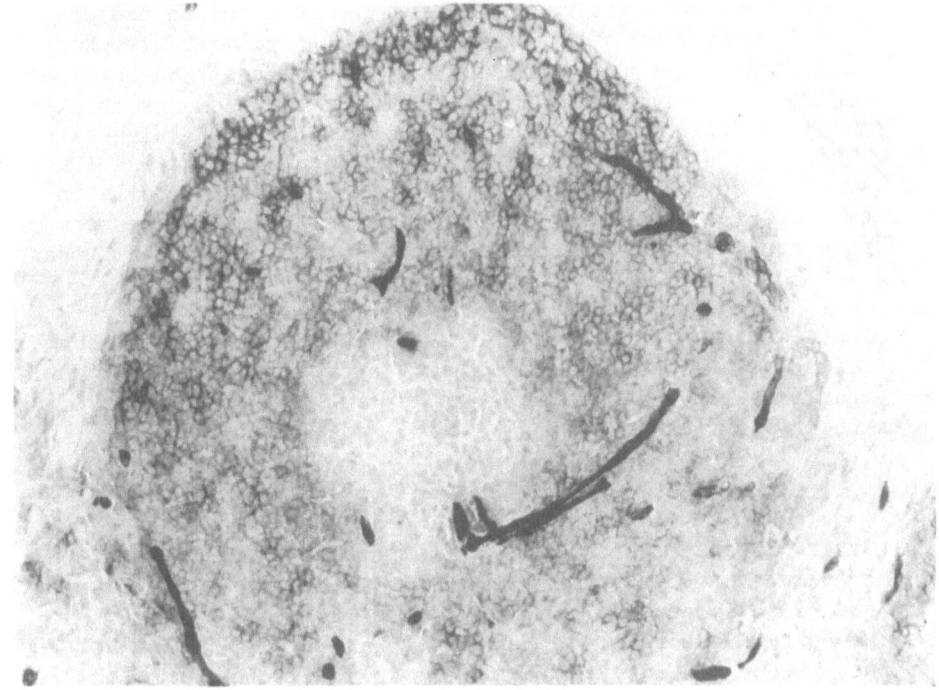

FIG. 4:   Alkaline phosphatase staining of follicle with beginning
germinal center reaction (x 200).

TAB. 1:   Immunologic markers of alkaline phosphatase positive
lymphomas.

ALKALINE PHOSPHATASE POSITIVE LYMPHOMA

membrane Ig	strong IgM with weak IgD or IgG
C3b receptor	?
C3d receptor	++
Fc receptor	−
E sheep receptor	−
E mouse receptor	−
cytoplasmic Ig	−

---

phosphatase positive lymphomas, including the positive Burkitt type
lymphomas are of B-cell origin.

In normal human lymph nodes alkaline phosphatase positive cells
can be found in primary follicles and in lower numbers in the mantle
zone of secondary follicles. These positive staining lymphocytes
should be carefully distinguished from strongly staining "reticu-
lumcells" in the paracortex and especially around the follicles. We
have never observed positive staining cells in germinal centers (Fig.
4). This localization of alkaline phosphatase positive lymphocytes
in normal lymph nodes is in accordance with a B-cell character of
these cells. In normal peripheral blood very low numbers of alkaline
phosphatase positive lymphocytes can be detected. The highest number
of positive cells in 5 normal lymphocyte concentrations was 1 per
1000 lymphocytes. The relatively high number of these cells in
primary follicles, the absence in germinal centers and the very low
number in peripheral blood is compatible with a virginal B lymphocyte
character.

The alkaline phosphatase positive lymphomas could represent a
maturation arrest before the germinal center reaction. The nodular
character in some of these lymphomas may indicate the preservation
of homing properties.

REFERENCES

1.   Gérard-Marchant, R., Hamlin, I., Lennert, K., Rilke, F.,
      Stansfeld, A.G., van Unnik, J.A.M.,: Classification of non-
      Hodgkin's lymphomas. Lancet ii:406, (1974).
2.   Lennert, K., Löffler, H., Leder, L.D.: Ferment histochemische
      Untersuchungen des Lymphknotens. I:Alkalische Phosphatase in
      Schnitt und Ausstrich. Virchows Arch. Path. Anat. 334 (1961)
      399.

3. Lukes, R.J., Collins, R.D.: Immunologic characterization of
    human malignant lymphomas. Cancer 34 (1974) 1488.

4. Nanba, K., Jaffe, E.S., Braylan, R.C., Soban, E.J., Berard,
    C.W.: Alkaline Phosphatase-positive malignant lymphoma. Am.
    J. Clin. Path. 68 (1977) 535.

5. Rappaport, H.: Tumors of the hematopoietic system. Atlas of
    Tumor Pathology, sect. 3, fasc. 8. Washington, D.C., A.F.I.P.,
    (1966).

DEFINITION OF GERMINAL CENTER CELL-DERIVED LYMPHOMAS BY ANALYSIS OF COMPLEMENT RECEPTOR SUBTYPES AND MORPHOLOGICAL CRITERIA

H. Stein, G. Tolksdorf and K. Lennert

Institute of Pathology

University of Kiel, 2300 Kiel, W. Germany

Previous studies by Lukes and Collins (8,9) and our own group (7,13) suggested that a large proportion of malignant non-Hodgkin's lymphomas are derived from germinal center cells (GCC) and there are different types of lymphomas in this group. In extension of our earlier studies, we compared the morphological and various immunological features of GCC and cells of malignant lymphomas of the B-cell type.

In reactive germinal centers two main types of lymphoid cells can be distinguished: (a) large cells with a large round nucleus poor in chromatin and with membrane-associated, medium-sized nucleoli and sparse intensely basophilic cytoplasm. These cells are called centroblasts. (b) Smaller cells with cleaved nuclei, small nucleoli, and pale cytoplasm, called centrocytes. These two types of GCC are outlined in Figure 1a.

FOLLICULAR HYPERPLASIA

Immunological studies of cells from lymphatic tissue rich in germinal centers (spec., hyperplastic tonsils) revealed that GCC bear surface immunoglobulin (SIg) and express complement receptors (CR) for both C3b and C3d (Fig.1a). We demonstrated the simultaneous presence of C3b receptors and C3d receptors on (a) suspended GCC by means of a rosette test and identified the GCC by cytology, and (b) frozen sections by means of the EAC adherence assay. The latter assay showed that the GCC and follicular mantle cells have both CR subtypes, whereas the parafollicular cells and, in many instances,

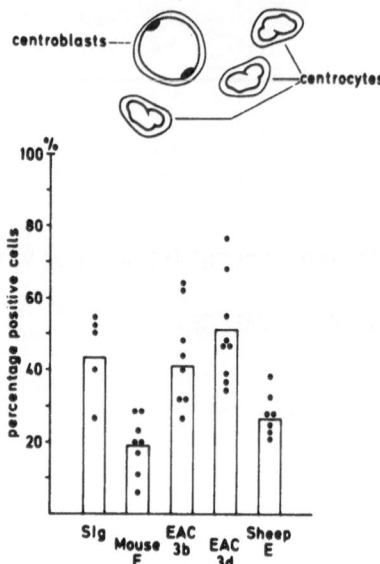

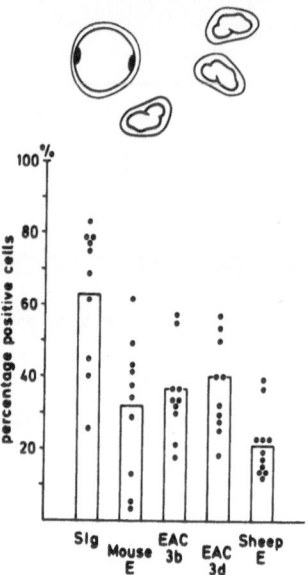

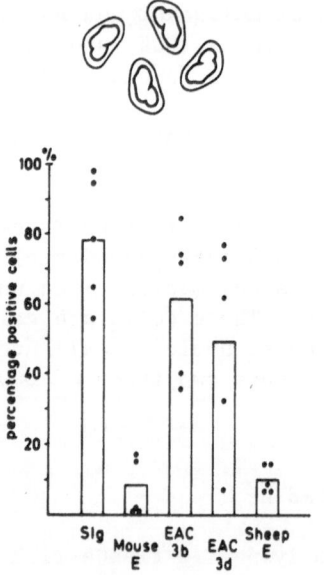

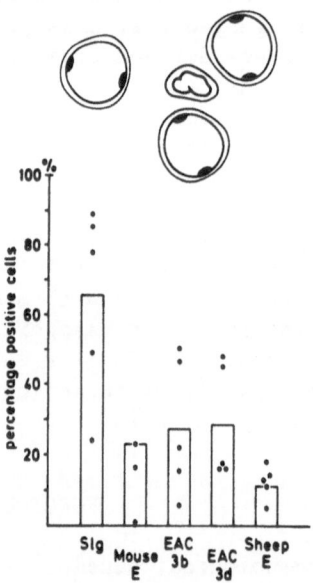

FIG. 1 a – d: Symbolic representation of the characteristic cells
and surface markers in (a) follicular hyperplasia, (b) centroblastic/
centrocytic lymphoma, (c) centrocytic lymphoma, and (d) centroblastic
lymphoma.   The immunological methods are described in detail elsewhere (14).   The IgM-EAC3b and IgM-EAC3d were prepared and tested
according to the procedures described by Bokisch and Sobel (1) and
Ross and Polley (12).   Height of columns is the mean value.

a large number of the interfollicular cells express the C3b receptor and lack the C3d receptor (15).

As shown in Figure 1a, 20% of the cells present in GCC-rich lymphatic tissue are capable of binding mouse erythrocytes. The average T-cell content was approximately 30%.

Among the malignant lymphomas of B-cell type, three types of lymphoma could be distinguished that show features of GCC.

CENTROBLASTIC/CENTROCYTIC LYMPHOMA
(FOLLICULAR LYMPHOMA)

The first type is follicular or nodular lymphoma. Until recently, many pathologists (cf., 11) did not regard a follicular or nodular growth pattern as corresponding to reactive follicles, but as merely an architectural variant that could be seen in any of the histological types of malignant lymphoma. Lennert, however, pointed out in several papers (4,5) the similarity between the cells of follicular lymphoma and germinal centers. Immunological studies (3,13) in recent years have also shown a great similarity in immunological markers between follicular lymphoma and germinal centers.

As outlined in Figure 1b, follicular lymphoma consistently contains both types of GCC, i.e., centroblasts and centrocytes, whereby the centrocytes always predominate in number. Since only the cytological composition, and not the growth pattern, proved to be a constant feature (the follicular growth pattern is missing in 5% of cases), the term "centroblastic/centrocytic lymphoma" was proposed (6) to replace "follicular lymphoma". The strongest argument for the close relationship between centroblastic/centrocytic lymphoma cells and reactive GCC comes from the finding that centroblastic/centrocytic lymphoma cells bear CR for both C3b and C3d, like GCC (15). The CR subtypes are not only simultaneously expressed on both centroblastic/centrocytic lymphoma cells and GCC, but they are also distributed in centroblastic/centrocytic lymphoma in the same manner as in follicular hyperplasia. As recently reported (15), EAC3d adheres to frozen sections from centroblastic/centrocytic lymphoma only in the central area of the neoplastic nodules, whereas EAC3b adheres not only to the central areas, but also to the parafollicular zone and often between the neoplastic follicles, although less densely.

Comparing other immunological markers, one finds T-cells in centroblastic/centrocytic lymphoma in a percentage similar to that in follicular hyperplasia. The proportion of mouse erythrocyte rosette-forming cells, on the other hand, was significantly higher in centroblastic/centrocytic lymphoma than in follicular hyperplasia, but clearly lower than in chronic lymphocytic leukemia (CLL) of the B-cell type.

CENTROCYTIC LYMPHOMA

We called the second type of malignant lymphoma that we believed to be derived from GCC "centrocytic lymphoma", because it is composed only of cells resembling reactive centrocytes (Fig.1c). Centroblasts are consistently absent. Beside their similar morphology, the close relationship between the tumor cells and the small GCC is supported by the demonstration of both CR subtypes on the centrocyte-like tumor cells.

The separation of centrocytic lymphoma from centroblastic/centrocytic lymphoma is justified not only by the differences in cytology, but also by the following immunological findings. (a) Centrocytic lymphoma contains no, or only a few cells capable of binding mouse erythrocytes. (b) In centrocytic lymphoma there are merely a few T-cells. Furthermore, the survival time of patients with centrocytic lymphoma is much shorter than that of patients with centroblastic/centrocytic lymphoma (2).

Centrocytic lymphoma cells differ immunologically from CLL cells by their higher density of SIg, the presence of both CR subtypes (CLL cells usually have only C3d receptors), and their inability to bind mouse erythrocytes.

CENTROBLASTIC LYMPHOMA

The third malignant lymphoma that we regard as a GCC-derived tumor is characterized by a predominance of cells resembling centroblasts, as outlined in Figure 1d. The assumption of a close relationship between this tumor and GCC is based not only on similarity in morphology, but also (a) on the observation that centroblastic lymphoma often supervenes on centroblastic/centrocytic lymphoma and (b) on the demonstration of both CR subtypes on the tumor cells. In centroblastic lymphoma, however, the expression of surface markers proved to be less constant than in the other types of GCC lymphoma. Centroblastic lymphoma has the poorest prognosis among the types of lymphoma discussed here. We have therefore grouped it with the malignant lymphomas of high-grade malignancy. An inconsistent expression of surface markers was also found in other malignant lymphomas of high-grade malignancy and thus appears to be a characteristic feature of high-grade malignant lymphomas.

OTHER MALIGNANT LYMPHOMAS PROBABLY
RELATED TO GERMINAL CENTER CELLS

A majority of the lymphoplasmacytic/-cytoid lymphomas (LP immunocytoma) appear to be related to GCC or their derivatives, since these tumors often contain cells resembling centrocytes and centroblasts.

The relationship to GCC conforms with the demonstration of both CR subtypes on the tumor cells. The remaining LP immunocytomas have a surface marker constellation resembling that of CLL of the B-cell type.

Lymphomas that are probably derived from cells of primary follicles or lymphoid cuffs are not included in the concept of classification of GCC-derived lymphomas presented here. The existence of such lymphomas was recently indicated by the demonstration of alkaline phosphatase in cells of primary follicles and mantle zones and in lymphoma cells that resembled' cells of primary follicles and mantle zones in cytology (10).

REFERENCES

1. Bokisch, V.A., Sobel, A.T. J. exp. Med. 140 (1974) 1336.
2. Brittinger, G., Bartels, H., Bremer, K., Dühmke, E., Gunzer, U., König, E., Stein, H. (Kieler Lymphomgruppe), in: Hämatologie und Bluttransfusion, Vol. 18, pp. 211-223. Löffler, H. Ed., München: Lehmanns (1976).
3. Jaffe, E.S., Shevach, E.M., Frank, M.M., Berard, C.W., Green, I. New Engl. J. Med. 290 (1974) 813.
4. Lennert, K. Pathologie der Halslymphknoten. Berlin-Göttingen-Heidelberg-New York: Springer (1964).
5. Lennert, K., in: GANN Monograph on Cancer Research, Vol. 15, pp. 217-231. Akazaki, K., Rappaport, H., Berard, C.W., Bennett, J.M., Ishikawa, E., Eds., Tokyo: University of Tokyo Press (1973).
6. Lennert, K., Mohri, N., Stein, H., Kaiserling, E. Brit. J. Haemat. 31 (Suppl.) (1975) 193.
7. Lennert, K., Stein, H., Kaiserling, E. Brit. J. Cancer 31 Suppl. II (1975) 29.
8. Lukes, R.J., Collins, R.D., in: GANN Monograph on Cancer Research, Vol. 15, pp. 209-215. Akazaki, K., Rappaport, H., Berard, C.W., Bennett, J.M., Ishikawa, E., Eds., Tokyo: University of Tokyo Press (1973).
9. Lukes, R.J., Collins, R.D. Brit. J. Cancer 31 Suppl. II (1975) 1.
10. Nanba, K., Jaffe, E.S., Braylan, R.C., Soban, E.J., Berard, C.W. Amer. J. clin. Path. 68 (1977) 535.
11. Rappaport, H. Atlas of Tumor Pathology, Sect. 3, Fasc. 8., Washington, D.C.: Armed Forces Inst. of Pathology (1966).
12. Ross, G.D., Polley, M.J. J. exp. Med. 141 (1975) 1163.
13. Stein, H. Immun. Infekt. 4 (1976) 52 and 95.
14. Stein, H. The immunologic and immunochemical basis for the Kiel classification, in: Malignant Lymphomas Other than Hodgkin's Disease, Lennert, K., in collaboration with Mohri, N.,Stein, H., Kaiserling, E., Müller-Hermelink, H.K., Berlin-Heidelberg-New York: Springer (1978) pp. 529-657.
15. Stein, H., Siemssen, U., Lennert, K. Brit. J. Cancer 37 (1978) 520.

SPLEEN CELL POPULATIONS IN HODGKIN'S DISEASE

A.M. Smithyman, G. Munn, B. Koziner, C.T.C. Tan and M. de Sousa

Sloan-Kettering Institute for Cancer Research, 1275 York Avenue, New York, New York 10021, U.S.A.

INTRODUCTION

Hodgkin's disease (HD) remains one of the most baffling and poorly understood of the human lymphomas. The number of theories advanced to account for the aetiology of this disease are legendary, ranging from the early attempts to line it to tuberculosis (1), to more recent searches for a viral agent (2). As regards the nature of the neoplastic cell, the last two years have seen proposals that the HD cell is a macrophage (3,4), a T cell (5), a B cell (6) and a dendritic cell (7).

In a preliminary study of the distribution of iron and the iron binding proteins, ferritin, transferrin and lactoferrin, in the spleen and lymph nodes of patients with HD, our results tended to support the view that the HD cell is a monocyte (8). In addition the results indicated that some of the typical large binucleated cells seen in HD tissues contain ferritin.

In the present paper we confirm these preliminary results and extend our observations to the analysis of cells in cell suspensions and short term cultures from HD spleens.

MATERIALS AND METHODS

Details of the procedures for preparing cell suspensions, iron staining, and immunofluorescence staining for ferritin, transferrin and lactoferrin have been published elsewhere (8).

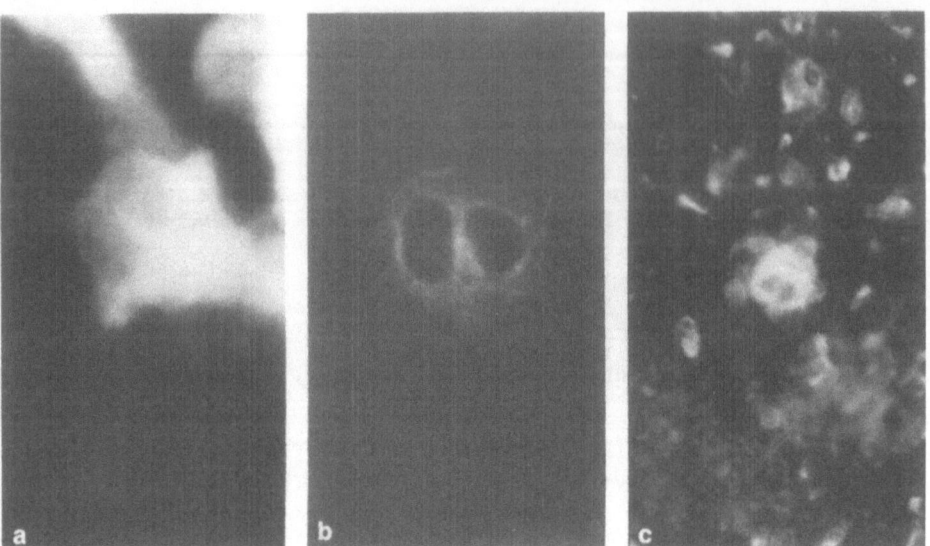

FIGS. 1 a, b and c: Fluorescence micrographs of atypical binucleate cells obtained from patients with HD and stained for ferritin (by the sandwich method).

a.   large brightly stained binucleate cell in frozen spleen section

b.   similar cell in pleural effusion fluid

c.   binucleate cell in short term spleen cell cultures

Spleen Cell Cultures

Short term spleen cell cultures were established according to the method of Treves, Feldman and Kaplan (9).

Patient Material

Splenic tissue was obtained from 12 pediatric and 6 adult patients at staging laparotomy. Of these only 4 were demonstrably involved by the disease according to conventional pathalogical classification. A total of 12 "control" spleens were obtained from patients with Gaucher's disease, chronic lymphocyte leukemia (CLL), hairy cell leukemia, acute lymphocyte leukemia (ALL) and splenic lymphoma.

RESULTS AND DISCUSSION

Spleen sections from all HD cases, whether involved or not, were found, using the fluorescent antibody technique, to contain elevated levels of ferritin compared to controls. Furthermore, in the involved spleens heavy deposits of ferritin were observed in a characteristic pattern at the periphery of the tumor nodules. These same areas stained heavily for iron, though in uninvolved tissues little iron was visible. The ferritin and iron deposits appeared to be associated with large polymorphous cells (Fig.1a) lying in the band of sclerotic tissue surrounding the tumor nodules.

These patterns were reflected in the staining of the spleen cell suspensions. We observed, as others have reported previously (10), considerable cell clustering in the HD but rarely in the control spleen cell suspensions. The cell clusters consisted of between 10 - 30 cells, formed of a large central cell surrounded by small lymphocytes and occasionally granulocytes. This large central cell, which has been identified as the Hodgkin's cell by Stuart and his colleagues (10) stained very brightly for ferritin. Large, binucleate cells staining brightly for ferritin were also observed in pleural effusions from two HD patients (Fig.1b). Similar large binucleate cells containing ferritin were found to persist, mostly as an adherent population in short term spleen cell cultures from HD patients (Fig.1c). These cells phagocytosed latex particles and iron added to the cultures (G. Munn - unpublished observations).

In view of the known capactiy of mononuclear phagocytes to synthesize large quantities of ferritin (11) the most likely candidate for the large atypical cells described would be a transformed macro-phage. This, in addition to the other observations above, supports the proposal of Long and his colleagues (3), and of Kaplan and Gartner (4), that the neoplastic cell in HD is monocytic in origin. Cells of the mononuclear phagocyte system are crucial to the body's iron cycle so the gradual expansion of a malignant clone of these cells would provide a logical explanation for the many abnormalities of iron metabolism associated with this disease, such as the lymph node siderosis (12), the failure to handle iron dextran (13), and the high serum and tissue ferritin levels (14).

Considerable control is necessary with such an interpretation, however, as staining of Reed-Sternberg cells for ferritin by the immunoperoxidase technique has proved negative (15).

REFERENCES

1.   Reed, D.M., On the pathological changes in Hodgkin's disease with special reference to its relation to tuberculosis. John Hopkins Hosp. Rep. 10 (1902) 133.

2.   Hirshaut, Y., Reagan, R.L., Perry, S., De Vita Jr., V., Barile, M.F. The search for a viral agent in Hodgkin's disease. Cancer 34 (1974) 1080.

3.   Long, J.C., Zamecnik, P.C., Aisenberg, A.C., Atkins, L. Tissue culture studies in Hodgkin's disease. Morphologic, autogenic, cell surface and enzymatic properties of cultures derived from splenic tumors. J. Exp. Med. 145 (1977) 1484.

4.   Kaplan, H.S., Gartner, S. "Sternberg-Reed" giant cells of Hodgkin's disease: Cultivation in vitro, heterotransplantation and characterization as neoplastic macrophages. Int. J. Cancer 19 (1977) 511.

5.   Order, S.E., Hellman, S. Pathogenesis of Hodgkin's disease. Lancet 1 (1972) 571.

6.   Boecker, W.R., Hossfeld, D.K., Gallmaier, W.H., Schmidt, C.G. Clonal growth of Hodgkin's cells. Nature 258 (1975) 235.

7.   Curran, R.C., Jones, E.L. Dendritic cells and B lymhpocytes in Hodgkin's disease. Lancet 2 (1977) 349.

8.   De Sousa, M., Smithyman, A., Tan, C. Suggested models in exotaxopathy in lymphoreticular malignancy. Am. J. Path 90(2) (1978) 497.

9.   Treves, A.J., Feldman, M., Kaplan, H.S. Primary cultures of human spleen macrophages in vitro. J. Immunol. Methods 13 (1976).

10.   Stuart, A.E., Williams, R.W., Habeshaw, J.A. Rosetting and other reactions of the Reed-Sternberg cell. J. Path. 122 (1977) 81.

11.   Munro, H.N., Linder, M.C. Ferritin: Structure, biosynthesis and role in iron metabolism. Physiol. Rev. 58(2) (1978) 317.

12.   Dumont, A.E., Ford, R.J., Becker, F.F. Siderosis of lymph nodes in patients with Hodgkin's disease. Cancer 38 (1976) 1247.

13.   Beamish, M.R., Jones, P.A., Trevett, D., Evans, I.H., Jacobs, A. Iron metabolism in Hodgkin's disease. Brit. J. Cancer 26 (1972) 444.

14.   Bieber, C.P., Bieber, M.M. Detection of ferritin as a circulating tumor-associated antigen in Hodgkin's disease. Natl. Cancer Inst. Monogr. 36 (1973) 147.

15.   Poppema, S. Personal communication.

ISOELECTRIC FOCUSING PATTERN OF ACID PHOSPHATASE IN NORMAL SPLENIC
TISSUE, IN THE LYSOSOMAL FRACTION OF VIABLE SPLENIC LYMPHOCYTES AND
IN CASES OF HAIRY CELL LEUKEMIA

D. Schmidt, M. Staudinger and M.R. Parwaresch

Institute of Pathology, University of Kiel

2300 Kiel, West Germany

INTRODUCTION

The activity of acid phosphatase (AcP) (E.C.3.1.3.2.) has been
claimed to show characteristic variations in different lymphoproliferative diseases (Yam and Mitus, 1968; Catovsky et al, 1974).
Recent results have established fairly specific electrophoretic
patterns of AcP - isoenzymes in some malignant lymphomas. A tartrate
resistant isoenzyme in polyacrylamide (PAA) disc electrophoresis
could be identified in cases of hairy cell leukemic by Yam et al.
(1971).

The present work represents a preliminary attempt towards an
analysis of lysosomal AcP from lymphocytes on the basis of their
different isoelectric points using isoelectric focusing (IEF) on
thin-layer PAA-slabs.

The aim of the study is to detect enzyme fractions as marker
proteins, specific to individual entities of malignant lymphomas.

MATERIALS AND METHODS

Three normal human spleens, ectomized due to trauma and two
substantially enlarged spleens in cases of hairy cell leukemia with
a tartrate resistant lymphocyte portion in blood of 18-25 per cent
were studied. Minced fresh tissue specimens were subjected to
lymphocyte separation (Bøyum, 1968).

Aliquot samples of the whole decapsulated splenic tissue were
lyophilized. Enzyme extraction was established as indicated in

589

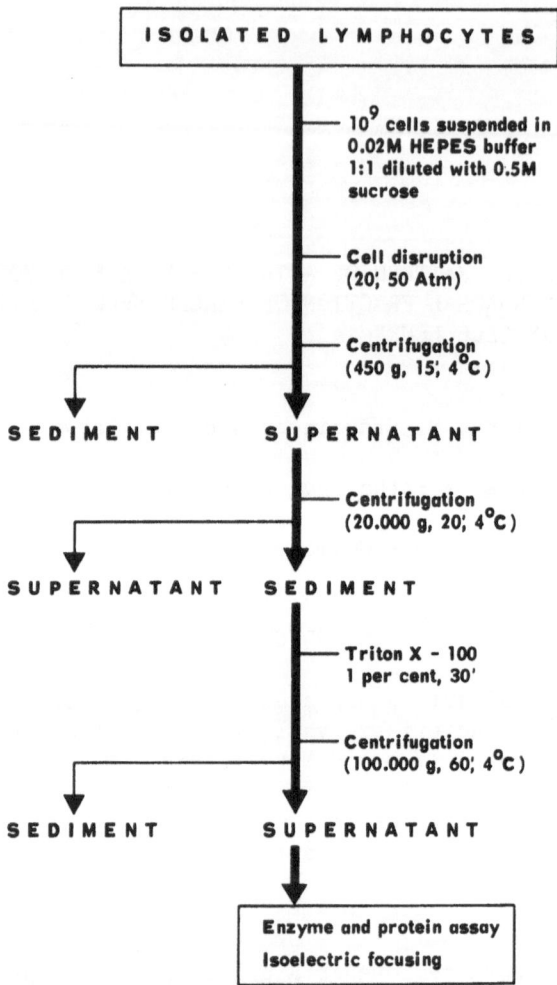

FIG. 1: Sequence of technical measures for the extraction of AcP from viable lymphocytes.

Figure 1. The 100 000 x g supernatant was used for protein (Haury, Munich) and enzyme assay (Andersch and Szczypinski, 1947; Fishman, 1953). AcP was visualized on PAA-slabs, using naphthol AS-B1 phosphoric acid and hexazotized pararosaniline (Goldberg and Barka, 1962). For each run, a minimum of eight mU enzyme per mg protein was utilized.

RESULTS AND DISCUSSION

Isoelectric focusing of AcP, gained from splenic tissue, showed twenty enzyme bands within a pH-range 6.5-3.89 (Fig.2). The band

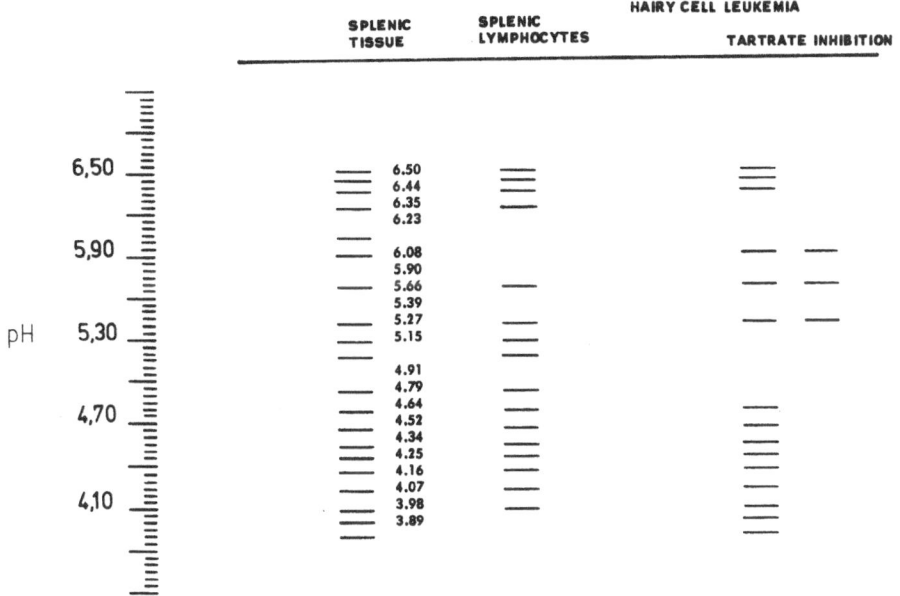

FIG. 2: AcP isoelectric focusing pattern of whole splenic tissue, purified splenic lymphocytes and hairy cell leukemia with three tartrate resistant bands.

next to the cathode was the most intensive one. In runs from separated splenic lymphocytes bands at pH-loci 6.08, 5.9, 3.98 and 3.89 were missing. In cases of hairy cell leukemia pH-loci 6.23, 6.08, 5.27, 5.15 and 4.91 were missing. On attempts to enzyme inhibition with 50 mM tartrate, all bands but those, precipitated at pH-loci 5.9, 5.66 and 5.39 disappeared. As expected, IEF-pattern of lyophilized whole splenic tissue covers a number of twenty clearly discernable bands, not all of lymphocytic origin. Bands derived from granulocytes, monocytes, platelets and from pulp cord macrophages as well as those derived from vascular and sinusoidal splenic cells are also included among this number.

Separated splenic lymphocytes showed only 16 enzyme bands, all detectable in the runs from whole splenic tissue. In the present work, an exact localization of these bands on the pH-scale could be established. It was however not possible to relate the four missing bands in lymphocyte extracts to a certain cell line. Though lymphocytes, separated from spleens thoroughly infiltrated by hairy cell leukemia, were far beyond from being free of impurities, the IEF-pattern achieved, missed five bands. After enzyme inhibition, only three bands proved resistant. All three fractions, occuring in the whole splenic tissue proved to resist tartrate inhibition only in cases of hairy cell leukemia.

The results so far achieved, appear to some extent promising and hold out the prospect of finding AcP subfractions specific to individual lymphoma entities or even to normal lymphocyte subpopulation.

REFERENCES

1. Andersch, M.A., Szczypinski, A.J., Amer. J. clin. Path. 17 (1947) 571.
2. Bøyum, A., Scand. J. clin. Lab. Invest. 21 Suppl. 97 (1968).
3. Catovsky, D., Galetto, J., Okos, A., Miliani, E., Galton, D.A.G., J. clin. Path. 27 (1974) 767.
4. Fishman, W.H., J. biol. Chem. 200 (1953) 89.
5. Goldberg, A.F., Barka, T., Nature (Lond.) 195 (1962) 297.
6. Yam, L.T., Li, C.Y., Lam, K.W., New Engl. J. Med. 284 (1971) 357.

A MOLECULAR APPROACH DELINEATING SURFACE MARKERS ON HUMAN T-LYMPHOCYTES[1]

Edwin W. Ades[2] and Charles M. Balch[3]

The Cellular Immunobiology Unit of the Tumor
Institute, Departments of Surgery and Microbiology,
The Veterans Hospital, and the Compreshensive
Cancer Center, University of Alabama in Birmingham,
Birmingham, Alabama 35294

INTRODUCTION

Isolation of human T-cell antigens is an important step in the biological characterization of T-cell subpopulations bearing these distinctive antigens. Since the outer plasma membranes of T-lymphocytes exhibit an array of protein markers, heterologous antisera raised against intact T-cells usually yield multiple antibodies against each of these cell surface constituents (1-6). These antisera can be rendered pecific for T-lymphocytes by repeated adsorptions; however, even adsorbed T-cell specific sera may be comprised of antibodies for more than one T-cell differentiation antigen (5,7). Monovalent antisera reacting with immunochemically purified surface antigens will be increasingly important for biological studies of human T-cells.

Previously, we characterized rabbit antisera raised against intact monkey thymocytes (AMT) and demonstrated its cross-reactivity with human T-cells using immunofluorescent techniques (8,9). As an initial step in T-antigen purification, we used this specific antiserum in the present study to immunochemically identify two distinct T-cell differentiation antigens (TDA) expressed on normal thymocytes, blood T-cells and three cultured T-cell lines.

MATERIALS AND METHODS

Lymphoid cell lines were maintained as suspension cultures in
RPMI 1640 supplemented with 10% heat inactivated fetal calf serum
(FCS), 0.05 mg/ml Gentamicin (Schering Corp., Kenilworth, N.J.) and
0.3 mg/ml glutamine. MOLT-3, MOLT-4 and HSB-2 are T-cell lines
(10, 11) and RAJI (PIR) is a B-cell line (12). Human peripheral
blood T-lymphocytes were prepared by E-rosette formation and
isolated on a Ficoll-Hypaque cushion as previously described (4).
Less than 1% of the cells in this preparation were surface immunoglobulin (sIg) positive. Human thymus was prepared as previously
described (4). Viability of all cell preparations was greater
than 98%.

To 1.5 x 10^7 cells in 130 μl of PBS and 100 μl of 10^{-5}M
potassium iodide were added ^{125}I - iodide (4 mCi), 50 ul of
lactoperoxidase (2.0 mg/ml) and 20 μl of 0.03% H_2O_2. The cells
were vigorously mixed, incubated at 30°C for 5 minutes and another
50 ul of lactoperoxidase and 20 ul of 0.03% H_2O_2 were added, mixed
and incubated. The reaction was stopped by adding 10 ml of chilled
PBS. The cells were centrifuged at 350 x G for 15 min. at 4°C and
washed twice with PBS.

Radioiodinated cells (1.5 x 10^7) were solubilized in 0.5%
sodium deoxycholate (DOC) in 10 mM Tris-HCl pH 8.2 containing 100 ul
of 1 mM phenylmethyl-sulphonylfluoride (PMSF) for 30 minutes on ice
with intermittent vigorous agitation. Following incubation the
lysate was centrifuged at 4,000 x G at 4°C for 15 minutes. The
supernatant was removed and reacted with adsorbed specific rabbit
anti-monkey thymocyte serum (AMT) (4,9) and co-precipitated with
formalin-fixed Staphylococcus aureus Cowan strain I (13). Conditions
for co-precipitation with S. aureus were optimized resulting in
greater than 90% of the AMT being precipitated.

Specific co-precipitates of radioiodinated cell-surface proteins
were resolved by either 5-20% gradient gel or 10 or 15% gels in a
discontinuous buffer system according to the method of Laemmli (14).
Relative mobilities (R_f) were expressed as the ratio of the length
of migration of the sample and a Bromphenol Blue dye marker. Gel
electrophoresis of molecules of known molecular weight were performed
simultaneously with the sample.

RESULTS

Two distinct T-lymphocyte antigens of approximately 25,000
daltons (p25) and 16,000 daltons (p16) were identified (Fig. 1). We
have designated these as TDA-1 and TDA-2 respectively. There was
no non-specific precipitation of membrane proteins from a human

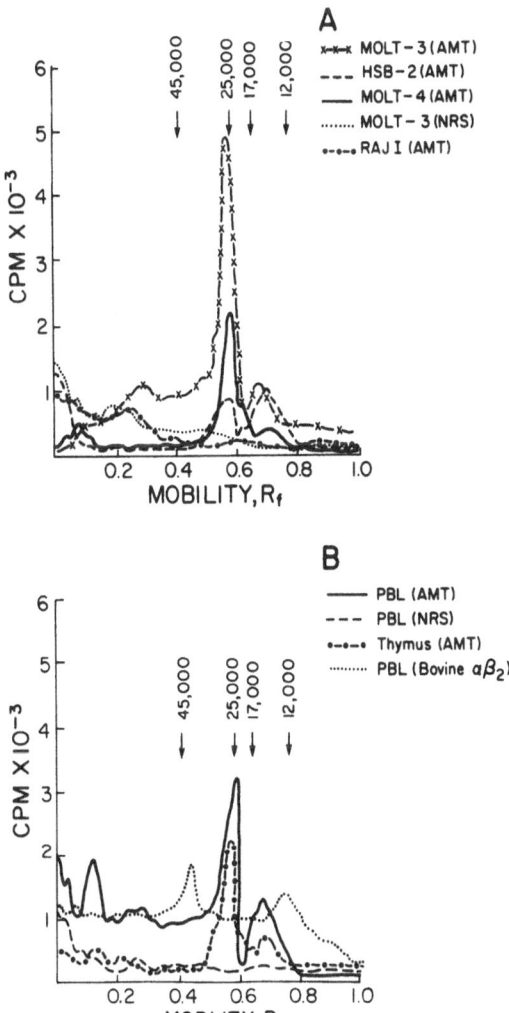

FIG. 1.   SDS-PAGE profiles of cultured lymphoblastoid cell lines
(1A) and normal lymphocytes (1B).   AMT identified two T-cell
differentiation antigens (TDA-1 and TDA-2).

B-lymphoblastoid cell line (RAJI) (Fig. 1a) using either AMT or
normal rabbit serum (NRS) and no precipitation of a T-cell line
(Fig. 1a) or adult E-rosette positive blood lymphocytes (Fig. 1b)
with NRS and Staph protein A. Immunodepletion experiments were
then performed to demonstrate that AMT was not reacting with B_2-
microglobulin. Solubilized membrane proteins reacting with bovine
anti-B_2-microglobulin (a generous gift from Dr. R. Reisfeld, Scripps
Clinic and Research Foundation, La Jolla, California) were first
removed by immunoprecipitation and the remaining proteins reacted
with AMT. The two antigen peaks reacting with AMT had different
migration profiles than B_2-microglobulin by SDS-PAGE (Fig. 1b).

Similar relative quantities of TDA-1 (p25) and TDA-2 (p16)
were detected on human peripheral T-cells and thymocytes. MOLT-4
cells contained less of the TDA-1 peak than did MOLT-3. HSB-2 cells
gave a small peak in the same location as the TDA-1 on MOLT-3 cells
and a relatively large peak of TDA-2. Adsorption of AMT with HSB-2
removed the capacity of the antiserum to precipitate TDA-2 from
MOLT-3, but did not eliminate reactivity with TDA-1 (data not shown).

DISCUSSION

Two antigen peaks with different molecular weights (25,000 and
16,000 daltons) were isolated from solubilized human T-lymphocyte
membranes using specific T-cell antiserum. These T-cell differentiation antigens (TDA-1 and TDA-2) were identified on normal as well
as cultured T-cells and are probably distinct determinants rather
than breakdown products of larger molecules since:

1.   there was different representation of the two antigens among
the cell lines tested,

2.   the migration of two peaks was essentially unchanged after
reduction with 2 mercapthoethanol, and

3.   the buffers contained proteolytic inhibitors during the
solubilization procedures.

The antigens precipitated by AMT had different patterns of
representation on normal and cultured T-cells. MOLT-3 cells, MOLT-4
cells, thymocytes and blood T-cells contained relatively more of
TDA-1, while the reverse relationship was observed with HSB-2 cells
(i.e. a greater relative amount of TDA-2). However, this type of
immunochemical analysis permits only a semi-quantitative comparison
of total antigen density from one cell source to another.

We analyzed the relationships of the two TDA peaks detected on
MOLT-3 and HSB-2 cells respectively by adsorption studies. Adsorption

of AMT with HSB-2 cells removed all of the antibodies reactive with the TDA-2 from MOLT-3, but only slightly reduced the quantity of detectable TDA-1. This observation suggests that the p25 proteins of HSB-2 and MOLT-3 may not be antigenitically identical. Alternatively, the p25 on MOLT and HSB may be identical, though sparsely represented on HSB-2, thereby reducing the efficiency of HSB to remove antibodies recognizing MOLT-p25.

It is likely that there are more than two antigens on PBL. Proteins of higher molecular weight were precipitated by AMT from blood T-cells but we have not yet established their specificity. Other investigators have also characterized membrane antigens from human T-cells with different molecular weights (15, 16) while these multiple antigenic determinants with different molecular weights may be distinct biological entities, the differences noted may be due to variations in solubilization techniques, the polyacrylamide gel system, or the different specificities of the antisera used. The probability of multiple human T-cell differentiation antigen(s) is analogous to similar findings in rodents (19-23).

The immunochemical characterization of TDA-1 and TDA-2 should facilitate their isolation as individual immunogens. Preparation of monovalent antisera against each of the human T-cell differentiation antigens should then enable a more precise understanding of T-cell subpopulations bearing these distinctive antigens. Human T-cell subsets may bear some functional analogies to T-cell subsets in mice bearing membrane alloantigens. Clearly, the identification of these patterns of antigenic expression will be important in defining functional and maturational properties of human T-lymphocyte subpopulations and their deviations from the normal in various disease states.

REFERENCES

1. Owen, F.L., Fanger, M.W., J. Immunol., 113 (1974) 1138.
2. Owen, F.L., Fanger, M.W., Immunochem. 13 (1976) 121.
3. Jondal, M., Wigzell, H., Aiuti, F., Transpl. Rev. 16 (1973) 163.
4. Balch, C.M., Dougherty, P.A., Dagg, M.K., Diethelm, A.G., Lawton, A.R., Clin. Immunol and Immunopath., 8 (1977) 448.
5. Ades, E.W., Gordon, D.S., Phillips, D.J., LaVia, M.F., Martin, L.H., Black, C.M., Hubbard, M., Reimer, C.B., Amer. J. of Path., In Press, (1978).
6. Aiuti, F., Wigzell, H., Clin. Exp. Immunol. 13 (1973) 171.
7. Balch, C.M., Dagg, M.K., Cooper, M.D., J. Immunol. 117 (1976) 447.
8. Ades, E.W., Bukacek, A., Zwerner, R., Dougherty, P.A., Balch, C.M., J. Immunol., In Press (1978)
9. Balch, C.M., Lawton, A.R., Cooper, M.D., IN "In Vitro Methods of Cell Mediated Immunity", ed. Bloom, B., David, J., Academic Press (1976) p.105.

10. Minowada, J., Ohnuma, T., Moore, G.E., J. Natl. Cancer Inst., 49 (1973) 891.
11. Foley, G.E., Lazarus, H., Farber, S., Uzman, B.G., Boome, B.A., McArthy, R.E., Cancer, 18 (1965) 522.
12. Pulvertaft, R.J.V., Lancet, 1 (1964) 238.
13. Kessler, S.W., J. Immunol. 117 (1976) 1482.
14. Laemmli, V.K., Nature (London), 227 (1970) 680.
15. Zimmerman, B., Chapman, M.L., Eur. J. Immunol. 3 (1976) 446.
16. Anerson, J.K., Metzgar, R.S., J. Immunol., 120 (1978) 262.
17. Letarte-Muirhead, M., Barclay, A.N., Williams, A.F., Biochem. J. 151 (1975) 685.
18. Barclay, A.N., Letarte-Muirhead, M., Williams, A.F., Biochem. J. 151 (1975) 699.
19. Vitetta, E.S., Boyse, E.A., Uhr, J.W., Eur. J. Immunol. 3 (1973) 446.
20. Esselman, W.J., Miller, H.C., J. Exp. Med., 139 (1974) 445.
21. Atwell, J.L., Cone, R.E., Marchalonis, J.J., Eur. J. Immunol. 3 (1973) 446.
22. Kuchich, U.N., Bennertt, J.C., Johnson, B.J., J. Immunol. 115 (1975) 626.
23. Zwerner, R.K., Barstad, P.A., Acton, R.T., J. Exp. Med. 146 (1977) 986.

ACKNOWLEDGEMENTS

1. This investigation was supported by grants from the Medical Research Service of the Veteran's Administration and from the National Institute of Health (CA 13148, CA 16673).

2. Recipient of a Special Fellowship from the Leukemia Society of America.

3. Recipient of a Faculty Fellowship in Oncology from the American Cancer Society.

EFFECT OF THYMIC HUMORAL FACTOR (THF) IN VITRO ON BONE MARROW AND BLOOD CELLS FROM B, T AND NULL CELL ACUTE LYMPHATIC LEUKEMIA (ALL)

B. Shohat and N. Trainin

Clinical Laboratory, Beilinson Medical Center, and

Weizmann Institute of Science, Rehovot, Israel

INTRODUCTION

The nature of null cell ALL is a matter of controversy. The findings of Topuz et al. (1) indicate a T cell lineage of the null cells whereas the studies of Fu et al. (2) and of Kaplan et al. (3) provide evidence for a possible B cell lineage. In the present study the nature of null cell lymphoblasts was further elucidated with the aid of a thymic humoral factor (THF), bone marrow cells and a local xenogeneic graft-versus-host reaction.

MATERIALS AND METHODS

The patient material comprised 5 children with null cell ALL (E^- $SMIg^-$ or EAC^-), 6 with T cell ALL (E^+) and one with B cell perinatal ALL (E^- $SMIg^+$). All of the patients were tested upon initial presentation and 6 of them were retested when in remission from 5 to 12 months later.

Cell isolation. Mononuclear cells obtained from heparinized peripheral blood and bone marrow were separated by the Ficoll Hypaque sedimentation technique and finally resuspended in phosphate-buffered saline (PBS).

Graft-versus-host reaction (GVHR). 0.1 ml of the above mononuclear cells, containing 20 x 10^6 cells, were injected intradermally into the closely-shaven abdominal skin of inbred Lewis rats weighing 100-180 gr which had been pretreated 24 hours previously with 100 mg/kg of cytoxan. On the 5th day the rats were injected

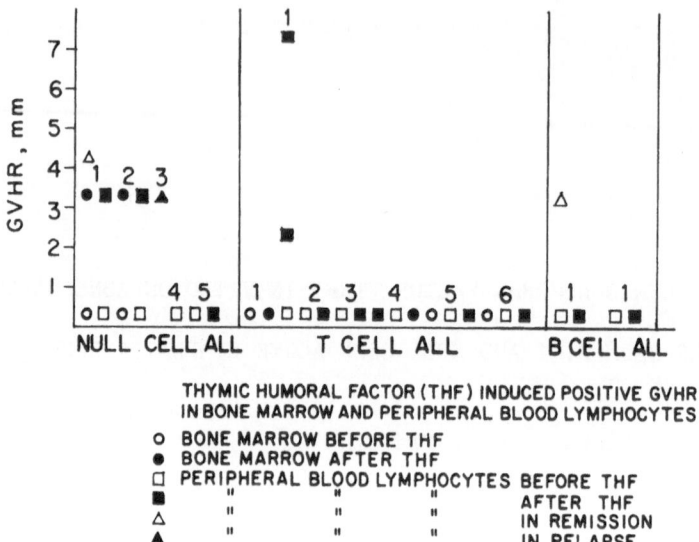

FIG. 1:   Effect of THF on local xenogeneic GVHR obtained with bone marrow and peripheral blood lymphocytes from null T and B ALL.

intravenously with 0.4 ml of 1% of Evan's blue and 5 hrs later the entire abdominal skin was excised and the blue stain measured with calipers. A mean diameter of 2 mm or more was assessed as positive and less than 1 mm as negative (4).

Incubation of mononuclears with THF.   20 x 10^6 mononuclear cells were incubated for 60 minutes at 37°C with 100 μg THF (control cells were incubated in PBS alone), washed 3 times in PBS and inoculated as described above.

Surface markers.   E rosettes were determined according to the technique of Jondal et al. (5), EAC rosettes by the technique of Bianco et al. (6) and surface immunoglobulins by that of Pernis et al. (7); E rosettes at 37°C were tested according to the method of Borella and Sen (8).

RESULTS

Bone marrow or peripheral blood lymphoblasts or lymphocytes obtained from all 12 children with ALL (null, B or T) gave a negative GVHR when tested at the initial presentation. THF was able to induce immunocompetence of bone marrow null lymphoblasts in 2 of the 3 cases of null ALL tested, with conversion of the negative ⌐

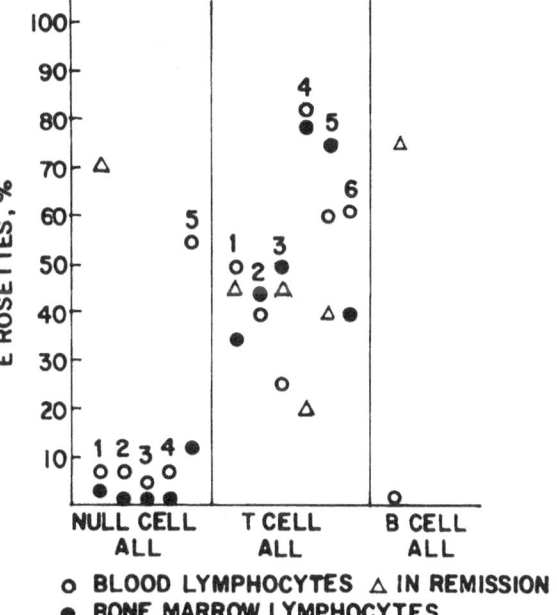

FIG. 2:   E rosette percentages obtained with bone marrow and peripheral blood lymphocytes from null T and B ALL.

to positive being observed only in these 2 children (Fig.1). In contrast, incubation of T lymphoblasts from the bone marrow of 2 children with T cell ALL had no effect on these cells, as demonstrated by the negative GVHR. Incubation with THF of the peripheral blood lymphocytes and lymphoblasts of the 6 patients with T ALL led to a reversion from negative to positive in only one patient (Fig.1). No effect of THF on B cell ALL lymphoblasts was observed in the child with perinatal B ALL. The peripheral T lymphocytes of 2 children tested during remission, the one with perinatal B ALL and the other with null ALL, mounted a normal GVHR.

Membrane surface markers.   Four of the 5 children with null cell ALL initially had E rosette values below 10% in bone marrow and blood; one of these, when tested in remission, showed a rise of 68%. In the group with T cell ALL the percentage of E rosettes in the specimen of bone marrow taken initially ranged from 36% to 80%; when tested in remission the blood of 4 of these children showed below normal percentages of E rosettes ranging from 21% to 42%, and low absolute number of T cells, from 297 to 403 cells/mm^3. The blood of the child with perinatal B cell ALL initially showed only

2% E rosettes but when he was in remission the E rosette value rose
to 77% (Fig.2).

DISCUSSION

Most important among the findings of this study is the demonstration that THF can induce differentiation of null cell blasts
from ALL bone marrow to functionally immunocompetent T cells.
Touraine et al. (9) showed that human marrow cells when treated
with thymic extracts acquired surface specific T antigen recognized
by anti-T cell serum but did not yield cells responsive to phytohaemagglutinin or allogeneic cells.

Tsukimo and Zampkin (11) were unable to induce the formation
of E receptors on null lymphoblasts from cases of ALL and therefore
suggested that lymphoblasts do not have the same surface properties
as normal stem cells. Recent experiments by Aiuti et al. (10) and
Topuz et al. (1) showed that this conception was not valid since
they were able to induce E receptors on null lymphoblasts obtained
from bone marrow and peripheral blood of ALL. Our experiments are
the first to provide evidence that null cell lymphoblasts can be
brought to a functional state of immunocompetent T_2 cells by THF.
The fact that one of the 3 cases of null cell ALL failed to respond
to THF may be explained by the findings of Fu et al. (2) that some
of the cells in null cell ALL express a human B lymphocyte antigen.

The GVHR model has already been used in experimental animals
by Goldstein et al. (12) in order to demonstrate the influence of
thymosin on normal bone marrow cells. The local xenogeneic GVHR
constitutes a simple, accurate method for testing the functional
integrity of human T lymphocytes and has been used by one of us to
assess cell-mediated immunity in cancer patients (4,13). A direct
relationship between the dose of lymphocytes injected and the
magnitude of the local xenogeneic GVHR has already been shown by us
(15). This reaction has been demonstrated to be very sensitive and
can be abolished by anti-T lymphocytic serum (14) or enhanced by THF
provided precursor T cells are present (15). The findings of the
present study constitute additional evidence that thymic hormone can
induce immunocompetence if the precursor target cells are present.
The method of induction of the ability to mount a local GVHR in
human lymphocytes may be of value in the differential diagnosis of
leukemia as well as in the measurement of thymic factors in body
fluids and their purification.

REFERENCES

1.   Topuz, U.O., Candar, A., Okcuoglu, Astaldi, G., Boll. Ist.
      Sierater, Milanese 56 (1977) 5.

2.   Fu, S.M., Winchester, R.J., Kunkel, U.G., J. Exp. Med. 142
     (1975) 1334.
3.   Kaplan, J., Ravindranath, X., Peterson, W.D. Jr., Blood 49
     (1977) 371.
4.   Shohat, B., Joshua, H., Clin. Exp. Immunol. 24 (1976) 534.
5.   Jondal, M., Holm, G., Wigzell, H., J. Exp. Med. 36 (1972) 207.
6.   Bianco, C., Patrich, R., Nussenzwek, V., J. Exp. Med. 132 (1970)
     1702.
7.   Pernis, B., Farni, J., Amante, L., J. Exp. Med. 132 (1970) 1001.
8.   Borella, Z., Sen, Z., Cancer 34 (1974) 646.
9.   Touraine, J.L., Incefy, G.S., Touraine, F., Rho, Y.M., Good,
     R.A., Clin. Exp. Immunol. 17 (1974) 151.
10. Aiuti, F., Schirmacher, V., Amerati, P., Fluorilli, M., Clin.
     Exp. Immunol. 20 (1975) 499.
11. Tsukimo, J., Zampkin, B.C., New Eng. J. Med. 293 (1975) 455.
12. Goldstein, A.Z., Gura, A., Howe, M.Z., White, A., J. Immunol.
     106 (1971) 773.
13. Shohat, B., Joshua, H., Kott, I., Urca, I., Isr. J. Med. Sci.
     12 (1976) 1462.
14. Shohat, B., Peled, I., Kessler, E., Cancer Immunology and
     Immunotherapy. In press.
15. Shohat, B., Spitzer, S., Topilsky, M., Trainin, N., Biomedicine.
     In press.

SERUM AND SECRETORY IMMUNOGLOBULIN LEVELS IN PRELEUKAEMIC AKR MICE

AND THREE OTHER MOUSE STRAINS

J.G. Mink and R. Benner

Dept. of Cell Biology and Genetics

Erasmus University, Rotterdam, The Netherlands

SUMMARY

Levels of IgM, IgG_1, IgG_2 and IgA were determined in serum and milk of AKR mice, which spontaneously develop lymphoma at 6-14 months of age. As a reference C3H, CBA and C57BL mice were studied. Of the four mouse strains studied AKR had the lowest serum and secretory IgA levels. The values of the other immunoglobulins in AKR mice were comparable to those of CBA mice. C3H and C57BL mice had significantly higher immunoglobulin levels. Serum of lactating mice showed fairly decreased IgG_1 and IgG_2 levels as compared with non-lactating mice, probably due to transudation into the milk. The serum IgM and IgA levels were not consistently affected by lactation.

INTRODUCTION

There are several indications that in animals and man IgA deficiency is related to autoimmunity and malignancy (1). Furthermore, people who have suffered from a congenital infection with rubella virus (2,3) have a relatively high incidence of selective IgA deficiency. The relationship between IgA deficiency, auto-immunity and malignancy is unclear at present.

AKR mice have a naturally occurring infection with an endogenous virus, the Gross murine leukaemia virus, which is present from birth (4,5). Infection with this virus causes lymphoma in all AKR mice between 6 and 14 months of age, but not necessarily in other mouse strains (4,5). In addition, AKR mice have been reported to have

very low serum IgA levels (6). Concerning immunoglobulin levels in
secretions of mice, there is a lack of data in the literature.
Serum and secretory IgA are reported to be produced by largely
separate populations of immunoglobulin-synthesizing cells (7,8).
Therefore, we decided to investigate whether the IgA deficiency of
AKR mice only holds for serum, or is general. This paper presents
quantitative data on levels of IgA and the other immunoglobulin
classes in serum and milk of AKR mice. For comparison similar
determinations were done in C3H, CBA and C57BL mice.

MATERIALS AND METHODS

Mice. Five months old female AKR/FuRdA, C3H/fA, CBA/Rij and
C57BL/Rij mice were used. The AKR ($H-2^k$) mice were bred at our own
department, the C3H ($H-2^k$) mice were purchased from the Laboratory
Animals Centre of the Erasmus University, Rotterdam, and the CBA
($H-2^q$) and C57BL ($H-2^b$) mice were purchased from the Medical Biological Laboratory TNO, Rijswijk, The Netherlands.

Collection of serum and milk. Blood was taken with a capillary
pipette from the orbital plexus. After isolation of the serum, the
samples were stored at -70^oC prior to use. Milk was collected
(0.3-0.5 ml during 15 min) 5 to 9 days after parturition, by aspar-
ation using a modification of the milking device described by
McBurney et al (9). The offspring was separated from the mothers
18 hr before milking. Lactating mice were intraperitoneally injected
with 0.4 u.i. Oxytosin (Piton-S$^{(R)}$; Organon, Oss, The Netherlands)
per kg body weight 30 min before milking, in order to stimulate
milk-flow. After collection the milk was centrifuged twice for 30
min at 27,000 g in order to collect clear milk-serum.

Quantitation of immunoglobulins. The levels of IgM, IgG_1, IgG_2
and IgA in serum and milk were determined by using the rocket electrophoresis method according to Laurell (10). The agarose solution was
supplemented with 1% polyethyleneglycol (MW 7000). Before electrophoresis the immunoglobulins were carbamylated according to Weeke (11).
For quantitations peak surfaces instead of peak heights were calculated. A large pool of normal mouse serum obtained from approximately
one-year-old CBA mice was used as a reference serum. The concentration of IgM, IgG_1, IgG_2 and IgA in the reference serum was determined by comparing with a mouse immunoglobulin reference standard
containing myeloma proteins (Meloy Laboratories, Inc., Springfield,
USA). The reference serum contained 38.5 mg IgM, 230.2 mg IgG_1, 432.8
mg IgG_2 and 178.8 mg IgA per 100 ml. The antisera to mouse IgM, IgG_1
and IgG_2 were raised in rabbits by Nordic Immunological Laboratories,
Tilburg, The Netherlands. The antiserum to mouse IgA was raised in
a goat by Meloy Laboratories. All antisera were found to be specific
for the respective mouse immunoglobulins as tested by immunoelectrophoresis and rocket electrophoresis.

TAB. 1:   Immunoglobulin concentrations in serum of 5-month-old AKR, C3H, CBA and C57BL mice.

Mouse strain	IgM	IgG_1	IgG_2	IgA	Total Ig[a]
AKR(8)[b]	18.1+1.7[c]	133.9+20.4	220.9+19.8	39.5+ 1.5	412.4+28.5
C3H (10)	32.7+3.1	258.2+47.2	311.6+19.3	177.5+20.8	780.0+55.2
CBA (7)	26.9+4.7	159.4+25.6	295.0+ 9.5	61.9+ 5.6	543.2+28.3
C57BL(8)	30.1+1.7	118.1+11.5	485.8+14.3	83.9+ 7.4	717.9+19.9

a)   Total immunoglobulin concentration was calculated by summing up the figures for the various classes and subclasses.

b)   Numbers of mice tested in parentheses.

c)   Figures represent the arithmetic mean $\pm$ 1 SEM in mg per 100 ml serum.   Total immunoglobulin levels of AKR and CBA mice were significantly lower than in C3H and C57BL mice ($p < 0.005$).

Quantitation of protein in milk.   Protein concentration in milk was determined by the Lowry assay, as modified by Bensadoun and Weinstein (12).

RESULTS

Serum IgM, IgG_1, IgG_2 and IgA levels were determined in 5-month-old AKR mice.   For comparison these Ig levels were also measured in H-2 compatible C3H mice and in CBA and C57BL mice of the same age. AKR serum contained 18.1 $\pm$ 1.7 mg IgM, 133.9 $\pm$ 20.4 mg IgG_1, 220.9 $\pm$ 19.8 mg IgG_2 and 39.5 $\pm$ 1.5 mg IgA per 100 ml serum (Tab.1).   These figures are within the range of the immunoglobulin levels found in CBA mice, except for IgA.   No consistent pattern in the relative amount of the different immunoglobulin (sub) classes was found in the four mouse strains tested.   C57BL mice were found to have a relatively high level of IgG_2, while C3H mice were proportionally high for IgG_1 and IgA.   Total immunoglobulin concentration was the lowest in AKR mice, while the highest immunoglobulin levels were found in C3H and C57BL mice.

In order to investigate whether the relatively low IgA level in AKR mice also holds for secretions, immunoglobulin levels were compared in the milk of the aforementioned four strains of mice.   The

TAB. 2: Immunoglobulin concentrations in serum and milk of 5-month-old lactating AKR, C3H, CBA and C57BL mice.

Mouse strain	Sample [a]	IgM	IgG$_1$	IgG$_2$	IgA	Total Ig [b]
AKR(5) [c]	serum	22.8+2.2 [d]	41.1+ 4.8	84.9+13.1	36.1+ 2.8	184.9+14.4
	milk	<0.9	15.3+ 2.6	34.8+ 6.7	84.3+14.2	134.4+15.9
C3H(5)	serum	31.0+3.7	64.9+11.9	82.2+19.5	50.4+11.3	228.5+25.7
	milk	<0.9	32.7+ 6.7	41.8+15.9	107.8+22.9	183.2+28.6
CBA(5)	serum	22.4+1.3	36.4+ 7.2	59.8+ 3.7	78.0+12.8	196.6+15.2
	milk	<1.2	12.1+ 3.0	24.2+ 3.8	118.5+12.9	154.8+13.8
C57BL(7)	serum	32.5+2.0	84.9+10.6	168.3+23.2	94.0+16.5	379.7+30.4
	milk	<2.0	39.1+ 5.7	78.2+16.1	201.5+15.7	318.8+23.2

a) Serum and milk were collected 5 to 9 days after parturition.

b) Total immunoglobulin concentration was calculated by summing up the figures for the various classes and subclasses.

c) Number of mice tested in parentheses.

d) Figures represent the arithmetic mean + 1 SEM in mg per 100 ml serum or milk.

effect of lactation upon the serum immunoglobulin levels was also
determined in these mice. It was found that the IgA level in milk
was the lowest for AKR mice (Tab.2). However, this value was nearly
as high as found in CBA mice. Also the IgG_1 and IgG_2 concentration
in milk of AKR and CBA mice were of about the same magnitude. The
levels of IgG_1, IgG_2 and IgA in milk of C57BL mice were about twice
as high as in AKR and CBA mice. In the milk of neither strain of
mice IgM was clearly present. Comparison of the concentrations of
various immunoglobulin classes and subclasses in milk and serum
showed that the ratio between secretory and serum immunoglobulin
level was the highest for IgA.

Lactation did not affect the serum IgM and IgA levels, as can
be deduced from comparison of Tables 1 and 2. Only in C3H mice the
serum IgA level was reduced during lactation. A relatively large
decrease of the serum IgG_1 and IgG_2 levels during lactation was a
consistent finding. This lowered the total serum immunoglobulin
level by at least 50 per cent.

Differences in secretory immunoglobulin levels between various
mouse strains might be related to the protein concentration in these
secretions. Therefore, the protein concentration was determined in
the various milk samples. Milk of AKR, CBA and C57BL mice appeared
to contain about equal amounts of protein, but the protein concentration in milk of C3H mice was clearly higher (Tab.3). Consequently,
relative immunoglobulin levels (calculated as milligram immunoglobulin
per gram protein) in milk of C3H mice (Tab.3) were less high than the
absolute immunoglobulin levels (Tab.2). These relative immunoglobulin
levels of C3H mice were the lowest of the four mouse strains tested.
C57BL mice on the other hand, appeared to have the highest relative
immunoglobulin levels.

DISCUSSION

AKR, NZB and SJL/J mice have a high incidence of spontaneously
occurring tumors. Since there is a relationship between immunocompetence and malignancy, these strains have been investigated for
a possible immunodeficiency at the humoral and cellular level (cf.
ref. 13 and 14). While most authors agree that leukaemic AKR mice
have a decreased immunocompetence, preleukaemic AKR mice have been
reported to have normal or somewhat decreased humoral and cellular
immune reactivity (cf. ref. 4 and 13). Potter and Liebermann (6)
reported that AKR mice are deficient for serum IgA. In view of these
data we considered it worthwhile to quantitate the serum and secretory
IgA levels of AKR mice, and to compare that with those of other, low
tumor incidence, mouse strains. Of the four mouse strains tested,
our AKR/FuRdA mice (which have a medium life span of 32 weeks) were
found to be the lowest for IgA in serum (Tab.1) and milk (Tab.2).

TAB. 3:   Protein concentration and relative immunoglobulin levels
in milk of 5-month-old AKR, C3H, CBA and C57BL mice.

Mouse strain	Protein (g/100ml)	IgM	IgG_1	IgG_2	IgA	Total Ig
AKR	$2.4+0.1^{a)}$	$<0.18^{b)}$	9.0+1.8	14.4+3.0	34.8+6.0	58.5+ 2
C3H	4.1+0.6	< 0.18	7.8+1.8	10.2+3.6	25.8+6.6	43.8+ 7.8
CBA	2.6+0.3	< 0.42	4.2+1.2	9.0+1.8	45.6+7.2	59.4+21.6
C57BL	3.0+0.2	< 0.78	12.6+1.8	25.8+5.4	66.6+7.2	105.6+ 9.0

a)   Figures represent the arithmetic mean + 1 SEM.

b)   Relative immunoglobulin levels were calculated as milligram
immunoglobulin per gram protein. For these calculations the immunoglobulin concentrations from Tab.2 were used.

However, these levels in AKR mice were not far below those of CBA
mice, which is a long-lived strain without specific immune pathology
(15). Therefore, the low IgA level of AKR mice is probably not a
major permitting factor in the development of lymphoma.

As most other mammalian species, mouse serum IgA consists predominantly of molecules sedimenting in the 9S range (16), indicating
that it has the dimer form, just like the majority of secretory IgA.
The origin of mouse serum IgA was thought to be predominantly the
gut associated lymphoid tissue (17). However, studies of Haaijman
et al. (18) have shown that the mouse bone marrow also contains
large numbers of IgA containing cells, indicating that this organ
might substantially contribute to the serum IgA level.

There is a lack of data in the literature concerning immunoglobulin levels in mouse colostrum and milk. It has been shown that
mouse colostrum contains IgA, IgG_1 and IgG_2, but no IgM (19,20).
Our results show that the same holds for milk, when collected 5-9
days after parturition (Tab.2). Quantitatively, IgA was predominant.
Similar results have been reported for milk of rats (21,22) and many
other mammals (8). In the neonatal mouse the IgG_1, IgG_2 and IgA from
milk are probably resorbed into the blood. This supposition is
supported by the observation that in newborn mice the serum IgG_1,
IgG_2 and IgA levels increase fastly after birth, and decrease after
weaning (20,23).

There is a large body of evidence that the majority of IgA in
secretions is synthetized locally. In vitro experiments have shown

that mouse mammary tissue can synthesize IgA (19). In how far
transudation of IgA from serum contributes to the secretory IgA in
mouse milk is unclear. If there is any contribution, this is not
consistently reflected in a decrease of the serum IgA level. On
the other hand, serum IgG_1 and IgG_2 level decrease by about 50%
during lactation (cf. Tables 1 and 2). This might be due to
transudation into the milk. Indeed, there is ample evidence that
IgG in milk is predominantly derived from serum (8). This even
holds for the large amounts of IgG in bovine colostrum and milk
(24).

REFERENCES

1.   Ammann, A.J., Hong, R., In: Immunologic disorders in infants
      and children (E.R. Stiehm, W.A. Fulginiti, Eds.)   pp. 199-214,
      Saunders, Philadelphia (1973).
2.   Soothill, J.F., Hayes, K., Dudgeon, J.A., Lancet i,(1966) 1385.
3.   Lawton, A.R., Royal, S.A., Self, K.S., Cooper, M.D., J. Lab.
      Clin. Med., 80 (1972) 26.
4.   Hays, e.F., In: Virus tumorigenesis and immunogenesis (W.S.
      Ceglowski, H. Friedman, Eds.,) pp. 321-334 Academic Press, New
      York (1973).
5.   Klein, J., In: Biology of the mouse histocompatibility-2
      complex, pp. 389-410, Springer-Verlag, Berlin (1975).
6.   Potter, M., Lieberman, R., Adv. Immunol. 7 (1967) 91.
7.   Benveniste, J., Lespinats, G., Adam, C., Salomon, J.C., J.
      Immunol. 107 (1971) 1647.
8.   Tomasi, T.B., In: The immune system of secretions (A.G. Osler,
      L. Weiss, Eds.,) pp. 57-86, Prentice Hall, Inc. Englewood
      Cliffs, N.J., (1976).
9.   McBurney, J.J., Meier, H., Hoag, W.G., J. Lab. Clin. Med. 64
      (1964) 485.
10.   Laurell, C.B., Scand. J. Clin. Lab. Invest. 29, suppl. 124,
      (1972) 21.
11.   Weeke, B., Scand. J. Clin. Lab. Invest., 21 (1968) 351.
12.   Bensadoun, A., Weinstein, D., Anal. Biochem., 70 (1976) 241.
13.   Melief, C.J.M., Schwartz, R.S., In: Cancer 1 (F.F. Becker, Ed.)
      pp. 121, Plenum Press, New York (1975).
14.   Stutman, O., In: Mechanisms of tumor immunity (I. Green, S.
      Cohen, R.T. McCluskey, Eds.,) pp. 27-53, Wiley and Sons, New
      York (1977).
15.   Smith, G.S., Walford, R.L., Mickey, M.R., J. Natl. Cancer
      Inst., 50 (1973) 1195.
16.   Nash, D.R., Vaerman, J.P., Bazin, H., Heremans, J.F., Int. Arch.
      Allergy 37 (1970) 167.
17.   Vaerman, J.P., Heremans, J.F., Immunology 18 (1970) 27.
18.   Haaijman, J.J., Hijmans, W., Mech. Ageing Develop. 7 (1978) 375.
19.   Asofski, R., Hylton, M.B., Fed. Proc. 27 (1968) 617.

20. Fahey, J.L., Barth, W.F., Proc. Soc. Exp. Biol. Med. 118 (1965) 596.

21. Michalek, S.M., Rahman, A.F.R., McGhee, J.R., Proc. Soc. Exp. Biol. Med., 148 (1975) 1114.

22. McGhee, J.R., Michalek, S.M., Ghanta, V.K., Immunochemistry 12 (1975) 817.

23. Kalpaktsoglou, P.K., Hong, R., Good, R.A., Immunology 24 (1973) 303.

24. Newby, T.J., Bourne, J., J. Immunol. 118 (1977) 461.

ACKNOWLEDGEMENTS

The authors thank Prof. O. Vos for his continuous support and interest, and Dr. J. Radl for critical reading of the manuscript.

ADULT T CELL LEUKEMIA. HISTOLOGICAL FEATURES OF THE LYMPHOID TISSUES

Masao Hanaoka, Shigeru Shirakawa[1], Junji Yodoi[1], Takashi Uchiyama[1] and Kiyoshi Takatsuki[1]

Department of Pathology, Institute for Virus Research
[1]   Department of Medicine, School of Medicine
Kyoto University, Kyoto, Japan

INTRODUCTION

Recently new classifications of non-Hodgkin lymphoma including leukemic forms have been proposed from the immunocytological point of view based on T and B cell identification (1-8). Surface marker analysis of lymphoid neoplastic cells revealed that B cell malignancy is more common than T cell malignancy in adults (9). Since our initial report on chronic lymphocytic leukemia of T cell type (T CLL) (10,11), over one hundred cases of "adult T cell leukemia" have been found in Japan. Adult T cell leukemia or leukemic T cell lymphoma shows characteristic clinical features and cytological findings of leukemic cells in the peripheral blood, bone marrow and lymph nodes. In this report, a variety of histological patterns of the lymphoid tissues in this disease will be presented.

MATERIALS AND METHODS

Patients

This study is based upon 14 patients. Lymph node specimens were obtained by biopsy on nine patients and autopsy was done on ten patients. These patients were admitted to the hospitals in Kyoto-Osaka-Kobe area. It is noteworthy that 11 of 14 patients were born in the south-western parts of Japan, especially nine in Kyushu (12, 13). The patients' clinical and hematological findings are summarized in Table 1.

TAB. 1:   14 Cases of Adult T Cell Leukemia.

Age 29 - 76 years old, Sex Male 6, Female 8	
Duration of disease	3 M - 38 M
Lymphadenopathy	14/14 (+ - +++)
Hepatomegaly	8/14
Splenomegaly	8/14
Skin affection	11/14

WBC	28,000 - 193,000
Leukemic cells	49 - 98%
Bone marrow lymphocytes	0.4 - 52.0%
Severe anemia	0/14
E-rosette forming cells*	62 - 86%
Percent killed by ATS and C*	63 - 96%

Autopsy cases	
Thymus atrophy	10/10
Spleen weight	366 + 358g
Liver weight	1427 + 362g

* Separated periperal lymphoid cells

TAB. 2:   Specificity of ATS Cells killed by ATS and C (%).

Thymus	97 - 100
Spleen	22 - 32
Bone marrow	22
Peripheral blood lymphocytes	
Normal	55
Macroglobulinemia	0
B CLL	0

Inhibition of rosette formation by ATS (1%)	
E rosette formation	100
EAC rosette formation	0

Identification of neoplastic T cells

Details were reported separately (12). Besides the routine surface marker study, blood or lymph node cells were examined by cytotoxicity test using complement and a rabbit anti-human thymocyte

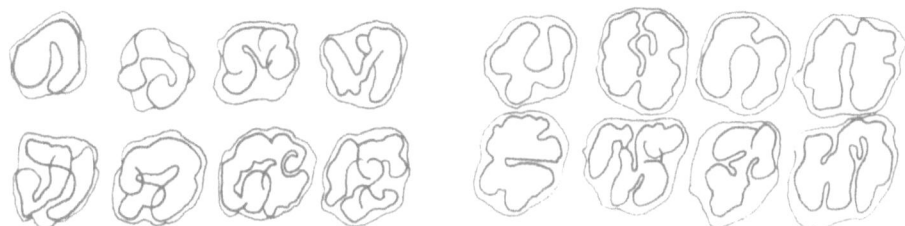

FIG. I: Nuclear Forms of T Cell Leukemic Cells in Smear Preparations of Peripheral Blood (Two cases of Reticulosarcoma Cell Predominant Type).

serum absorbed with human erythrocytes, liver powder, bone marrow cells, and unsolubilized serum proteins (ATS). The specificity of this ATS was confirmed as shown in Table 2. ATS also killed cells of cultured Sézary cell line (14). The percent killed by ATS showed a good correlation with E-rosette formation while the surface immunoglobulin bearing cells or EAC-rosette forming cells were not affected by ATS.

RESULTS

Leukemic cells in smear preparations
of blood and bone marrow

Details were reported in the previous paper (11). In May-Giemsa staining, peroxidase negative leukemic cells showed generally pleomorphic nuclear forms (Fig.I). The nuclei are lobulated, convoluted and notched.

Histological features

The neoplastic cells which proliferated diffusely in the lymphoid tissues, skin, liver, lungs and other organs were generally pleomorphic, occasionally admixing bizarre giant cells. No nudular pattern was formed by these neoplastic cells. The thymus was atrophic in all cases and the leukemic cells infiltrated into the medulla in some cases. The bone marrow was infiltrated by leukemic cells, but to a lesser degree than in the case of T ALL in childhood. The leukemic cells infiltrating into the skin in 11 cases did not usually affect the epidermal basement membrane, but Pautrier microabscess involving the upper dermis was seen in two cases of pleomorphic leukemia cell predominant type as mentioned later. The histological variety of the lymphoid tissues was also one of the characteristics of adult T cell leukemia. The histological findings of the lymph nodes and other

TAB. 3:   Histological Classification of Lymph Nodes in 42 Cases of
Adult T Cell Leukemia.

Type	Biopsy	Autopsy
Well-differentiated,		
lymphocytic predominant	9	2
Poorly-differentiated		
leukemic cell predominant	5	9*
Pleomorphic leukemic cell predominant	1	3
Lymphosarcoma	10	1
Reticulosarcoma cell predominant	8	2
Others	1**	0
Total	34	17

* Reticulosarcoma in lung   **   Histocytes increased

lymphoid tissues were tentatively classified into the following five
types.

  Well-differentiated, lymphocytic predominant type. Among five
cases in this group, an autopsy case showed findings which were
histologically indistinguishable from those in typical B CLL. In
the lymph node in two biopsy cases, well-differentiated lymphocytes
were predominant, whereas many small leukemic cells in the peripheral
blood in these cases had a lobulated nucleus. Another case showed
findings resembling Hodgkin granuloma in all of the lymph nodes
obtained from the autopsy and biopsy done on four occasions during
the follow-up period of three years. In this case, histiocytic cells
possessing nucleoli increased in number in the mass of well-differentiated lymphocytes and also the infiltration of eosinophils was
remarkable, but no typical Reed-Sternberg's cell was observed during
the course. A lymph node biopsy obtained from a patient with Sézary
syndrome showed dermatopathic lymphadenitis with well-developed B
cell zones (marginal cortex and germinal centers). A small number
of leukemic cells infiltrated into the paracortical area where dendritic reticulum cells with a long twisted and pale nucleus proliferated. The leukemic cells have a variously deformed hyperchromatic
nucleus.

  Poorly-differentiated leukemic cell predominant type. All five
cases were autopsied. Normal structure of the lymphoid tissues was
partially destroyed. The leukemic cells were mainly of poorly-differentiated lymphocytic type, accompanying some well-differentiated cells

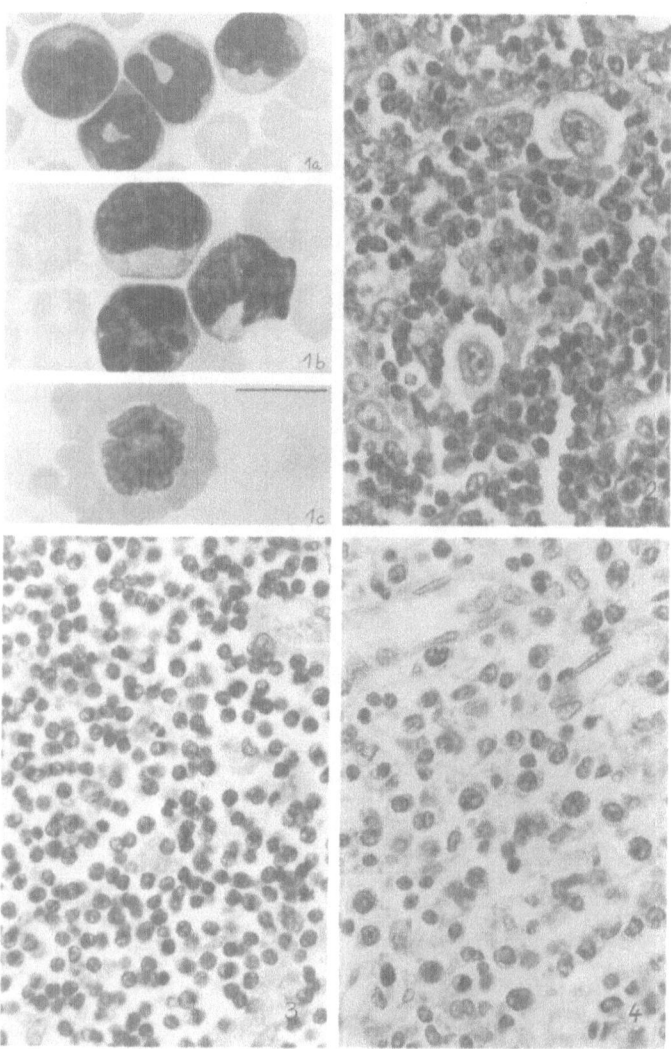

FIGS. 1 - 4:

1: Leukemic cells in the peripheral blood from patients with adult
T cell leukemia. 1 a-c: An E-rosette forming cell, bar shows 10 μ.
2 - 8: Lymph nodes from patients with adult T cell leukemia, H.E.
staining. Magnifications are 2/5 of those in 1-a c. 2: U.S.,
57 years of age, female, biopsy, well-differentiated lymphocytic
predominant type resembling Hodgkin granuloma. 3: U.Y., 42 years of
age, female, autopsy, well-differentiated lymphocytic, predominant.
4: M.K., 61 years of age, male, autopsy, poorly-differentiated
leukemic cells predominant.

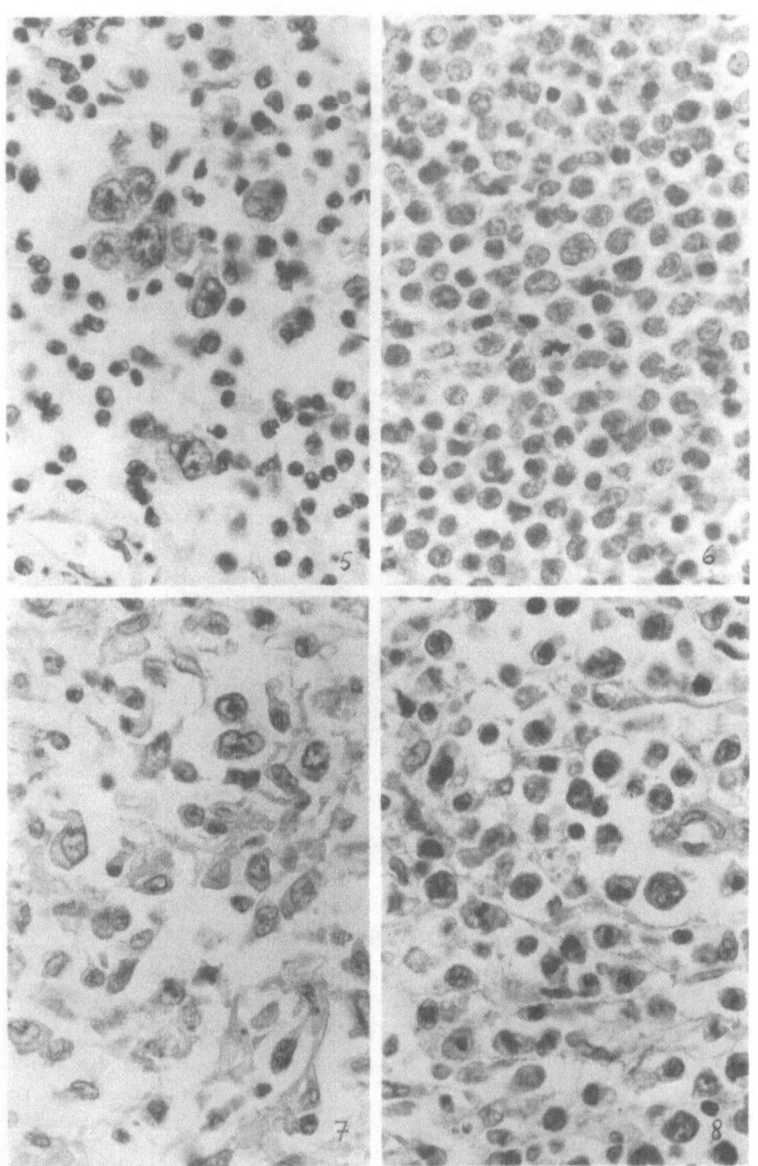

FIGS. 5 - 8:

5: H.Y., 65 years of age, male, autopsy, pleomorphic leukemic cells
predominant. 6: M.D., 71 years of age, female, biopsy, lymphosarcoma. 7 and 8: Z.M., 30 years of age, male, autopsy. 7: reticulosarcoma cell predominant region. 8: pleomorphic leukemic cell
predominant region.

and a few bizarre giant cells. Leukemic cells with smooth surface appeared to float separately each other in the sinusoidal structure. A lymph node biopsy interpreted as dermatopathic lymphadinitis showed the infiltration of poorly-differentiated lymphocytes in the paracortical area where dendritic reticulum cells proliferated.

Pleomorphic leukemic cell predominant type. Three cases of this type included one which was considered to have transformed from lymphosarcoma type at the time of biopsy. The normal structure of the lymphoid tissues was destroyed, and an increase in fine networks of reticulin fibrils was marked. Pleomorphic large neoplastic cells infiltrated diffusely and separately each other in pseudosinusoid (15) in the lymph nodes and other lymphoid tissues accompanying small and large leukemic cells, bizarre giant cells and ones resembling Reed-Sternberg's cells. No neoplastic phagocytes were observed as seen in the case of so-called malignant histiocytosis (15,16).

Lymphosarcoma type. One case studied by both biopsy and autopsy and one of each biopsy and autopsy case showed the findings consistent with typical lymphosarcoma. Poorly-differentiated lymphocytes were densely distributed in the lesion.

Reticulosarcoma cell predominant type. A lymph node biopsy showed the findings of reticulosarcoma admixing well- or poorly-differentiated leukemic cells (diffuse lymphoma mixed lymphocytic-histiocytic (17)). Another autopsy case showed various changes from tissue to tissue, including the findings of typical reticulosarcoma of reticular or pleomorphic subtype and pleomorphic leukemic cell predominant type. The leukemic cells in the surrounding fat tissue were composed of round poorly-differentiated lymphocytic leukemic cells infiltrated there. In the tissues of these cases, cells transformed from large reticulosarcoma cells to round leukemic cells were observed. In the peripheral blood in both cases, the leukemic cells were mostly round and large having a lobulated nucleus.

COMMENTS

It was demonstrated that adult T cell leukemia in Japan showed a variety of histological features. Including our own series of 14 patients, we had an opportunity to study 34 biopsy and 17 autopsy specimens from a total of 42 patients with this disease by the courtesy of the many hospitals and several pathologists. The results were summarized in Table 3. Both poorly-differentiated and pleomorphic leukemic cell predominant types and found in almost all autopsy cases, while most of the biopsy specimens obtained before treatment showed the findings of reticularsarcoma, or lymphosarcoma. Only four biopsy cases showed poorly-differentiated or pleomorphic leukemic cell predominant types. This result suggests the possibility that the therapeutic procedures might be responsible for the changes in the histological findings during the follow-up periods.

REFERENCES

1.   Lukes, R.J., Collins, R.D. Br. J. Cancer 31 (suppl.2) (1975) 1.
2.   Lennert, K., Stein, H., Kaiserling, E. Br. J. Cancer 31
     (suppl.2) (1975) 29.
3.   Green, I., Jaffe, E., Shevach, E.M., Edelson, R.L., Frank, M.M.,
     Berard, C.W. International Academy of Pathology Monograph, N.
     16, eds. J.W. Reback et al., pp. 282, Williams & Willkins Co.
     Baltimore (1975).
4.   Lukes, R.J., Taylor, C.R., Chir, B., Phil, D., Parker, J.W.,
     Lincoln, T.L., Pattengale, P.K., Tindle, B.H. Am. J. Pathol.
     90 (1978) 461.
5.   Siegel, F.P., Fillippa, D.A., Koziner, B. Am. J. Pathol. 90
     (1978) 451.
6.   Seligman, M., Preud'Homme, J.L., Vrout, J.C. Progress in
     Immunology III, eds. T.S. Mandel et al., pp. 618, Australian
     Acad. Sci., Canberra (1977).
7.   Shimoyama, M., Minato, K. Rec. Adv. RES. Res. 16 (1978) 119.
8.   Minato, K., Shimoyama, M. Rec. Adv. RES. Res. 17 (1978) in
     press.
9.   Ederson, R.L., Kirkpatrick, C.H., Shevach, E.M., Shein, P.S.,
     Smith, R.W., Green, I., Lutsner, M. Ann Intern. Med. 80 (1974)
     685.
10. Yodoi, J., Takatsuki, K., Masuda, T. N. Engl. J. Med. 296
     (1974) 572.
11. Yodoi, J., Takatsuki, K., Aoki, N., Masuda, T. Acta. Haem. Jap.
     37 (1974) 46.
12. Uchiyama, T., Yodoi, J., Sagawa, K., Takatsuki, K., Uchino, H.
     Blood 50 (1977) 481.
13. Takatsuki, K., Uchiyama, T., Sagawa, K., Yodoi, J. Topics in
     Hematology, eds. S. Seno et al., pp. 73. Excerpta Medica
     Amsterdam (1978).
14. Ishii, K., Yodoi, J., Hanaoka, M., Furuyama, J. J. Cell. Physiol.
     94 (1978) 93.
15. Warnke, R.A., Kim, H., Dorfman, R.F. Cancer 35 (1975) 215.
16. Bryne, G.E., Rappaport, H. GANN Monograph on Cancer Research,
     eds. K. Akazaki et al., pp. 145, Tokyo Univ. Press Tokyo (1975).
17. Rappaport, H. Tumors of the Hematopoietic System. Atlas of
     Tumor Pathology, Sec. III, Fasc. 8, Armed Forces Inst. of Pathol.
     Washington (1966).

ACKNOWLEDGEMENTS

     The authors are deeply grateful to the following pathologists
for their contribution to this study: Dr. M. Sasaka (Osaka Red Cross
Hospital), H. Yamabe (Tenri Hospital), H. Tankawa (Amagasaki Hospital),
K. Matsumoto (Shinko Hospital), K. Tomimoto (Shizuoka Central Hospital), T. Tasaka and H. Fujiwara (Kyoto Univ.).

We wish to thank the following organizations who gave us the chance to observe the specimens of this disease: Dept. of Pathology and Cancer Institute, Kagoshima Univ.; Atomic Disease Inst., Nagasaki Univ.; Aichi Cancer Center; National Cancer Center; Dept. of Pathology, Keio Univ.; Dept. of Pathology, Tohosu Univ.

MEMBRANE GLYCOPROTEIN PATTERNS OF NORMAL AND MALIGNANT HUMAN LEUKOCYTES

Leif C. Andersson and Carl G. Gahmberg

Department of Pathology and Transplantation Laboratory
and Department of Bacteriology and Immunology
University of Helsinki, SF 00290 Helsinki 29, Finland

INTRODUCTION

Human leukocytes descend from common pluripotent hematopoietic stem cells. During the sequence of functional differentiation the various leukocytes express characteristic surface structures, recognized as surface markers, antigens and receptors. Most of these are cell membrane glycoproteins (1). By mapping the glyco- proteins of defined leukocyte populations a deeper insight into the structural/functional relationships of surface molecules may be obtained. Moreover, comparison of the surface glycoprotein patterns of normal leukocytes with those of cells in various disorders might give information about the molecular changes that occur in different dysfunctional states and malignancies.

The surface glycoproteins of different lymphoid cells have recently been studied by the use of radiolabeling and polyacrylamide slab gel electrophoresis (2,3). These investigations have shown that the main populations of human and murine lymphocytes express different and characteristic surface glycoprotein patterns (4,5). Analysis of the membrane glycoprotein profiles also allowed the identification of human hematopoetic cell lineages with high accuracy (6,7).

In this report we summarize some recent results with special emphasis on the usefulness of the selective surface labeling method for the classification and differential diagnosis of human hemato- poietic malignancies.

MATERIALS AND METHODS

Isolation of normal and malignant leukocytes

The procedures for the isolation of the main lymphocyte populations, monocytes and granulocytes from fresh human blood have
been reported in detail (5). Leukemic cells were obtained from
patients with newly diagnosed acute lymphocytic leukemia (ALL) or
acute myeloid leukemia (AML), and from patients with chronic
lymphocytic leukemia (CLL) or chronic myeloid leukemia (CML)
undergoing blast crisis. The cells were isolated from heparinized
blood or bone marrow aspirates by Ficoll-Isopaque density centrifugation. If the leukemic cells were contaminated by more than
10% morphologically normal cells they were further purified by
density gradient centrifugation and/or by velocity sedimentation
at one-g (5).

In vitro activation and isolation of T-lymphocytes

Nylon wool-purified blood T-lymphocytes were cultivated with
optimal concentrations of phytohemagglutinin (PHA) or concanavalin-A
(ConA) or with mitomycin-C-treated allogeneic mononuclear blood
cells in mixed lymphocyte culture (MLC). Blast cells were isolated
to a purity exceeding 95% from the cultures by velocity sedimentation
at one-g (5).

Radiolabeling of cell surface glycoproteins

The membrane glycoproteins were labeled by reduction with
NaB^3H_4 after treatment of intact cells with neuraminidase and
galactose oxidase (5). After labeling the cells were solubilised
in 0.15M NaCl-1 % Triton-X-100 containing a protease inhibitor,
the nuclei were pelleted and the supernatants used for slab gel
electrophoresis.

Polyacrylamide slab gel electrophoresis

Electrophoresis was performed on 8% polyacrylamide slab gels
with ^{14}C-labeled marker proteins in the peripheral slots. The gels
were fixed and treated for fluorography as described (4).

RESULTS AND DISCUSSION

Surface glycoprotein patterns of normal lymphocytes

The fluorographic patterns of surface labeled blood T, B and
null lymphocytes (cells with lymphocytic morphology but lacking T

FIG. 1:   Fluorographic eletrophoresis patterns of galactose-
oxidase-NaB^{3}H$_4$ labeled lymphocytes and T blasts. A = T lymphocytes,
B = B lymphocytes, C = null lymphocytes, D = PHA blasts, E = ConA
blasts, F = MLC blasts (3 days of culture), G = T cells kept in
unstimulated cultures for 6 days, H = PHA blasts, I = ConA blasts,
J = MLC blasts (6 days of culture), K = 14C-labeled marker proteins,
TH = thyroglobulin, TR = transferrin, HA = human serum albumin,
OA = ovalbumin, HB = hemoglobin. GP210 indicates a protein with an
apparent MW of 210.000 etc.

and B cell markers) are shown in Fig. 1A-C. The T lymphocytes
express four closely spaced labeled bands in the high molecular
weight region, GP200, 180, 165 and 160. B lymphocytes and null
cells have one major band in this region with an apparent molecular
weight of 210.000. The major band, GP120, is expressed on T and B
lymphocytes but only weakly labeled in null cells. These patterns
of the main lymphocyte populations are constant for corresponding
cells obtained from different donors.

Glycoprotein patterns of in vitro-activated T blasts

     The fluorographic patterns of PHA-, ConA- and MLC-activated
T lymphoblasts show similarities with those of resting T lymphocytes
(Fig. 1D-J). The patterns of mitogen-stimulated T blasts differ
from those of MLC T blasts. The MLC blasts express a major band,
GP130, which was evident already after three days in culture (Fig.1F),
and strongly labeled after six days in culture (Fig. 1G). This is

only weakly present on PHA and ConA-activated cells and on T
lymphocytes kept in unstimulated cultures. The GP120, on the
other hand, is apparently absent from the MLC blasts while it is
the major protein in this MW-range of resting T lymphocytes and
mitogen-activated T cells (8) (Fig. 1G-I). This finding of a
prominent "new" band, GP130, in the fluorography pattern of MLC
T blasts parallels that earlier reported in the mouse system (4)
where a certain glycoprotein was found on the MLC-activated killer
T cells but not on proliferating "helper" T cells (9). The GP130
was detectable on MLC-blasts cultivated for 3-4 days but required
5-7 days to reach maximal expression which suggests that this
particular membrane protein represents a differentiation marker
for human killer T cells. The GP130 was also heavily labeled on
blood T lymphoblasts from patients with acute infectious mononucleosis, which shows that T blasts may also express this surface
protein in vivo (10).

Surface and glycoprotein patterns of leukemic cells (Fig. 2)

    Acute lymphocytic leukemia (ALL). The fluorographic patterns
of cells from four patients with ALL are shown in Fig. 2A-D. The
cells run in slots A, B and C were "null" cells according to
surfact marker analysis, while the case shown in 1D was a T-ALL
(sheep red blood cell rosette-positive). The ALL cells of non-B
non-T cell type are characterized by a distinct labeling of the
GP210 which is also found on "null" lymphocytes and B lymphocytes
but not on mature T cells. On the other hand, ALL cells with the
ability to bind sheep erythrocytes did not express the GP210 but
instead some of the "T cell" characteristic bands of GP160-200.
Intermediate forms of differentiation towards T cells can also be
seen as shown in Fig. 2C. In this particular case there is
expression of some of the T cell bands in the upper molecular
weight region. These cells were unable to bind sheep erythrocytes
but the clinical course was highly malignant. This finding
indicates that within the group of common or "null" ALLs cases
with incomplete T cell differentiation can be observed. The
heavy labeling of the GP120-130 seems to be a common feature for
undifferentiated leukemias of lymphoblastic or myeloblastic type.
Moreover, the distinct expression of GP210 coincided with the
presence of GP42 (which is the heavy chain of HLA) and GP31 and 24
(HLA-D). Based on our experience from extensive studies on ALL and
AML cells we suggest that this represents the real "null" cell or
stem cell pattern.

    The fluorography patterns of three cases with CLL are shown in
Fig. 2E-G. These are different and easily distinguishable from
those of ALL. Two basic patterns can be seen in the group of CLLs:
one with heavy labeling of the GP210 and frequently clear expression
of GP42, 31 and 24 while the GP120 region is relatively weakly

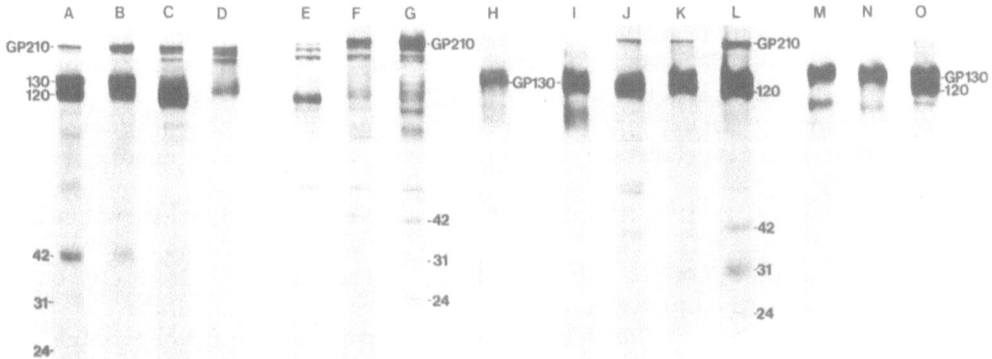

FIG. 2:   Fluorographic electrophoresis patterns of galactose-
oxidase-NaB^{3}H$_4$ labeled leukemic cells: A -D = ALL cells, E - G
= CLL cells, H = normal granulocytes, I - L = AML cells and M - O
= CML cells.

labeled (2F-G). This pattern is found on the "typical" CLL cells
of B cell type which carry surface Ig. The other basic pattern is
shown in Fig. 2E which is characterized by a narrow distinct band
in the 120 MW region and the absence of GP210 and GP31 and 24.
This type constitutes about 1/5 of the cases, they neither bind
sheep erythrocytes nor stain for surface Ig.

    The surface glycoprotein patterns of undifferentiated acute
myeloid leukemias (AML) are similar to those of "null" ALL, that
is prominent expression of GP210, heavy labeling of the GP120,
GP31 and 24 (Fig. 2J-L). This indicates that both of these
disorders represent malignant transformation of the very early
stage of the hematopoietic differentiation chain, maybe of a common
stem cell. When the AMLs are morphologically differentiated (promyelocytic leukemia) the corresponding changes are seen in the
glycoprotein patterns (Fig. 2I); they are the disappearance of
the GP210 and diffuse labeling of proteins in the molecular weight
range of 100.000. This pattern is rather similar to that seen on
normal granulocytes (Fig. 2H).

    The fluorographic pattern of CML cells shows similarities with
that of granulocytes as could be expected (Fig. 2M-O) During blast

crisis the patterns resembling those obtained with cells from acute
promyelocytic leukemias are obtained (Fig.2I). A clearly distinguishable labeling of the GP31 and GP24 is, however, not found on the
CML cells. This indicates that although the blast crisis indicates
a dedifferentiation of the malignant clone (or lack of differentiation), it doesn't seem to involve the very early stages where the
HLA-D molecules (GP24 and 31) are expressed. No clear differences
have been found between the surface glycoprotein profiles of
morphologically mature granulocytes from patients with Philadelphia-
chromosome positive CML and those isolated from healthy donors (11).

In conclusion the analysis of the surface glycoprotein pattern
after selective radiolabeling is a sensitive method for identification of different cell types. Although the clinical implications
of the surface glycoprotein analysis for individual cases of
leukemias are still to be seen, this method offers a new approach
to classify hematopoietic malignancies and to estimate their degree
of differentiation. Moreover, the mapping of the membrane glycoproteins provides the basis for search of surface molecular changes
associated with malignancy.

REFERENCES

1.   Gahmberg, C.G., In:Poste, G., Nicholson, G.L., (eds) (1976)
      "Dynamic aspects of cell surface organization" vol. 3, North
      Holland, Amsterdam.
2.   Gahmberg, C.G., Hakomori, S., J. Biol. Chem., 248 (1973) 4311.
3.   Gahmberg, C.G., Andersson, L.C., J. Biol. Chem., 252 (1977)
      5888.
4.   Gahmberg, C.G., Häyry, P., Andersson, L.C., J. Cell. Biol. 68
      (1976) 642.
5.   Andersson, L.C., Gahmberg, C.G., Blood (1978) in press.
6.   Andersson, L.C., Gahmberg, C.G., Nilsson, K., Wigzell, H.,
      Int. J. Cancer 20 (1977) 708.
7.   Nilsson, K., Andersson, L.C., Gahmberg, C.G., Wigzell, H.,
      Int. J. Cancer 20 (1977) 702.
8.   Andersson, L.C., Gahmberg, C.G., Kimura, A.K., Wigzell, H.,
      Proc. Nat. Acad. Sci. (1978) in press.
9.   Kimura, A.K., Wigzell, H., J. Exp. Med. 147 (1978) 1418.
10.   Andersson L.C., Gahmberg, C.G., J. Clin. Immunol. Immunopathol.
      10 (1978) 41.
11.   Gahmberg, C.G. et al., submitted.

ACKNOWLEDGEMENTS

Supported by The Finnish Cancer Society and the Finnish Academy.

IN VIVO ACTIVITY OF LYMPHOCYTES SENSITIZED IN VITRO BY ANTIGEN-FED

MACROPHAGES: INHIBITION OF LYMPHOMA GROWTH

[1]Abraham J. Treves, [2]Michael Feldman, [3]Cyril Honsik and [3]Henry S. Kaplan

[1]Department of Radiation & Clinical Oncology, Sharett
Institute of Oncology-Hadassah University Hospital
Jerusalem, Israel
[2]Department of Cell Biology, The Weizmann Institute of
Science, Rehovot, Israel
[3]Department of Radiology, Stanford University School of
Medicine, Stanford, California, USA

ABSTRACT

In previous studies, we have shown that macrophages fed with
radiation leukemia virus could induce primary in vitro sensitization
of lymphocytes which could be measured by their cytotoxic activity
against target cells. In the present study, we tested the in vivo
influence on tumor growth of such lymphocytes. We found that macro-
phage-mediated sensitized lymphocytes could protect mice against
tumor growth if injected into normal recipients four days prior to
challenge with lymphoma cells. The protective function of such
lymphocytes was not affected by their irradiation, but no protection
occurred in sublethally irradiated recipients. This indicated that
the sensitized lymphocytes did not inhibit tumor cell growth directly
but recruited an effector protective response in the recipient mice.
This protective activity was different from the one elicited by
lymphocytes which had been sensitized directly against cells carrying
antigens cross-reacting with RadLV. The protective activity of the
directly sensitized lymphocytes was radiosensitive and was probably
mediated by their direct cytotoxic activity against tumor cells.

INTRODUCTION

In vitro sensitization of unprimed lymphocytes against tumor
specific antigens could be achieved by direct interaction of lympho-

cytes with syngeneic tumor cells (1-4). Recently, we have described
a method for in vitro sensitization in which the tumor specific
antigens were presented to lymphocytes by antigen-fed macrophages
(5). Splenic lymphocytes, which had been sensitized by macrophages
fed with radiation leukemia virus (RadLV), caused specific target
cell injury in vitro (6,7). Such sensitized lymphocytes could also
inhibit lymphoma tumor growth in vivo when administered intraperitoneally (i.p.) four days before the inoculation of tumor cells (8).
In the present study, we tested the possibility that effector lymphocytes induced in vitro by virus-fed macrophages, affect tumor growth
in vivo indirectly, by recruitment of host defense response.

MATERIALS AND METHODS

Specific pathogen-free 8-10 weeks old (C57BL/Ka xBALB/c)F_1 mice
were used.

Two in vitro established cell lines were used in this study:
BL-5, a non-infected line derived from C57BL/Ka embryo fibroblasts
(9) was used for direct sensitization of lymphocytes. BL/VL$_3$, a
line of neoplastic lymphoid cells derived from a RadLV induced
C57BL/Ka lymphoma and producing a leukemogenic thymotropic RadLV
(10) was used for challenging test mice with tumor cells. The virus
preparation used as antigen for feeding macrophages was the RadLV,
a cell free extract of RadLV induced C57BL/Ka lymphoma cells prepared
as described (11).

The method for in vitro sensitization of lymphocytes by antigen-
fed macrophages has been described (5,6). Briefly, peritoneal
exudate cells were obtained from mice which had been injected with
peptone medium. The cells, $2 \times 10^6/3$ ml, were plated in 6 cm petri
dishes with or without the addition of RadLV preparation. Three
hours later, the media were replaced with virus-free medium. On the
next day, 30×10^6 syngeneic spleen cells (SC) were plated on the
macrophage monolayers in 4 ml of medium and incubated for four days.
Direct sensitization of lymphocytes against BL-5 cells was performed
by incubating 30×10^6 sc on monolayers of 3000 rads irradiated BL-5
fibroblasts in similar conditions. In both methods of sensitization,
after the sensitization period, the lymphocytes were collected and
residual macrophages were removed by adherence to plastic surface
which was followed by adherence to nylon wool columns. The sensitized
cells were injected i.p. into normal mice. Control groups of mice
received either no lymphocytes or lymphocytes sensitized by macrophages without antigen. Four days after the injection of the lymphocytes, the mice were challenged i.p. with $4-5 \times 10^4$ BL/VL$_3$ lymphoma
cells. The mice were followed for three months and at that time all
surviving mice were killed and dissected. The proportions of

<u>TAB. 1:</u> Survival of mice inoculated with sensitized lymphocytes and lymphoma cells. *

Sensitization of lymphocytes	Irradiation	Time of Inoculation of sensitized lymphocytes	Survival of mice %
No lymphocytes	-	-	20 (17/87)
Macrophages	-	-4 days	25 (22/89)
Macrophages + RadLV	-	-4 days	82 (80/97)**
Macrophages + RadLV	-	day 0	38 (6/16)
Macrophages + RadLV	3000 rads of sensitized lymphocytes	-4 days	81 (13/16)**
Macrophages + RadLV	450 rads of recipient mice	-4 days	8 (2/24)
BL-5 Fibroblasts	-	-4 days	50 (12/24)**
BL-5 Fibroblasts	3000 rads of sensitized lymphocytes	-4 days	0 (0/16)

* Sc were sensitized either by macrophages, by RadLV-fed macrophages or against BL-5 fibroblast monolayers. Two-5×10^6 sensitized cells were inoculated i.p. into syngeneic mice 4 days prior to the i.p. inoculation of $4-5 \times 10^4$ VL_3 lymphoma cells. In one group (line 4) the sensitized lymphocytes were inoculated together with tumor cells. In other groups, either the sensitized lymphocytes or the recipient mice were irradiated before the injection.

** This group is significantly different from the control group (first line). $p < 0.01$.

surviving mice in the different experimental groups were compared to the one in the medium injected control group by the Chi-square test. The results of 12 experiments are summarized in Table 1. Each experimental group was repeated at least twice in independent experiments.

RESULTS

Spleen lymphocytes, which had been sensitized by RadLV-fed macrophages, were tested for their in vivo activity. The sensitized lymphocytes were injected i.p. into normal mice four days prior to the injection of BL/VL_3 lymphoma cells (third line, Tab.1). The

results indicated that lymphocytes sensitized by RadLV-fed macrophages protected the mice against lymphoma growth as compared to the
activity of control lymphocytes. They also suggest an active role
for the immunogenic material presented to the lymphocytes by the
macrophages. The requirement for four days interval between the
injection of the lymphocytes and the tumor cells was tested by
injecting the sensitized lymphocytes into normal recipients together
with BL/VL$_3$ tumor cells. (Fourth group, Tab.1). In this combination,
no inhibition of lymphoma growth was observed. Hence, a time interval
was required for the sensitized lymphocytes to express their protective activity. The requirement for time interval between the
injection of the sensitized lymphocytes and the tumor cells could
be explained by the possibility that the injected lymphocytes did
not interact directly with the cells but rather recruited a host
defense response. To test this possibility, we irradiated either
the sensitized lymphocytes (fifth group, Tab.1) or the recipient
mice (sixth group, Tab.1) before their injection. We found that
whereas irradiation of the lymphocytes did not affect their protective activity, irradiation of the recipient mice abolished the
protective response of the injected cells. These results indicated
that the sensitized lymphocytes were radioresistant and required
host radiation sensitive cells for exerting their protective effect.
The activity of the lymphocytes sensitized by RadLV-fed macrophages
was compared to that of lymphocytes which were sensitized directly
against BL-5 cells. The BL-5 cells were found to cross-react with
antigens in the RadLV preparation as tested by the cytotoxic activity
of lymphocytes which had been sensitized by antigen-fed macrophages
(6,7). Spleen cells which had been sensitized directly against BL-5
cells protected the recipient mice against tumor development (seventh
group, Tab.1). This protection, which was weaker than the protection
conferred by macrophage mediated sensitized lymphocytes, was completely abolished if the sensitized cells were irradiated prior to
their injection. Hence, the protective activity of the directly
sensitized lymphocytes was radiosensitive.

DISCUSSION

In vitro sensitization of lymphocytes against virus associated
antigens was performed by two different methods: macrophage mediated
and direct sensitization. In the first method, the antigen was
presented to lymphocytes by macrophages and in the second method, the
cellular antigen was introduced into spleen cell suspensions. Both
methods of sensitization resulted in the induction of cytotoxic
lymphocytes, which caused target cell injury in vitro (6,7). When
tested for their in vivo effect on tumor growth, the lymphocytes
sensitized directly against BL-5 cells were less efficient in their
protective activity from the lymphocytes sensitized by RadLV-fed
macrophages. The main difference between the effector cells elici

in these two methods of sensitization was their sensitivity to irradiation. The lymphocytes sensitized by antigen-fed macrophages could induce their protective activity in vivo even after their irradiation, whereas the lymphocytes sensitized directly did not protect against tumor development after their in vitro irradiation. This phenomenon could be explained by different mechanisms of protective activity elicited by each of these effector populations. The requirement for time interval for the expression of the protective activity elicited by the macrophage mediated sensitized lymphocytes and their resistance to irradiation suggest that this effector population did not affect tumor growth directly; they mediate this function by recruiting effector cells from the host immune system. This possibility was supported by our finding that sublethal irradiation of the recipient host before the inoculation of the lymphocytes, abolished their ability to be protected. Hence, a radiosensitive response in the host was required for the induction of protective response by the macrophage mediated sensitized lymphocytes.

The protective activity induced in vivo by the macrophage mediated sensitized lymphocytes, correlated with their in vitro cytotoxic activity and had shown similar specificity pattern. The cytotoxic activity of this population of sensitized lymphocytes was demonstrated in vitro by the terminal labeling assay in which the remaining target cells were labeled after the effector phase (5,6,7). However, it was difficult to demonstrate their cytotoxic activity by the prelabeling assay, in which radiolabeled release from prelabeled target cells was measured (12). The activity of the directly sensitized lymphocytes could be measured equally well by both assays of cytotoxicity (12). These results may be explained by the inability of macrophage mediated sensitized lymphocytes to cause direct cytolysis of target cells, which might be the reason for their lack of competence in inhibiting tumor growth when injected simultaneously with tumor cells.

In a different system, it was shown that guinea-pig lymphocytes which had been sensitized by antigen-fed macrophages, reacted in a proliferative response to a second challenge with the antigen (13). Considering these phenomena, we suggest that the macrophage mediated sensitization results in the induction of initiator lymphocytes. These initiator lymphocytes may be equivalent to the responding cells in mixed lymphocyte cultures and different from the killer cells induced by direct sensitization. The initiator lymphocytes mediated the inhibition of tumor development in vivo by recruitment of an additional defense response. Thus, different conditions of in vitro sensitization may result in the induction of different effector populations which can inhibit tumor growth by different mechanisms.

Analysis of cell surface alloantigens of the effector population and characterization of the immune defense response recruited in the host will help in testing the possibility of in vitro induction of initiator lymphocytes by antigen-fed macrophages and their possible difference from the killer lymphocytes induced by direct sensitization.

REFERENCES

1. Schechter, B., Treves, A.J., Feldman, M. J. Nat. Can. Inst. 56 (1976) 975.
2. Ilfeld, D., Carnaud, C., Cohen, I.R., Trainin, N. Int. J. Can. 12 (1973) 213.
3. Schechter, B., Segal, S., Feldman, M. J. Immunol. 20 (1977) 1268.
4. Treves, A.J., Cohen, I.R., Feldman, M. J. Nat. Can. Inst. 54 (1975) 777.
5. Treves, A.J., Schechter, B., Cohen, I.R., Feldman, M.J. Immunol. 116 (1976) 1059.
6. Treves, A.J., Feldman, M., Kaplan, H.S. J. Nat. Can. Inst. 58 (1977) 1527.
7. Treves, A.J., Decleve, A., Lieberman, M., Feldman, M., Kaplan, H.S. J. Immunol. In press (1978).
8. Treves, A.J. Immunol. Rev. 40 (1978) 205.
9. Lieberman, M., Niwa, D., Decleve, A., Kaplan, H.S. Proc. Nat. Acad. Sci. 70 (1973) 1250.
10. Lieberman, M., Kaplan, H.S., Decleve, A. In: Biology of Radiation Carcinogenesis (J. Yuhas, R. Tennant, J. Regan, Eds.) p. 237, Raven Press, N.Y. (1976).
11. Lieberman, M., Kaplan, H.S. Science 130 (1959) 387.
12. Treves, A.J., Honsik, C., Lieberman, M., Decleve, A., Feldman, M., Kaplan, H.S. In: "The Macrophages and Cancer", Proceeding of Eures. Meeting, Edinburgh.
13. Thomas, D.W., Shevach, E.M. J. Exp. Med. 144 (1976) 1263.

SUMMING-UP - IMMUNOLOGIC MARKERS IN HUMAN MALIGNANT LYMPHOMAS

Maxime Seligmann

Laboratory of Immunochemistry and Immunopathology
(INSERM U 108), Research Institute on Blood Diseases
Hôpital Saint-Louis, Paris 10e, France

Most human lymphoid malignancies are of monoclonal origin. This
conclusion has been supported by three main lines of evidence: 1)
the presence in all the cells of a tumor of a marker chromosome; 2)
the uniform expression among the tumor cell population of a single
form of an X-linked enzyme such as glucose-6-phosphate-dehydrogenase
in heterozygous females; 3) the homogeneous nature, in B cell proliferations, of membrane-bound or secreted immunoglobulin molecules.
These lymphoid malignancies vary considerably with respect to the
differentiation capabilities of the proliferating cells. Whereas in
some instances the malignant cells pursue uninterrupted maturation,
in other cases, they appear to be "frozen" at a given stage along the
differentiation pathway of the B or T line. As we heard in the first
papers of this session, the study of immunologic markers has provided
new information on the nature of lymphoma cells and may lead to a
more rational categorization of these diseases. However the relia-
bility of the results of such studies depends upon an awareness of a
number of problems and pitfalls.

CRITICAL EVALUATION
OF IMMUNOLOGIC MARKERS

Most of the techniques commonly used for the identification of
human B and T cells by their membrane properties are now reasonably
well standardized. It is obvious that one has to study the immunologic markers of the tumor cells themselves and not those of the
presumably normal surrounding cells. Therefore the methods applied
to frozen sections are reliable only in cases with a nodular pattern
or to tissues with an overwhelming homogeneous population of lymphoma

cells. The study of cell suspensions has the advantage of allowing
to assess the morphology of individual cells with given surface
markers.

The existence of subpopulations of B and T cells with distinct
markers and functions which has been well established in mice becomes
increasingly important in man. For instance two broad human T cell
subpopulations are defined by the presence of receptors for IgM or
IgG, the former including T cells with helper activity and the latter
T cells with suppressor activity. Moreover human B and T cells
express different markers according to the successive steps along
their differentiation pathway. This applies to many currently
available immunologic markers for which the precise sequence of
expression is not yet definitely known, to surface glycoproteins as
shown by Andersson and to some enzymes such as terminal deoxynucleotidyl transferase(TdT) which, as discussed by Mertelsmann, is a
useful marker in the study of lymphomatous leukemic cells. This
enzyme is normally found in thymocytes and in their bone marrow precursors but lost as the cell further matures to peripheral T lymphocyte. It should however be noted that it may be present in small
amounts in lymphoid stem cells and early B cell precursors. In view
of these considerations, it is obvious that lymphomatous cells which
arise from a single clone and which have limited capabilities to
undergo further differentiation may lack some markers of other subsets of normal lymphoid cells or of peripheral cells belonging to the
same subset and that conversely the malignant cells may express some
markers which are not detected on the corresponding peripheral cells.

Membrane bound Ig detectable by immunofluorescence or other
procedures constitute the most reliable marker of B cells. They
give also evidence for the genetic commitment of the cell when truly
monospecific antisera to various Ig chain subclasses are used. It
should however be emphasized that the mere presence of Ig molecules
on the surface of a cell does not necessarily mean that they are
produced by that cell. The main sources of extrinsic surface Ig
leading to erroneous interpretations are the presence of labile cyto-
philic IgG, the attachment of Ig aggregates or immune complexes to an
Fc receptor and the binding of antibodies to membrane antigens. The
importance of using Fab'2 reagents of proven monospecificity, the
necessity of proper identification of positive cells and the procedures required to insure that surface Ig are indeed synthesized by
the cells under study have been outlined. The detection of surface
IgG with both types of light chains argues strongly in favour of
extrinsic Ig. By contrast the simultaneous presence of several heavy
chain classes of membrane bound truly produced Ig molecules (most
frequently IgD combined with IgM) with identical light chains and
variable regions can be observed and occurs at some stages during the
development of a B cell clone and during ontogeny. Intracytoplasmic
Ig is of course also a reliable B cell marker since only B cells

produce Ig molecules. Intracytoplasmic Ig is not only found in the late stages of the B cell differentiation pathway since pre-B cells contain a small amount of intracytoplasmic IgM in the absence of detectable surface Ig. Obviously, here again, the presence of Ig molecules with both light chain types argues against the hypothesis that they are synthesized by the cell under study.

The demonstration of truly produced Ig molecules is of paramount importance for the identification of B cells since it is now established that several other B cell markers are found only on some subsets of B cells and since several other markers are not specific for B cells. For instance receptors for complement components or for the Fc of IgG are expressed not only by monocytic cells but also by subsets of T cells. The Ia-like B cell antigens revealed by allo- or hetero-antisera are also present on normal precursors of the granulocytic series and on activated T cells. Similarly some markers previously thought to be specific for a subset of T cells, such as the receptor for Fc_μ, have been recently found on some human B lymphocytes.

Hetero-antisera raised against human (or monkey) normal or foetal B and T cells and against various leukemic cells of known phenotype are now widely used to identify malignant lymphoid cells. Immunofluorescence is by far a safer procedure than cytotoxicity which does not allow simultaneous checking of other markers and direct examination of positive cells, but truly specific antisera are not easy to obtain. As discussed by Ades, some of the reactive antigenic molecules are now in the process of being characterized. Monoclonal antibodies produced by hybridomas will surely be of great help in this field. Some antisera react only with subsets of B or T cells. When used for identification of lymphomatous cells they may lead to false negative results if the monoclonal malignant cells under study do not arise from this reactive subset. Lymphomatous cells which are frozen at early stages along the differentiation pathways may not have acquired some membrane antigens of mature B or T cells and may therefore be devoid of reactivity with antisera to such antigens. Conversely lymphomatous cells may express some antigenic determinants absent on normal peripheral B and T cells. Such determinants include foetal and other derepressed antigens, virus-associated antigens and "differentiation" antigens. Most, if not all, so called leukemia-specific antigens may fall in these categories. Antisera raised against foetal or leukemic cells may contain antibodies which react with such antigenic determinants of lymphomatous cells.

HUMAN LYMPHOMAS

Immunologic studies have provided definite confirmation of pathologic and clinical findings in some groups of lymphomas such as well-differentiated diffuse lymphocytic, nodular, and Burkitt's lymphomas which are all monoclonal B-cell malignancies.

The same membrane markers were found on lymphocytes from patients with "well-differentiated diffuse lymphocytic lymphoma" and with the common B derived chronic lymphocytic leukemia, thus confirming the close relationship between these two conditions. In "immunocytomas with plasmacytoid features", the pattern of membrane markers is similar to that found in Waldenström's macroglobulinemia, suggesting the proliferation of an IgM producing B cell clone with persistent differentiation up to the secreting plasma cell.

The results of immunologic studies in the "nodular" lymphomas have supported the views of Lennert and of Lukes, who proposed, on the basis of morphologic studies, that these lymphomas arise from follicular center cells. Practically all such tumors studied thus far in various laboratories, regardless of the cytologic subtype and of the degree of nodularity, have proved to be B-derived malignancies with usually a high density of Ig molecules bound to the membrane of the lymphomatous cells. The malignant cells of nodular lymphomas also bear C3 receptors similar to the predominant cell of the lymphoid follicle and Stein gave you his latest results in this field.

The neoplastic cells from African cases of Burkitt's lymphoma were evaluated for surface markers and glucose-6-phosphate dehydrogenase, and this disease was shown to be a monoclonal B-cell proliferation. Similar surface characteristics were found on Burkitt's tumor cells in French and American patients whose disease presented as lymphoma or as acute leukemia.

The investigation of immunologic markers in "diffuse poorly differentiated lymphocytic" lymphomas in adults has led to similar results in various laboratories. Most cases are B cell malignancies. This appears to be the rule when these diffuse lymphomas are recognized morphologically to be of follicular center cell origin. In roughly 10% of the patients, the neoplastic cells had T-surface characteristics and in a similar percentage no membrane markers were detectable.

Immunologic studies have helped to define the subgroup of childhood lymphoblastic lymphoma. In most of these cases, T lymphocytic markers were demonstrated on the neoplastic cells, as well as complement receptors. These lymphomatous cells also contain TdT. They appear to be of thymic origin and they have the same cytochemical, enzymatic and immunological phenotype as cells of the T derived subgroup of acute lymphoblastic leukemia. On the basis of both clinical and immunologic data, these two diseases are closely related and probably represent different manifestations of the same neoplastic process.

Diffuse large cell ("histiocytic") lymphomas appear immunologically to represent a heterogeneous group. Only occasional cases may be truly related to the monocytic series. The study of membrane markers and mainly the data obtained after in vitro culture of such lymphomatous cells have provided evidence in favour of this hypothesis in a few patients. Fifty to 60% of large cell lymphomas appear to originate from B cells. Burkert et al. discussed their most recent results obtained by isoelectric focusing of the Ig molecules produced by such lymphomatous cells. T cell derived large cell lymphomas appear to be infrequent since they account for less than 10% of the cases. In more than 30% of the patients, the large lymphomatous cells are devoid of the usual immunologic markers of mature B or T lymphocytes, including antigenic determinants revealed by heteroantisera.

Taylor et al. discussed cases where two different histological types of lymphoma occur in a single patient. It should be stressed that large cell immunoblastic lymphomas arising in patients previously affected with chronic lymphoproliferative diseases of well-documented B cell origin such as chronic lymphocytic leukemia, Waldenström's macroglobulinemia, α chain disease or follicular lymphoma are always monoclonal B cell derived tumors. In all such cases, but one studied by the Amsterdam group, the results of the characterization of the membrane bound Ig showed that the supervening large cell lymphoma did not represent the emergence of a second malignant clone but was related to the original B cell proliferation. Similarly when a large cell immunoblastic lymphoma occurred in patients affected with T derived chronic lymphoid proliferations such as T derived CLL or Sezary syndrome, the lymphomatous cells were of the T nature.

Altogether the immunological phenotype of non Hodgkin's lymphomas is most often B derived. There are some indications that those patients with diffuse lymphomas with malignant cells demonstrating B membrane markers may survive longer than the other patients. However the study of more patients is warranted in order to evaluate the possible prognostic significance of the membrane markers. This evaluation is of special importance for the large cell lymphomas where long survivals are obtained in about 30% of the cases after intensive chemotherapy. Further studies should indicate whether or not the lymphomas of these patients belong to a specific immunologic subgroup.

T derived lymphomas are mainly observed in childhood and are quite rare in adults. Peripheral T cell neoplasia in adults include the Sezary syndrome and mycosis fungoides and the rare T derived chronic lymphocytic leukemia. As recalled in this session by Hanaoka T derived CLL occurs in Japan where the common B derived CLL is very rarely observed. In most of the 25 cases of T derived CLL studied by our group in Paris, the disease displayed peculiar clinical and hematological features.

In a number of cases and in a fair percentage of large cell
lymphomas, the malignant cells lack the usual immunologic markers of
B and T cells. An analogous situation exists in the major subgroup
("non T non B") of acute lymphoblastic leukemias which is clearly
heterogeneous with respect to the level of differentiation of the
leukemic cells which include presumably lymphoid stem cells, pre B
and pre T cells. This latter possibility is supported by some of
the results reported by Shohat.

It should be stressed that the membrane phenotype of the proliferating lymphomatous cells does not necessarily identify the
target cell for the neoplastic event which may hit a precursor cell.
For instance, multiple myeloma obviously corresponds to the proliferation of the most mature cells of the B cell series. However, in
a fair number of untreated myeloma patients, the presence in the
blood and/or bone marrow of "monoclonal" populations of B lymphocytes
expressing (and synthesizing) the same immunoglobulin isotypic and
idiotypic determinants as those of the serum myeloma protein, has
been demonstrated. These findings suggest that in such patients the
target for the neoplastic transformation is not a plasma cell but a
B lymphocyte or a B lymphocyte precursor. Moreover recent data from
our laboratory indicate the presence in one patient of a homogeneous
population of T lymphocytes synthesizing identical receptors which
share the antigen binding activity and the idiotypic (but not isotypic) determinants of the myeloma globulin produced by the malignant
B cells, suggesting that T cells may be involved in myeloma. Some of
the data reported by Schedel may have a similar meaning.

The cellular origin of the Reed-Sternberg cell has been much
disputed. Some investigators consider that its morphological features
argue in favour of a lymphoid origin and suggest a transition between
lymphocytes, transformed lymphoid cells and Reed-Sternberg cells. On
the basis of the presence of intracellular immunoglobulin, most often
detected by the immunoperoxidase technique, several authors have
claimed that Reed-Sternberg cells may be related to the B cell axis.
It should however be emphasized that most often polyclonal IgG immunoglobulin molecules with both light chain types were found within the
cytoplasm of a single cell. Since such a finding is hardly compatible
with the hypothesis of an actual cell product, these immunoglobulin
molecules may have been phagocytised. Indeed intracytoplasmic Ig was
no more found in these cells after short term in vitro cultures. Few
data are available on immunologic markers of Reed-Sternberg cells
since it is difficult to obtain a sufficient number of such cells from
lymph node biopsies. The presence of receptors for complement components and for the Fc of IgG does not solve the problem since it is
consistent with either a lymphoid or monocytic origin. The latter
hypothesis is strongly supported by the data obtained after in vitro
culture.

SESSION   B 2

IMMUNOPATHOLOGY OF PARASITIC DISEASES

CHAIRPERSONS:

A.C. Allison

V. Houba

INTRODUCTION - IMMUNOPATHOLOGY OF PARASITIC DISEASES

V. Houba

WHO-Immunology Research and Training Centre

Nairobi, Kenya

Mechanisms involved in immunopathology of parasitic diseases are the main subjects for presentations and discussions of this session.

Many parasitic diseases are characterized by a long-term persistence of parasites in the hosts, due to not fully effective therapy on one hand and to less effective (non-sterile) immunity on the other hand. These conditions have created a special and rather complicated host-parasite relationship supported by escape mechanisms of parasites to immune response, such as coating of parasites by self-substances of the host, antigenic variations and others.

Although principally both humoral and cellular mechanisms of the immune response participate at the development of immunopathological lesions in parasitic diseases, more attention has been given in the past to humoral components, especially immune complexes and complement.

Immune complexes (IC) are formed when antibodies bind with relevant antigens: in parasitic diseases this can happen at the site of parasite penetration, in circulation and in tissues. One should remember that binding of antibody with antigen is a physiological protective function of antibody. Most of the IC formed are removed by physiological routes and, therefore, their presence in the circulation and/or in phagocytic cells should not always be regarded as pathological feature. Unfortunately, IC may under certain conditions initiate harmful effects leading to tissue injury or to impairment of otherwise protective immunological mechanism. These conditions may be due to multivalent properties of IC (such as their size, antigen-antibody ratio, affinity of binding between both components, activation of complement etc.); some of these properties undergo a change

during the course of infection: a typical example is a release of
enormous amounts of antigens from dying parasites which can substantially influence the ratio between antigen and antibody in favour of
antigen excess. Another reason may be failure of the reticuloendothelial system to remove IC from circulation; again, a typical
example can be the saturation of this system by parasites and their
products in patients exposed to several parasitic infections in the
tropics; in which case IC of even larger sizes circulate for
prolonged periods of time.

IC preformed in circulation may localize in the walls of vessels
in different organs as described in kidney lesions in malaria, trypanosomiasis, schistosomiasis and other infections. Local formation of
IC has been also quite intensively studied and the findings indicate
that this mechanism may play a significant role in the pathogenesis
of lesions, as has been shown in heart lesions in trypanosomiasis,
kidney lesions in schistosomiasis and others.

Complement has been always regarded as an important humoral
effector of IC induced lesions; the alternate pathway of its activation by different products of micro-organisms, and parasites themselves, has stimulated further research in this field. Although
complement induced damage is the most frequent cause of IC injury in
human pathology, other mediators should be also considered.

Increased levels of IgE in hosts infected with different parasites have been known for long time and sometimes have been used as
helpful diagnostic criteria. Their significance in pathology was
usually attributed to hypersensitivity reactions of type I; more
recent data have shown that the biological importance of IgE extends
to other mechanisms.

Cell-mediated mechanisms of immunopathological lesions in parasitic diseases are mainly represented by delayed type hypersensitivity.
A typical example here is the granulomatous reaction around eggs
trapped in the liver, gut and other tissue in schistosomiasis; there
is quite good evidence that this reaction is due to soluble egg antigens passing through the pores of the egg shell.

A combination of humoral and cellular mechanisms seems to play
a significant role in damage to parasites as demonstrated by antibody-
dependent, cell-mediated reactions in vitro. The relevance of these
mechanisms to in vivo situations is still questionable and should be
further studied. Recent data have shown that a blockade of Fc
receptors of effector cells by IC may be responsible for the failure
of these reactions in vivo in some situations, but obviously many
other factors could be involved. This interference of IC with cellular effectors represents a harmful effect; on the other hand,
local formation of IC within delayed hypersensitivity reactions

(granulomata) in schistosomiasis represents a beneficial effect as
it minimizes the pathological consequences caused by the cellular
mechanisms.

Prolonged persistence of parasites, with frequent relapses, and
their contact with host cells and tissues obviously influence the
spectrum of responses of the host. Auto-immune reactions quite often
appear to perpetuate the lesions originated by parasites or their
products, and in some situations stimulate a "vicious circle".
Similarly, other conditions may cause differences in reactivity of
the host leading to impairment of coordination, immunosuppression,
polyclonal activation of cells and other features, some of which will
be presented in this session. It seems that a disturbance or a
failure of regulatory functions may be one of the important factors
for inadequate immune response in parasitic diseases leading to the
development of immunopathological lesions.

MALARIA INFECTION IN MICE.   PLASMODIUM BERGHEI INFECTION IN MICE:

A MODEL FOR IMMUNE COMPLEX DISEASE AND AUTOIMMUNITY

Lambert G. Poels, Catherine C. van Niekerk, Christoph
R. Jerusalem, J. Agterberg* and E.H. van Elven*

Division Malaria Research Center; Department of Cytology
and Histology, Faculty of Medicine, University of Nijmegen
Nijmegen, The Netherlands

*Central Laboratory of the Netherlands Red Cross Blood
Transfusion Service and Clinical Immunology, University
of Amsterdam, Amsterdam, The Netherlands

INTRODUCTION

The malaria parasite Plasmodium berghei can produce profound
impairment of immune responses to unrelated antigens (1). The
infection, however, is also associated with hypergammaglobulinemia
(1). A minor part of these immunoglobulins is specific for parasitic antigens, and is precipitated in renal glomeruli as immune
complexes (2). The major part of the immunoglobulins during
infection is of unknown specificity. Chemotherapeutic elimination
of parasitemia did not inhibit the synthesis of "non-specific"
immunoglobulins; proliferation of plasma cells in the spleen went
on (1), and deposition of a "second type" of I.C. in renal glomeruli,
free of plasmodial antigens, did not cease (2). This phenomenon
might be explained in terms of autoimmunity. In the present study
we investigated the involvement of autoantibodies in the formation
of immune complexes, and their possible relationship to renal
lesions.

RESULTS

Autoantibodies and Mode of Induction

Sera, diluted 1:10, were assayed for autoantibodies on cryostat-
sections of gastric tissue, liver, kidney, heart muscle, and on
suspensions of erythrocytes and thymocytes with immunofluorescence
technique.

TAB. 1:

		immunization	autoantibodies		percentage
			SMA	ANA	parasitemia
A	1	malarious serum	–	–	0
	2	parasite extract	–	–	0
B*	1	intact p. osyphilic RBC	–	–	0
	2	intact p. reticulocytes	–	–	0
C	1	infection cured on d. 4	+	–	1 – 3
		" " " d. 7	+++	+	10 – 15
		" " " d.14	+++	+	45 – 60
D		hyperimmune serum	+++	+/+++	0

Groups A and B were immunized over a period of 6 weeks once a week.
Group B/C received chloroquine (300 mg/L) in drinking water.

The autoantibodies detected by this technique were direct
against smooth muscle (SMA) and nuclear factors (ANA). Data in
Table 1 show that the formation of autoantibodies could not be
induced by immunizing mice with soluble parasitic antigens (group
A 1 and A 2), or "particulate antigen" (group B 1 and B 2, intact
parasitized erythrocytes under chloroquine protection). Chemotherapeutic treatment of the infection at varying times after
inoculation (group C 1-3) shows that a short term infection with
low parasitemia (C 1) is sufficient to induce the formation of SMA.
Apparently a proliferating, metabolizing parasite is required for
the induction of autoimmunity.

Germinal Centers in the Thymus

Although the thymus involutes during severe malaria infection
(3), cured hyperimmune mice were found to develop germinal centers
in the "reconstituted" thymus (Fig.1) comparable to splenic architecture. This observation provides supportive evidence for the
existence of autoimmunity (4).

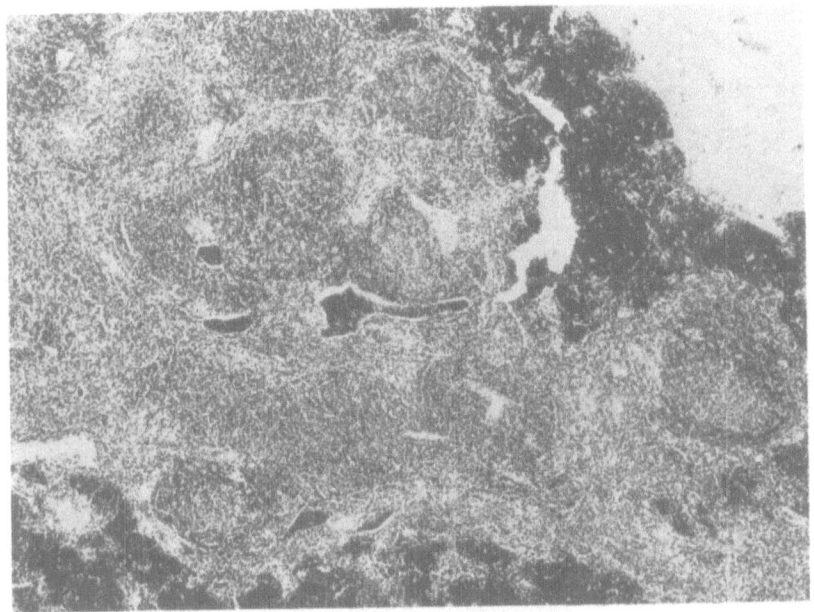

FIG. 1:   Thymic germinal centers in recovered hyperimmune mice
(magn. X 400).

Localization of I.C. in renal glomeruli

Using peroxydase conjugated antibodies to mouse IgG and to
parasitic antigens, the deposited I.C. were localized in renal
glomeruli electronmicroscopically. The results confirmed our
previous findings that no relevant differences in localization of
I.C. were observed in infected or in hyperimmune mice.

Circulating Soluble I.C. in
Serum in Infected and Cured Mice

Quantity of I.C.   The content of circulating I.C. in sera was
estimated using 3.5% PEG (polyethylene glycol) precipitation
technique (5). The method has been found to correlate fairly well
with the C_1q binding test and not to be interferred with significantly
by free IgG or IgM (5).

I.C. were present in severely infected mice (day 14-21) and in
cured hyperimmune mice. The data are in agreement with the detection
of I.C. in renal glomeruli in infected and hyperimmune mice.

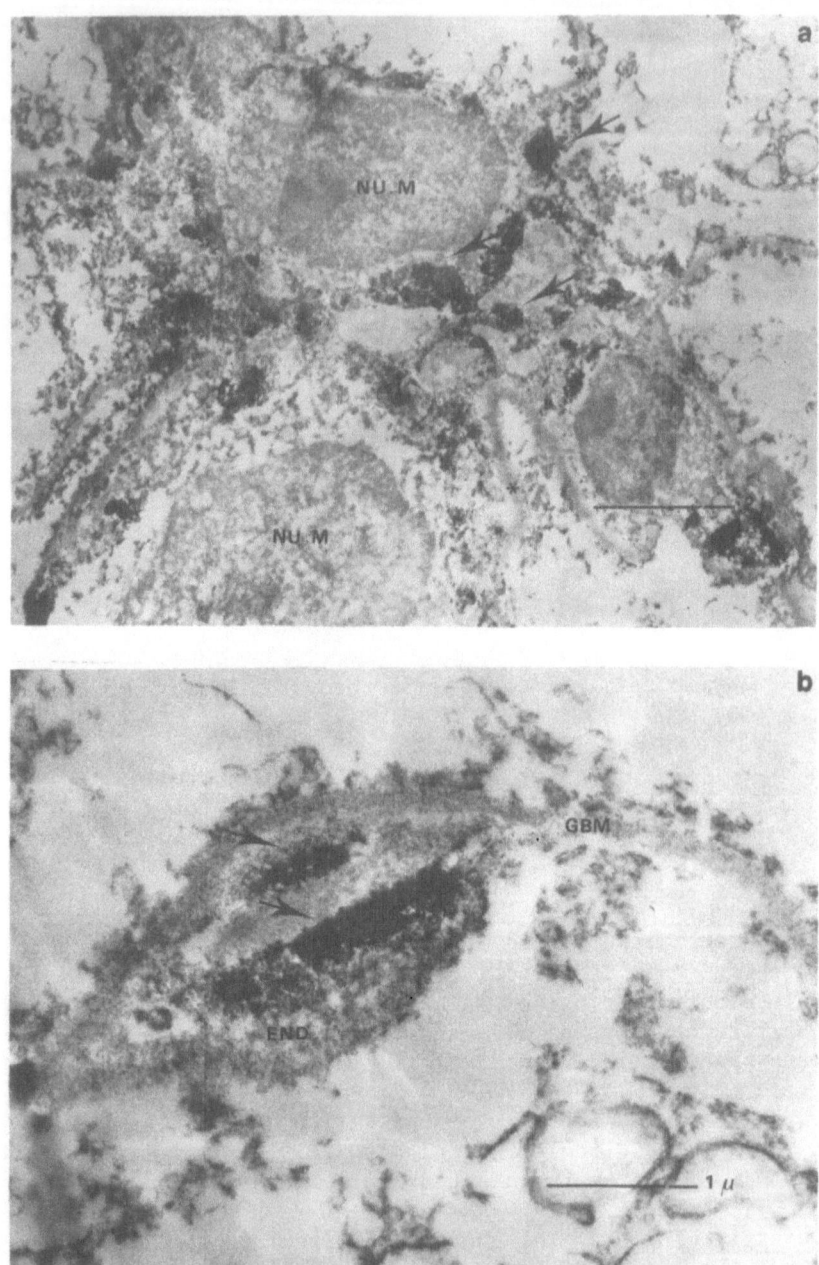

FIG. 2: Detection of IgG in the deposited I.C. (arrows) in mesangial cells (a) and subendothelial location (b) in malaria infected mice. GBM = glomerular basement membrane; END = endothelium; NU.M = nucleus mesangial cell.

TAB. 2:   I.C. content in serum.

days after infection	0	7	14	21	hyperimmune serum
O.D. 280 nm	0.06	0.09	0.49	0.52	0.32
$\overline{SD}$ +	0.01	0.02	0.04	0.05	0.04

Precipitate was obtained from 0.75 ml serum at 3.5% PEG.

Quality of I.C.   Sera were fractionated according to molecular size on Biogel A-0.5 m column (6).   The first fraction (B I), containing high molecular weight compounds was analyzed on DE-52 ion exchange columns with phosphate buffer, pH 8.0 at a strength of 0.01 M and 0.3 M.

Complement Activity (CH 50)

Elimination of parasites by chloroquine caused increased binding of complement (C3/C4) to the deposited I.C. in renal glomeruli, while at the same time proteinuria gradually ceased (2).

As the infection progresses complement activity falls down to a low level, while returning to normal level after chloroquine treatment.

DISCUSSION

Direct and circumstantial evidence has been presented that malaria infection (P. berghei) in mice is associated with an auto-immune process. Actively metabolizing, proliferating parasites seem to be a requirement for the induction of autoantibodies (SMA and ANA). Autoimmunity can be viewed as a problem of immunologic regulation. P. berghei has been shown to be an excellent example of immune deregulation (1,2). A combination of several phenomena, like reduced T cell function (thymic involution, 8,9); depressed response to PHA (10), imbalance between T helper - T suppressor cells (11), and the presence of overwhelming amounts of parasitic antigens, some of which have B cell mitogenic activity (12) may favor the development of autoimmunity. In addition one could suggest that self antigens of erythrocyte membranes have been altered by the incorporation of parasitic antigens (6), or have been demasked by interaction with the parasite and

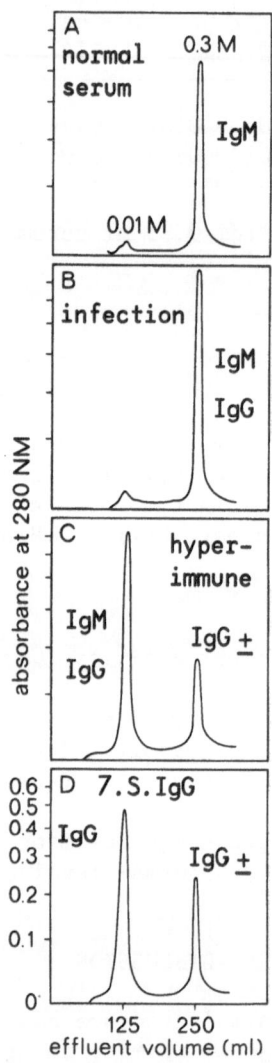

FIG. 3: shows the DE-52 elution profiles of the HMW fraction obtained from (A) normal serum; (B) 14 days after infection; (C) = hyperimmune serum; D = the third Biogel fraction (B III, containing IgG from normal serum). The figures show that during infection IgG molecules have appeared in HMW-fraction and that it is more tightly bound to the DE-52 than free IgG (Fig.D). In hyperimmune sera IgG has also migrated to a HMW fraction, in addition both IgM and IgG have lost binding affinity and become eluted predominantly at 0.01 M.

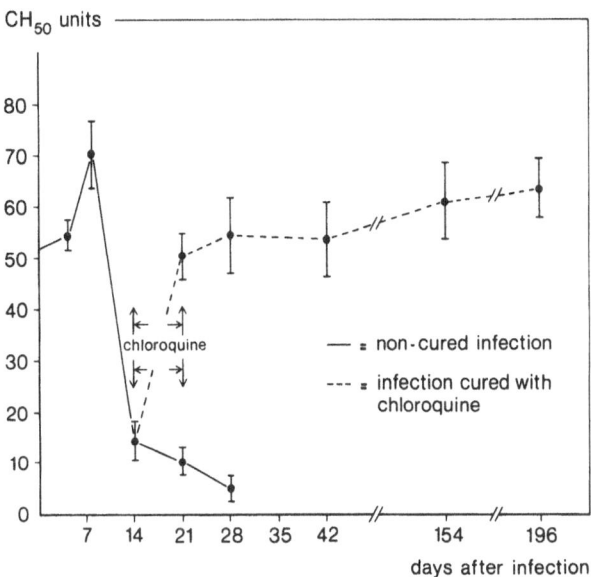

FIG. 4: Complement activity (CH 50) in sera of P. berghei infected Balb/c mice, and after chloroquine therapy (7).

become autoreactive. Evidence has been presented for the existence of different types of circulating immune complexes in infected and in hyperimmune mice. It is likely that autoantibodies participate in the formation and subsequent deposition of I.C. in the renal glomeruli. Some preliminary results obtained with acid elution of kidney tissue suggest that at least SMA can be recovered. Data presented in this paper and previously do not support a hypothesis that complement, though bound to I.C., is responsible for renal lesions. The low CH 50 level in malarious serum possibly affects the size and composition of immune complexes and their solubility in the glomerular deposits (13,14), as well as their half life in serum and glomeruli. The different quantities of circulating soluble I.C. in malarious and in hyperimmune sera might also contribute to their deposition rates.

REFERENCES

1. Poels, L.G., van Niekerk, C.C., Exp. Parasitol. 42 (1977) 235.
2. Poels, L.G., van Niekerk, C.C., Pennings, L., Agterberg, J., van Elven, E.H., Exp. Parasitol. 43 (1977) 255.
3. Kretschmar, W., Jerusalem, C., Z. Tropenmed. Parasitol. 14 (1963) 279.
4. Hayward, A.R., Soothill, J.F., in "Contemporary Topics in Immunobiology 2 (1975) 351.

5. Digeon, Mr., Laver, M., Riza, I., Bach, J.F., J. Immunol.
    Methods 16 (1977) 165.
6. Poels, L.G., van Niekerk, C.C., Franker, M.A.M., van Elven,
    E.H., Exp. Parasitol. 42 (1977) 182.
7. Berden, J.H.M., Hagemann, J.F.H.M., Koene, R.A.P., J. Immunol.
    Methods, in press.
8. Jerusalem, C., Isr. J. Med. Sci., in press.
9. Jerusalem, C., de Wit, J., Proceedings 3rd Int. Congress of
    Parasitology 2 (1974) 1115.
10. Spira, D.T., Golenser, J., Gery, I. Clin. Exp. Immunol. 24
    (1976) 139.
11. Jayawardena, A.N., Am. J. Trop. Med. Hyg. 26 (1977) 223.
12. Freeman, R.R., Parish, C.R., Clin. Exp. Immunol., in press.
13. Takahaski, M., Czop, J., Ferreira, A., Nussenzweig, V.,
    Transpl. Rev. 32 (1976) 121.
14. Izui, S., Lambert, P.H., Miescher, P.A., Clin. Exp. Immunol.
    30 (1977) 384.

ACKNOWLEDGEMENTS

The cooperation of Ms. J. Hagemann is gratefully acknowledged.

SUPPRESSOR CELLS IN TRYPANOSOMA CONGOLENSE-INFECTED MICE

Terry W. Pearson, Georges E. Roelants, Lena B. Lundin
and Kathleen S. Mayor-Withey

International Laboratory for Research on Animal
Diseases (ILRAD), P.O. Box 30709, Nairobi, Kenya

SUMMARY

Spleen cells from mice infected with T. congolense strongly
suppressed lymphocyte stimulation induced in normal spleen cells by
incubation with mitogens or allogeneic cells. Cell dilution studies
showed that suppressor activity was extremely strong. Suppressor
cell activity was markedly reduced by treatment of spleen cell
populations with mitomycin-C and was unaffected by treatment with
anti-Thy.1 sera and complement. Removal of cells which bound
carbonyl iron or which bound to nylon columns, decreased but did
not abolish suppressor activity.

INTRODUCTION

The reduced lymphocyte responses seen in Trypanosoma congolense-
infected mice cannot be explained simply by dilution of T or B
lymphocytes in spleens of infected animals (1). For this reason we
decided to test for suppressor cell activity in spleen cells from
mice infected with T. congolense.

MATERIALS AND METHODS

Spleen cells from uninfected female 6-8 week old C3H-Tif mice
were used as a source of responding lymphocytes whereas spleen cells
from both uninfected and infected mice were the source of "suppressor"
cells. Mitomycin-C treated spleen cells from females 6-8 weeks old
BALB/c mice were used as stimulator cells in mixed lymphocyte

TAB. 1:   Suppression of Mitogen-Induced Lymphocyte Stimulation by Addition of Spleen Cells from Mice Infected with T. Congolense.

Culture Combination			CPM	Stimulation Ratio a)	Percent Suppression b)
A C3H+MED+C3H$_m$			550		
" " +C3H			2,092		
" " +C3H$_m$	INFECTED$^{c)}$		447		
" " +C3H	INFECTED		225		
C3H+LPS$^{d)}$+C3H$_m$			27,907	50.7	
" " +C3H			31,020	56.4	
" " +C3H$_m$	INFECTED		16,010	29.1	43
" " +C3H	INFECTED		3,555	6.5	90
B C3H+MED+C3H$_m$			266		
" " +C3H			922		
" " +C3H$_m$	INFECTED		218		
" " +C3H	INFECTED		317		
C3H+ConA+C3H$_m$			47,822	178.8	
" " +C3H			41,811	157.2	
" " +C3H$_m$	INFECTED		42,723	160.6	11
" " +C3H	INFECTED		17,513	65.8	58

a)   Calculated as: $\dfrac{\text{mean CPM in mitogen-stimulated cultures}}{\text{mean CPM in medium controls (C3H+MED+C3H)}}$

b)   Difference in stimulation above background (between control and infected spleen) expressed as percent of stimulation above background obtained with control spleen cells as suppressors.

c)   Mice were infected for 39 days before removal of spleens.

d)   Although a wide range of LPS and ConA dilutions were used in each experiment, only maximum responses are shown regardless of mitogen dilution.

reactions (MLR). Infection of C3H-Tif mice was performed by injection 10^3 T. congolense strain 5E-12 into the peritoneum as previously described (2).

Mitogen stimulations were performed in flat-bottomed micro-plates. Microwells received 2.5×10^5 responder cells, medium or mitogen dilutions, and 2.5×10^5 cells as "suppressors" in a total volume of 0.3 ml. After 48 hours lipopolysaccharide (LPS) or 72 hours concanavalin A (Con A), ^{125} IUDR was added to each microwell. Cultures were harvested 4 hours later.

TAB. 2:   Suppression of Lymphocyte Stimulation in Normal Mixed
Lymphocyte Cultures by Addition of Spleen Cells from Mice Infected
with T. Congolense.

MLR Combination		CPM	Stimulation Ratio[a]	Percent Suppression[b]
C3H x C3H$_m$		1,710	1.0	
C3H x $\swarrow$BALB/c$_m$ $\nwarrow$C3H$_m$		17,656	10.3	
C3H x $\swarrow$BALB/c$_m$ $\nwarrow$C3H		11,087	6.5	
C3H x $\swarrow$BALB/c$_m$ $\nwarrow$C3H$_m$	INFECTED[c]	8,099	4.7	60
C3H x $\swarrow$BALB/c$_m$ $\nwarrow$C3H	INFECTED	1,519	0.9	100

a)   Calculated as: $\dfrac{\text{mean CPM in allogeneic cultures}}{\text{mean CPM in syngeneic cultures (C3H x C3H}_m)}$

b)   As in footnote b) in Tab.1.

c)   Mice were infected for 27 days before removal of spleens.

     Mixed lymphocyte reactions were also performed in flat-bottomed
microplates. Microwells received 5 x 10^5 responder lymphocytes,
2.5 x 10^5 mitomycin-C treated stimulator cells and unless otherwise
indicated, 2.5 x 10^5 cells as "suppressors" in a total volume of
0.2 ml. After 100 hours incubation ^{125} IUDR was added to each well
and cultures harvested 16 hours later. Cells added as "suppressors"
were often treated with mitomycin-C. Cells so treated are designated with the subscript $_m$.

     Separation of spleen cells into adherent and non-adherent
populations (3), treatment with AKR anti-C3H serum and guinea pig
complement (4), enrichment of T and B lymphocyte populations on
nylon wool columns (5) and removal of macrophages with carbonyl iron
and a magnet (6) were all performed essentially as described.

     The numbers of T and B lymphocytes, null cells and macrophages
in the various cell preparations were determined using fluorescence
microscopy techniques as previously described (2,7).

TAB. 3:   Titration of "Suppressor" Cell Activity in MLR.

Number of Suppressors/Well[a] (X10³)		Stimulation Ratio[b]	Absolute Cell Number Per Well[c] (X10³)			
			B Lymphocytes	T Lymphocytes	Null	Macrophages
250	CONTROL	8.5	103	130	17	2
	INFECTED	0.2	2	15	217	15
125	CONTROL	8.6	52	65	9	1
	INFECTED	1.3	1	8	109	8
62.5	CONTROL	8.5	26	33	5	.5
	INFECTED	1.7	0.5	4	55	4
31.2	CONTROL	8.6	13	17	3	.25
	INFECTED	2.5	0.3	2	28	2

a)   MLR combinations were as in Tab.2. The total cell number per well was kept constant by addition of mitomycin-C treated (C3H$_m$) control spleen cells. "Suppressors" were not mitomycin treated in this experiment and were from spleens of 38 day infected C3H-Tif mice.

b)   As in footnote (a) in Tab.2.

c)   Determined by fluorescence microscopy.

RESULTS AND DISCUSSION

     The effect of adding spleen cells from the trypanosome-infected mice to cultures containing normal spleen cells and varying concentrations of LPS or Con A, is shown in Tab.1. Lymphocyte stimulation was markedly suppressed when spleen cells from infected (but not when from uninfected) mice were added. Treatment of the suppressor cell populations with mitomycin-C reduced their suppressive activity but did not abolish it. Strong suppression was also seen when spleen cells from infected mice were added to normal MLR (Tab.2). Again, mitomycin-C treatment markedly reduced the degree of suppression. Treatment of suppressor cell populations with 2500 RADS from a Cesium source similarly reduced their activity (data not shown).

     Titration of suppressor cell activity was performed by decreasing the number of spleen cells added as suppressors (Tab.3). Strong suppression was seen even when the spleen cells were diluted 8 fold. Addition of spleen cells from normal (uninfected) mice did not suppress normal MLR stimulation at any dilution tested (data not shown). In this experiment, the proportions of T lymphocytes,

TAB. 4: The Effect of Various Treatments on Suppressor Cell
Activity of Spleen Cells from Mice Infected with T. Congolense.

	NUMBER OF EXPERIMENTS	CELLS/ TREATMENT[a]	MEAN PERCENT SUPPRESSION[b]	% CELLS REMOVED BY TREATMENT[c]
A	5	UNTREATED	88	NOT
		MITOMYCIN-C	42	DETERMINED
B		UNTREATED	95	72 (MACROPHAGES) NOW
	3	ADHERENT	86	IN NON-ADHERENT PORTION
		NON-ADHERENT	87	
C		UNTREATED	84	51 (T LYMPHOCYTES)
	3	ANTI-THY.1	88	31 (MACROPHAGES)
D		UNTREATED	100,75	90 (T LYMPHOCYTES)
	2	CARBONYL-IRON	62,23	100 (MACROPHAGES)
E		UNTREATED	74	60 (T LYMPHOCYTES)
	1	NYLON EFFLUENT	60	BOUND TO NYLON
		NYLON BOUND	82	

a)   Treated or untreated spleen cells were added as "suppressors"
in MLR as in Tab.2. Mice were infected for 21-32 days.

b)   As in footnote b) in Tab.1. The individual values are given
for the experiments "D" and for experiment "E".

c)   Determined by fluorescence microscopy.

B lymphocytes, null cells and macrophages present were determined
by immunofluorescence techniques. The number of cells of each type
present in each well was then calculated. At the highest dilution
of suppressors, the ratios of responder lymphocytes to B lymphocytes,
T lymphocytes, null cells or macrophages in the suppressing
population were 1666:1, 250:1, 18:1 and 250:1 respectively. Thus
if the suppressor cells were of a single cell type then they suppress
strongly. The numbers and types of cells present in the cultures at
the end of the 5 day incubation were not determined however and in
the absence of mitomycin treatment could have changed markedly during
incubation. We therefore treated the suppressor cells in various
ways in order to define the type(s) of suppressor cell involved.

Tab.4 summarizes the experiments performed to define the nature
of the suppressor cell(s).

Mitomycin-C treatment reduced suppressor activity greatly
although it did not abolish it. Both adherent and non-adherent cells
suppressed nearly as well as unfractionated cells. The non-adherent

populations were slightly enriched in macrophages, contrary to expectations and perhaps due to their state of activation. Anti-Thy.$1^+c'$ treatment did not reduce suppressor activity at all but in fact did not kill all Thy.1 bearing cells as it did not control (uninfected) spleen populations.

Removal of cells which took up carbonyl iron or bound to nylon columns markedly decreased suppression but did not eliminate it. Carbonyl iron treatment removed T cells as well as macrophages. However the failure to reduce suppression with anti-Thy.$1^+c'$ and the number of T lymphocytes in "nylon bound" suppressing populations suggests that some T cells as well as macrophages are suppressor cells in this system. This issue will probably be resolved by using slightly less crude methods for separation of the cell populations involved.

REFERENCES

1. Roelants, G.E., Pearson, T.W., Mayor-Withey, K.S., Lundin, L.B., (Preceeding paper).
2. Morrison, W.I., Roelants, G.E., Mayor-Withey, K.S., Murray, M., Clin. Exp. Immunol. (1978) (In Press).
3. Mosier, D.E., Science 158 (1967) 1573.
4. Parthenais, E., Lapp, W.S., Scand. J. Immunol. 7 (1978) 215.
5. Julius, M.H., Simpson, E., Hertzenberg, L.A., Eur. J. Immunol. 3 (1973) 645.
6. Corsini, A.C., Clayton, C., Askonas, B.A., Ogilvie, B.M., Clin. Exp. Immunol. 29 (1977) 122.
7. Loor, F., Roelants, G.E., Ann. New York Acad. Sci. 354 (1975) 226.

IMMUNE DEPRESSION IN TRYPANOSOMA CONGOLENSE-INFECTED MICE

G.E. Roelants, T.W. Pearson, K.S. Mayor-Withey and
L.B. Lundin

International Laboratory for Research on Animal Diseases
(ILRAD), P.O. Box 30709, Nairobi, Kenya

The capacity of spleen cells from Trypanosoma congolense-
infected mice to respond to the mitogens concanavalin A and bacterial lipopolysaccharide and to allogeneic lymphocytes is severely
depressed or abolished. Moreover these cells cannot serve as
stimulators of DNA synthesis in mixed lymphocyte reactions. The
lack of responsiveness or of stimulation cannot be attributed to
the dilution of appropriate B or T lymphocytes by the large number
of "null" cells found in the spleen of infected mice. These "null"
cells bear approximately ten times more H-2 antigen than normal
lymphocytes but are devoid of Ia antigen.

INTRODUCTION

Animals infected with African trypanosomes show decreased
immune responsiveness (reviewed in 1). Studies on experimental
animals have focussed mainly on B cell responses in Trypanosoma
brucei infections. We have studied a variety of T cell responses
in CBA/J and C3H/Tif mice infected with Trypanosoma congolense
strain 5E-12. This strain causes a long lasting infection (2) and
thus mimics human and bovine disease better than the usually highly
virulent Trypanosoma brucei.

MATERIALS AND METHODS

Mice: female 6-8 week old CBA/J or C3H/Tif mice (G. Bomholtgard)
were used throughout. Infection was performed by injecting 10^3
Trypanosoma congolense strain 5E-12 into the peritoneum (2).

TAB. 1:   Depression of Mitogen-Induced Lymphocyte Stimulation in
Spleen Cell Suspensions of Trypanosoma Congolense-Infected Mice (a).

DAYS AFTER INFECTION		STIMULATION INDEX		ABSOLUTE CELL NUMBER PER WELL ($\times 10^{-3}$)						
		LPS	CON A	SMALL LYMPHOCYTES			BLAST CELLS			MACRO-PHAGES
				B	T	NULL	B	T	NULL	
9	CONTROL	31.4	84.0	144	72	14	0	0	0	0
	INFECTED	2.4	12.5	120	30	22	6	6	8	8
17	CONTROL	33.5	63.0	136	48	16	0	0	0	0
	INFECTED	2.1	14.0	28	20	124	8	0	14	6
23	CONTROL	39.6	123.3	138	54	2	4	0	0	2
	INFECTED	0.9	2.6	82	22	38	28	6	12	12

a)   These results are from one representative reproducible experiment.

b)   Calculated as: $\dfrac{\text{mean CPM in mitogen-stimulated cultures}}{\text{mean CPM in medium controls}}$

Mitogen stimulations were performed in flat-bottomed microplates.
Microwells contained 5×10^5 viable cells in 0.25 ml. Full titrations
to find the optimal stimulatory dose of mitogen were carried out in
each case. After 48 hours (LPS) or 72 hours (Con A), [125] IUDR was
added and the cultures harvested 4 hours later.

Mixed Lymphocyte Reactions (MLR) were also performed in flat-
bottomed microplates. Microwells contained 5×10^5 responder and
5×10^5 mitomycin-C treated stimulator cells in a total volume of
0.2 ml. After 100 hours [125] IUDR was added and the cultures
harvested 16 hours later. The generation of cytotoxic lymphocytes
was determined in a ^{51}Cr-release cell mediated lympholysis (CML)
assay as described (3). Detailed conditions for mitogen, MLR and
CML assays will be reported in detail (T.W. Pearson et al., submitted
for publication).

Characterization of Cells: the proportions and absolute number of
B (Ig^+), T ($Thy.1^+$) and null ($Ig^-Thy.1^-$) cells were determined by
immunofluorescence procedures (2,4). Quantitation of cell surface
H-2 antigens was performed by quantitative absorption of a titrated
cytotoxic alloantiserum (5).

TAB. 2: Depression of Lymphocyte Stimulation in MLR Using Spleen Cells from Trypanosoma Congolense-Infected Mice as Responder or Stimulators.

DAYS AFTER INFECTION	STIMULATION INDEX		ABSOLUTE CELL NUMBER PER WELL $(\times 10^{-3})$						
	CELLS AS RESPON- DERS	CELLS AS STIMU- LATORS	SMALL LYMPHOCYTES			BLAST CELLS			MACRO- PHAGES
			B	T	NULL	B	T	NULL	
9 CONTROL	6.9	16.0	270	195	35	0	0	0	0
INFECTED	1.5	4.5	230	75	50	5	15	5	10
17 CONTROL	28.6	6.1	340	120	40	0	0	0	0
INFECTED	2.2	0.5	70	50	310	20	0	35	15
23 CONTROL	10.1	11.1	345	135	5	10	0	0	5
INFECTED	2.2	2.0	205	55	95	70	15	30	30

a) These results are from one representative reproducible experiment.

b) Calculated as: mean CPM in allogeneic cultures
                    ─────────────────────────────────
                    mean CPM in syngeneic cultures

RESULTS AND DISCUSSION

Mitogen-induced stimulation of spleen cells from uninfected or 9, 17 and 23 day infected mice is shown in Tab.1. LPS stimulation is almost completely abolished by day 9 of infection. Con A stimulation is reduced but is still appreciable 9 and 17 days after infection (13% and 22% of normal, respectively) and is practically abolished at day 23 after infection.

The capacity of spleen cells from infected mice to serve either as responders or as stimulators in MLR across a major histocompatibility barrier is shown in Tab.2. The responder capacity is practically abolished by day 9 after infection. At that time 28% of the stimulatory capacity was still present but it was abolished by day 17 of infection.

Under the conditions used, LPS stimulates B cells while Con A stimulates T cells (reviewed in 6). The MLR responder cells are a subset of T cells while stimulator cells are Ia bearing B cells (reviewed in 7). It is known that spleen cell populations of Trypanosoma congolense-infected mice undergo drastic changes with a

TAB. 3:   Mixed Lymphocyte Reaction Using Various Numbers of Normal Responder T Lamphocytes.

CELL NUMBERS PER WELL			NUMBERS OF RESPONDER T CELLS/ WELL	MLC CMP	BACK- GROUND CPM	STIMU- LATION INDEX (a)
CBA	CBA_m	$C57BL/6_m$				
$5x10^5$	$2.5x10^5$	$2.5x10^5$	150,000	13,866	3,385	4.1
$2.5x10^5$	$5.0x10^5$	$2.5x10^5$	75,000	2,810	447	6.3
$1.25x10^5$	$6.25x10^5$	$2.5x10^5$	37,500	700	185	3.8

a)   Calculated as: $\dfrac{\text{mean CPM in allogeneic cultures}}{\text{mean CPM in syngeneic cultures}}$

large increase in B and especially "null" cells (2). Thus the absence of responder or stimulatory capacity could possibly be due to the lack of appropriate number of B or T cells in the spleen suspensions assayed.

The composition of the spleen cells suspensions used is also reported in Table 1 and 2. For LPS stimulation enough B cells were certainly present 9 days after infection to give a normal response. At later days the B cell numbers were decreased. At all days studied the number of T cells in the spleens of infected mice was less than half that in spleens of control mice (Tab.1). This was also the case for the MLR responder T cells (Tab.2). In MLR, the number of B cells in the spleen suspensions from 9 and 23 day infected mice was not much different from the number in spleens of uninfected controls. Thus the decreased response to LPS and reduced stimulator capacity in MLR could not be explained by reduced numbers of B lymphocytes. The effect of the decrease in the number of T cells had to be evaluated further.

T lymphocytes from spleens of normal uninfected mice were diluted in MLR to give numbers comparable to those found in the spleen of infected mice (50,000 to 75,000). It is shown in Table 3 that reducing the number of T cells in responder populations from 150,000 to 75,000 and 37,500 dramatically reduces the number of CPM incorporated in the allogeneic MLR and in the control syngeneic culture. However the stimulation ratios were not reduced. Thus the decrease in T cell numbers was not responsible for the decreased responses from infected mice.

TAB. 4:   Stimulation of 5 x 10^5 C57BL/6 Cells by Purified C3H B Cells.

UNINFECTED		INFECTED	
STIMULATION INDEX (a)	NUMBER OF B CELLS/ WELL($x10^{-3}$)	STIMULATION INDEX (a)	NUMBER OF B CELLS/ WELL($x10^{-3}$)
5.4	245	7.8	186
5.9	122	9.1	93
4.3	61	6.3	46
3.5	31	4.7	23
2.2	15	2.4	13
1.4	8	1.9	6
0.9	4	1.4	3

a)   Calculated as: $\dfrac{\text{mean CPM in allogeneic cultures}}{\text{mean CPM in syngeneic cultures}}$

Since the number of B cells appeared to be adequate for stimulation in MLR it was decided to investigate whether there was an intrinsic defect in the MLR stimulatory property of B cells from spleens of infected animals. Populations enriched in B cells can be obtained by sequential agglutination of spleen cells with soybean agglutinin, Ig passage through foetal calf serum and treatment with anti Thy.1 serum and complement (G.E. Roelants et al., unpublished). In this way normal spleen cells consisting of 99% B lymphocytes and 1% null cells were compared (for their stimulatory capacity in MLR) to spleen cells from 30 day infected mice consisting of 74% B lymphocytes, 18% null cells and 8% macrophages. The results presented in Table 4 show that the B lymphocyte population enriched from infected mice had a comparable or better stimulatory capacity in MLR when compared with a similar population of B lymphocytes from uninfected animals.

CONCLUDING REMARKS

The functions of B and T lymphocytes in spleens from Trypanosoma congolense-infected mice are drastically reduced or abolished. This phenomenon is not due to the dilution of adequate responder or stimulator cells by null cells. Rather it will be shown in a companion paper (T.W. Pearson et all., herein) that there is an active suppression caused by one or several types of suppressor cells.

REFERENCES

1. Murray, M., Urquhart, G.M., in:Immunity to blood parasites of animals and man (Miller, L.H., Pino, J.A., McKelvey, J.H. eds), Plenum Press, New York (1977) p.209.
2. Morrison, W.I., Roelants, G.E., Mayor-Withey, K.S., Murray, M., Clin. Exp. Immunol. (1978) in press.
3. Stern, P., Pearson, T., Transplantation (1978) in press.
4. Loor, F., Roelants, G.E., Ann. New York Acad. Sci. 354 (1975) 226.
5. Kohler, G., Pearson, T., Milstein, C., Somatic Cell Genetics, 3 (1977) 303.
6. Greaves, M.F., Janossy, G., Transplant. Rev. 24 (1975) 177.
7. Nabholz, M., Miggiano, V.C., in: B and T cells in immune recognition (Loor, F., Roelants, G.E., E.E. eds.) Wiley, London, (1977) p.261.

RELEVANCE OF POLYCLONAL ANTIBODY FORMATION TO THE DEVELOPMENT OF AUTOIMMUNITY : THE MODEL OF AFRICAN TRYPANOSOMIASIS

Jacques A. Louis, Paul-Henri Lambert, Takatoshi Kobayakawa and Shozo Izui

WHO Immunology Research and Training Centre, Lausanne/ Geneva

Institute of Biochemistry, Epalinges and Hopital Cantonal Geneva, Switzerland

The ability of bacterial lipopolysaccharides (LPS) to trigger the proliferation and differentiation of B lymphocytes in mice, is a well documented phenomenon (1). Administrated in conjunction with antigens, they are also powerful adjuvant of humoral immune responses (2). The possibility that LPS plays a role in the development of autoantibodies is supported by several reports (3,4). However, the precise mechanism(s) by which LPS induce the formation of auto-antibodies remains unclear. It could be that LPS modulate an auto-antigen driven immune response or alternatively, that LPS induce the differentiation of autoantigen reactive cells. The formation of auto-antibodies with various specificities and the production by the host of large quantities of immunoglobulins have been described during African trypanosomiasis. It is therefore possible that the mechanism(s) operational in the formation of autoantibody after LPS administration are similar to those involved in the development of autoantibody seen during African trypanosomiasis. The mechanism by which LPS induce, in mice, the formation of anti-DNA and other auto-antibodies has been investigated and the possible role of polyclonal B cell activation in the development of autoantibodies has been analysed during the course of African trypanosomiasis.

INDUCTION OF ANTI-DNA ANTIBODIES BY POLYCLONAL B CELL ACTIVATORS

The injection of LPS (10 to 100 μg) into mice of various strains induced the formation of anti-DNA antibodies which were already

detected after 3 days (3,5). The maximal response was observed on
day 8. Such injection also led to the appearance of DNA in circulating blood 4 to 24 hours later. Such results could suggest that
the development of anti-DNA antibodies, in this system, would reflect
an enhancement by LPS of an immune response to the released DNA.
However, recent experiments indicate that the induction of anti-DNA
antibodies by LPS is a direct consequence of its ability to trigger
polyclonal B lymphocyte activation.

First, advantage was taken from the existence of the C3H/HeJ
strain of mice which are resistant to most of the biological effects
of LPS including adjuventicity and mitogenicity. It was observed
that the injection of 50 μgr of LPS into C3H/HeJ mice failed to
induce neither the release of DNA in circulation nor the formation
of anti-DNA antibodies (6). In contrast, both phenomena were seen
in similarly treated congenic LPS-high responder C3HeB/FeJ mice.
Since the cellular defect accounting for the lack of mitogenicity of
LPS on C3H/HeJ lymphocytes is confined to the B cell compartment,
the release of DNA and the formation of anti-DNA antibodies after
LPS injection was investigated in C3H/HeJ mice previously transferred
with 50×10^6 C3HeB/FeJ spleen cells. In those mice, there was no
detectable release of DNA in circulation but high titers of anti-DNA
antibodies were measured (6). The reconstitution of the responsiveness to LPS of C3H/HeJ mice was not affected by the removal of T
lymphocytes from the spleen cells inoculum. These results indicate
that the formation of anti-DNA antibodies after LPS does not require
release of DNA in circulation.

Secondly, the ability of various substances to induce polyclonal
antibody synthesis was compared to their capacity to trigger the
formation of anti-DNA antibodies and to provoke the release of DNA
in circulation. It was observed that the injection of more than
0.1 μg LPS, 200 μg of Dextran sulfate (DS) or 10 μg Poly I-poly C
led to the appearance of DNA in circulating blood. While doses as
high as 2 mg of purified protein derivative of tubercule bacteria
RT 32 (PPD) were inefficient in that respect. Anti-DNA antibodies
were found in the serum of mice injected with more than 10 μg LPS,
1 mg DS and also in mice receiving 2 mg PPD. However, there was
no detectable anti-DNA in mice injected with Poly I-poly C. The
ability of various doses of LPS, DS, PPD and Poly I-poly C to induce
in vivo polyclonal antibody synthesis was studied by measuring the
number of splenic antibody producing cells (PFC) against sheep red
blood cells (SRBC) or trinitrophenylated-SRBC (TNP-SRBC) and by
titrating serum antibodies to dinitrophenylated bovine serum albumin
(DNP-BSA). Values obtained in these three test systems increased
significantly after the injection of at least 10 μg LPS, 1 mg DS or
2 mg PPD but not in mice injected with Poly I-poly C. A further
point which merits emphasis is that the kinetic of anti-DNP antibodies in serum after injection of 50 μg of LPS was similar to that

of anti-DNA antibodies. Anti-DNA and anti-DNP antibodies were shown
by sephadex G-200 gel filtration analysis to belong mainly to the
IgM class. These results indicate that doses of LPS, DS or PPD which
induce polyclonal antibody synthesis, in mice, also trigger a parallel
formation of anti-DNA antibodies. In contrast, there was no correlation between the ability of the tested substances to provoke the
release of DNA in circulating blood and to induce anti-DNA antibodies
(7).

Therefore, the formation of anti-DNA antibodies in mice injected
with LPS seems to be the direct result of the stimulation of polyclonal antibody synthesis. Recently, antilymphocyte antibodies were
also detected in the serum of mice injected with LPS (8).

It is possible that polyclonal B cell activation induced by a
variety of, naturally occuring, triggering events would lead to the
development of various autoantibodies. The intensity and the specificity of the autoimmune response are likely dependent on the number
of B cells specific for the corresponding autoantigen. This hypothesis is in agreement with the demonstration of the genetic control
of the formation of anti-DNA antibodies after stimulation with LPS
in various strains of mice (3).

POLYCLONAL ANTIBODY SYNTHESIS AND
FORMATION OF AUTOANTIBODIES IN AFRICAN TRYPANOSOMIASIS

The possible association of polyclonal antibody synthesis with
autoimmune responses has been investigated in mice infected with
trypanosomes. Indeed, this disease represents a model of infection
in which there is an increased level of serum immunoglobulins and a
concomittant occurrence of some autoantibodies (9).

The activation of polyclonal antibody synthesis was tested after
infection of mice with T.brucei by measuring the number of splenic
PFCs against SRBC, TNP-SRBC or fluorescinated-SRBC (FITC-SRBC) (10).
The values obtained in these 3 test systems began to increase 3 days
after the injection of 10^5 trypanosomes. The number of PFCs per
spleen progressively reached a maximum by day 17 while a peak was
observed on day 6 when these values were expressed as PFC per 10^6
spleen cells. It should be noted that the total number of lymphocytes
in the spleen of infected mice is increased by 15 times 3 weeks after
the onset of the disease.

The requirement for T cells in this non specific induction of
proliferation and differentiation of B lymphocytes was investigated
using Balb/c athymic nude (nu/nu) mice. Since the number of PFCs
against TNP or SRBC in nu/nu mice was similar to that observed in
nu/+ mice, the B lymphocyte activation associated with trypanosomiasis

does not appear dependent on a negative or a positive influence from T cells.

In view of this evidence for an intense polyclonal B cell activation during the early stages of trypanosomiasis, the possibility of a concomittent formation of autoantibodies has been investigated (10). First, it was observed that mice infected with 10^5 T. brucei developed a significant anti-DNA response. The titers of anti-SSDNA reached a peak by day 10 and then decreased slowly. These antibodies were of the IgM class. Secondly, during such infection, a sharp increase in the number of antibody-producing spleen cells directed to bromelain-treated syngeneic mouse red blood cells was observed. Since treatment of mouse red blood cells with bromelain reveals hidden autoantigens, these PFCs are the expression of an autoimmune response. Thirdly, antibodies cytotoxic for syngeneic and allogeneic thymocytes were detected using a complement mediated cytotoxicity assay (10). A maximal thymocytotoxic activity was observed in the serum of mice infected 30 days previously; it was still detectable at a dilution of 1/64 and was due to IgM antibodies. It should be stressed that the formation of anti-DNA, anti-Br MRBC and antithymocyte autoantibodies follow the same kinetics. It is also parallel to the development of anti-SRBC, anti-TNP and anti-FITC antibodies indicating the polyclonal B cell activation.

These results suggest that in experimental African trypanosomiasis the development of autoantibodies is an expression of a generalized polyclonal B cell activation.

SUMMARY

There is an induction of anti-DNA antibodies in mice following the administration of bacterial lipopolysaccharides, Dextran sulfate and PPD, which is closely associated with the property of these substances to trigger a polyclonal B cell activation.

In the experimental model of African trypanosomiasis there is also an intense polyclonal antibody synthesis paralleled by the formation of several autoantibodies : anti-DNA, anti-bromelain treated mouse red blood cells and antithymocyte antibodies.

REFERENCES

1.   Coutinho, A., Möller, G. Adv. Immunol. 21 (1975) 113.
2.   Johnson, A.G., Gaines, S., Landy, M. J. Exp. Med. 103 (1956) 225.
3.   Fournié, G.J., Lambert, P.H., Miescher, P.A. J. Exp. 140 (1974) 1189.

4. Primi, D., Hammarström, L., Smith, C.I.E., Möller, G. J. Exp.
    Med. 145 (1977) 21.
5. Izui, S., Lambert, P.H., Fournié, G., Türler, H., Miescher, P.A.
    J. Exp. Med. 145 (1977) 1115.
6. Izui, S., Zaldivar, N.M., Scher, I., Lambert, P.H. J. Immunol.
    119 (1977) 2151.
7. Izui, S., Kobayakawa, T., Zryd, M.J., Louis, J., Lambert, P.H.
    J. Immunol. 119 (1977) 2157.
8. Izui, S., Lambert, P.H., Louis, J., Miescher, P.A. Manuscript
    in preparation.
9. Houba, V., Allison, A.C. Lancet i (1966) 848.
10. Kobayakawa, T., Lambert, P.H., Louis, J. Manuscript in prepa-
    ration.

ACKNOWLEDGEMENTS

This work has been supported by the Swiss National Research
Foundation, the Dubois Ferrière Dinu Lipatti Foundation and the
World Health Organisation. We thank Mrs. Lynn Rose, Ms Catherin
Hug and Edith Mödder, Mr. Guy Brighouse for their excellent technical
assistance, and Mrs. Francoise Ruffet for her contribution in typing
this manuscript.

IN VIVO AND IN VITRO INTERACTION OF TRYPANOSOMA CRUZI WITH MOUSE

MACROPHAGES AND HEART MUSCLE CELLS - FILM PRESENTATION

W. Ax, J. Dyonysius and K.D. Hungerer

Research Laboratories of Behringwerk A.G.

Marburg, West Germany

FILM COMMENTARY

In research on the immunopathology of Chagas infection in the mammalian host, the study of the interaction of Trypanosoma cruzi with host cells is of specific interest. We have shown in a new mouse footpad model that processing of T. cruzi inside macrophages depends on the immune status of the host animal. Macrophages from normal mice act as host cells while macrophages from specifically sensitized (immunocompetent) animals act as active phagocytes. It is demonstrated in nude mice and reconstituted nude mice that this "switch" from host to phagocyte is T-lymphocyte dependent.

The film presents, using time-lapse cinematography, cultures of mouse peritoneal macrophages of immune and non-immune animals infected with blood (trypomastigote) and culture (epimastigote) form of T. cruzi. Contact of parasite with macrophages and penetration was studied to elucidate the process of phagocytosis. Intracellular multiplication of parasites, resulting in death of the host cell and escape, by vigorous rupture of the cell membrane, of newly formed parasites, can be seen in macrophages and heart cells (Fig.1).

INFECTION OF MACROPHAGE
CULTURES WITH ISOLATED BLOOD FORMS

After only a few minutes, trypomastigote blood forms establish contact with the surface of the macrophages; this behavior is clearly different from that of the culture forms. The flagellae remain free in every case. The trypanosome "rubs" several times on the cell surface with the side on which the undulating membrane is

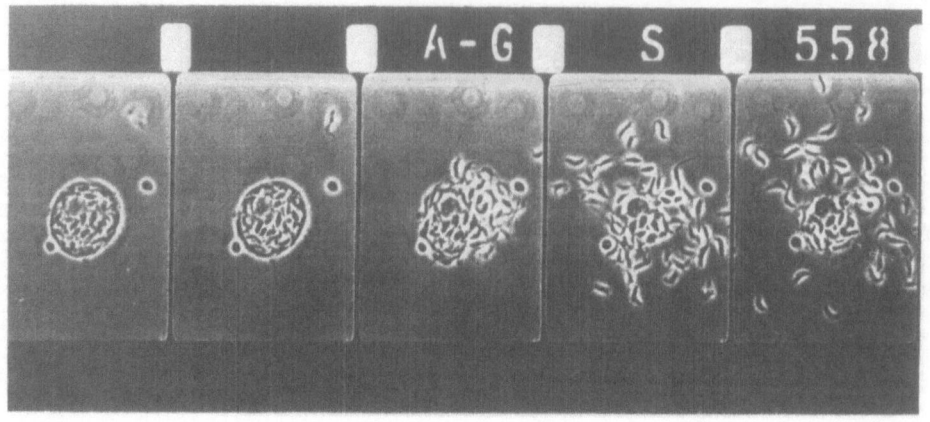

<u>FIG. 1</u>:   Sequence of events of rupture of a macrophage releasing
numerous parasites, developing inside the host cell (strong magnification of a 16 mm film sequence).

located, and then presses itself, rear end first, onto or into the
membrane. The latter draws back at first. Whether in doing this
it encloses the trypanosome cannot be clearly ascertained under a
light microscope. No particular reaction can be detected in the
interior of the macrophage at this point. But immediately after
entering the cell, the trypanosome moves freely and actively inside
the plasma. Up to 40% of the cells are infected, the number depending
upon the trypanosome/macrophage ratio and the duration of incubation.
After an average of 72 to 100 hours, the pseudocysts are mature, and
burst.

In regard to the primary interaction between blood forms and
macrophages from mice which were pretreated in various ways, no
qualitative difference can be found in their mutual behavior. Animals
were pretreated specifically by 1) a living vaccine attenuated by
ethidiumbromide, 2) by lyophilized dead T. cruzi, or non-specifically
with 1) complete Freund's Adjuvans or 2) dead lyophilized L. donovani.

INFECTION OF MACROPHAGE
CULTURES WITH ISOLATED CULTURE FORMS

When a cultured trypanosome (epimastigote) touches the surface
of a macrophage, it frequently and very rapidly adheres to the latter
and is passively surrounded by invaginated macrophage plasma membrane
and engulfed into a vacuole. This represents a typical phagocytosis

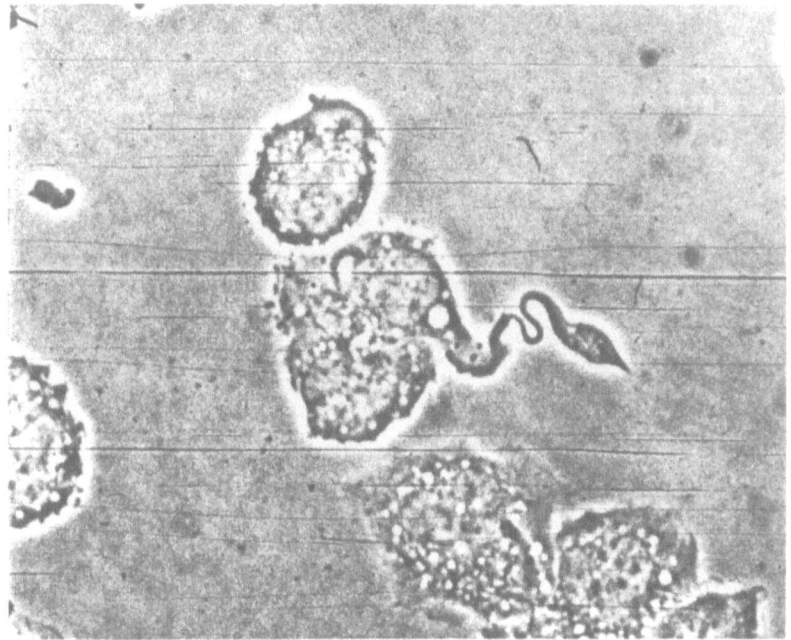

FIG. 2:   Phagocytosis of culture form of T. cruzi. Macrophage
"captures" parasite via the flagellum by plasma protrusion, (strong
magnification from 16 mm film).

process on the part of the macrophage. A short time later numerous
phase-optically dense particles (lysosomes?) start flowing in the
direction of the phagocytic vacuole. Most frequently the trypanosomes are captured at their flagellar end and engulfed by plasma
protrusions that are sometimes extremely elongated (Fig.2).

If the interaction between these trypanosomes and macrophages
is observed, no difference can be seen between it and other culture
forms. The trypanosomes are passively phagocytized, preferentially
via their flagellae, regardless of whether they are trypomastigote
or epimastigote in their morphological character. If epimastigote
trypanosomes obtained from cultures that have been repeatedly passaged
on a synthetic medium are used for infecting macrophage cultures,
pseudocysts are also found inside some of the macrophages, the extent
depending upon the concentration used. When the pseudocysts burst,
mainly trypomastigote forms emerge, i.e. a form qualitatively
different from that used for the infection.

The result of this investigation is the in vitro demonstration
of the markedly reduced ability of the macrophages to actively

phagotize blood forms of T. cruzi, a system which probably acts in
vivo in a comparable way, as one of the possible escape mechanisms
for the parasites. The reason for this remarkable behavior has to
be elucidated now.

COMPARISON OF THE ABILITY OF EOSINOPHILS AND NEUTROPHILS, AND OF
EOSINOPHILS FROM PATIENTS WITH S. MANSONI INFECTION AND NORMAL
INDIVIDUALS, TO MEDIATE IN VITRO DAMAGE TO SCHISTOSOMULA OF S.
MANSONI

Mathew Vadas, John David, Anthony Butterworth, Vaclav
Houba, Lisa David and Nancy Pisani

Robert B. Brigham Hospital, Harvard Medical School and
the Wellcome Trust Research Laboratories, Nairobi

A major step in the understanding of immune effector mechanisms
operating against the larval form of S. mansoni (schistosomula) was
the description by Butterworth et al. (1) of the in vitro damage
caused by antibody dependent cell-mediated mechanism to schistosomula.
The experimental system involved mixing schistosomula with serum from
infected patients (antibody) and buffy coat cells (mixed leucocytes)
from peripheral blood and assaying the damage to schistosomula either
microscopically or by the release of ^{51}Cr from labelled organisms.
Studies with purified cells from patients with S. mansoni infection
and eosinophilia suggested that the eosinophils were the active cell
component in the buffy coat preparations (2,3).

It is of interest to compare cells from normal and infected
individuals in the above systems. Unfortunately the methods of
purification of eosinophils available did not allow the recovery of
pure eosinophils in reasonable numbers from non-eosinophilic
individuals. Thus, in an effort to develop a method of purification
of eosinophils from non-eosinophilic blood, we attempted to adapt a
method developed by Ross and his colleagues (4,5) for the separation
of bone marrow components.

In this paper we shall describe this method, show the effect of
the separated cell components in three in vitro systems on schistosomula and compare cells from patients with S. mansoni infection and
normal individuals in one of the assay systems.

The method for purification of eosinophils and neutrophils has
been described in detail elsewhere (6). Briefly, it involves the
centrifugation at 1200 g for 45 min of buffy coat cells obtained by

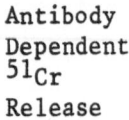
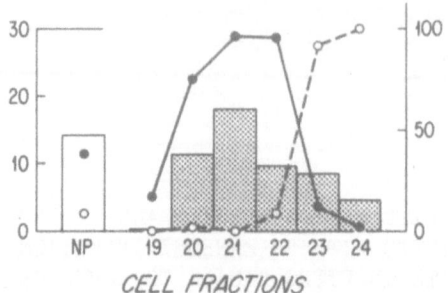

Antibody
Dependent
^{51}Cr
Release

Percent
eosinophils
(o) and
neutrophils
(●)

CELL FRACTIONS

FIG. 1:   Antibody dependent ^{51}Cr release by nonpurified (NP) buffy
coat cells (open bar) and by Metrizamide discontinuous gradient
purified fractions (stippled bars). The difference between the sum
of the percentages of eosinophil and neutrophil and 100 gives the
percent mononuclear cells in each fraction. Cell fraction numbers
indicate the percent of M used in the gradient step from the top of
which cells were collected.

dextran sedimentation of heparinized blood over discontinuous
gradients of either Ficoll-Hypaque (F-H) or slightly hypertonic
Metrizamide (M). F-H gradients are made by diluting with water a
stock solution of 15% Ficoll and 20% Hypaque, M ones by diluting
with Tyrodes gel a stock solution of 30% M in Tyrodes gel. After
centrifugation, the cells are collected from each density interface,
cell numbers are estimated on a Coulter counter, and a differential
is counted on cytocentrifuged slides stained with Giemsa.

The cell recovery from F-H gradients is about 75% and from M
ones in the excess of 95%. The high recovery in the latter instance
insures that no major cell component is lost during the separation
procedure. The purity of eosinophils was greater than 90% and often
100% (in 22 out of 29 separations using F-H and in 21 out of 26
separations using M). In the cases when the purity of eosinophils
was less than 90% the content of eosinophils in blood was less than
2%. This method also yielded more than 95% pure preparations of
neutrophils and of monocytes.

Next we examined the effect of these purified components in the
^{51}Cr release assay. The release of ^{51}Cr was estimated after a 7 hr
incubation of labelled somula, antibody and equal numbers of either
unpurified buffy coat cells or one of the cell fractions obtained
after a M gradient. The result of a typical experiment is shown in
Figure 1. Both practically pure neutrophils and eosinophils caused

TAB. 1:

Cell fraction*	NP	1.08	1.09	1.11	1.12
Composition (N/E)**	60/5	85/5	96/0	5/97	4/94
Percent adherence***	45	15	15	70	55

*   Numbers indicate density of F-H gradient from top of which cells were removed. NP-non purified.

**   Percentage of neutrophils (N) and eosinophils (E) in fraction.

*** Adherence in the absence of antibody was 3-4%.

antibody dependent ^{51}Cr release, but the highest level was seen in the neutrophil preparations. These findings have been obtained in over 20 experiments and are consistent over a wide range of effector target ratios and durations of incubation. The inferior performance of eosinophils in this assay was not due to the stress of the separation procedures. Microscopically and electron-microscopically the cells are intact after separation and are 100% viable. The above finding differs from our earlier observations that neutrophils were ineffective in this in vitro system. The most likely explanation is that the separation procedure in our earlier experiments involved 2 gradients, and the recovery of neutrophils was very low. This small subpopulation of neutrophils, which have a low density, have again been shown not to be effective in this system.

Next we attempted to compare eosinophils and neutrophils from patients with S. mansoni infection with those from individuals in the ^{51}Cr release assay. Technically satisfactory experiments were performed on 11 patients. The average eosinophila in these patients was 11.8% and the average S. mansoni egg count in their stools was 620 per g. This group was compared to 6 normals with an average of 3% eosinophils in their peripheral blood. The mean neutrophil mediated antibody dependent ^{51}Cr release in the group with infection was similar to that in the normals (16.9 vs 17.8 respectively). In contrast, the mean eosinophil mediated antibody dependent ^{51}Cr release was 10.6 in the infected and 5.6 in the normal group. These latter figures differ at a $p < 0.05$. We have not yet established if eosinophils from patients with eosinophila not due to S. mansoni infection also perform better than those from normal individuals.

Another assay measuring the interaction of cells with antibody coated schistosomula involves the measurement of adherence of these cells to the organism. Adherence is quantitated as the percent of

TAB. 2:

Cell fraction[*]	NP	20	22	Mix	23	24
Composition (N/E)[**]	65/3	80/0	98/0	80/20	30/70	5/95
Percent death[***]	4	3	0	6	42	48

[*]   Numbers indicate percentage of M gradient from top of which cells were collected. NP - nonpurified. Mix mixture of 22 and 24 in ratio of 4:1.

[**]   Percentage of neutrophils (N) and eosinophils (E) in fractions.

[***] Death in the absence of antibody was 1-2%.

organisms which bear 3 or more cells on their surface after an incubation period of 3 hr. The results of a typical experiment are shown in Table 1. Both neutrophil and eosinophil rich cells adhered to antibody coated schistosomula, but the highest degree of adherence was seen in the eosinophil rich fraction. These findings were reproducible in more than 10 experiments using blood from either normal individuals or patients with S. mansoni infection. It was now of interest to determine if either of these cell populations are able to kill the parasite in vitro. In order to see parasite death, it was necessary to extend the incubation period to 7 or 24 hr. Parasites were counted as dead if they did not wriggle and took up methylene blue dye. Some of these organisms were surrounded by many layers of cells ('coffins'). The antibody dependent death of parasites after 7 hr of incubation with various cell fractions is shown in Table 2. Purified eosinophils caused parasite death roughly in proportion to their numbers. Pure neutrophils were not effective. This experiment was repeated 5 more times with similar findings.

The increased ability of eosinophils over neutrophils to adhere to schistosomula was surprising in view of the paucity of Fc receptors detected on their surface (7,8,9). Using our purified cell preparations the percentage of Fc receptor bearing eosinophils (as determined by rosetting techniques) was considerably less than neutrophils and the rosettes which did form were less dense. In addition depletion of eosinophils with the ability to form rosettes did not lead to a decrease in their capacity to adhere to antibody coated schistosomula.

The findings in this paper raise several interesting questions. First, does the ^{51}Cr release assay detect an early phase of damage to the parasite, which, given the appropriate circumstances, can be repaired? Secondly, is the relative inability of neutrophils to adhere to schistosomula an intrinsic property of the cell, or is it due to an active process by the parasite ridding itself of attached cells? Finally, does the adherence of eosinophils to antibody coated schistosomula involve a structure different from the Fc receptor or does a second event stabilize the weak union formed by eosinophil Fc receptor and antibody coated schistosomula? We are currently trying to resolve these three questions in our laboratory.

SUMMARY

A reliable and reproducible method that produces separate fractions of pure eosinophils and neutrophils from normal peripheral blood was described.

The interaction of eosinophils and neutrophils with antibody coated schistosomula was examined in vitro.

Neutrophils were highly active in the ^{51}Cr release assay and most formed rosettes with antibody coated red cells, but they adhered poorly to schistosomula and did not kill the organisms.

Eosinophils, although they were less active in the ^{51}Cr release assay than neutrophils and few formed rosettes, adhered strongly to schistosomula and, in the presence of antibody, were able to kill organisms.

Organisms from patients with S. mansoni infection and eosinophilia were more effecient than eosinophils from normal individuals in their capacity to release ^{51}Cr from labelled somula in the presence of antibody.

REFERENCES

1. Butterworth, A.E., Sturrock, R.F., Houba, V., Rees, P.H. Nature (Lond.) 252 (1974) 503.
2. Butterworth, A.E., Sturrock, R.F., Houba, V., Mahmoud, A.A.F., Sher, A., Rees, P.H. Nature(Lond.) 256 (1975) 727.
3. Butterworth, A.E., David, J.R., Franks, D., Mahmoud, A.A.F., David, P.H., Sturrock, R.F., Houba, V. J. Exp. Med. 145 (1977) 136.
4. Ross, G.E., Jarowski, C.I., Rabellino, M.E.M., Winchester, R.J. J. Exp. Med. 147 (1978) 730.
5. Winchester, R.J., Ross, G.D., Jarowski, C.I., Wang, C.Y., Halper, J., Broxmire, H. Proc. Nat. Acad. Sci. USA 74 (1977) 4012.
6. Vadas, M.A., David, J.R., Butterworth, A.E., Pisani, N.T., Siongok, T.A. (To be published)
7. Tai, P.C., Spry, C.J.F. Clin. Exp. Immunol. 24 (1976) 415.
8. Gupta, S., Ross, G.D., Good, R.A., Siegal, F.P. Blood 48 (1976) 755.

9.   Ottesen, E.A., Stanley, A.M., Gelfand, J.A., Gadek, J.E.,
      Frank, M.M., Nash, T.E., Cheever, A.W. Amer. J. Trop. Med.
      Hyg. 26 (1977) 134.

ACKNOWLEDGEMENTS

    Supported by a grant from the Clark Foundation and by the
Wellcome Trust.

SIGNIFICANCE OF LOCAL FORMATION OF IMMUNE COMPLEXES WITHIN GRANULOMATA IN SCHISTOSOMIASIS

V. Houba, R.F. Sturrock and A.E. Butterworth

WHO-Immunology Research and Training Centre and Wellcome

Trust Research Laboratories, Nairobi, Kenya

The formation of granulomata around the eggs trapped in different tissues (mainly liver and gut) in hosts infected with A. mansoni or S. japonicum is a typical example of a cell-mediated mechanism resulting in immunopathological lesions in parasitic diseases; it also represents the main pathological consequence of these infections, leading to the hepatosplenic form of the disease. The eggs themselves cause little damage to the tissue, but the granulomatous host reaction around each egg may destroy a volume of tissue equal to 100 times that of the egg alone (Bloch et al., 1972).

It is now quite well documented that granuloma formation is an immunological reaction of the cell-mediated (delayed hypersensitivity) type to soluble antigens released from the eggs (Warren et al., 1967; Boros and Warren, 1970; Warren 1974a; Warren 1974b). The size of granulomata increases with time, reaching a peak with subsequent diminution; the time sequence depends on strains of parasite and hosts studied. It is important to note that diminution in the size of newly formed granulomata is accompanied by a marked improvement in hepatosplenic disease (Warren, 1974).

The phenomenon of diminishing granulomata was originally called "endogenous desensitization" (Domingo and Warren, 1968), and was later explained by "immunological blockade" (Warren, 1974), probably mediated by antibodies.

We have studied this phenomenon in baboons infected by S. mansoni, on liver samples obtained from serial biopsies and autopsies, using immunofluorescence technique (Sturrock et al., 1976, 1978; Houba, 1976; Houba, 1977). At the beginning of granuloma formation (about 6 weeks after infection) we were able to demonstrate soluble

egg antigens around the eggs in tissue, but no antibody or complement.
Later on, and especially around the time of maximum granuloma size
(8-16 weeks), the precipitates positive for egg antigens, IgM and
complement were found between the cells or phagocytozed inside the
cells, usually on the periphery of the granulomas. This finding
suggested local formation of immune complexes within granulomata:
egg antigens coming from the eggs, antibodies from the circulation.
These complexes were phagocytozed by neutrophils, eosinophils and,
perhaps, other cells approaching from the periphery of granuloma.
Positive immunofluorescence findings of immune complexes were also
seen during the later stage of infection (after 20 weeks) in smaller
granulomata, but, in these specimens, the phagocytes were usually
distributed within the whole granuloma; in some of the specimens we
were also able to demonstrate the plasma cells, suggesting that at
this later stage antibodies could be produced locally.

The time sequence between formation of immune complexes and
diminution of granuloma size suggests that competition for egg
antigens is an explanation for the diminution in size of the new
granulomas. This interference of humoral mechanisms with cellular
reactions would represent a rather rare example of a beneficial
mechanism in immunopathology.

It was interesting that the antibody to soluble egg antigens
in the deposits was always IgM, even at later stages of infection.
IgG was not present during the early stage of granuloma formation,
but it was detected at later stages when, however, it did not have
egg antigen specificity and was always found in a fibrous pattern
between the cells. Topographically, in double immunofluorescence
staining, it corresponded more to collagen fibres than to fibrin.
It seemed, therefore that this IgG may simply adhere to newly formed
collagen fibres or, perhaps, that it might be an autoantibody to
collagen.

In conclusion, local formation of immune complexes between
egg antigens and IgM antibodies may explain the diminution of granuloma size due to competition for the antigens; this interference of
a humoral mechanism with a cellular (delayed type) reaction represents
a rather rare example of a beneficial mechanism in the immunopathology
of parasitic diseases.

REFERENCES

1.   Bloch, E.H., Abdel Wahab, M.F., Warren, K.S. Am. J. Trop. Med.
      Hyg. 21 (1972) 546.
2.   Boros, D.L., Warren, K.S. J. exp. Med. 132 (1970) 488.
3.   Domingo, E.O. Warren, K.S. Am. J. Pathol. 52 (1968) 369.

4. Houba, V. In: Pathophysiology of parasitic infection. Ed.
    E.J.L. Soulsby, Academic Press, New York, pp. 221-232 (1976).
5. Houba, V. In: Progress in Immunology III. Eds. T.E. Mandel,
    C. Cheers, C.S. Hosking, I.F.C. McKenzie, G.J.V. Nossal.
    Australian Academy of Science, pp. 681-687 (1977).
6. Sturrock, R.F., Butterworth, A.E., Houba, V. Parasitology 73
    (1976) 239.
7. Sturrock, R.F., Butterworth, A.E., Houba, V., Karamsadkar, S.D.,
    Kimani, R. S. mansoni in the Kenyan baboon (Papio anubis):
    The development and predictability of resistance to homologous
    challenge. Trans. Roy. Soc. Trop. Med. Hyg., accepted (1978).
8. Warren, K.S. In: Parasites in the host; mechanisms of survival.
    Ed. Ciba Foundation, Elsevier-North Holland, pp. 243-261, (1974a).
9. Warren, K.S. Adv. Biosc. 12 (1974b) 637.
10. Warren, K.S., Domingo, E.O., Cowan, R.B.T. Am. J. Pathol. 51
    (1967) 735.

ACKNOWLEDGEMENTS

The authors are indebted to Mrs. J.E. Houba and Mrs. M.
Kinyanjui for their excellent technical help. This study was
supported by World Health Organization and Wellcome Trust.

THYMUS-DEPENDENCE AND KINETICS OF INTESTINAL MAST CELLS AND GLOBULE LEUCOCYTES

E.J. Ruitenberg, Anneke Elgersma and C.H.J. Lamers

Laboratory for Pathology, National Institute of Public

Health, P.O. Box 1, Bilthoven, The Netherlands

INTRODUCTION

The numbers of mast cells and intra-epithelially located globule leucocytes in the gut mucosa of various animal species, including laboratory rodents and ruminants, increase during the intestinal phase of nematode infections (1,2). Both cell types are characterized by metachromatic intracytoplasmatic granules. Although the cellular response is connected with the immune expulsion of worms from the gut, the function of these cells is still unclear.

Based on the absence of mast cell globule leucocyte proliferation in congenitally athymic (nude) $B_{10}LP$ mice infected with the nematode Trichinella spiralis we suggested that intestinal mast cells represent a separate population of mast cells which is thymus (T) dependent (3). The cellular response was restored after thymus transplantation. This clearly indicated that the thymus plays a crucial role in the appearance of these cell types. Theoretically this may be due to 1) the presence of an intact thymus, 2) thymus serum factor(s), 3) T dependent serum antibodies, or 4) T dependent cellular reactions and/or their products. In this report we studied the second and third possibility in athymic mice.

MATERIALS AND METHODS

Reconstitution studies were performed in male Balb/c nude (nu/nu) mice (Gl.Bomholdtgaard, Aarhus, Denmark). Comparisons were made with age-matched mice heterozygous for the nude gene (+/nu).

Mice were infected by oral inoculation with 300 T.spiralis larvae. Groups of infected or uninfected nude mice were a) treated twice with normal Balb/c +/nu serum (N.M.S.), by intraperitoneal injection of 0.5 ml at days 0 and 5; b) treated twice with hyper-immune serum (HIS), collected from 14-week old male Balb/c +/nu mice, infected orally with 300 T.spiralis larvae at 10 and 13 weeks of age. An amount of 0.5 ml HIS (72 h. PCA titer $\geqslant 1 : 40$) was injected intraperitoneally in the recipient mice at 0 and 5 days after injection, or c) controls for the treatment.

Groups of infected and uninfected +/nu mice were included as well. All groups were autopsied at 7 days post infection (p.i.). The presence of intestinal mast cells and globule leucocytes was studied in a 10 cm portion of the proximal jejunum with a Swiss roll technique. Tissues were processed as described previously (3).

RESULTS

In uninfected +/nu and nu/nu mice very few intestinal mast cells were present in the villus stroma. They were localized subepithe-lially or scattered both in the core of the villus from tip to bottom, and in the lamina propria between the crypts of Lieberkühn. Globule leucocytes were localized in the epithelium of both the crypt and the base of the villus.

At day 7 p.i. the number of intestinal mast cells in +/nu mice was increased (Tab.1). The localization was the same as in the uninfected animals. The number of globule leucocytes in +/nu mice at day 7 was increased as well. Now, the cells were also observed in the epithelium of the mid-villous and occasionally in the tip region. Both in the uninfected and infected +/nu mice the number of globule leucocytes was higher than that of intestinal mast cells.

The results of the effect of serum transfer on the appearance of intestinal mast cells and globule leucocytes in infected nu/nu mice at day 7 after infection are presented in Table 1.

In infected NMS-treated nude mice an increase in intestinal mast cells as compared to non-infected NMS-treated mice was observed. No increase was seen in untreated or HIS-treated infected nude mice.

The number of intestinal globule leucocytes increased three to four-fold in all three infected groups, irrespectively of the transfer of NMS or HIS. After infection globule leucocytes were also found in the mid-villous region. Very few metachromatic intra-epithelially located cells in the crypts of Lieberkühn and the base of the villus showed mitotic figures. These cells were believed to be globule leucocytes. Furthermore, metachromatic cells were observed twice within the lumen of the gut.

TAB. 1: Effect of serum transfer on appearance of intestinal mast cells and globule leucocytes in the small intestine of male Balb/c nude mice, 7 days after oral infection with 300 Trichinella spiralis larvae each (compared with non-treated +/nu mice).

Group	Status	T.spiralis	Treatment	Intestinal mast cells mean ± s.d.	p**	Globule leucocytes mean ± s.d.	p**
1	nu/nu	-	-	0.89 ± 0.60*	N.S.	1.60 ± 2.07*	N.S.
2	nu/nu	+	-	0.89 ± 0.60		5.40 ± 3.71	
3	nu/nu	-	NMS +/nu***	0.80 ± 0.45	< 0.02	1.00 ± 1.73	< 0.02
4	nu/nu	+	NMS +/nu	2.80 ± 1.30		5.80 ± 3.03	
5	nu/nu	-	HIS +/nu***	1.20 ± 1.64	N.S.	3.00 ± 2.12	< 0.05
6	nu/nu	+	HIS +/nu	0.40 ± 0.55		9.60 ± 4.72	
7	+/nu	-	-	0.40 ± 0.90	< 0.02	6.60 ± 1.70	< 0.001
8	+/nu	+	-	6.20 ± 3.80		117.60 ± 46.30	

* : mean number of intestinal mast cells or globule leucocytes per 20 villus/crypt units per animal (groups of 5 animals).

** : statistical analysis (Student's t test).

*** : normal serum (NMS) from male Balb/c +/nu mice, 10-15 weeks of age, injected intraperitoneally (0.5ml) in the recipient mice at days 0 and 5 post infection

**** : hyperimmune serum (HIS) collected from Balb/c +/nu mice, 14 weeks of age, infected orally with 300 T.spiralis larvae at 11 and 13 weeks of age, and injected intraperitoneally (0.5 ml) in the recipient mice at days 0 and 5 post infection. 72 h-passive cutaneous anaphylaxy (PCA) reaction performed with HIS, yielded a PCA titer of ≥1:40.

DISCUSSION AND CONCLUSIONS

Although in infected NMS treated nude mice an increase in mast cells was observed the conclusion that a thymus serum factor played a role was invalidated by the results of the HIS treated group. Therefore it can be concluded that the intestinal mast cell response to a T.spiralis infection is T-dependent, but not dependent on thymus serum factor(s) or specific T-dependent antibodies. So far, only thymus reconstitution yielded results comparable to those of intact +/nu mice (3). With regard to the origin of the mast cell recent unpublished studies in rats showed that as yet unidentified precursor cells (from thymus origin?) proliferate in the intestinal mucosa under the influence of a parasitic (T.spiralis) stimulus to "mastoblasts" and mature into mast cells. This observation supports earlier findings in N. brasiliensis infected rats (1).

The T.spiralis infection in nude mice induced a minor increase in the number of globule leucocytes which is thus thymus-independent and occurs in the absence of a mast cell response. The major increase in numbers of globule leucocytes in infected animals with an intact thymus is paralleled by an increase in intestinal mast cells, which was lower than that of globule leucocytes. On the basis of these data it can be concluded that the dramatic increase in numbers of globule leucocytes is presumably a consequence of the presence of a thymus or of thymus-dependent reactions, excluding thymus-dependent antibodies, induced by a Trichinella infection. Together with the observed mitotic activity of globule leucocytes, these conclusions lead to the hypothesis that globule leucocytes are intra-epithelial cells independent of mast cells. The presence of some metachromatic cells within the gut lumen suggests an extrusion of globule leucocytes form the villus epithelium. The latter hypothesis is further supported by recent observations in T.spiralis-infected rats in which globule leucocytes were observed to shift from a predominantly infra- to a mainly supra-nuclear position in relation to the post infection time (Ruitenberg and Elgersma, unpublished results).

The origin of the globule leucocyte has been the subject of debate since its first description in the intestinal mucosa of various mammals (4). In contrast to most authors, who described the globule leucocyte as a cell derived from another cell type (mast cells, eosinophils, plasmacells, lymphocytes), Takeuchi and co-workers (5) believed globule leucocytes to be a specific cell type of mesenchymal origin. Our observations would support the idea that the globule leucocyte is a cell sui generis.

The conclusions of this experiment are therefore:

1. the intestinal mast cell response to T.spiralis is dependent on an intact thymus or T-dependent cellular reactions.

2. globule leucocytes represent an independent cell population.
3. a minor globule leucocyte response to a T.spiralis infection
is T-independent.
4. a major globule lecucoyte response to a T.spiralis infection
is T-dependent, but independent of thymus serum factor(s) or
specific T-dependent antibodies.

REFERENCES

1. Miller, H.R.P., Jarret, W.F.H., Immunology 20 (1971) 277.
2. Gregg, P., Dineen, J.K., Rothwell, T.L.W., Kelly, J.D., Vet.
   Parasit. 4 (1978) 35.
3. Ruitenberg, E.J., Elgersma, A., Nature, Lond., 264 (1976) 258.
4. Weill, P., Arch. Mikrosk. Anat. Entw. Mech. 93 (1919) 1.
5. Takeuchi, A., Jervis, H.R., Sprinz, H., Anat. Rec., 164 (1969)
   79.

INHIBITION OF LYMPHOCYTE PROLIFERATION DURING PARASITIC INFECTION WITH NIPPOSTRONGYLUS BRASILIENSIS

H. Stockinger and W. König[1]

Institute of Medical Microbiology, Johannes Gutenberg University, Mainz, West Germany

[1]Correspondence: Dr. W. König, Inst. of Med. Microbiology 6500 Mainz, Hochhaus Augustusplatz, W. Germany

INTRODUCTION

It is now well established that parasitic infections can lead to the production of high titers of IgE anti parasitic antibodies in experimental animals and in man (1,2). One of the best studied experimental systems involves the ability of the nematode parasite Nippostrongylus brasiliensis (N.B.) to stimulate a high titer re- aginic antibody response to worm antigens in the rat. These studies were extended by the reports of Orr and Blair that parasitic infec- tions can cause non specific proliferation of IgE antibody response against antigens unrelated to those of the parasite (3). The amplification of an already existing IgE antibody response can be induced before infection by inoculating the antigen together with a conventional adjuvant (2). IgE responses against different antigens may be simultaneously potentiated, while the IgE response remains largely unaffected. The indications that larvae produce factors which stimulate the previously programmed IgE response has been confirmed recently (4). It has been demonstrated that serum of infected rats contains a factor which leads to the maturation of IgE-B cells in the bone marrow. While all these data are in favour of a highly differentiated immune response, as is determined by the production of a minor antibody class, recent data in several parasite models emphasize the role of suppressive events on the stimulation of lymphocytes with mitogens. Wicher et al. described the inhibition of the lymphocyte response to phytohaemagglutinin in treponema pallidum infected rabbits and further demonstrated that the serum of infected rabbits contains inhibitors which suppressed the mitogenic and allo- geneic lymphocyte response (5-7). An impairment of the capacity to

generate alloantigen specific cytotoxic T lymphocytes (CTL) was
observed in mixed lymphocyte cultures (MLC) established with spleen
cells from mice infected with schistosoma mansoni (8). Inhibitors
of lymphocyte proliferation can be produced by factors released
from the parasite as well (9). In contrast, Bloch et al. demonstrated
a stimulation of ^{3}H-thymidine uptake by mesenteric lymph-node and
spleen cells to Concanavalin A during the primary infection of rats
with Nippostrongylus brasiliensis (10). We studied the mitogenic
responsiveness of rats after primary and secondary infection with
N.B. towards PHA and investigated the effect of serum derived from
infected rats on normal lymphocytes with regard to their proliferative functions.

MATERIALS AND METHODS

Infection of rats with N.B. was carried out as described by
Ogilvie (1,11) and the radioimmunoassay (RIA) for IgE was performed
as has been published (12). The parasite directed IgE antibody in
the serum of rats infected with N.B. was determined by the passive
cutaneous anaphylaxis (PCA) reaction with a sensitization period of
48 hrs. Serial dilutions of the antiserum were injected intracutaneously into the back of normal rats and the animals received an
intravenous injection of worm extracts and 1 ml of 1% Evans blue.
Single cell suspensions were obtained from mesenteric lymph-node
and spleen cells by teasing them through a stainless sieve in cold
RPMI 1640 containing 100 U penicillin and streptomycin per ml.
Cells were washed, resuspended in TC-199 medium containing 5% AB$_6$
serum, 2 mM glutamine and 100 U penicillin-streptomycin. 1 x 10^6
cells were suspended in 200 μl medium and cultured in microtiter
plates for 72 hours. 1 μCi ^{3}H-thymidine was added; 18-24 hours
later, cells were collected by a cell harvester and the filterbound
radioactivity was measured. Unless mentioned otherwise, data are
expressed as standard index (SI % = mean experimental counts/min
divided by counts of the control/min). Enrichment of T cells was
performed on nylon wool columns as has been described by Julius and
Herzenberg (13).

RESULTS AND DISCUSSION

For parasite infection Wistar rats were inoculated with 2500
larvae of N.B. and reinfected with 5000 larvae after 28 days. Serum
was obtained every third day and the IgE-antibody titers determined
by RIA and PCA reaction. The non parasite IgE-antibody titer
increased from day 5 and peaked at day 14, while the parasite specific IgE antibody was almost negligible; after reinfection specific
IgE antibody increased at day 5 showing a peak at day 13-16 and then

TAB. 1:   Pattern of mitogenic responsiveness of mesenteric lymph-node (MLN) and spleen cells to PHA, during primary and secondary infection of rats with N.B. (+: = enhancement;   -: = suppression).

| days after | 1. infection | | 2. infection | |
infection	MLN-cells	spleen cells	MLN-cells	spleen cells
		stimulatory index		
1	+3.7+0.8	+4.5+0.2	+ 7.5	-1.2
3	n.d.	+1.3	+ 2.3	+1
7	-4	+1	- 4	-4
12	n.d.	n.d.	+18.9	+1
14	-4	-2	n.d.	n.d.
28	+1	n.d.	n.d.	n.d.

$$\text{stimulatory index} = \frac{\text{mean experimental cpm + PHA}}{\text{PHA control of normal rats}}$$

declined rapidly. Its pattern paralleled the IgE antibody response measured by the RIA. While the total IgE antibody content in unin-fected sera was about 0.3μg/ml, the IgE antibody titer increased up to 150-300 μg/ml during infection. With many groups of animals it could be demonstrated that the IgE antibody response was non persistent but transitory. Using the fluorescent technique, the occurence of IgE-B cells was studied in Wistar rats. It was observed that IgE-B cells could be detected in spleen and mesenteric lymph-node cells already at day 7 after infection. About 8% of the total lymphocytes revealed fluorescence which increased at day 14 and revealed background levels at day 28 after infection. On the whole, more IgE-B cells were detected in MLN cells as compared to spleen cells. While these results have been demonstrated by others as well (4), it was a necessary tool in our studies to correlate the mito-genic responsiveness of lymphocyte to a characteristic immunological feature during the course of parasite infection.

The preferential production of a minor antibody class represents a highly differentiated immune response. Therefore, it was of particular interest to study the mitogenic responsiveness of the lymphocytes during the infection of rats with N.B.

Spleen and mesenteric lymph-node cells were obtained at days 1, 5, 7 and 14 after primary infection. The mitogenic responsiveness to PHA (16 μg) was studied and compared to that of non infected rats. Table 1 demonstrates that spleen and mesenteric lymph-node cells show a significant enhancement of ^{3}H-thymidine uptake as compared to normal

TAB. 2:   Effect of normal and infected serum on the lymphocyte
proliferation of MLN-cells obtained from normal rats to PHA.

serum during infectious days	stimulatory index MLN-cells
0	3.5+0.3
1	4.0
5	-1.5
7	-2+0.3
8	+1
10	-2
14	-2+0.3
28	1.5+0.5

$$\text{stimulatory index} = \frac{\text{mean experimental cpm + serum + PHA}}{\text{control cpm + PHA}}$$

rats at day 1, which is followed by a rapid decline at day 5 and
leads to a marked suppression of the ^{3}H-thymidine uptake at days
7 and 14.   The suppression is more easily demonstrated in mesenteric
lymph-node cells as in spleen cells.   When rats were infected after
5-6 weeks and the time course of the mitogenic responsiveness was
carried out, the following results were obtained : With mesenteric
lymph-node cells an enhancement of the mitogenic responsiveness was
observed at day 1, followed by a significant suppression at day 8
and a second enhancement at day 12.   This pattern was reproducible
although the degree of enhancement and suppression varied in different experiments.   With spleen cells, the mitogenic responsiveness
equals the control,   i.e. uninfected rats;   they show a suppression
at day 7 and reach normal levels at day 12.   These data indicate
that during primary infection an enhancement of the mitogenic
responsiveness is followed by a long lasting suppression of spleen
and mesenteric lymph-node cells, while in reinfected animals these
effects are not as pronounced.   Currently, experiments are in
progress to clarify which cell might be responsible for the suppressive effect.

The infection with N.B. does not only affect the cells, but
induces serum derived inhibitors as well.   Normal mesenteric lymph-
node cells were incubated either with normal rat serum or with sera
obtained at various days after infection and their responsiveness
towards PHA was studied (Tab.2).   It is apparent that the presence
of normal rat serum increases the mitogenic responsiveness up to 4
fold as compared to the control which shows the responsiveness in

the presence of medium. When the sera of infected rats were added to the culture, it was demonstrated that from day 5, the responsiveness of the cells decreased and was less than the control (PHA + cells + medium). The loss of enhancing activity of normal rat serum and even the suppression could be demonstrated with infected sera for more than 4 weeks. The inhibitory factors could be enriched in fractions obtained at 40 and 50% salt saturation.

It appears from our data that these factors act on the cells and not on mitogenic stimulus. The serum derived inhibition is a reversible phenomenon and can be removed by washing the cells. While the inhibitors have not been characterized biochemically until now, it appears from our data that soluble worm antigen exerts its inhibitory effects on the stimulation of lymphocytes as well. These data combined support the idea that during parasitic infection a highly differentiated immune response is initiated. The differentiation leads to a loss in the lymphocyte responsiveness resulting in suppression and inhibition of the immune functions towards stimuli unrelated to the antigens of the parasite.

REFERENCES

1. Ogilvie, B.M., Jones, V.E. Immunity in the parasitic relationship between helminths and host. Progr. All. 17 (1973) 93.
2. Bloch, K.J., Ohman, J.L., Waltzin, J., Cygan, E.W. Potentiated reagin response: initiation with minute doses of antigen and mitogens followed by infection with N. brasiliensis. J. Immunol. 110 (1973) 197.
3. Orr, T.S.C., Blair, A.M.J.N. Potentiated reagin response to egg albumin and conalbumin in N. brasiliensis infected rats. Life Sci. 8 (1969) 1073.
4. Ishizaka, T., Urban, J., Ishizaka, K. IgE formation in the rat following infection with N. brasiliensis. Cell.Immunol. 22 (1976) 248.
5. Wicher, V., Wicher, K. In vitro cell response of treponema pallidum infected rabbits. I. Lymphocyte transformation. Clin. exp. Immunol. 24 (1977) 480.
6. Wicher, V., Wicher, K. In vitro cell response of treponema pallidum infected rabbits. II. Inhibition of lymphocyte response to phytohaemagglutinin by term of t. pallidum infected rabbits. Clin. exp. Immunol. 29 (1977) 487.
7. Wicher, V., Wicher, K. In vitro cell response of treponema pallidum infected rabbits. III. Impairment in production of lymphocyte mitogenic factor. Clin. exp. Immunol. 29 (1977) 496.
8. Coulis, P.A., Lewert, R.M., Fitch, F.W. Splenic suppressor cells and cell mediated cytotoxicity in murine schistosomiasis. J. Immunol. 120 (1978) 58.

9.   Dessaint, J.P., Cannis, D., Fisher, E., Capron, A. Inhibition
     of lymphocyte proliferation by factor(s) produced by schisto-
     soma mansoni. Eur. J. Immunol. 7 (1977) 624.

10. Bloch, K.J., Towle, Ch., Mills, J.A. Stimulation by mitogen
     and metabolic antigen of DNA synthesis by mesenteric lymph
     node and spleen cells obtained during primary infection of
     rats with N. brasiliensis. Cell. Immunol. 28 (1977) 181.

11. Ogilvie, B.M., Love, R.J., Jarra, W., Brown, K.N. Nippostongylus
     brasiliensis infection in rats. Immunology 32 (1977) 521.

12. Ishizaka, T., König, W., Kurata, M., Mauser, L., Ishizaka, K.
     Immunologic properties of mast cells from rats infected with
     Nippostrongylus brasiliensis. J. Immunol. 115 (1975) 1078.

13. Julius, M.H., Simpson, E., Herzenberg, L.A. A rapid method
     for the isolation of functional thymus-derived murine lympho-
     cytes. Eur. J. Immunol. 3 (1973) 645.

ACKNOWLEDGEMENTS

This study was supported by DFG, SFB 107, A 6.

IMMUNOPATHOLOGY OF M. LEPREMURIUM (MLM) INFECTION IN B6 C3AN AND

(C3HxB6) F1 MICE

R. Nayak[1], T. Holden, M. de Sousa and R.A. Good

Sloan-Kettering Institute for Cancer Research

New York, N.Y. 10021, USA

INTRODUCTION

Experimental studies of infection with M. lepremurium have revealed the existence of differences in the cellular reaction to lesions of murine leprosy in outbred and inbred strains of mice differing at the H-2 locus (1-6).

The present paper is the first of a series in which we shall examine in detail the question of a possible association between the major histocompatibility complex and susceptibility to the experimental form of the infection. We examine the histopathological and bacteriological features of MLM infection in C3H AN (C3H), C57B1/6 (B6) and (C3H x B6) F1, male and female mice.

MATERIALS AND METHODS

Experimental animals: B6 mice were obtained from Jackson Laboratories, Bar Harbor, Maine. C3H and F1 mice were purchased from Cumberland Farms, Clinton, Tennessee.

Inoculum and Inoculation: MLM of Hawiian Strain was generously given to us by Dr. Soo Duk Lin of Seoul University, S. Korea. The bacilli were propagated in C3H mice by subcutaneous inoculation in

---

[1]   Present address: Dept. of Pathology, Rhode Island Hospital, Brown University Division of Biological and Medical Sciences, Providence, Rhode Island, USA.

the axilla. When the axillary inflammatory nodules were 5 - 10 mm
in diameter, the animals were killed and the nodules excised under
sterile conditions. The nodules were finely minced with sterile
scissors and diluted in Hanks BSS or RPMI 1640. The suspension was
ground in a Mickle homogenizer to liberate intracellular bacilli.
The suspension was allowed to settle for 5 minutes and the bacteria
enriched supernate withdrawn. This was diluted further and the
bacteria counted. The bacterial concentration was finally adjusted
to 10^9 bacilli/ml. The mice received 0.1 ml (containing 10^8 bacilli)
of the inoculum into the tail vein. Thirty to forty animals per
group were inoculated at 8-12 weeks of age; groups of 10-12 mice
were killed at 2 and 3 months after inoculation. The remaining
mice were followed daily and killed when found sick at the terminal
stages of the disease.

Bacteriology: Samples of liver and spleen were weighed. The
spleens were finely minced and suspended in 2 ml of RPMI 1640. The
suspension was homogenized to liberate intracellular bacilli,
allowed to settle and the supernate withdrawn. The final volume of
the suspension was made up to 4-10 ml depending on the stage of the
disease.

The livers were homogenized in glass tissue grinders with 2 ml
of RPMI 1640. The suspension was diluted and centrifuged at 1,000
RPM for 10 mins. The supernate was withdrawn and the pellet
containing liver tissue discarded. The supernate was then centrifuged at 10,000 for 20 mins, to sediment the bacilli. The bacterial
pellet was re-suspended in 5-10 ml of RPMI 1640 depending on stage
of disease.

Bacteria in these suspensions were counted by the method of
Shepard and McCrae (7) and the results expressed as numbers of MLM
microorganisms per mg of tissue.

Histology: The tissues were immediately fixed in formol
alcohol and subsequently processed by standard methods. Sections
were stained with Zeel-Nielson stain for detection of acid fast
bacilli (AFB) and with Hematoxylin-Eosin.

RESULTS AND DISCUSSION

AFB Counts: Some degree of individual variation was seen in
each group examined. In general, however, within each group, the
bacterial counts in spleen and liver were lower in female mice than
in male mice, and in both female and male mice, lower numbers of
bacilli were found per mg of tissue in the liver than in the spleen.

B6 males had the highest liver bacterial load at 2 months
(161.72 x 10^3 AFB/mg) and three months (3652.1 x 10^3 AFB/mg) post
inoculation, in contrast with the lower numbers found in male C3H
livers at 2 months (27.4 x 10^3 mg) and 3 months (291.85 x 10^3/mg)
and the much lower recoveries from the (C3H x B6) F1 livers
(2.09 x 10^3/mg at 2 months and 23.62 x 10^3/mg at 3 months). A
similar pattern of bacterial load was observed in the female
livers, i.e. B6>C3H>F1.

The differences in spleen bacterial counts between the three
groups of mice studied were not as clearcut as those seen in the
liver. At 3 months post-inoculation, however, the highest spleen
counts in males and females were found in B6 mice, the lowest in
(C3H x B6) F1 and intermediate numbers of AFB were recovered from
the C3H spleens.

The finding of highest bacterial counts in the organs of B6
mice was accompanied by the poorest clinical progression of the
disease in this group of mice.

Histopathology: In the two-parent strains the liver lesions
observed were similar to those previously reported by Closs (5).
Little or no mononuclear cell reaction was seen surrounding the MLM
loaded macrophages, whereas the lesions in B6 liver contained a
clearcut mononuclear infiltrate. In spite of this, the bacterial
counts in the B6 livers were significantly higher than those in C3H
mice.

In the spleen and lymph nodes, the MLM infection was found to
have a very precise ecology. Mycobacteria in the C3H mice were
first seen to proliferate in the splenic thymus dependent areas,
mostly at the boundary with the B cell region. The microorganisms
expanded within these areas and were also found in the red pulp.
Except for the animals killed at the terminal stages, they did not
proliferate in the B cell areas of the white pulp. Likewise in
the lymph nodes, mycobacteria were found in the endothelium of the
post-capillary venules in the outer section of the thymus dependent
area, but not so conspicuously in the B cell areas. In addition,
much higher numbers of MLM were seen in the inguinal than in the
mesenteric lymph nodes.

In conclusion, we have confirmed that different strains of
mice differ in susceptibility to MLM infection. We failed to
confirm, however, previous reports indicating that B6 are less
susceptible than C3H mice (5). In the present study we found the
highest bacterial counts in B6 organs and a poorer clinical progression in this group of mice. Furthermore, we have observed differences in susceptibility between males and females and F1 hybrid
resistance at least in the early stages of infection. In previous

reports of MLM infection female mice were used.

F1 hybrids of certain inbred mouse strains are known to be able to reject parental hemopoietic tissue grafts (8). This reaction is immunogenetically specific, thymus-independent resistant to lethal irradiation and abrogated by antimacrophage agents. It is tempting to speculate that a similar genetically determined but non-specific heightened macrophage activity accounts for the antimycobacterial resistance in the F1 hybrid mice. Finally, we found that mycobacteria showed very precise environmental preferences for growth within the lymphoid tissues. Further clarification of the mechanism underlying the preferential proliferation of MLM in inguinal lymph nodes, in post-capillary venule endothelium and in splenic thymus dependent area macrophages, should provide clues for identification of the cell populations responsible for resistance or susceptibility within one host and clues for the conditions of growth necessary for culture of the microorganisms in vitro.

REFERENCES

1. Closs, O., Haugen, O.A., Acta. Path. Micro. Scand., Section A. 81 (1973) 401.
2. Closs, O., Haugen, O.A., Acta. Path. Micro. Scand., Section A. 82 (1974) 459.
3. Closs, O., Haugen, O.A., Acta. Path. Micro. Scand., Section A. 83 (1975) 51.
4. Closs, O., Haugen, O.A., Acta. Path. Micro. Scand., Section A. 83 (1975) 59.
5. Closs, O., Infection and Immunity 12 (1975) 480.
6. Closs, O., Infection and Immunity 12 (1975) 706.
7. Shepard, C.C., MacRae, D.H., Int. J. Leprosy 36 (1968) 78.
8. Cudkowicz, G., Bennett, M., J. Exp. Med. 134 (1971) 1513.

ACKNOWLEDGEMENT OF FINANCIAL SUPPORT

This work was done with support from NIH Grants CA 08748, CA 10267.

GENETICS AND MECHANISMS OF RESISTANCE OR SUSCEPTIBILITY TO MURINE LISTERIOSIS

Christina Cheers[1], T.E. Mandel[2] and I.F.C. McKenzie[3]

[1]Department of Microbiology, [2]Walter and Eliza Hall Institute, [3]Department of Medicine, Austin Hospital University of Melbourne, Parkville, Victoria 3052, Australia

INTRODUCTION

Surprisingly little is known about the detailed genetics and immunological or physiological mechanisms which govern resistance or susceptibility to bacterial infection, although considerable information exists on the response of various inbred mouse strains to different infections (1). Frequently the observed effects are multigenic, but more often they have not been analysed. An exception to this is resistance of mice to Salmonella typhimurium which appears to be due to a single gene controlling the strength of delayed type hypersensitivity responses to a number of antigens, including salmonella (2).

In order to examine the genetics of cell mediated, rather than humoral, immunity to a bacterium, Listeria monocytogenes was chosen as an ideal model organism. It induces an acute infection of mice and can be lethal. The mechanism of acquired immunity in mice has been studied in detail (3) and does not involve antibody (4). We found that different strains of mice fell distinctly into two categories of resistant or susceptible to intravenously administered listeria (5). C57B1/6, C57B1/10, SJL and NZB were resistant. Balb/c, CBA, DBA/1, C3H, A/WySn, WB/Re, LP.RIII and 129/J were susceptible. Of these we chose to study in detail the genetics and mechanisms of resistance/susceptibility in two strains, C57B1 and BALB/c. The first results of these investigations have already been reported (5,6). The present paper deals largely with further attempts to elucidate the number of genes involved and differences in the inate ability of the cells of the two strains to handle the organism.

TAB. 1:   Resistance of backcross and F_2 mice to approximately 1 x 10^4 listeria

Strain	% resistant	Number tested
BALB/c	2	45
(BALB/c x C57Bl/6)F_1	96	45
BALB/c x F_1 backcross	52	131
C57Bl/6 x F_1 backcross	96	45
BALB/c	5	20
(BALB/c x C57Bl/10)F_1	93	27
(BALB/c x C57Bl/10)F_2	79	154

METHODS

The strains of mice used, method of infecting and assaying infection have been described (5,6).

Microscopy: Tissues were fixed in buffered formalin for light microscopy or with Karnovsky's fixative (7) for electron microscopy and then processed by conventional techniques. The ultra thin sections were stained with uranyl acetate and lead citrate, and paraffin sections with haematoxylin and eosin or with Gram stain.

RESULTS AND DISCUSSION

Three approaches have been used to determine the number of genes governing resistance or susceptibility. The F_1 hybrid between C57Bl and BALB/c mice was found to be intermediate in its resistance (5), suggesting either incomplete penetrance of interaction between resistance and susceptibility genes in the two parents. Nevertheless it was possible to chose a dose of listeria which was uniformly lethal for BALB/c and non-lethal for (BALB/c x C57Bl)F_1. This dose, approximately 1 x 10^4 was used to distinguish resistant and susceptible individuals in backcrosses to either parent, or amongst (BALB/c x C57Bl)F_2. The results of a number of experiments are pooled in Tab. 1.

If a single gene governs resistance, it is expected that 50% of the backcross onto the susceptible strain will be susceptible, 50% resistant, while the backcross onto the resistant strain will be

TAB. 2:   Listeria in livers of susceptible or resistant mice

Dose of Listeria	Log_{10} listeria/g of liver $\pm$ S.E.			
	3 hours		24 hours	
	BALB/c	C57B1/10	BALB/c	C57B1/10
1×10^3	-	-	5.28+0.10	4.00+0.28
1×10^5	3.91+0.12	3.80+0.10	6.84+0.03	5.79+0.09
1×10^7	5.70+0.18	5.81+0.11	9.68+0.10	8.00+0.13
1×10^9	7.61+0.14	7.43+0.09	-	-

100% resistant (1). The observed figures, 52% of the BALB/c x F_1 backcross and 96% of the C57B1/6 x F_1 backcross being resistant conform closely to these expectations. Similarly with the F_2 mice, a single gene would be expected to produce 75% of resistant progeny. The observed figure was 79%.

This evidence strongly suggests that the different behaviour of resistant C57B1 mice and susceptible BALB/c mice is governed by a single gene or group of linked genes. Earlier work (5) showed that the resistance gene was not linked to MHC, Ig allotype, H-1, H-3, H-4, H-8, Thy-1, Hc or coat colour genes. Efforts to produce a line, congenic with BALB/c but carrying the genes for resistance to listeria, have reached the third generation backcross. The mice are still approximately 50% resistant, 50% susceptible.

We have found that acquired immunity was equally efficient in C57B1 and BALB/c (6), but the infection differed in two main respects. The bacterial numbers initially reaching spleen and liver were identical in C57B1 and BALB/c mice, but normal macrophages from resistant mice were better able to suppress early progress of infection than were those of susceptible mice. The difference was evident particularly in the liver within the first 24 hours (Tab.2). Secondly the resistant mice developed acquired immunity and marked bactericidal activity more than 24 hours before the susceptible mice (Fig.1).

In view of the strong suggestion of a single gene, it may be that the two observations are inter-related. Therefore we examined events in the liver during the first 24 hours by light and electron microscopy. Light microscopy of the livers of mice 24 hours after 1×10^7 listeria showed foci of infection associated with Kupffer cells. These cells were crammed with gram positive organisms.

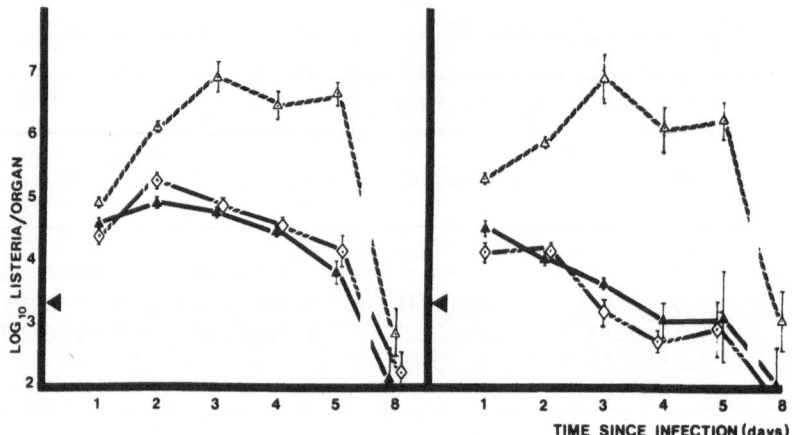

FIG. 1:   Growth of 2 x 10^3 listeria in the spleens (left) and
livers (right) of BALB/c (Δ --- Δ), C57Bl/10 ($\blacktriangle$———$\blacktriangle$) and
(BALB/c x C57Bl/10)F$_1$ ($\Diamond$___. .___ $\Diamond$) mice. Groups of 5 mice.
Vertical bars represent standard errors.

Fewer foci were apparent in C57Bl/10 mice than in BALB/c mice, but
numbers of bacteria in individual C57Bl/10 or BALB/c cells were
indistinguishable. Electron microscopy showed bacteria unbounded
by phagocytic membranes (Fig.2) in the Kupffer cells of both strains.
Other membranes in the cells were satisfactorily delineated. Furthermore in livers of mice infected for only 3 hours with 1 x 10^9 listeria
(the dose necessary in order to see any bacteria) the bacteria were
seen within phagocytic vacuoles (Fig.2). Often there were many
bacteria within a single vacuole, either because they were ingested
as a group or possibly because of fusion of vacuoles. Although
numbers of bacteria were indistinguishable between the two strains
at three hours by light or electron microscopy or by viable counts,
electron microscopy revealed a higher percentage of apparently
damaged electron transparent bacteria in the BALB/c mice.

Both strains showed a well-developed polymorph response 24 hours
after injection of low doses of listeria, but this was lacking in
BALB/c mice given 1 x 10^7 bacteria. Although listeria were rarely
seen in polymorphs, this curious observation led us to investigate
the effect of a polymorph exudate in the peritoneal cavity on the
lethality of intraperitoneally injected listeria. An exudate
comprising 70-80% polymorphs did not alter the LD$_{50}$ or time to death
in either strain (Chan and Cheers, unpublished).

In conclusion, it seems that resistance to L. monocytogenes in
mice is governed by a single gene or group of linked genes. Differences in the handling of L. monocytogenes organisms by the macrophages of resistant and susceptible strains of mice become evident
within 24 hours of infection. Polymorphs, although prominent in the

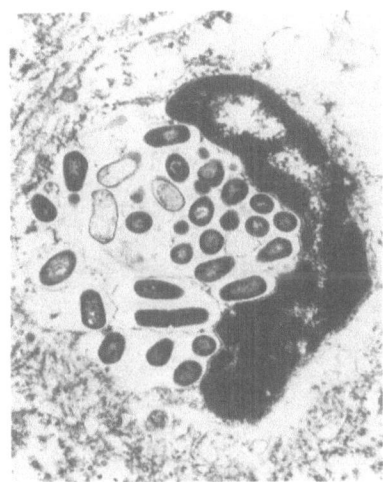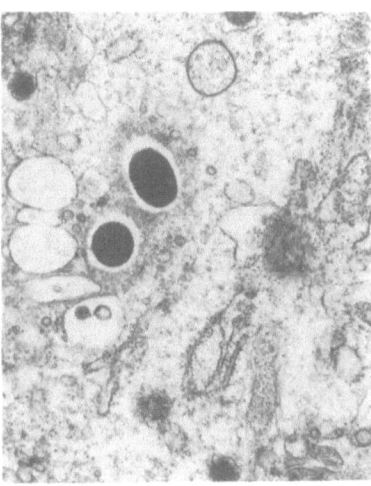

FIG. 2:   Electron micrographs of listeria within Kupffer cells of BALB/c mice. Left: Section taken 3 hours after infection showing many bacteria, some apparently damaged, within a phagocytic vacuole. Magnification 12,000X. Right: Section taken 24 hours after infection showing bacteria free within cytoplasm. Magnification 23,000X. (Reduced 30% for purposes of reproduction.).

early exudate, apparently do not protect against listeria. The mechanism whereby the liver Kupffer cells suppress early growth of listeria, and whether early macrophage handling also explains the differences in the time of onset of immunity in the resistant and susceptible strains remain to be seen.

REFERENCES

1. McDevitt, H.O., Landy, M., Genetic control of immune respon-
    siveness. Academic Press, New York. (1972).
2. Plant, J. Glynn, A.A., J. inf. Disc. 133 (1976) 72.
3. North, R.J., in Mechanisms of Cell Mediated Immunity, ed. R.J.
    McClusky, S. Cohen. John Wiley & Sons, New York. (1974).
4. Miki, K., Mackaness, G.B., J. exp. Med. 120 (1964) 93.
5. Cheers, C., McKenzie, I.F.C., Inf. Imm. 19 (1978) 755.
6. Cheers, C., McKenzie, I.F.C., Pavlov, H., Waid, C., York, J.,
    Inf. Imm. 19 (1978) 763.
7. Karnovsky, M.J., J. Cell. Biol. 27 (1965) 137A.

ACKNOWLEDGEMENTS

This work is supported by the National Health and Medical Research Council of Australia.

GENETIC CONTROL OF SUSCEPTIBILITY TO T. CONGOLENSE INFECTION IN

INBRED STRAINS OF MICE

W.I. Morrison, G.E. Roelants, T.W. Pearson and Max Murray

International Laboratory for Research on Animal Diseases

(ILRAD), P.O. Box 30709, Nairobi, Kenya

INTRODUCTION

In recent years much attention has been focussed on the possible genetic control of susceptibility to disease. In the case of livestock diseases, the use of certain breeds or lines of animals which show increased resistance, may have potential application. Thus in trypanosomiasis of cattle certain breeds such as the West African Ndama have been shown to be less susceptible than Zebu or European breeds to the disease (1). In parallel with studies in cattle we have examined the susceptibility of different inbred strains of mice to Trypanosoma congolense infection. Having established that differences in susceptibility occur between strains of mice, an attempt has been made to determine the underlying mechanism and to characterise its genetic basis.

MATERIALS AND METHODS

Unless stated otherwise, infection of mice was performed by intraperitoneal inoculation of 5×10^3 T. congolense, strain 5E-12, as previously described (2). All mice used were females of 10-12 weeks of age. Susceptibility of the various strains was determined by measuring levels of parasitaemia and duration of survival (2). Groups of at least 30 mice were used with a minimum of 12 animals from each group being monitored daily for levels of parasitaemia over 24-26 days of infection.

Spleen cell suspensions prepared from infected and control mice

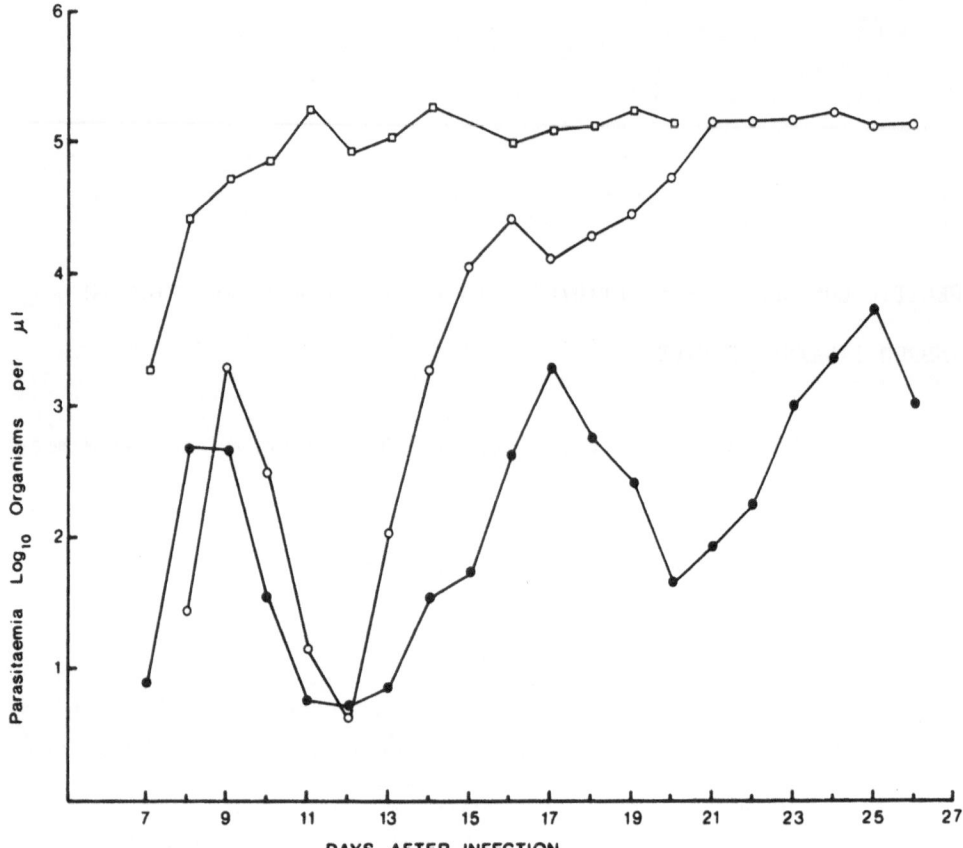

FIG. 1:   Daily mean parasitaemia in groups of 12 A/J (□), C3H/He
(o) and C57B1 /6 (●) mice infected with T. congolense.

were tested for response to the mitogens lipopolysaccharide (LPS)
and concanavalin A (Con A) and in mixed lymphocyte reaction (MLR)
with allogeneic spleen cells.   In addition, the suppressor activity
of infected spleen cells on an ongoing MLR of syngeneic control
responder cells with allogeneic targets was tested.   Details of these
procedures are described in a companion paper (3).

RESULTS AND DISCUSSION

T. congolense infection was compared in 8 inbred strains of
mice.   Marked differences in survival were found between the 8
strains ranging from the highly susceptible A/J all of which had
died by day 30 after infection, to the much less susceptible C57B1/6
most of which survived beyond day 80 (Tab.1).   There was not a clear
cut differentiation into strains of high and low susceptibility but

TAB. 1:   Duration of survival in inbred strains of mice infected
with T. congolense.

| Mouse Strain | Percentage Deaths | | | | | Mean Survival Time |
| | Days After Infection | | | | | |
	20	40	80	120	160	(Days)
A/J	85.7	100				15.8
SWR/J	88.0	100				16.9
129/J	58.5	90.2	100			22.6
BALB/c/A	20.0	28.8	100			49.5
DBA/1J	0	62.2	100			36.3
C3HeJ	0	12.5	100			59.0
AKR/A	0	7.9	45.4	97.7	100	81.7
C57BL/6J	0	2.8	13.8	61.1	100	110.2

rather a gradation between the A/J and C57B1/6 strains. A similar
pattern of relative susceptibility has been found using 5 other
isolates of T. congolense. However, the differences in susceptibility are very much dependent on the virulence of the trypanosomes.
Thus, using a relatively virulent trypanosome the differences in
survival between strains are much smaller. Susceptibility was
closely related to the levels of parasitaemia at least during the
early stages of infection. Thus, in A/J mice, consistently high
levels of parasitaemia in excess of 10^5 organisms per μl were found
from day 9 onwards (Fig.1). By comparison C57B1/6 mice showed a
characteristic series of parasitaemic peaks between which the level
of parasitaemia was extremely low or undetectable. C3H/He mice
which were of intermediate susceptibility initially showed a pattern
of parasitaemia similar to C57B1/6 but later showed sustained high
levels of parasitaemia.

Infectivity titrations carried out in A/J and C57B1/6 mice have
shown similar ID_{50} values for the strains. Thus there does not
appear to be a difference in susceptibility to infection per se but
rather a difference in the ability of the different strains of mice
to limit the numbers of parasites in the circulation (2).

To test the effects of infection on the immune system of 4 of
the mouse strains (A/J, C3H/Tif, AKR and C57B1/10) we measured
splenic lymphocyte responses to mitogens and to allogeneic cells
and also measured suppressor cell activity of spleen cells at

TAB. 2:   Suppression of response to mitogens and allogeneic cells
and suppressor activity (*) on a normal MLR of spleen cells from 4
strains of mice infected with T. congolense.

Mouse Strain	Percentage Suppression							
	Day 9		Day 17		Day 24			
	Con A	LPS	Con A	LPS	Con A	LPS	MLR	Sup- pressor*
A/J	95	90	100	100	100	95	100	100
C3H/Tif	98	88	99	100	96	100	91	98
AKR	87	86	81	71	82	100	69	56
C57BL/10	13	4	87	80	91	82	52	38

various intervals after infection (Tab.2). Mice were infected by
intraperitoneal inoculation of 5 x 10^3 organisms of T. congolense
13E-1. This isolate was derived by mouse passage from 5E-12 and
was found to be slightly more virulent than 5E-12 so that the C3H/Tif
mice showed higher levels of parasitaemia and died at an earlier
stage of infection than the C3H/He mice in previous experiments.
However both AKR and C57Bl/10 mice showed longstanding infections.
In general the responses to Con A and LPS were more depressed in
the strains of highest susceptibility. With the exception of
C57Bl/10 mice at day 9, depression was always greater than 70%. At
day 24 of infection, the depression of response of infected spleen
cells in MLR and their suppressor activity on normal MLR both
appeared to be related to mouse strain susceptibility. That is,
spleen cells from the more susceptible strains showed greater
depression and suppressor activity (Tab.2).

A comparison of susceptibility was made between C57Bl/10 mice
and the congenic resistant strains B10A, B10.BR and B10.D2/new. No
significant differences in levels of parasitaemia or in survival
were found. Thus it would appear that H-2 haplotype does not
obviously influence susceptibility to T. congolense infection.

A comparison of susceptibility was also carried out in A/J and
C57Bl/6 mice, (A/J x C57Bl/6) F1 hybrids and the corresponding backcrosses. This experiment is still in progress and is now at day 60
after infection. All of the A/J and 20% of the (F1 x A/J) mice have
died while no deaths occurred in the other groups. All of the F1
hybrids and the (F1 x C57Bl/6) backcross mice showed a cyclical
pattern of parasitaemia similar to the C57Bl/6. However the peak

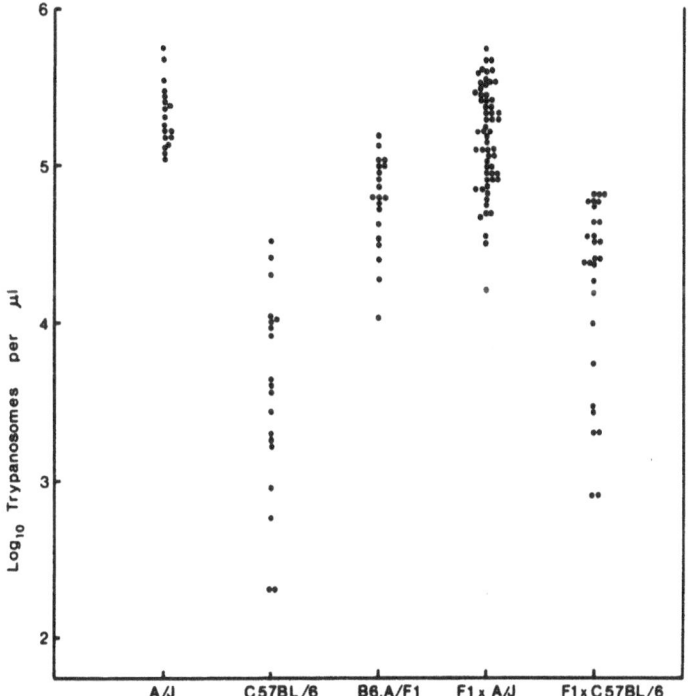

FIG. 2:   First peak of parasitaemia in individual mice infected
with T. congolense.

levels of parasitaemia in the Fl hybrids were significantly higher
than in the C57B1/6;   the (Fl x C57B1/6) backcross mice generally
showed a level of parastiaemia intermediate between the parental
strains (Fig.2) The levels of the initial peak of parasitaemia in
Fl x A/J) backcross mice were found to overlap those found in the
A/J and Fl hybrid mice. As in the A/J parents, in some of the
backcross mice this high level of parasitaemia was maintained;
however, in approximately 70% of the animals the level of parasitaemia dropped dramatically by at least 2 log_{10} units before
rising to a second peak. Thus it would appear that the relative
resistance exhibited by the C57B /6 mice is inherited as a partially
dominant trait under complex genetic control involving at least 2
genes.

REFERENCES

1.   Murray, P.K., Murray, Max, Morrison, W.I., Wallace, M., McIntyre,
     W.I.M. International Scientific Council for Trypanosomiasis
     Research and Control, 15th Meeting (1978) in press.

2.   Morrison, W.I., Roelants, G.E., Mayor-Withey, K.S., Murray,
      Max, Clin. Exp. Immunol. (1978) in press.
3.   Pearson, T.W., Roelants, G.E., Lundin, L.B., Mayor-Withey, K.S.,
      (1978) (These proceedings).

SESSION   C

IMMUNOLOGICAL REACTIONS AND
IMMUNOTHERAPY OF MALIGNANT DISEASES

CHAIRPERSONS:

Eva Klein
M.D. Hanna, Jr.

INTRODUCTION - IMMUNOLOGICAL REACTIONS AND IMMUNOTHERAPY OF MALIGNANT DISEASE

Eva Klein

Department of Tumor Biology, Karolinska Institute

S-104 01 Stockholm 60, Sweden

In the beginning of the development of tumor immunology, when experiments were already conducted with well defined systems excluding the influence of histocompatibility antigens, the accumulation of important information was explosive. During the latest years our understanding about the oncogenic viruses and the immune system increased. As usual with increasing knowledge the number of unanswered questions increased. It may seem disappointing that progress has been relatively slow in two important areas of intense activity with many investigators involved. They deal with the following questions: 1. Are there immune parameters in the tumor patient which can be exploited for diagnosis or anti tumor activity response?

2. What is the relevance of the in vitro tumor related immune reactivities for the anti tumor response in vivo? Before we can design meaningful attempts to influence autologous tumor growth we have to know more about these questions.

A number of papers in the morning program deal with cell mediated immunity towards tumor cells. I will also address myself to this question. In addition, I shall tell about some experiments conducted in our laboratory which deal with anti tumor autoimmunity in patients with solid tumors.

Initially lymphocytotoxicity studies in both experimental systems and in patients with different tumor types, were interpreted to show tumor specific selective reactivities (15). However, frequent cytotoxicity obtained with lymphocytes of healthy donors and untreated animals led to the recognition that the capacity to attack certain

tumor cell lines is a regularly occurring, not a disease related
phenomenon.

The discovery initiated intensive studies in several laboratories motivated mainly for two reasons: 1. characterization of a
new cytotoxic phenomenon and 2. in order to achieve a test condition
which could be used for tumor immunity studies, revealing disease
related effects, it is necessary to characterize and perhaps eliminate
this effect.

At present, in vitro cytotoxicity tests aimed to demonstrate
disease related selective recognition are performed with the awareness
that at least three known effector mechanisms exist in which lymphocytes participate. 1. T-cells equipped with antigen recognizing
receptors (8). 2. ADCC-antibody dependent cytotoxicity; cells affect
targets which have been selected out by the recognition of antibodies
(25). 3. NK - natural killing - cells destruct on seemingly indis-
criminative bases by unknown mechanisms (28).

The NK effect is a general, in experimental animals, age-related
phenomenon (16,22). Because of the lack of knowledge about its initiation it was designated with the attribute "natural" - natural
killer - though it is not excluded that it might be generated by
classical immunization.

The active lymphocytes are not the mature T or B cells and in
contrast to T cell mediated killing the effect is not histocompatibility restricted (5,22). In man the activity of a certain lymphocyte subset is correlated to the enrichment in Fc positive cells (1,
2).

There is a considerable interest presently in the NK effect of
the animal systems since one of the important questions is the in
vivo relevance of the phenomenon. Transplantation tests with a
lymphoma line showed that the rejection of small inocula by semi-
syngeneic mice paralleled the in vitro reactivity of the strain (23).

When an in vitro carried NK sensitive lymphoma line, YAC-1, was
retransplanted and propagated in mice its sensitivity declined (6).
This experiment and the rule that cultured lines are highly sensitive
would indicate that only such cells can be established for longer
time in the host which lack the sensitivity to this mechanism.
Consequently, the NK system may represent a potent surveillance
mechanism. While sensitivity is not an obligatory feature of tumor
derived cell lines it may be assumed that if during oncogenesis
malignant cells with sensitivity to the NK arise, these are eliminated

Indicative for the role of NK cells in immune surveillance is
the low incidence of naturally occurring tumors in nude mice (30),

expected to be unprotected since they lack T cell mediated and T cell dependent mechanisms considered to be crucial in graft rejection. Spleen cells of nude mice have efficient NK activity when tested in vitro (16,22).

While our knowledge about the characteristics of the NK effect is steadily increasing there are still many important unclarified aspects. Among this is the nature of the cell surface target which is responsible for the sensitivity to the killing. It has been proposed that virally determined antigens have this role, however, in view of recent results this may not be the case (5,38).

Somatic cell hybrids usually express the allo- and virus determined surface antigens derived from both partners unless subjected to selective pressure. The behaviour of hybrid lines made from high and low NK sensitive partners would therefore be expected to follow the highly sensitive one if the killing effect would be directed against such cell surface antigens or surface macromolecules the determination of which are regulated similarly. In contrast, if sensitivity is determined by surface properties related to differentiation it may be absent in the hybrid cells since differentiation products are usually suppressed in the hybrids. We have therefore tested hybrid lines available in our laboratory for sensitivity to the lytic effect of spleen cells derived from unmanipulated mice. In all cases hybrids between high and low sensitive cells were weakly sensitive (38).

It may be possible that the killer cells do not operate on the basis of a conventional antigen recognition. During certain stages of differentiation or activation, thymus dependent lymphocytes may acquire cytotoxic potential. Cytotoxicity would be manifested against target cells toward which the lymphocytes carry recognition receptors. The efficiency of killing would be determined by the target cell, depending on its inherent sensitivity. This assumption is strengthened by the finding that thymocytes and activated T cells recognize and attach to cells of the same species (12). This recognition may be an important factor also in cytotoxicity of mitogen activated T lymphocytes which act preferentially on cells of their own species (29).

NK activity was found to be relatively decreased in the spleen of tumor bearing animals (murine sarcoma virus and methylcholanthrene-induced tumors and nude mice carrying grafts from human lymphoblastoid cell lines) (7) and in the blood of tumor patients (27). In our series 47% of cancer patients (the majority with lung carcinoma) failed to exert cytotoxicity towards the highly NK sensitive K562 cell line while all the healthy donors tested in parallel had strong reactivity (35).

Since specific cellular killing is known to be effected by the
T cell population and mature T cells have no NK effect - either in
man or mice and rats - detection of disease related cytotoxicity on
cell lines is expected to be possible by using characterized lymphocyte subsets. The T cell mediated effects can be investigated either
directly or after in vitro sensitization, achieved in culture when
the effecter population is exposed to antigen carrying cells for
several days (10).

In view of the histocompatibility restrictions of the T cell
mediated killing (19) it is questionable whether established cell
lines can be used as prototype targets in man. It is likely that
in search for tumor specific reactivities the experiments have to
be performed in autologous systems. However, at least in one human
disease - infectious mononucleosis - T cell mediated cytotoxicity
was demonstrated in short term assay on allogeneic target cells (4,
31). On the other hand experiments with breast cancer patients
using similar lymphocyte subsets failed to reveal selective cytotoxicity towards breast cancer derived lines (3).

In an effort to eliminate at least some of the factors which
hamper interpretation of results with cell lines two tests have been
designed in our laboratory for measuring cell-mediated anti-tumor
recognition in man, the autologous tumor stimulation, ATS, and autologous lymphocyte cytotoxicity, ALC. In both tests, tumor cells
separated from biopsy specimens were allowed to react with autologous
lymphocytes.

We considered that the advantage of using biopsy cells is that
the antigen source is not subjected to the modification and selective
conditions of tissue culture. The disadvantages are the variability
of the quality, the quantitative limitation and the laboriousity of
tumor cell separation.

The autologous tumor stimulation (ATS)-test registers DNA
synthesis of lymphocytes following 6-day cultivation with mitomycin-
treated biopsy cells (33). At least part of the responding cells
belongs to the T subset. Lymphocytes attached to the tumor cells
during the early period of cocultivation were shown to rosette with
SRBC. Moreover when prefractionated populations were used, the T-
enriched fraction reacted while the T-depleted fractions did not (34).

In our initial series ATS was obtained in 30% of 197 patients
with solid tumors (the majority with lung carcinomas or osteosarcomas).
Improvement of the test conditions by using exclusively tumor cell
enriched populations of good viability as stimulators, the incubation
of tumor cells prior to the test (this step was introduced to allow
resynthesis of putative cell surface antigens if removed by the
procedure of preparation of tumor cell enriched suspensions) and the
use of T cell enriched responder population has given considerably

increased positive cases (60%). Thus according to this test the
majority of patients seem to recognize immunologically their own
tumor cells (34). In criss cross tests lymphocytes were stimulated
for DNA synthesis when confronted with autologous tumor cells and
only exceptionally when confronted with allogeneic ones. In 36
tested combinations only 2 biopsies stimulated allogeneic lymphocytes (34).

The autologous lymphocytotoxicity (ALC) test was worked out
recently (36). Short term ^{51}Cr-release microtest was used to
register the killing of biopsy cells.

In experiments performed until present, lymphocytes were cytotoxic for autologous tumor cells in 16/29 cases. The specificity
was investigated by criss cross tests. ALC positive lymphocytes
reacted with allogeneic tumor cells only in 4/52 combinations.
Lymphocytes from healthy donors were negative in 13 experiments.

ALC positivity required blastogenesis. The opposite was not
true i.e. not all cases with blastogenesis had cytotoxic activity.

In a further step, generation of cytotoxic cells was attempted
by cocultivating the lymphocytes and autologous tumor biopsy cells
for 6 days, a procedure which has been shown to be efficient in some
experimental tumor systems (26). In 12/20 cases (3 also showed
primary ALC) secondary ALC was obtained (37). The targets were
frozen stored biopsy cells. Reactivity with allogeneic tumors was
rare. In 12 tests in which 2° ALC was generated, only 1 among 22
allogeneic tumor suspensions were killed.

The reactivities registered in autologous combinations, the
effect of cocultivation leading to blastogenesis and the generation
of cytotoxicity with maintained autologous reactivity strongly
suggest genuine tumor specificities. Because biopsy cells are only
exceptionally affected by NK cells such effect does not disturb the
experiments. It has to be emphasized that the cocultivations were
performed in human serum. This is of major importance because
cultivation of lymphocytes in fetal calf serum is known to generate
non-discriminative cytotoxicity.

Comparison of our results with the earlier extensive material
on human tumors shows an important difference because the latter
indicated tissue specific tumor specificity. With various tumor
types using short term cultured cells as targets cross reactivities
between tumors originating in the same tissue were reported (15).
These studies may have been devoid of NK effects because the target
cells were cultured only during a short time. Apart from technical
factors (48^{h} microcytotoxicity or colony inhibition in the experiments of Hellströms and short term Cr^{51} release test in our series)

the nature of target cells is the main difference.

The preferential if not absolute autologous reactivity may be
indicative for individual antigens or reflects the influence of
histocompatibility on T cell mediated cytotoxicity. The earlier
cross reactivities, indicating tissue related specificities may be
reconciled with the duration of the cytotoxic test. In animal tumor
systems with strong antigenicity long term tests have overridden the
histocompatibility restriction, however there was still a stronger
effect if the effector and target cells were histocompatible (32).

Recently attention is directed to the functional characterization
of in situ immunity. It is likely that lymphoid infiltration of tumor
tissue is a manifestation of immunological recognition. If so, it can
be expected that the infiltrating lymphocytes bear the characteristics
of immunologically active cells and even express specific function
directed against tumor cells. The latter has not been demonstrated
however in the strictly autologous condition. In experiments in which
tumor derived lymphocytes were shown to be cytotoxic, the target cells
carrying relevant antigens were selected for high sensitivity to
cellular attack (17,21,24). In fact there is no compelling evidence
for the growth inhibitory function of tumor infiltrating lymphocytes.
The assumption first to be considered would be that if a host response
occurs, the growing tumor is made up of cells selected for immuno-
resistance. This might not be generally true since in some tumor
cases blood lymphocytes were cytotoxic for autologous biopsy cells
but only seldom was such activity demonstrated with tumor derived
lymphocytes.

According to the histopathology of tumor tissue the extent
lymphoid infiltration varies with the type of tumor but also with the
individual case. It is uncertain whether the stromal reaction correlates with the clinical course. For some tumor types such a correlation might exist. In lung carcinomas the degree of cellular
infiltration was shown to be more extensive in the differentiated
tumors, which have usually a better prognosis also (19). We have
attempted to dissociate tumor and infiltrating stroma cells in order
to study certain functions of the latter. There was a great variation
in the success of obtaining lymphocytes in sufficient amounts in
various tumor types. Superimposed to this was the variation between
individual cases. In nasopharyngeal carcinoma (20), adenocarcinoma
and squamous cell carcinoma of the lung and seminoma the majority of
infiltrating lymphocytes are T cells (13). This is not true for all
tumor types however. In thyroid carcinomas mammary carcinoma most of
the infiltrating cells were "null" cells and in ovarial carcinoma and
uterine carcinosarcoma equal amount of T, B and "null" cells were
detected (18). When tested for natural killer effect or cytotoxicity
against the tumor cells separated from the biopsy the lymphocytes were
ineffective in most cases (35,36).

On the other hand the characteristics of the tumor infiltrating
T cells were found to be similar to in vitro activated T cells (13).
The signs of activation were: formation of "stable" rosettes (11) and
the ability to attach to a number of cell lines of human origin;
natural attachment, NA phenomenon (12). In addition a proportion of
T cells were seen attached to tumor cells in the biopsy suspensions.
This attachment was firm enough not to be dissociated under the
conditions used for dispersion of the tumor tissue.

The biological significance of these in situ tumor cell attached
T lymphocytes is unclear.

We have recently discovered that activated T cells, derived from
MLC, moreover thymocytes and neuraminidase treated blood lymphocytes
could attach to a variety of cells. The phenomenon was demonstrated
with human and murine cells and was restricted to the species i.e.
there was no cross reaction (12). Since it occurred with thymocytes
and neuraminidase treated blood T cells of unmanipulated animals and
healthy donors we have denoted it natural attachment, NA.

When such T cells attached to target cells they enhanced the
cytotoxic activity of added monocytes and macrophages (14). While
it is unknown whether these in vitro events reflect in vivo activities,
in the present context it is of importance that the tumor infiltrating
T cells exhibit characteristics of in vitro activated T cells, and of
T cells separated from arthritic synovial fluid (14).

The autoimmunity of patients with solid tumors is still not
proven beyond doubts. No evidence withstanding scrutiny is available
for immunological recognition of tumor cell surfaces. On the other
hand the claims for such response are convincing enough to proceed
with the hypothesis that in a high number of cases this is a reality.
It is of importance therefore to provide evidence that signs for
active immunity can be detected in situ. This would provide a ground
for the aim to divert the seemingly unsuccessful, unsatisfactory
reaction into an efficient one.

REFERENCES

1. Bakács, T., Gergely, P., Cornain, S., Klein, E. Int. J. Cancer
    19 (1977) 441.
2. Bakács, T., Gergely, P., Klein, E. Cellular Immunol. 32 (1977)
    317.
3. Bakács, T., Klein, E., Ljungström, K.G. Cancer Letters 4 (1978)
    191.
4. Bakács, T., Svedmyr, E., Klein, E., Rombo, L., Weiland, D.
    Cancer Letters 4 (1978) 185.
5. Becker, S., Fenyö, E.M., Klein, E. Europ. J. Immunol. 6 (1976)
    882.

6. Becker, S., Kiessling, R., Klein, G. To be publ.
7. Becker, S., Klein, E. Europ. J. Immunol. 6 (1976) 892.
8. Cerottini, J.C., Brunner, K.T. Adv. in Immunol. 18 (1974) 67
    New York, Academic Press.
9. Doherty, P.C., Blanden, R.V., Zinkernagel, R.M. Transpl. Rev.
    29 (1976) 28.
10. Engers, H.D., MacDonald, H.R. Contemp. Topics in Immuno-Biology.
    Plenum Press, N.Y. 5 (1976) 145.
11. Galili, U., Schlesinger, M. J. Immunol. 117 (1976) 730.
12. Galili, U., Galili, N., Vánky, F., Klein, E. Proc. Natl. Acad.
    Sci. USA 75 (1978) 2396.
13. Galili, U., Vánky, F., Rodrigues, L., Klein, E. To be publ.
14. Galili, U., Rosenthal, L., Galili, N., Klein, E. To be publ.
15. Hellström, K.E., Hellström, I. Adv. Cancer Res. 12 (1969) 167.
16. Herberman, R.B., Nunn, M.F., Lavrin, D.H. Int. J. Cancer 16
    (1975) 230.
17. Holden, H.J., Haskill, J.S., Kirchner, H., Herberman, R.O. J.
    Immunol. 117 (1976) 440.
18. Háyry, P., Tötterman, T.H. In press (1978).
19. Ioachim, H.L. J. Nat. Cancer Inst. 57 (1976) 465.
20. Jondal, M., Klein, G. Biomedicine 23 (1975) 163.
21. Jondal, M., Svedmyr, E., Klein, E., Singh, S. Nature (Lond.)
    266 (1975) 405).
22. Kiessling, R., Klein, E., Wigzell, H. Eur. J. Immunol. 5 (1975)
    230.
23. Kiessling, R., Petrányi, G., Klein, G., Wigzell, H. Int. J.
    Cancer 15 (1975) 933.
24. Klein, E., Becker, S., Svedmyr, E., Jondal, M., Vánky, F. Ann.
    N.Y. Acad. Sci. 276 (1976) 207.
25. MacLennan, I.C.M. In: Clinical Tumor Immunology. Ed. J. Wybran,
    M. Staguet. Pergamon Press, Oxford (1976) p.47.
26. Plata, F., McDonald, H.R., Engers, H.D. J. Immunology 117 (1976)
    52.
27. Pross, H.F., Baines, M.G. Int. J. Cancer 18 (1976) 593.
28. Pross, H.F., Baines, M.G. Cancer Immunol. Immunotherap. 3 (1977)
    75.
29. Stejskal, V. Scand. J. Immunol. 5 (1976) 479.
30. Stutman, O. Science 183 (1974) 534.
31. Svedmyr, E., Jondal, M. Proc. Natl. Acad. Sci. 72 (1975) 1622.
32. Ting, C.-C., Law, L.W. J. Immunol. 117 (1977) 1259.
33. Vánky, F., Stjernswärd, J. In: In vitro methods in cell mediated
    and tumor immunity. II.Eds. B. Bloom, J.R. David. Acadamic Press
    Inc. N.Y. (1976) p.597.
34. Vánky, F. To be published.
35. Vose, B., Vánky, F., Argov, S., Klein, E. Eur. J. Immunol. 7
    (1977) 753.
36. Vose, B., Vánky, F., Klein, E. Int. J. Cancer 20 (1977) 512.
37. Vose, B., Vánky, F., Fopp, M., Klein, E. Int. J. Cancer 21 (1978)
    588.

38. Ährlund-Richter, L., Klein, E. To be published.

ACKNOWLEDGEMENTS

The authors' work mentioned in this publication was performed pursuant to Contract N01-CB-64023 and N01-CB-74144 with the Division of Cancer Biology and Diagnosis, and Welfare. Grants have also been received from the Swedish Cancer Society.

PREGNANCY-ASSOCIATED GLYCOPROTEIN (α_2-PAG) IN THE SERA OF CHILDREN WITH MALIGNANCIES

H.U. Schwenk, E. Steigenberger, S. Trincsek

University Childrens' Hospital

Erlangen, W. Germany

Tumor markers, in the basic sense, are substances which are produced by tumors and released into the blood. They include the tumor-associated antigens, hormones and enzymes. The α_2-pregnancy-associated glycoprotein, or α_2-PAG, (synonyms: SP_3, pregnancy-zone protein, xm factor) is one of the "pregnancy proteins", substances regularly demonstrable in the sera of pregnant women, which, however, are not pregnancy specific, but appear also as acute-phase glyco-proteins in several diseases. It has been shown in several publi-cations (1,2) that the detection of α_2-PAG is of no significance for the initial diagnosis of tumors in adults, but may be used in the follow-up of the post-operative course of the disease. The first investigations of α_2-PAG in connection with malignant diseases in children will be published (3). α_2-PAG can therefore be counted as a tumour-associated protein in the wider sense.

PATIENTS AND METHODS

Four groups of subjects were examined: healthy, newborn infants from whom blood was taken in the 6-10th day of life for phenylketonuria screening; normal siblings of children with tumors; hospitalised infants and children up to 15 years of age with miscellaneous non-malignant diseases; children older than one month, with malignant tumors.

α_2-PAG was determined with the electro-immunodiffusion method of Laurell (4) using an antiserum supplied by Behringwerke, Marburg, and an electrophoresis chamber supplied by Degasa, Heidelberg. To set up a standard curve, a standard serum was provided of 159 mg/100 ml

TAB. 1:   Increased α_2-PAG levels in children.

Probands	Patients with α_2-PAG >0.5 mg/100 ml
healthy newborns (n = 200)	0
newborns, with non-malignant diseases (n = 50)	0
healthy children (n = 58) (from 1 month - 14 years)	3
Children with non-malignant diseases (n = 350)	91
children with malignant diseases (n = 60)	32

by Behringwerke, Marburg, which was run with each determination at appropriate dilutions. The agarose (1%) was diluted in Veronal buffer ph 8.6, the antiserum was used in a concentration of 0.5 ml per 25 ml agarose. The limit of detection of this method was about 0.5 mg/100 ml.

RESULTS

α_2-PAG Levels in Non-Malignant Diseases of Childhood

In infancy, levels of α_2-PAG of over 0.5 mg/100 ml are probably very unusual (Tab.1), since none of the 50 patients of this age with miscellaneous diseases, and none of the 200 healthy infants showed such levels. With increasing age raised concentrations were determined in children, especially those with chronic infections. The mean value was 2.84 mg/100 ml, the standard deviation $\pm$ 2.1.

α_2-PAG Levels in Malignant Diseases in Childhood

a) before treatment. Infants with a manifest malignant tumor could not be examined in the 2 years of our investigation. For the malignant tumors, in particular the neuroblastomas and Wilms tumors, there was a fairly consistent rise in the levels of α_2-PAG; the values measured were within the same range of concentrations as those found for the non-malignant diseases, with a mean value of 4.11 mg/100 ml and a standard deviation of $\pm$ 2.0. Malignant lymphomas were nearly always negative at the beginning of therapy.

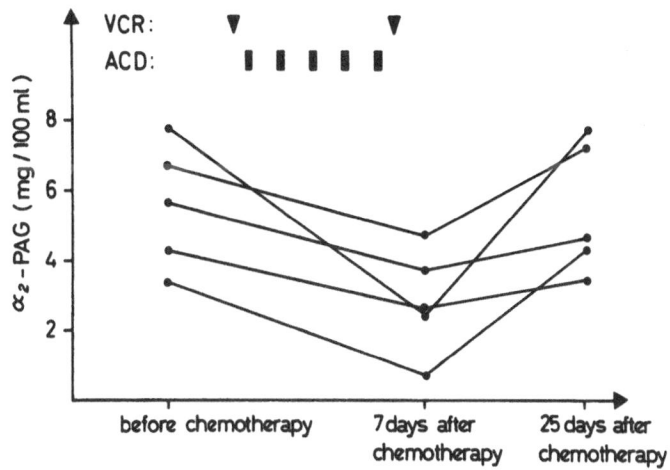

FIG. 1:   The effect of chemotherapy of 2 x 1.5 mg/m^2 Vincristine
and 5 x 450 µg/m^2 Actinomycin D on the level of α_2-PAG.

b)   post-operative.   Although increased levels of α_2-PAG could
be determined in Hodgkin disease patients during radiotherapy, these
values fell during chemotherapy (Fig.1). Despite complete removal
of the tumors, these levels rose again in the treatment-free period
with the increase of peripheral leucocytes.

After complete removal of the tumor the fall in α_2-PAG values
was very slow, for 5 Wilms' tumors stage 1 it was still over the
limit of detection after 12 months, even though the biological half-
life of this protein is given as 5-7 days (5) (Fig.2).

DISCUSSION

This investigation was made in order to clarify whether the
determination α_2-PAG can be used as a tumor marker for :

1.   the initial diagnosis of malignant diseases, i.e. in a tumor
screening programme. (As yet, such trials have been uniformly

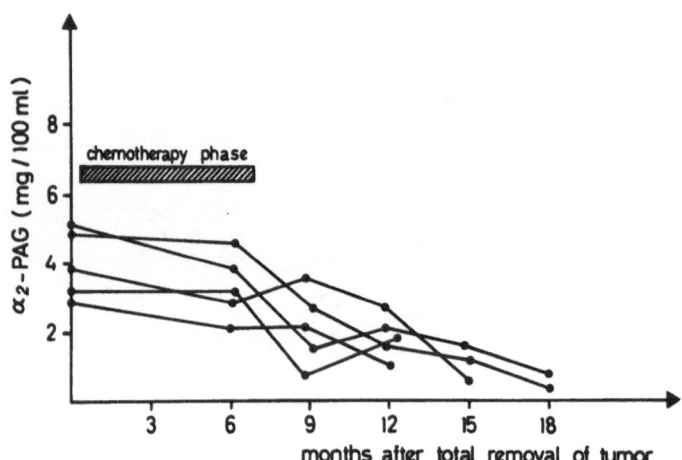

FIG. 2:   The fall of α_2-PAG after complete removal of a Wilms'
tumor in 5 patients.

unsuccessful since, so long as the tumour mass is small, the concentration of tumor antigen in the serum is below the limit of detection
or, with very sensitive methods of detection, the specificity is
lost).

2.   post-operative follow-up and monitoring of therapy in cancer
patients.

The repeated determination of α_2-PAG has been shown not to be
of any use in the monitoring of the post-operative progress in
children. On the one hand, the necessary chemotherapy reduces the
α_2-PAG concentration, on the other hand the level of this glycoprotein may be many months detectable even though the tumor has
been completely removed. This indicates, however, that this tumor-
associated protein is not produced by the tumor itself.

This production of α_2-PAG, probably occurring in the leucocytes
(6), suggests that this protein may be present even when the tumor
is very small. This is in contrast to carcino-embryonic antigen and
alpha foetoprotein, increased levels of which are not usually found
with very small tumors. The protein would seem to be especially
useful for the diagnosis of tumors in newborn infants; our investigation of 250 infants showed that increased levels of this protein

are very seldom found, unless a tumor is present. To avoid the
misinterpretation of a materno-foetal transfusion, IgA determination
should also be carried out. Screening tests for congenital tumors
in the newborn are not yet possible, but may be more promising when
more tumor markers can be determined simultaneously.

REFERENCES

1. Bauer, H.W., Gropp, C., Sieber, A., Bohn, H., Thoraxchirurgie
    25 (1977) 139.
2. Stimson, W.H., Lancet I (1975) 755.
3. Schwenk, H.U., Steigenberger, E., Klin. Paediat. (in press).
4. Laurell, C.B., Anal. Biochem. 15 (1966) 45.
5. Bohn, H., Arch. Gynäk. 217 (1974) 219.
6. Stimson, W.H., Blackstock, J.C., Behring. Inst. Mitt. 57 (1973)
    92.

CIRCULATING HUMAN T CELL SUBSET WITH A REVERSIBLE E-ROSSETTING CAPACITY IN CANCER AND NORMALS-HYPOTHESIS ON THE REGULATORY MECHANISM INFLUENCING THEIR ROLE IN CMI

C. Moroz, B. Kupfer and Sh. Giler

Rogoff-Wellcome Med. Res. Inst., Tel-Aviv University
Medical School, Beilinson Medical Center
Petah-Tikva, Israel

INTRODUCTION

It is generally accepted that the immune response is depressed in patients with neoplastic diseases. One of the paramenters for evaluation of cell mediated immunity is the identification of T-lymphocytes in peripheral (PBL) blood by spontaneous rossette formation with SRBC (1,2). Patients bearing tumor tend to have lower percentages of RFC than patients with no evidence of the disease (3). This type of discrimination of disease status is best demonstrated if suboptimal incubation temperatures are used in the rossette procedure (1,3,4). In the current peper we would like to summarize the experimental evidence for the existence of a circulating T cell subset with a reversible capacity to form E-rossettes. The inhibited state of rosette formation of this T cell subset is accompanied by a decrease in cell mediated immunity.

Experimental

In recent studies on PBL of patients with Hodgkin's disease and with breast cancer, we identified a subpopulation of T-lymphocytes (10-20%) reacting with anti-T cell serum which do not form E-rossettes (E⁻). In both types of cancer, ferritin was bound to the surface of these T-cells (5-7). It is noteworthy that in Hodgkin's disease as well as in breast cancer ferritin was identified as a tumor associated antigen (8,9), and was demonstrated in elevated amounts in patients sera (8,10). Incubation of PBL derived from these cancer patients with Levamisole or with fetal calf serum (FCS), but not with adult serum resulted in restoration

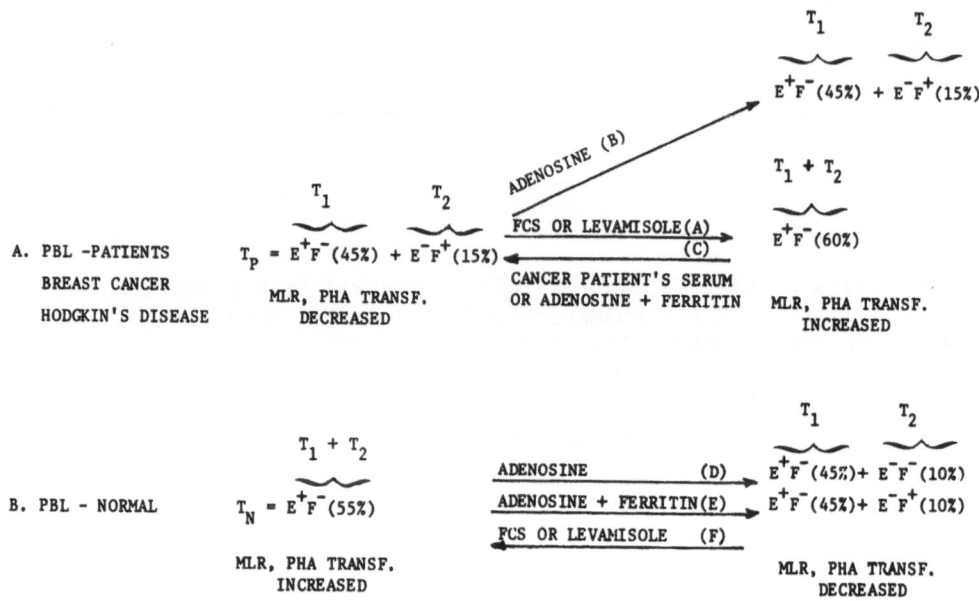

T = T LYMPHOCYTES REACTING WITH ANTI-T CELL SERUM.

E = CELLS FORMING E-ROSSETTES.

F = CELLS REACTING WITH ANTI-FERRITIN.

FIG. 1: Summary of experimental data exhibiting the existence of reversible ERFC subpopulation.

of the capacity of E^- cells to form rossettes and in the removal of ferritin from the cell surface (E^+F^-) (5,7,11) (Fig.1A).

The restoration is reversible (Fig.1C), the rossette formation of this T cell subpopulation can be inhibited again by incubating the cells with the patient's serum (11) (Tab.1) or by incubation with adenosine (50 μM) (12,13). Incubation of PBL derived from breast cancer patients with adenosine does not further decrease the number of ERFC thus, not affecting the rossetting capacity of the E^+F^- T cell subpopulation (Fig.1B). However, it does inhibit the rossetting capacity of the FCS or Levamisole "restored" (E^+F^-) T subpopulation, resulting in the appearance of (E^-F^-) subpopulation (13). If spleen ferritin is added to the adenosine lymphocyte incubation mixture, ferritin is absorbed to the surface of the inhibited T cell subpopulation to form T (E^-F^+) (Fig.1C). In normal subjects, a small population of PBL (10%) with a reversible capacity to form E-rossettes (Fig.1) is evident following their incubation with adenosine (Tab.2). This T cell subpopulation in normals can bind ferritin (Fig.1E) only following pretreatment with adenosine or by incubation with serum from breast cancer patient (Tab.2) This

TAB. 1:   The reversible effect of FCS and breast cancer serum on
the number of ERFC and ferritin bearing lymphocytes from breast
cancer patients.

Breast Cancer Patient No.	Untreated PBL		FCS Treated PBL[a]			
			Incubated in Normal Serum[b]		Incubated in Breast Cancer Serum[b]	
	ERFC	F[+] Cells[c]	ERFC	F[+] Cells[c]	ERFC	F[+] Cells[c]
	%	%	%	%	%	%
1.	35	23	53	0	35	15
2.	37	16	56	1	37	7
3.	47	13	62	0	48	0
4.	45	18	60	0	45	18
5.	47	12	65	0	45	10

[a]   Lymphocytes (5×10^6/ml) were incubated in RPMI-1640 containing
20% FCS for 18 h at $37^{\circ}C$.

[b]   FCS treated lymphocytes were washed twice and resuspended
(5×10^6/ml) in RPMI-1640 containing 30% breast cancer serum or
normal human AB serum for 1 h at $4^{\circ}C$.

[c]   Percentage specific killing by anti-human spleen ferritin and
complement.

inhibition can be reversed (Fig.1F) by treatment with Levamisole
(12) or FCS (14).

DISCUSSION AND CONCLUSIONS

In conclusion a subpopulation of T cells with a reversible
capacity to form E-rossettes has been demonstrated in patients with
Hodgkin's disease (12), breast cancer (7,13) and in normals (12).
The inhibition of E-rossette formation by factors in the patient's
serum or by adenosine may reflect membranal changes in this T cell
subpopulation, which may influence their function. Indeed, a
depressed mixed lymphocyte reactivity (MLR) of breast cancer
lymphocyte is increased following restoration of the lymphocytes
by treatment with Levamisole or FCS (14). On the other hand
Hirschorn and Sela (15) have recently demonstrated that the addition
of adenosine to normal human PBL inhibited their response to PHA.
This effect could be reversed by treatment of the suppressed

TAB. 2:   Induction of a non rossetting ferritin bearing T cell
subset (E^-F^+) by incubation of normal PBL with adenosine and
ferritin or breast cancer serum.

Expt. No.	Untreated PBL		PBL Incubated With					
			Ferritin[a]		Adenosine Ferritin[b]		Breast Cancer Serum[c]	
	ERFC	F^+ Cells[d]	ERFC	F^+ Cells[d]	ERFC	F^+ Cells[d]	ERFC	F^+ Cells[d]
	%	%	%	%	%	%	%	%
1.	61	0	61	1	54	14	ND	ND
2.	63	0	64	0	57	7	ND	ND
3.	54	0	56	0	50	10	49	16
4,	54	0	55	0	48	6	47	9
5.	63	0	ND	ND	ND	ND	43	11

[a]   PBL (5×10^6/ml) were preincubated in RPMI-1640 containing
human spleen ferritin (5 µg/ml) for 60 min at 4°C. The cells were
washed twice prior to further testing.

[b]   PBL were incubated with RPMI-1640 containing adenosine (50 µM)
and ferritin (5 µM) as in a.

[c]   PBL were incubated in RPMI-1640 containing 30% breast cancer
serum as in a.

[d]   Percentage specific killing by anti-human spleen ferritin and
complement.

lymphocytes with FCS but not with adult serum (15). It was suggested
that adenosine inhibits the activity of adenosine deaminase (ADA),
resulting in a decrease in cellular immunity which may be similar to
that observed in patients suffering from inherited ADA deficiency.
The authors suggested that the addition of external ADA, found in
high level in fetal serum, caused the restoration of the capacity to
respond to PHA. In-vitro studies have demonstrated that inhibition
of ADA has a profound effect upon maturation of T-cell precursors,
as defined by E-rossetting and proliferation in the presence of PHA,
while not affecting differentiation of B-cell precursors (16).

On the above observations we base the following working
hypothesis. The small circulating T cell subpopulation, characterized
by low affinity E-rossetting capacity, is representing immature T
lymphocytes. Low concentrations of adenosine or its metabolites

may trigger metabolic events which are ultimately responsible for inhibition of maturation and proliferation of this T cell sub-population. The metabolic events are currently unknown. One of the possible mechanism may include elevation of cAMP which is known to arrest the cell at one stage of the cell cycle (17) and inhibit lymphocyte proliferation (18). This is in agreement with the observed restoration of the E-rossetting capacity and the immune function of these lymphocytes by Levamisole, a drug known to increase cGMP and thereby decrease cAMP (19).

In cancer patients (like Hodgkin's disease or breast cancer), adenosine or its metabolites, originating in the fast growing tumor tissue and found in elevated amounts in the serum, may trigger metabolic events affecting purine metabolism in the immature, low affinity ERFC- T cell subpopulation, resulting in the immuno-suppressive effect observed in these cancer patients. In addition, tumor associated antigen like ferritin, may play a secondary regulatory role. Further studies are carried out to test this hypothesis.

REFERENCES

1. Wybran, J., Fuderberg, H.H., J. Clin. Invest. 52 (1973) 1026.
2. Hersh, E.M., Gutterman, J.V., Mavligit, G.M., Patholobiol. Ann. 5 (1975) 133.
3. West, W.H., Sienknecht, C.W., Townes, A.S., Herberman, R.B., Clin. Immunol. Immunobiol. 5 (1976) 60.
4. Dieu, J., Payne, S., Alford, C., Heim, W., Pomeroy, T., Cohen, M., Oldham, R., Herberman, R.B., Clin. Immunol. Immunopathol. 8 (1977) 405.
5. Kaplan, H.S., Bobrove, A.M., Fuks, Z., Strober, S., N. Engl. J. Med. 290 (1974) 971.
6. Moroz, C., Giler, Sh., Kupfer, B., Urca, I., New Engl. J. of Medicine 296 (1977) 1173.
7. Moroz, C., Giler, Sh., Kupfer, B., Urca, I., Cancer Immunol. and Immunotherapy 3 (1977) 101.
8. Eshhar, Z., Order, S.E., Katz, D.H., Proc. Natl. Acad. Sci. 71 (1974) 3956.
9. Marcus, D.M., Zindberg, N., Arch. Bioch. Biophys. 162 (1974) 493.
10. Marcus, D.M., Zindberg, N., Clin. Res. 23 (1975) A447.
11. Fuks, Z., Strober, S., King, D.P., Kaplan, H.S., J. Immunol. 117 (1976) 1331.
12. Di-Perri, I., Auteri, A., Laghi, Pasini, F., Mattioli, F., Volpi, L., Proc. Symp. on Immunotherapy of Malignant Disease (1977) in press.
13. Moroz, C., Kupfer, B., Giler, Sh.N. Engl. J. of Medicine Letter to Editor. In Press.

14. Moroz, C., Kupfer, B., Giler, Sh. Proc. 12th Int. Leukocyte culture conference (1978) in press.
15. Hirschorn, R., Sela, E., Cell Immunol. 32 (1977) 350.
16. Ballet, J.J., Insel. R., Merler, E., Rosen, F.S., J. Exp. Med. 143 (1976) 1271.
17. Millis, A.J.T., Forrest, G., Pious, D.A., Biochem. Biophys. Res. Commun. 49 (1972) 1645.
18. Hadden, J.W., Ann. N.Y. Acad. Sci. 256 (1975) 352.
19. Hadden, J.W., Coffey, R.G., Hadden, E.M., Cell Immunol. 20 (1975) 98.

A TUMOR T CELL LINE WHICH CAN BE SPECIFICALLY ACTIVATED BY ANTIGEN

John C. Roder, Judy K. Ball and Sharwan K. Singhal

The Department of Microbiology and Immunology, and The
Cancer Research Laboratory, University of Western
Ontario, London, Ontario, N6A 5C1, Canada

INTRODUCTION

It is generally assumed that tumors of the lymphoid system are
"frozen" in permanent states of differentiation and cellular
activation. However, recent evidence suggests that appropriate
triggering signals induce H-chain gene switching in B lymphoblastoid
cell lines (1) and myeloma cells may undergo differentiation in vivo
(2).

It is well established that non-lymphoid tumors, such as
erythroid leukemia, can be induced to produce hemoglobin (3) and in
addition the specific protein inducer, MGI, can induce normal cell
differentiation in some types of myeloid leukemic cells (4). It is
not unreasonable to expect, therefore, that some T cell lymphomas
will be found which can be triggered immunologically by antigens
which combine with their corresponding receptor on these cells.

Although T cells are known to express antigen binding receptors
consisting in part of antibody variable regions (5,6), which may be
translated from mRNA in the cytoplasm (7), the mechanisms controllin
the induction of these V region genes remains unknown. Furthermore,
the events controlling the antigen dependent activation of T cells
expressing specific receptors is also poorly understood due largely
to the unavailability of homogeneous, monoclonal T cells. It is
likely that the production of antigen specific T cell lines will be
useful for investigations into the molecular biology of T cell
activation and differentiation just as the myelomas have been
indispensable in elucidating B cell function and control.

TAB. 1:   Tumorgenicity of In Vitro Cultured Thymic Lymphoma Cell
Line 485-2.

Number of Cells Injected[a]	Route of Injection	% Takes	Average latent period to death (days)
1×10^6	IP	100	10.2
1×10^5	IP	100	14.3
5×10^3	IP	100	20.5

[a]   Newborn, syngeneic mice were injected with 485-2 cells from
passage 6.

In this report we describe a thymine lymphoma which maintains
its immunocompetence and can be specifically activated upon contact
with antigen in an analogous manner to normal, non-transformed T
cells.

RESULTS AND DISCUSSION

The leukemia virus used in this study was originally isolated
from a thymic lymphoma induced by the neonatal injection of 7, 12-
dimethylbenzanthracene into CFW/D mice (8).   The virus was then
injected into newborn thymus 7 days after grafting under the kidney
capsule of adult mice and the cell lines (485-2,485-10,485-16) were
established from the resulting lymphomas. After 53 passages the
485-2 line had 41 stable chromosomes, a doubling time of 14.5 hr,
and induced 100% takes in vivo when as few as 5×10^3 cells were
injected (Tab.1).   Supernatant fluids from the cell line contained
infectious C-type virus particles which had a buoyant density of
1.6 gm/cc and contained reverse transcriptase activity as well as
60 - 70 S viral RNA (Ball, J.K., in preparation).   In addition almost
100% of these cells were killed by treatment with specific anti-
thymocyte serum and complement.

In a previous study (9) cell transfer experiments revealed that
virus induced thymomas contained functional helper T cells.   When
thymoma cells were tranferred together with SRBC and normal, syngeneic bone marrow cells into lethally irradiated recipients the
anti-SRBC response was several fold higher than when either bone
marrow or thymoma cells were transferred alone.   This experiment
suggested that transformed T cells from the thymoma might possess
normal immunocompetent function and further experiments were designed
to test this possibility.

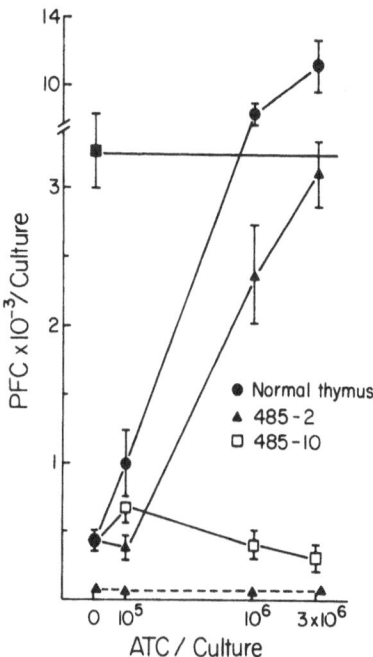

FIG. 1:   The specific, cell dose dependent, restoration of the PFC
response in T depleted cultures by activated tumor cells. Spleen
cells were cultured alone with SRBC (■) or were pre-treated with
anti-thymocyte serum and complement prior to culture (◗). Normal
thymocytes (●), 485-2 cells (▲) or 485-10 cells (□) were
activated 7 days with SRBC in lethally irradiated, syngeneic recipients and then added to T-depleted cultures together with SRBC.
Solid lines, anti-SRBC response; dashed lines, anti-HRBC response.
The response of normal spleen cell cultures to immunization with
HRBC was 1,330 PFC/culture.

TAB. 2:   The Activation of Tumor Cells with Sheep Erythrocytes.

Additions to T cell deprived spleen cell cultures[x]:	Plaque forming cells/10^6				% RFC vs SRBC
	anti-SRBC	p value[xx]	anti-HRBC	p value	
None	600± 52	-	516± 86	-	<1.0
485-2 cells activated with SRBC[++]	1,800±130	.01	549± 43	N.S.	32.0
485-2 cells activated with HRBC	715± 68	N.S.	n.t.[xxx]	-	n.t.
485-2 cells (non-activated)	540± 75	N.S.	n.t.	-	n.t.
Normal thymocytes activated with SRBC	2,530±210	.001	890±187	.05	10.8
Normal thymocytes activated with HRBC	720± 91	N.S.	2,021±110	.001	n.t.
485-10 cells activated with SRBC	500± 99	N.S.	n.t.	-	n.t.
485-16 cells activated with SRBC	300±120	N.S.	n.t.	-	n.t.

[x]   Normal CFW/D spleen cells were treated with anti-thymocyte serum and complement and then cultured 5 days with horse or sheep erythrocytes. Non-treated control cultures developed 3010 PFC/10^6 versus SRBC and 1935 PFC/10^6 versus HRBC.

[++]   4 x 10^7 normal thymocytes, 485-2, 485-10 or 485-16 cells were injected alone (non-activated) or together with 4 x 10^8 SRBC or HRBC into lethally irradiated (850 R), syngeneic recipients and the spleens were used as a source of activated cells 6 days later. A pre-determined optimum dose (10^6) of these cells was added, to culture.

[xx]   P values were determined by a student's t-test. N.S., not significant (p $\geqslant$.05).

[xxx] not tested,

It has previously been shown that T cells pre-exposed to the appropriate antigen in irradiated recipients are capable of cooperating with B cells in T cell deprived cultures, thereby restoring the antibody response (10,11). As shown in Tab.2, 485-2 cells activated with SRBC restored the anti-SRBC PFC response to almost the same level as normal, activated thymocytes. This restoration was specific since the use of horse erythrocytes (HRBC), or no antigen, during the activation step did not result in a PFC response significantly above background levels. Furthermore 485-2 cells activated with SRBC did not restore the anti-HRBC response whereas, normal thymocytes activated with HRBC did restore this response (anti-HRBC). The "helper" effect of activated 485-2 was cell dose dependent as shown in Fig.1. In addition, activated 485-2 cells bound to SRBC as shown in Tab.2. Two similar cell lines 485-10 and 485-16 failed to respond in the activation procedure (Tab.2, Fig.1) which suggests that the virus itself did not induce specificity changes but rather transformed a T cell which was by chance pre-programmed for anti-SRBC specificity.

Although these results firmly establish the specificity of the 485-2 line at the level of T cell triggering the specificity of the "helper" effect must also be established since activated T cells have non-specific effects when actived T cells are specifically triggered in the afferent limb of the response, the actual signal delivered to the B cell in the efferent limb could be specific or non-specific. Under the widely accepted 2 signal model of immune inducation (antigen = signal 1; T cell help = signal 2. 1 + 2 sequence = B cell induction; 2 alone no effect), the specificity of the actual T helper factor is largely irrelevant (unless macrophage signal focusing is involved). A more important point which we have addressed in this paper is the specificity at the level of T cell triggering which presumably occurs via a membrane bound, V region containing receptor. Although additional antigens should be tested, we feel that our control is the best one possible, namely the use of another erythrocyte (HRBC) which did not trigger these (SRBC) activated cells.

These results suggest that T cells in leukemic hosts maintain immunocompetence, but they do not explain the generalized and progressive immunodepression which occurs in mice injected with DMBA-LV. This effect was shown to result from tumor induced, non-T suppressor cells which non-specifically inhibited B cell function (12). The balance between these two coexisting phenomena of help and suppression could conceivably influence the course of tumor development and might help explain the increasing number of mechanisms postulated to account for tumor dependent immunosuppression.

SUMMARY

We have shown that permanently transformed T cells of a leukemic line (485-2) maintain their immunocompetent function and can be specifically activated by antigen. This cell line should facilitate investigations into the biochemical mechanisms of T cell activation and may help elucidate the nature of the T cell receptor.

REFERENCES

1. Kishimoto, T., Hirano, T., Kuritani, T., Yamamura, Y., Ralph, P., Good, R.A., Nature (In press) (1978).
2. Rohrer, J.W., Vaser, K., Lynch, R.G., J. Immunol. 114 (1977) 861.
3. Friend, C., Scher, W., Holland, J.G., Sato, T., Proc. Nat. Acad. Sci. (USA) 68 (1971) 378.
4. Sacho, L., Israel J. Med. Sci. 13 (1977) 654.
5. Binz, H., Wigzell, H., In: Contemp. Top. Immunobiol. 7 (1977) 11 (Ed. M.G. Hanna) (Plenum Press, New York).
6. Krawinkel, U., Cramer, M., Imanishi-Kari, T., Jack, R.S., Rajewsky, K., Mäkelä, O., Eur. J. Immunol. 8 (1977) 566.
7. Rabbits, T.H., Forster, A., Smith, M., Gillam, S., Eur. J. Immunol. 7 (1977) 43.
8. Ball, J.K., McCarter, J.A., J. Nat. Cancer Inst. 46 (1971) 751.
9. Roder, J.C., Ball, J.K., Singhal, S.K., Nature (In press) (1978).
10. Chan, E.L., Mishell, R.I., Mitchell, G.F., Science 170 (1970) 1215.
11. Roder, J.C., Bell, D.A., Singhal, S.K., J. Immunol. 115 (1975) 466.
12. Roder, J.C., Tyler, L., Ball, J.K., Singhal, S.K., Cellular Immunol. 36 (1978) 128.

A MODEL OF TARGET CELL RECOGNITION AND LYSIS BY NATURAL KILLER CELLS

John C. Roder[1] and Rolf Kiessling

The Dept. of Tumor Biology, Karolinska Institute

S 104 01 Stockholm 60, Sweden

INTRODUCTION

A population of naturally occurring, "null" lymphocytes in unimmunized mice has been shown to play a decisive role in tumor resistance in vivo (1). These cells, called natural killer (NK) cells, pre-exist at high levels in the host (2) and might be expected therefore to provide a first line of defense against newly arising malignancies. Recent investigations in our laboratory have focused on questions of specificity, control and mechanisms of target-effector interaction in the NK system.

RESULTS AND DISCUSSION

The problems under investigation required an assay to measure the contact or "recognition" phase of the interaction at the single cell level since (i) cytolytic or cytostatic assays measure events at the entire population level and (ii) lysis may be the final step in a complex series of independently controlled events and therefore yields little information concerning the "recognition" phase of target-effector contact.

As summarized in Tab.1, we have found two subpopulations of target binding cells (TBC) in the various lymphoid organs of normal, non-immunized mice. The first cell type is not adherent to nylon wool columns and binds in a selective fashion to a large number of

---

[1]   Scholar of the Canada Council, Killam Program.

TAB. 1:   A Comparison of Target Cell Binding by Nylon Adherent
and Non-Adherent Spleen Cells.

Characteristic	Nylon Non-Adherent TBC	Nylon Adherent TBC	Reference
Follows NK genotype pattern	Yes	No	2
Shows H-2 linkage in backcross	Yes	No	2
Follows age pattern of NK cell	Yes	No	2
Organ distribution follows NK cell	Yes	No	2
Correlates well with NK lysis in kinetics experiments (r=0.86)	Yes	No	4
Blocking by target cell sonicates	Yes	No	2,3
Time requirement for max. target cell binding	30 min	1 min	4
Mean number of targets bound per effector	1.3	3.27	2,5
TBC disrupted by EDTA	Yes	Yes	4
Binding at 0°C	Yes	Yes	4
Kills attached target	Yes	No	4
Frequency in whole spleen population	0.6-2.4%	15%	2

tumor cell targets which are susceptible to lysis (2). The rise
and fall in the frequency of these TBC, with age, closely parallels
the NK cell activity in these mice and TBC were specific since they
could be inhibited by cell surface glycoproteins of sensitive but
not insensitive targets (3). The genes controlling the frequency
of these TBC are inherited in a dominant fashion and are linked to
the H-2 region of chromosome 17 (2).

The strong correlation (r=.95) between the frequency of TBC in
various populations and the level of lysis provides strong indirect
evidence that the TBC may be related to the NK cell (2). This
suggestion was supported by the observation that the majority of
single target-effector conjugates contained lysed targets when
isolated in droplets under oil and incubated for several hours at
37°C (4).

In contrast, the second cell type, a nylon adherent population,
was not subject to any genetic control and bound to targets in a
non-specific manner (Tab.1). Furthermore, these nylon adherent cells
differered from nylon non-adherent TBC in their lack of correlation
with lysis, age variations, organ distribution and kinetics of
formation.

Depletion and enrichment of NK cytolytic activity according to various surface markers has revealed that the NK cell is Ig^-, $C3R^-$, $FcR^{\pm weak}$, $\theta^{\pm weak}$, possesses low affinity receptors for the lectin helix pomatia and has a high density (1.07 gm/cm^3) and a unique electrophoretic mobility midway between B and T cells (1, 6-8). Using a more direct approach we have stained TBC directly with various reagents and preliminary results confirm that the NK cell is a small lymphocyte by electron microscopy and reveal that the cell is negative in the ANAE, peroxidase and acid phosphatase reactions suggesting that it is not a monocyte or mature T cell. Further studies are in progress to examine other markers such as θ and FcR. Morphological examination of TBC by scanning and transmission E.M. revealed areas of "dynamic" membrane specialization and interdigitations in the area of cell contact (4).

As shown in Tab.2, binding to the target was found to be a necessary prerequisite for lysis to occur. If cell contact was inhibited by EDTA, lysis was not observed and in kinetics experiments target cell binding was detectable 5 to 10 min prior to measureable cell damage. In addition, when both target cell binding and lysis were abolished by trypsinization of the effector, both functions regenerated in a parallel time course which is compatible with the suggestion that binding occurs prior to lysis and is mediated by "protein like" cell surface "recognition" structures. Target-lymhpocyte contact alone, irrespective of the effector cell properties, was not a sufficient condition for lysis since nylon retained spleen cells did not lyse the targets to which they attached. Further experiments revealed that nylon non-adherent cells form stable contacts with targets in the presentce of DNP and NaN_3, whereas lysis was clearly inhibited. This suggests that energy is required for lysis but not binding in the NK system in contrast to cytotoxic T lymphocytes which require energy for binding and lysis (9,10). Inhibitors of serine proteases and colchicine, a microtubule disrupter, also prevented lysis but not binding by NK cells. One could speculate therefore, that the lytic unit on the NK cell involves an enzymatic activity which is triggered by an energy dependent pathway upon the binding of the target and effector via a separate "recognition" structure. One could further speculate that the energy is required to (i) expose the active site of the enzyme to the cells exterior or (ii) create a "dynamic" interaction with the target. The essential feature of this model which is shown schematically in Fig.1, is that target cell binding and lysis by NK cells are independently controlled events. This suggestion was supported by the observation that mice injected with tilorone, an interferon inducer, had greatly augmented NK activity with no effect on the frequency of TBC (4,11). This suggests that interferon may not act by expanding clone size but rather increases intrinsic lytic potential at the single cell level.

TAB. 2:   Independent Regulation of Target Cell Binding and Lysis.

Experimental Treatment[a]	Effect[b]		Reference
	TBC	lysis	
Trypsin	↓	↓	4
Trypsin + regeneration	↑	↑	4
Trypsin + cycloheximide	↓	↓	4
EDTA (1-10 mM)	↓	↓	4
NaN$_3$ (10-100 mM)	-	↓	4
DNP (0.1-1.0 mM)	-	↓	4
PMSF (0.01-1.0 mM)	-	↓	4
DIFP (0.1-10 mM)	-	↓	4
Colchicine	ND	↓	unpublished
Cytochalasin B	ND	↓	unpublished
Interferon inducers	-	↑,↑↑	4
0°	-	↓	4
4°	-	↓	unpublished
15°	-	↓	unpublished
20°	-	↑	unpublished
37°	-	↑↑	4

[a]   The effect of various inhibitors on target cell binding and lysis. Nylon wool column passed spleen cells pooled from 10 CBA mice were incubated together with ethylenediaminotetraacetic acid (EDTA), sodium azide (NaN$_3$), dinitrophenol (DNP), phenylmethylsulfonyl fluoride (PMSF) or diisopropylflorophosphate (DIFP) during a 2 hr cytolytic or TBC assay or spleen cells were pre-treated with trypsin.

[b]   ↑increase;   ↓decrease;   (-), no change.

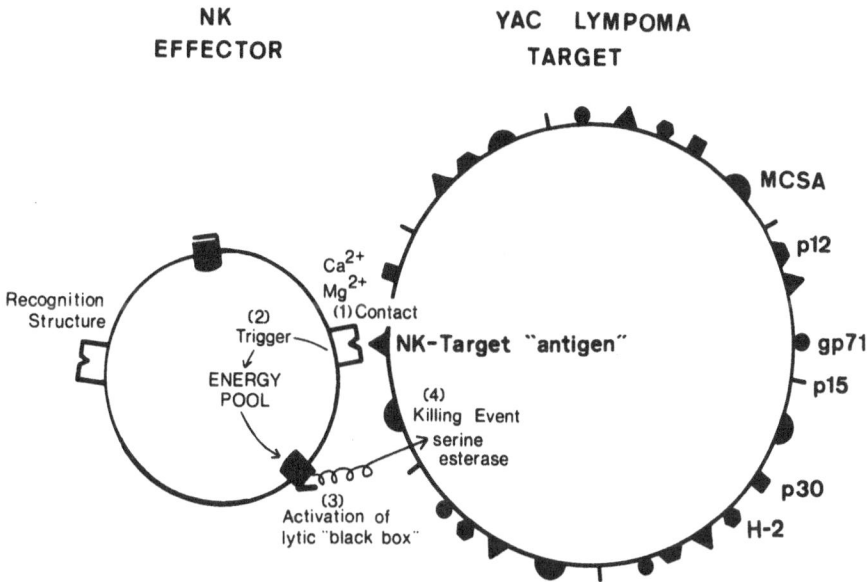

FIG. 1:   A schematic model of NK killing. The target structure
has been isolated and described whereas the NK receptor is inferred
and the "black box" activation of the serine esterase is entirely
speculative. Step 1 involves a divalent cation dependent and
specific contact between the target and effector. The interaction
between the NK receptor and target structure triggers an energy
dependent intrinsic arming of the NK cell. In step 2 this arming
involves the activation of a lytic "black box" which is shown by
the opening of the lid on this "box", step 3. The interaction of
the lytic moiety (serine esterase?) released from the box with the
target, step 4, and the subsequent death of the target is not
defined. Step 1 is blocked by EDTA, step 3 by DNP and NaN_3 and
step 4 by inhibitors of serine proteases such as PMSF and DIFP.

These observations should provide a rational basis for the
elucidation of the recognition structures and target "antigens"
involved in the NK system.

SUMMARY AND CONCLUSIONS

The results show that a subpopulation of nylon non-adherent
lymphocytes binds specifically to an NK sensitive target. Physical
separations and an analysis of co-variance indicate that this target
binding cell (TBC) represents the NK cell. In addition, it is shown
that binding is a necessary but not sufficient condition for target

cell lysis and furthermore, target cell binding and lysis are
independently controlled events. Target cell binding is under H-2
linked genetic control and varies with the age of the animal or
the organ site. The recognition structure is sensitive to trypsin
and the target "antigen" on one murine lymphoma has been isolated.
Problems concerning the polyclonality and specificity repertoire of
the NK cell are now amenable to investigation using the techniques
described. These observations may be of crucial importance to our
eventual understanding of natural resistance to tumors.

REFERENCES

1.   Kiessling, R., Haller, O., In: Contemporary Topics in Immuno-
      biology. (ed. by N. Warner, M. Cooper) in press (1978).
2.   Roder, J.C., Kiessling, R., Scand. J. Immunol. in press (1978).
3.   Roder, J.C., Rosen, A., Fenyö, E.M., Troy, F.A., Klein, G.,
      Proc. Nat. Acad. Sci. USA, in press (1978).
4.   Roder, J.C., Kiessling, R., Biberfeld, P., Andersson, B.,
      submitted for publication (1978).
5.   Roder, J.C., Kiessling, R., In: Current Trends in Tumor Immu-
      nology. Garland STPM Press, New York. in press (1978).
6.   Herberman, R.B., Holden, H.T., West, W.H., Bonnard, G.D.,
      Santoni, A., Nunn, M.E., Kay, H.D., Ortaldo, J.R., In:
      Proceedings of the International Symposium on Tumor-Associated
      Antigens and Their Specific Immune Response, in press (1978).
7.   Kärre, K., Becker, S., Haller, O., Örn, A., Andersson, L.C.,
      Ranki, A., Kiessling, R., Hayry, P., submitted for publication
      (1978).
8.   Haller, O., Gidlund, M., Hellstrom, U., Hammarstrom, S.,
      Wigzell, H., submitted for publication (1978).
9.   Berke, G., Gabison, D., Europ. J. Immunol. 5 (1975) 671.
10.   Martz, E., J. Immunol. 115 (1975) 261.
11.   Gidlund, M., Örn, A., Wigzell, H., Senik, A., Gressor, I.,
      Nature, in press (1978).

THE STIMULATION OF A T CELL RESPONSE IN THE SYNGENEIC HOST BY THE P-815 MASTOCYTOMA CELL AND THE ISOLATION OF A TUMOR-ASSOCIATED ANTIGEN WHICH HAS SOME H-2 ANTIGEN CHARACTERISTICS

M. Bertschmann, K.J. Clemetson and E.F. Lüscher

Theodor Kocher Institute, University of Berne
Berne, Switzerland

INTRODUCTION

Most spontaneous human tumors are non- or only weakly immunogenic. This situation differs from that in experimental tumor
systems, where unequivocal immune reactions have been described
for many syngeneic tumor-host combinations. In order to obtain
information from animal experimental systems, which is more relevant
to human cases, it seems important to select weakly immunogenic
systems, although such tumors may be more difficult to study
experimentally and give less profuse results than strongly immunogenic systems. We chose the P-815 tumor cell in the syngeneic
DBA/2 mouse as a model for the characterization of the hosts
reactions against this tumor and for the isolation and characterization of the relevant antigens - tumor specific or tumor
associated - from this cell. Although this tumor is generally
cited as being induced by methylcholanthrene this is by no means
certain. Dunn and Potter (1) originally describing the tumor,
refer to the P-815 tumor as a "second tumor mass, overlying the
sternum", which they characterized as a mastocytoma. The primary
tumor originating at the site of the methylcholanthrene painting
was a squamous cell carcinoma. Regardless of the way in which this
was actually induced, it is clear that it is very weakly immunogenic.

RESULTS

As described earlier (2) the immunogenicity of the P-815 tumor
in the DBA/2 mouse can best be demonstrated by injecting the tumor
cells intradermally (i.d.). By doing this many more tumor cells
are spontaneously eliminated before they form visible tumors than

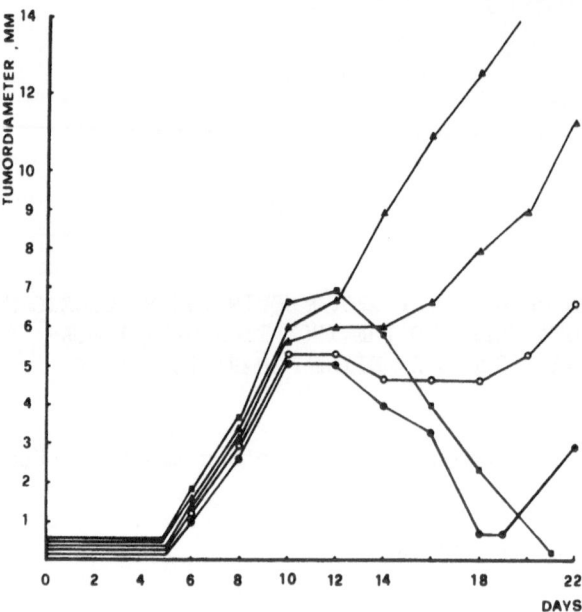

<u>FIG. 1:</u>   Intradermal growth of 10^4 P-815 cells in DBA/2 mice.
Typical growth curves indicated for individual animals.

when given intraperitoneally (i.p.) or subcutaneously (s.c.).   The
cell number for 100% tumor takes is 10^2 for i.p. or s.c. injection
and this cell number is also 100% lethal. With the i.d. injection
10^4 cells are needed to produce tumors in all animals and a variable
number of animals survive indefinitely after they have spontaneously
rejected their tumors. Animals which do not survive show more or less
pronounced phases of tumor regression or growth inhibition.

Typical growth curves are shown in Fig.1.

During an appreciable period of the early tumor growth, namely
between day 6 and 15 (or longer), a measurable immunity exists against
the P-815 tumor. This is demonstrable by the elimination before tumor
formation of a second P-815 tumor cell injection (10^4 cells), when
this second injection is made between day 6 and 15 (Fig.2). When
the second tumor cell injection is given on day 3, second tumors
develop. A second tumor cell injection of 10^6 cells can be suppressed
when injected between days 9 and 12 only, thus indicating a peak of
immune reactivity at that time (not shown in Fig.2).

At the time when the peak of concomitant immunity is reached
(day 10-12), the draining lymph node, i.e. the axillary node, is
grossly enlarged. Lymphoid cells from such nodes are able to exert
a cytotoxic effect <u>in vitro</u> against P-815 as target cells. When
tested in serial double dilutions against $[^3H]$ -TdR labeled targets a

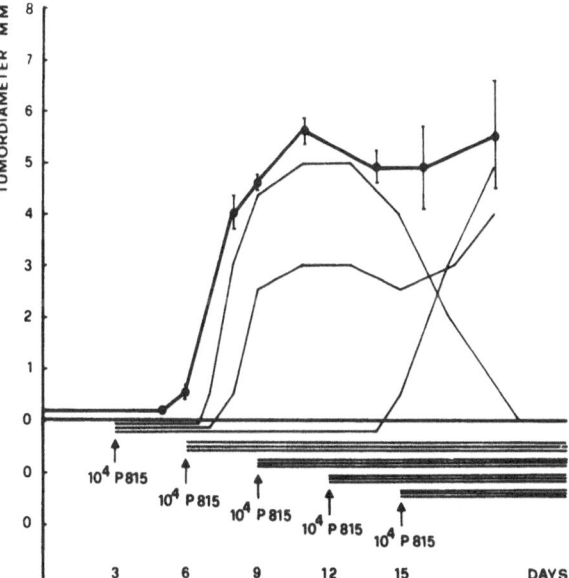

FIG. 2:   Development of concomitant immunity during the growth of
the primary tumor. •——• Size of the first tumor. Mean value per
group and standard error indicated.   ⊢——⊣ Size of second tumors.
Individual tumor-diameters indicated.

cell dose-dependency is apparent, as shown in Fig. 3. Strong target
cell killing is produced by cells from the draining node, whereas
cells from the non-draining nodes of tumor bearers showed the same
low cytotoxicity as lymph node cells from tumor-free animals.

The in vitro cytotoxicity of lymph node cells could be abrogated
completely by treatment of the effectors with anti-Thy-1.2 antibody
and complement, just as the transient or definitive periods of
regression of tumors were wiped out when animals were treated with
Cyclosporin A from day -1 to 5 after tumor cell injection. Cyclosporin A is an anti-lymphocytic compound, which affects T cell
stimulation (3).

These data together indicate that in vivo as well as in vitro
the immune reactivity of the DBA/2 host against its syngeneic P-815
tumor is a T cell effect. T cell effects can be demonstrated for a
short period of tumor development. It is not yet clear which cell-
type is responsible for the elimination of subtumorigenic cell
numbers, nor why in most cases the effectively initiated T cell
killing is abrogated and most animals die from tumors despite the
immunogens present on the tumor cell.

Tumor antigens were also demonstrated on the P-815 cell by

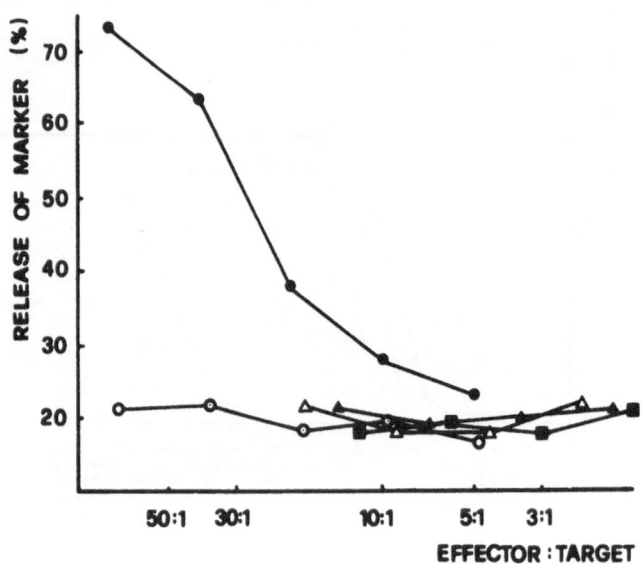

FIG. 3:   Cytotoxicity of lymph node cells from a tumor bearing
DBA/2 mouse (as indicated by percentage of release of the radioactive marker from previously labeled P-815 target cells). o——o
draining (axillary) node; ●——● pooled nodes of normal animal;
△ ▲ ■ non-draining nodes of tumor bearing animal.

cytolysis by antibody and complement (^{51}Cr-release assay). Antibody
formation cannot be demonstrated in the syngeneic host. Two antibodies, one an allo-antibody (C3H anti P-815), the other a xenoantibody (sheep anti P-815) were therefore rendered specific for the
P-815 cell by in vivo absorption in DBA/2 mice (4). By means of
these antibodies two distinct antigens were shown to be present on
the P-815 but not on normal DBA/2 cells. The lectin-binding
properties of these two and of the H-2 antigens are illustrated in
Fig. 4.

    Affinity chromatography was carried out with a membrane fraction
after solubilization by deoxycholate and papain (5). The figure
shows that H-2 antigens bind to the lectin from Lens culinaris and
can be eluted from the column by the corresponding sugar and the
antigen detected by the in vivo absorbed alloantibody(TS_A antigen)
also does so. The tumor associated antigen detected by the in vivo
absorbed xenoantibody (TS_X antigen) also binds to the Lens culinaris
lectin, however, it also binds to wheat germ agglutinin whereas the
two other antigens do not bind. The molecular weight of TS_X is
approximately 70 000 daltons, whereas H-2 and the TS_A antigen have
similar molecular weights of approximately 44 000. Nevertheless

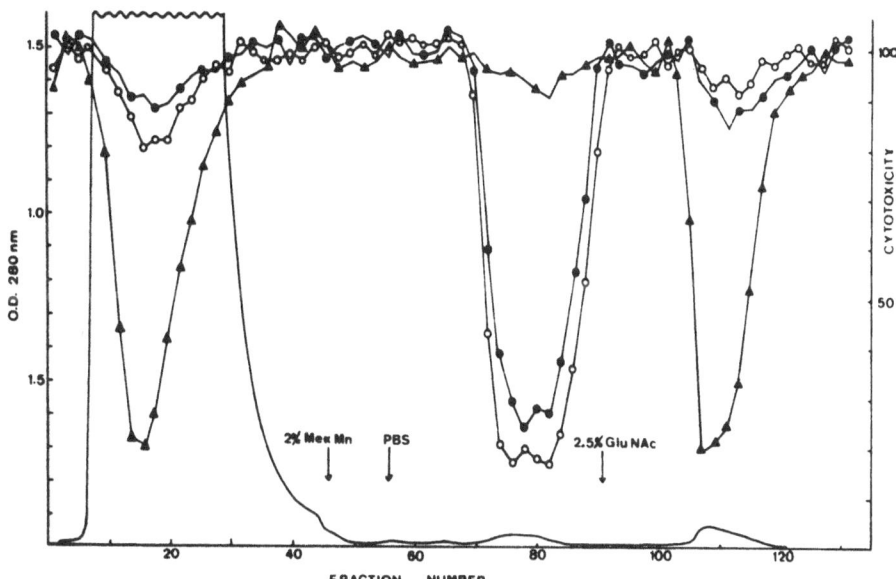

FIG. 4: Fractionation of deoxycholate/papain solubilized P-815 membranes on coupled Lens culinaris/wheat germ agglutinin affinity columns. Antigen activity measured by the inhibition of the cytotoxicity of the corresponding antibodies. o——o H-2 antigens. ●——● TS_A antigen (determined by a C3H anti P-815 antibody in vivo absorbed in DBA/2). ▲——▲ TS_X antigen (determined by a sheep anti P-815 antibody in vivo absorbed in DBA/2).

there are facts which point to TS_A being different from H-2 : 80% of TS_A is lost during cell fractionation procedures whereas only about 20% of H-2 is lost. It is generally more labile than H-2 and it does not coprecipitate with the H-2 antigens when immunoprecipitation is carried out using a C3H anti DBA/2 antibody and Staphylococcus aureus Cowan I as an Fc-binding agent.

SUMMARY

Although not obviously immunogenic when developing intraperitoneally or subcutaneously, the P-815 mastocytoma cell induces a significant immune response when injected intradermally into the syngeneic host. In some animals the immune reaction leads to spontaneous tumor regression and survival of the animals, but in most cases the effectively initiated immune-reaction is abrogated by as yet unknown mechanisms. The T cell is identified as the killer cell both in vivo and in vitro during the described period of immune reactivity.

By means of two antibodies from two different species, rendered specific for the P-815 tumor cell by in vivo absorption in DBA/2 mice, two distinct antigens have been identified, isolated and partially purified from P-815 cell membranes. One of them is obviously different from H-2 antigens, the other one shows striking similarities with H-2 antigens (molecular weight, lectin binding properties), but does not coprecipitate with H-2 antigens in an indirect precipitation assay, using Staph. aureus Cowan I as the Fc-binding agent.

REFERENCES

1. Dunn, T.B., Potter, M., J. Natl. Cancer Inst. 18 (1957) 587.
2. Bertschmann, M. et al., Schweiz. Med. Wschr. 102 (1972) 1197.
3. Borel, J.F., Immunol. 31 (1976) 631.
4. Bertschmann, M., et al., Europ. J. Cancer 12 (1976) 255.
5. Clemetson, K.J., et al., Europ. J. Cancer 12 (1976) 263.

ACKNOWLEDGEMENTS

This work was supported by the Swiss National Science Foundation, grant number 3.752.76.

CYTOTOXIC T CELL RESPONSES TO A SYNGENEIC TUMOUR: CONDITIONS FOR

PRIMARY ACTIVATION IN VITRO AND BIOLOGICAL ACTIVITY IN VIVO

Hilary S. Warren, J.A. Woolnough, C.P. Denaro and K.J. Lafferty

Department of Immunology, John Curtin School of Medical Research, Australian National University, P.O. Box 334 Canberra City, A.C.T., Australia

INTRODUCTION

In vitro T cell activation against alloantigens requires antigen presentation to the responsive cell in combination with an inductive signal, termed the lymphocyte costimulator. This inductive signal can be provided by allogeneic stimulator cells or can be provided exogenously using the supernatant from Con A-activated spleen cells (CS) as a source of the costimulator (1,2). Unlike responses to alloantigens, cocultivation of the P815 tumour of DBA/2 mice with syngeneic lymph node cells results in the generation of little cytotoxic activity which is detected only at high effector to target cell ratios and after long incubation times (3,4). We have recently reported that the addition of CS to in vitro cultures allows significant cytotoxic T cell activation of DBA/2 lymphocytes to the syngeneic tumour P815 (5). In this report the requirement for CS in the generation of P815 reactive cells is further characterized and preliminary studies on the biological effectiveness of these activated cells in controlling the growth of P815 in DBA/2 mice are presented.

MATERIALS AND METHODS

Preparation of Con A-activated cell supernatant (CS): This was as described previously (2,6). Briefly, 300×10^6 spleen cells were pulsed with 5 µg/ml Con A for 2 hrs in serum-free medium in 75 cm^2 surface area plastic flasks. The cell monolayer was washed, 30 mls serum-free medium was added and the cells incubated at 37^0 for 16-18 hrs. The supernatant was concentrated 10-fold over a PM-10 Diaflo membrane, sterile filtered and stored at -20^0.

TAB. 1:   The syngeneic response to P815.

Stimulator cell	CS	cytotoxic units CU/culture x 10^{-4}		
		$H-2^d$ P815	$H-2^d$ DBA/2 spl	$H-2^b$ C57Bl/6 spl
P815 γ -irradiated	−	< 0.5	<1.0	<1.0
P815 γ -irradiated	+	14.0	2.7	<1.3
none	+	2.4	1.5	<1.3
DBA/2 spleen blasts γ -irradiated	+	1.6	1.3	<1.3

Cell cultures and cytotoxic assays: Cultures contained 10^6 responding lymph node cells and 1.6×10^5 stimulator cells in 1 ml volumes in plastic multiwell trays (Falcon 3008).   Culture medium was Eagles medium containing 0.1mM 2-mercaptoethanol and 10% heat inactivated foetal calf serum.   10% CS was added on day 0 unless otherwise indicated.   Stimulator cells were γ -irradiated P815 (5000 r) or 2-day Con A-spleen cell blasts (2000 r).   Cultures were maintained for 5 days at 37° in an atmosphere of 10% CO_2, 7% O_2 and 83% N_2.   Cytotoxic activity was assayed against ^{51}Cr-labelled target cells, and is expressed as cytotoxic units (CU)/culture, where 1 CU is that activity required to lyse 1 target cell during a 4 hr incubation period (7).   Replicate assays have a standard deviation of $\pm 20\%$.   Cells from cultures with an activity of $10^{5.0}$ CU/culture cause 33% lysis of target cells at an effector target cell ratio of 1:1.

Testing the biological effect of in vitro generated cytotoxic cells in vivo: Groups of 4 mice were injected intraperitoneally (i.p.) with 10^3 P815.   Cells from in vitro culture were washed and 5×10^6 cells were injected i.p. 1 ml cell cultures yielded 0.8 to 1.2×10^6 cells on day 5 with activities for different experiments ranging between 30×10^4 and 70×10^4 CU/10^6 cells.   Cell numbers of P815 in the peritoneal cavity were determined after a complete peritoneal washout and estimating the proportion of P815 by Leishmans staining of cytocentrifuge preparations.

RESULTS

Activation of DBA/2 lymph node cells to P815:   As shown in Table 1, DBA/2 lymph node cells cultured with γ -irradiated P815 did not generate any cytotoxic activity unless CS was present.   80% of the cells were killed and more than 90% of the cytotoxic activity

TAB. 2:   Dose of CS and the magnitude of the syngeneic response to
P815.

final dilution of CS in culture*	$\frac{1}{20}$	$\frac{1}{40}$	$\frac{1}{60}$	$\frac{1}{80}$	0
CU/culture x 10^{-4}	65	47	24	10	<0.4

*   CS used in this experiment was concentrated 50-fold.

generated was destroyed after treatment with anti Thy 1.2 serum and
complement providing evidence that the effector cells in vitro are
T cells. The response obtained is not polyclonal as no killing of
C57B1/6 targets could be detected. However there was some killing
of DBA/2 targets over and above that of control cultures of DBA/2
lymph node cells, Υ -irradiated DBA/2 spleen cell blasts and CS.
This anti H-2^d response is small even when it is taken into account
that P815 is three times more easily lyzed than DBA/2 spleen cell
blasts (5). We can conclude from this data that the response generated is mainly directed against P815 associated antigens.

Requirement for CS in the generation of the syngeneic response
to P815:   As shown in Table 2, the magnitude of the cytotoxic
response generated in DBA/2 lymph node cells to P815 depended on
the amount of CS added to the cultures. The maximum cytotoxic
response was obtained if CS was added in the first 24 hours (Tab.3).
These results are similar to those obtained for the CS requirement
in allogeneic T cell activation to P815 (2,8).

Biological effect of in vitro generated syngeneic cytotoxic
cells: P815 is lethal for DBA/2 mice. 10^3 P815 injected i.p.
results in death of the mice by day 16-17. Preliminary experiments
showed that injection of 10^6 cells from syngeneic cultures i.p. on
day 0 led to a 98% reduction in P815 cell numbers in the peritoneal
cavity of DBA/2 mice on day 8. Subsequent experiments (Tab.4) showed
that injection of 5 x 10^6 cells from syngeneic cultures on days 0 and
1 or 0, 1 and 2 led to a 50-70% increase in mean survival time (MST)
of the mice. Multiple doses on subsequent days 8, 9, 15, 16 did not
increase the MST of the mice although the development of the massive
ascites prior to death was significantly delayed. The effect was
specific in that injections on days 0, 1 and 2 of medium alone, DBA/2
lymphocytes activated to allogeneic (C57B1/6) cells, or cells from
control cultures of DBA/2 lymph node cells and CS, did not increase
the MST of the mice.

TAB. 3:   Day of addition of CS and the syngeneic response to P815.

Day of addition	0	1	2	3	not added
CU/culture x 10^{-4} assayed on day 5	10	9	0.9	<0.2	<0.2

TAB. 4:   The effect of in vitro generated DBA/2 responsive cells on the mean survival time of mice injected with P815.

	Mean Survival Time in Days $\pm$ S.E.		
Treatment*	Expt 1	Expt 2	Expt 3
none	17.3+2.0	16.7+1.0	15.8+0.5
DBA/2 anti P815 cells	29.8+1.6	24.5+0.3	23.3+1.5
DBA/2 anti C57B1/6 cells	-	-	16.0+1.0

*   mice were injected with 10^3 P815 and 5×10^6 cultured cells on days 0 and 1 (Expt 1) or 0, 1 and 2 (Expts 2 and 3).

DISCUSSION

In the case of in vitro cytotoxic T cell responses to allo-antigens we have shown that a source of costimulator is an absolute requirement for lymphocyte activation (1,2,6,8). CS added to such cultures acts at an early stage of T cell induction, and has a continuing effect throughout the culture period (8). CS addition to cell cultures can also magnify ongoing responses (1). In the case of in vitro cytotoxic T cell activation of DBA/2 lymphocytes to the syngeneic tumour P815, the responses generated are weak and cannot be detected under the same conditions of culture and assay as allogeneic T cell activation. The addition of CS to the cultures causes a marked increase in the cytotoxic T cell response to P815. The effect requires the presence of P815 in the culture and cannot be accounted for by polyclonal activation induced by CS.

We have shown that cells generated in cultures of DBA/2 lymph node cells, γ-irradiated P815 and CS can delay the time of death of DBA/2 mice inoculated with P815. This biological effect is specific for DBA/2 lymphocytes activated to P815. We do not know whether the in vivo effector cells are T cells as they are in vitro and what influence other cells from the culture might have in this system. These studies are a preliminary step in determining conditions for a more effective immunotherapy of the P815 tumour in DBA/2 mice.

REFERENCES

1.   Lafferty, K.J., Woolnough, J.A.   Immunol. Rev. 35 (1977) 231.
2.   Talmage, D.W., Woolnough, J.A., Hemmingsen, H., Lopez, L., Lafferty, K.J.   Proc. Natl. Acad. Sci. USA 74 (1977) 4610.
3.   Lundak, R.L., Raidt, D.J.   Cell Immunol. 9 (1973) 60.
4.   Takei, F., Levy, J.G., Kilburn, D.G.   J. Immunol. 116 (1976) 288.
5.   Warren, H.S., Woolnough, J.A., Lafferty, K.J.   Aust. J. Exp. Biol. Med. Sci. 56 (1978) 247.
6.   Lafferty, K.H., Warren, H.S., Woolnough, J.A., Talmage, D.W. Blood cells.(1978) In press.
7.   Lafferty, K.J., Bootes, A., Dart, G., Talmage, D.W.   Transplantation 22 (1976) 138.
8.   Lafferty, K.J., Warren, H.S., Woolnough, J.A.   This volume. (1978).

OPPOSITE EFFECTS OF T-CELLS ON SYNGENEIC TUMOR GROWTH IN VIVO:
TUMOR INHIBITION BY MATURE LYMPHOCYTES AND ENHANCEMENT OF THE
SAME TUMORS BY IMMATURE CELLS

Myra Small

Department of Cell Biology
The Weizman Institute of Science
Rehovot, Israel

Our studies during the past few years on the interactions
between host lymphocytes and several syngeneic tumors in mice have
revealed that T-cells with opposing reactivities toward the same
tumor can be activated by exposure to the neoplastic cells. While
one population of sensitized T-cells is capable of inhibiting tumor
growth in vivo, a second T-cell population can abolish this effect
and bring about tumor enhancement. We have been investigating the
T-cells involved in each of these responses in order to understand
the cell characteristics required for each reactivity and to
selectively inactivate the tumor-enhancing T-lymphocytes in situ.
Our experiments indicate that these two reactivities of T-cells do
not involve parallel classes of mature T-cells but rather that they
represent responses characteristic of different stages in T-cell
maturation. Our hypothesis is that interaction between mature T-
cells and a tumor can lead to development of anti-tumor reactivity
while exposure of immature T-cells to the same tumor can trigger the
tumor enhancement process. Secondly we envisage that as tumor growth
progresses early thymocytes with tumor enhancing activity are
released from the thymus to the periphery where they counteract the
activity of the tumor-inhibiting T-cells. Evidence in support of
these two notions is presented below.

The first step in identification of the lymphocytes with opposite
effects on tumor growth was the physical separation of two spleen cell
fractions, one involved in tumor enhancement (in vivo) and the other
causing tumor inhibition (also in vivo). Such a separation was
achieved by taking spleen cells either from tumor-bearing mice (with
advanced tumors) or from cultures of spleen cells exposed to tumors
in vitro and submitting them to velocity sedimentation (1). One of

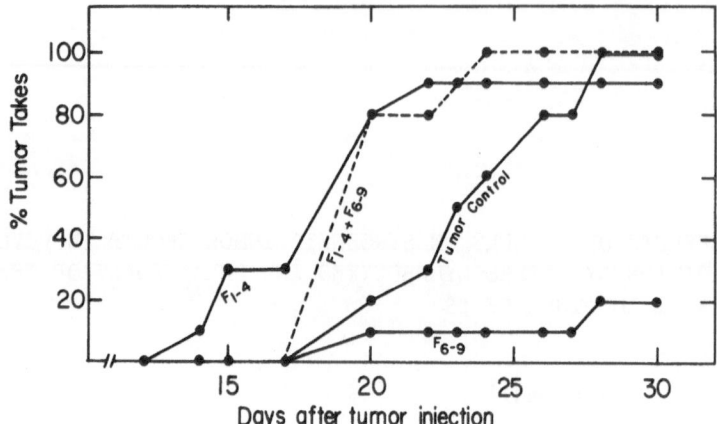

FIG. 1:   Fractionation of spleen cells from a tumor-bearing mouse
by velocity sedimentation. Cells taken from a C_3H mouse with a
syngeneic fibrosarcoma were separated into fraction F_{1-4} which
enhanced tumor growth in a Winn test with the same tumor (in comparison to the tumor control) and fraction F_{6-9} which inhibited
tumor growth in vivo (1).

the fractions recovered showed strong anti-tumor reactivity when
transferred with the same tumor to syngeneic mice (Fig.1). It is
important to note that this activity was apparent only in the
absence of the tumor-enhancing cells (1,2). A second fraction
recovered both from tumor- bearing mice with advanced tumors or
from cultures of spleen cells sensitized to tumors in vitro brought
about enhanced growth of the same tumors (1) (Fig.1). Since the
enhancing cells were dominant both in the unseparated population
and after mixture of the two fractions, these experiments suggested
that the tumor-inhibiting lymphocytes could be overwhelmed by the
tumor-enhancing lymphocyte population.

Further characterization of the tumor-inhibiting lymphocytes
(which appear to be specific for the tumor of sensitization (2))
revealed that they are depleted by a single low dose of ALS (a
procedure affecting recirculating mature peripheral T-cells (3))
(Fig.2). On the other hand, increased anti-tumor reactivity was
found (4) after treatment of spleen cell suspensions during sensitization with THF (thymic humoral factor) which brings about T-cell
maturation (5).

In contrast, the tumor-enhancing lymphocytes could be depleted
by thymectomy of adult mice (Fig.2). Since tumor-enhancing cells

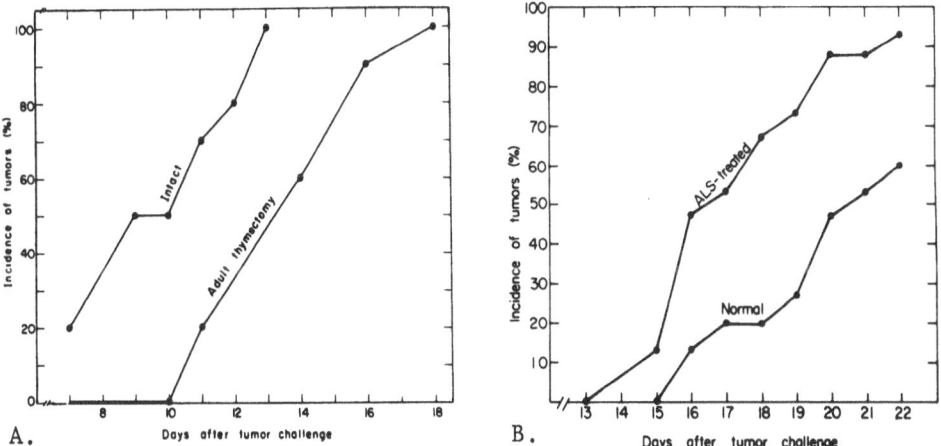

FIG. 2:   Depletion of either recent thymic migrants or mature recirculating peripheral T-cells with opposite effects on syngeneic
tumor growth. A.   5 x 10^4 3LL tumor cells were injected into the
footpad of $C_{57}Bl$ mice, intact or thymectomized 2 months before. B.
1 x 10^5 3LL tumor cells were injected into the footpad of $C_{57}Bl$
mice, normal or 2 days after ip injection of 0.03 ml ALS.

could also be detected in the thymus by assay without prior exposure
to the tumor (6,7), we could investigate characteristics which are
inherent to these cells and not a result of the sensitization
process. Tumor-enhancing cells in the thymus appeared to be in the
very early stages of thymic processing (6,7), (Fig.3). Thus they
are rapidly dividing thymocytes found in the subcapsular region of
the cortex, cells which are sensitive to the parenteral effects of
cortisone and repopulate the cortisone-depleted thymus. These early
thymocytes also express a low level of H-2 antigens on their surface
and lack PHA reactivity. Treatment of the tumor-enhancing thymocytes
with THF abolished this reactivity vis-a-vis tumor growth suggesting
that the cell characteristics involved in tumor enhancement are
repressed as the T-cells mature.

When we followed the kinetics of each of these opposing subpopulations in the spleen during the course of tumor growth (2), tumor
inhibiting cells appeared first and as tumor growth progressed their
activity declined and gave way to tumor enhancement by splenocytes
from the mice with advanced tumors. Both of these reactivities were
eliminated by anti-theta serum and complement (2) (Fig.4,5).

Finally, we have investigated whether premature release of early
thymocytes to the periphery occurs in parallel to this loss of anti-
tumor reactivity during tumor growth. As a marker characteristic of

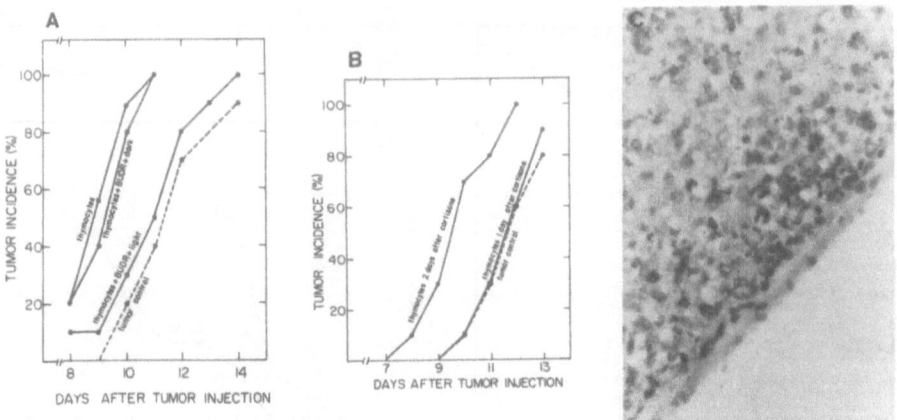

FIG. 3:   Characteristics of the early thymocytes involved in tumor
enhancement.   A.   BUdR plus light is lethal for the tumor-enhancing
thymocytes.   B.   These cells are cortisone sensitive and also repopulate the cortisone-depleted thymus.   C.   Location in the outer
thymic cortex of dividing repopulating thymocytes as shown by autoradiography.   3LL tumor cells with or without the thymocytes assayed
were injected into the footpad of $C_{57}Bl$ mice (6).

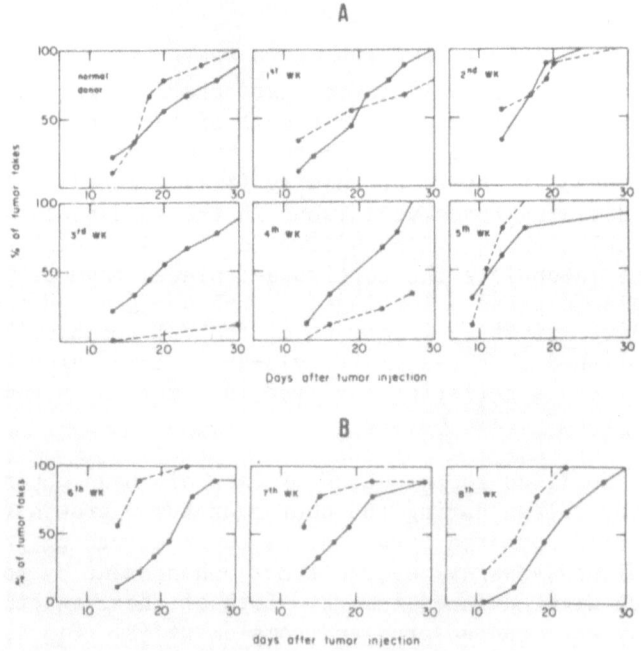

FIG. 4:   Detection of tumor inhibiting cells (A---) and tumor enhancing cells (B---) in spleen of C_3H mice after s.c. injection of
5×10^4 fibrosarcoma cells.   Lymphocytes were assayed in a Winn test
in comparison to tumor cells alone (———) (2).

EFFECT OF ANTI-THETA SERUM ON THE PROTECTIVE
AND ENHANCING ACTIVITIES OF SPLEEN CELLS
FROM TUMOR-BEARING MICE [1]

Spleen cells	Mean day of tumor appearance ±SE		
	Tumor cells only	Tumor cells + non-treated spleen cells	Tumor cells + $\alpha\theta$ + C'-treated spleen cells
Protective period	23.7±1.5	28.3±2.5	23.5±1.3
Enhancing period	27.5±2.2	22.3±0.8	30.6±2.5

[1] 5×10^4 fibrosarcoma cells injected alone or together with spleen cells at a 1:100 ratio. Recipients were normal syngeneic animals. —

FIG. 5:   Evidence that both reactivities measured in Fig.4 involved T-lymphocytes (2).

Accumulation of cells with TdT activity in the spleen during syngeneic tumor growth*

Mice	Cells assayed	TdT activity	
		pmoles dGTP incorporated per hr/10^8 cells	enzyme units per 10^8 cells
Normal	Thymus	1150 900 1100	1.05
	Spleen	10 18 30	0.02
Tumor bearing	Spleen Tumor-inhibiting period	100 400	0.25
	Spleen Tumor-enhancing period	900 500 900 500	0.70

* Chemically-induced fibrosarcoma in C3H/eb mice

Thymic origin of cells with TdT activity in spleens of mice with advanced syngeneic tumors*

Mice	Cells assayed	TdT activity	
		pmoles dGTP incorporated per hr/10^8 cells	enzyme units per 10^8 cells
Normal	Thymus	1400 1100 1200 1400	1.25
	Spleen	140 0 150 0	0-0.15
Tumor bearing	Spleen of intact mice	950 650 550	0.70
	Spleen of thymectomized mice	170 0	0-0.17

* Lewis lung carcinoma in C57B1/6J mice

FIG. 6:   Migration of thymocytes during the course of tumor growth (9).

thymocytes and not found in T-cells of normal spleen, lymph node or peripheral blood (8), we assayed for the enzyme TdT (terminal deoxy-nucleotidyl transferase). TdT activity was clearly detected in the spleen of mice with advanced tumors (when spleen cells enhanced tumor growth) but such enzyme activity was absent from the spleen when the mice were thymectomized before tumor challenge (9). Thus release of immature T-cells from the thymus does not seem to occur during the course of tumor growth (Fig.6).

REFERENCES

1.   Small, M., Trainin, N., J. Immunol. 117 (1976) 292.
2.   Gabizon, A., Small, M., Trainin, N., Int. J. Cancer 18 (1976) 813.
3.   Araneo, B.A., Marrack, P.C., Kappler, J.W., J. Immunol. 114 (1975) 747.
4.   Small, M., Trainin, N., Int. J. Cancer 15 (1975) 962.
5.   Trainin, N., Small, M., Kook, A.I., in: B and T Cells in Immune Recognition. F. Loor and G.E. Roelants, eds. John Wiley and Sons, Ltd. p.83 (1977).
6.   Small, M., J. Immunol. 118 (1977) 1517.
7.   Small, M., J. Immunol. (1978) in press.
8.   Baltimore, D., Silverstone, A.E., Kung, P.C., Harrison, T.A., McCaffrey, R.P., Cold Spring Harbor Symp. on Quantitative Biology XLI (1976) 63.
9.   Small, M., Lasser, M., Daniel, V., Israel J. Med. Sci. (1978) in press.

TUMOR METASTASES AND CELL-MEDIATED IMMUNITY IN A MODEL SYSTEM IN DBA/2 MICE. 2. CHARACTERISTICS OF A METASTASIZING VARIANT OF A CHEMICALLY INDUCED LYMPHOMA

Volker Schirrmacher and Geraldine Shantz

Institute of Immunology and Genetics, Deutsches

Krebsforschungszentrum, D 69 Heidelberg, W. Germany

Tumor Origin

A model system is presented suitable to study mechanisms of immunity against metastasizing tumors. It is a syngeneic system consisting of a non-metastasizing methylcholanthrene induced lymphoma of DBA/2 ($H-2^d$) mice (L 5178-YE, now designated Eb) and a metastasizing variant which arose spontaneously in 1968 during routine i.p. transplantation of Eb in syngeneic mice in Prof. P. Alexander's laboratory (L 5178-YES, now designated ESb) (1). The cause of the variant formation is not known at present. Events like mutation, chromosomal aberration, change in chromosome numbers, activation (derepression) of silent genes or cell-cell fusion (2) could be considered. It appears unlikely that ESb represents a de novo spontaneous tumor not related to Eb because it grew out as an ascites tumor within 7-10 days. Spontaneous tumors usually grow slowly at the beginning and do not grow as ascites.

The tissue origin of these tumors was investigated by studying the expression of lymphoid differentiation antigens, such as Ig and Thy 1.2. Using direct cytotoxicity and absorption assays, we demonstrated that both tumor lines were surface Ig negative and Thy 1.2 positive. This suggests that both tumors are of lymphoid origin, in particular of T lymphoid origin (3).

ESb, a Tumor Variant with Increased Malignancy and Metastasizing Capacity

Some of the properties in which ESb cells differ from Eb cells have been described previously (1,4) and are therefore only summarized in Table 1.

TAB. 1: Differences between the Non-Metastasizing Tumor Eb and Its Metastasizing Variant ESb. [1]

I.	TUMORS		
	1. Old designation	L 5178 Y-E	L 5178 Y-ES (1)
	2. New designation (Heidelberg lines)	Eb	ESb
II.	OBSERVATIONS AFTER 10^6 TUMOR CELLS s.c.		
	1. Death	4-5 weeks	7-10 days
	2. Tumor size	large	small
	3. Metastases	none	mainly in liver
III.	IMMUNOGENICITY IN VIVO	strong	weak
IV.	SHEDDING OF H-2 ANTIGENS	low	high
V.	STABILITY IN TISSUE CULTURE	good	poor

[1] Previous observations from P. Alexander's group (1,4).

We will begin the characterization with the cells morphology, then describe functional aspects relevant to malignancy in an in vitro test for invasive growth and finally analyze in vivo local tumor growth and dissemination.

Morphology.   The morphology of the two cell lines was studied by transmission electron microscopy (TEM), immuno-electron microscopy (IEM) and scanning electron microscopy (SEM) (3). ESb cells were found to differ from Eb cells typically (i) in the shape of the nucleus (TEM, see Fig.1) and (ii) in the structure of the cell surface (TEM, IEM and SEM). ESb cells are mostly covered with many long and thin membrane extrusions (microvilli) while Eb cells are smoother and carry microvilli which are lower in number, smaller and thicker. The expression of microvilli certainly changes and should be seen as a dynamic process which may be easily influenced by environmental factors. The electronmicrographs obtained with 3 different techniques, using various fixation procedures, however always demonstrated similar differences in membrane structure of ESb and Eb cells (further pictures are presented in 3), so that they may be considered as significant.

Invasion of normal tissue in vitro.   When ESb tumor cells were co-cultivated in vitro with syngeneic normal tissue, for instance from the lung, they could be shown (i) to firmly attach to these organ cultures and (ii) to be able to destroy the outer layers of normal cells. When Eb cells were used instead of ESb, no attachment of the tumor cells and no damage of the normal tissue could be seen (3, Lohmann-Matthes and Schleich, to be published).

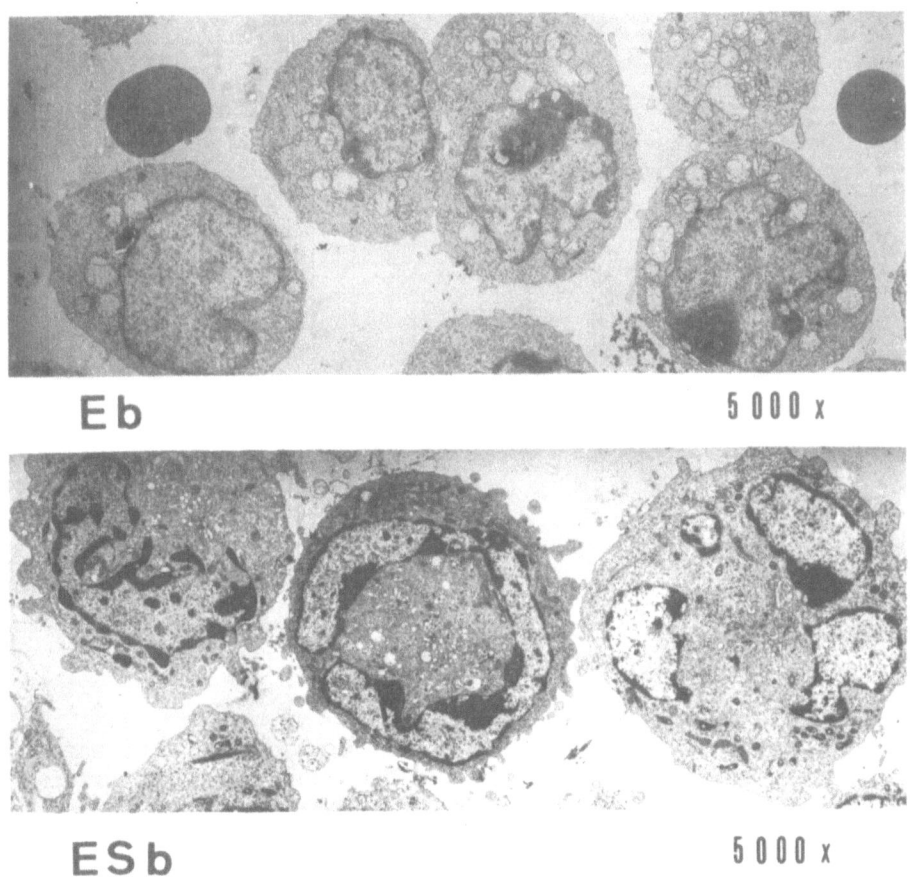

FIG. 1:   Electronmicrographs (TEM) of the non-metastasizing tumor and its metastasizing variant ESb.

In vivo local tumor growth and dissemination.   The increased malignancy of ESb cells demonstrated by the invasive growth in vitro was also obvious from the behaviour in vivo.   While less than 10 ESb tumor cells inoculated s.c. were sufficient to cause tumors in over 50% of the animals, the TD_{50} of Eb cells was about 1 000 times higher.   In addition to their increased tumorigenicity, ESb cells had a strikingly increased ability to disseminate and form metastases in internal organs, in particular the liver.   As a consequence, animals receiving ESb cells died much quicker than those receiving Eb cells.   As can be seen from Fig.2, Eb tumor-bearing animals started to die when the primary tumor had reached a size of about 2 cm in diameter (that is after about 4 weeks), while ESb tumor-bearing animals started to die already when the local tumor was just palpable (after about 10 days).

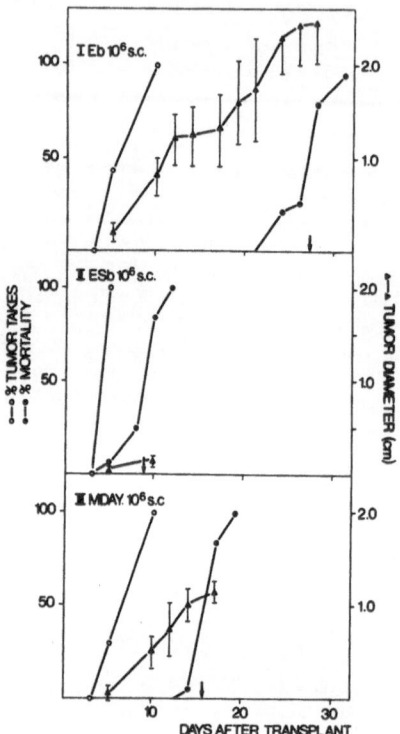

<u>FIG. 2</u>:   In vivo local tumor growth and mortality of mice which
received either the non-metastasizing tumor Eb, its metastasizing
variant ESb or an unrelated syngeneic chemically induced tumor,
MDAY, which also has metastasizing properties.

Escape from Immune Control as a Factor
Facilitating Metastases Formation by ESb Cells?

<u>Decreased immunogenicity</u>.   It has been shown previously that
DBA/2 animals can be protected against Eb tumor growth by preimmunization with irradiated Eb cells.   In contrast, preimmunization with
irradiated ESb cells resulted in only marginal protective immunity
against ESb cells (1).   It was inferred from this observation that
ESb cells had in comparison to Eb cells a much decreased immunogenicity.

<u>Decreased infiltration by macrophages</u>.   Histological sections
through local primary Eb or ESb tumors revealed one quite significant
difference, namely the extent to which these two tumor lines were
infiltrated by host-derived mononuclear macrophage-like cells,
mainly histiocytes.   While Eb tumors were heavily infiltrated, ESb

TAB. 2:   Rejection of ESb tumor cells in allogeneic mice.

Strain	H-2	Mls	H barrier to DBA/2	% mortality (at 4 weeks)	rejection
DBA/2	d	a	none	100	−
BALB/c	d	b	minor (multiple)	80	(+)
B10.D2	d	b	" "	0	+++
(DBA/2x B10.D2)F$_1$	d	axb	none	90	(+)
C57BL/6	b	b	major + minor	0	+++
CBA/j	k	d	" "	0	+++

tumors contained only few of these cells (3). From similar observations in other model systems and with human tumor material (5), an inverse relationship between macrophage content of primary tumors and metastatic spread has been postulated (6). It would be important to know whether infiltration of tumors by macrophages is a T cell dependent phenomenon and, if so, whether mestastasizing tumors suppress such T cells or lack the ability to activate them.

   Increased shedding of histocompatibility antigens.   As reported by Cavey et al. (4), ESb cells release histocompatibility antigens in vivo and in vitro at a greater rate than the non-metastasizing tumor Eb. In addition, using a complement-dependent cytotoxicity assay, it was shown that antigen-antibody complexes formed by the addition of anti H-2 serum to intact cells disappeared more repidly from the surface of ESb than from Eb cells (antibody-induced modulation). From these and other studies (7) it was proposed (i) that the instability of surface antigens may be an integral feature of malignant cells and (ii) that shedding of membrane antigens may represent a mechanism of escape from immune control (8). Shed membrane antigens, in particular tumor-specific antigens, could be considered either to block potential immune effector mechanisms (antibody or T cell mediated) and/or to induce suppressor cells. It remains to be shown whether any of these possible escape mechanisms is operative in vivo in the ESb tumor-bearing animal.

Rejection of the Metastasizing ESb Tumor Cells Across Major or Minor Histocompatibility Barriers

   Having shown that ESb cells (i) have the potential to destroy and invade normal tissue in vitro and (ii) shed histocompatibility antigens at an increased rate, it was of interest to find out whether immune cells would be able to destroy or otherwise control these

highly malignant cells. This question was investigated by testing
the growth or rejection of ESb cells after inoculation into various
kinds of allogeneic hosts. Some of the results obtained are
summarized in Table 2.

Allogeneic mice differing at the major H-2 complex (C57BL/6 and
CBA/j) were able to reject a s.c. inoculum of 10^6 ESb cells. Allogeneic mice differing only at minor histocompatibility (H) loci and
being H-2 identical with DBA/2 were found to be either susceptible
(e.g. BALB/c) or resistant (e.g. B10.D2) to the metastasizing
lymphoma. F_1 hybrids between the syngeneic DBA/2 and the resistant
strain B10.D2 were susceptible.

These results show that the immune system (of allogeneic mice)
is principally capable of rejecting a highly malignant metastasizing
tumor. Further immunogenetic studies are under way to characterize
the gene(s) important for resistance to metastasizing DBA/2 tumors.

The mechanism of tumor resistance will be elucidated by studying
cellular immunity reactions. Immune spleen cells from allogeneic
regressor mice, after restimulation in vitro with inactivated ESb
tumor cells, could be shown to be able to kill ^{51}Cr labeled ESb cells
within a 4 h assay (unpublished results). The capacity of such
immune cells to transfer protective immunity against metastases in
syngeneic recipients is presently being investigated. Preliminary
results look promising indeed.

REFERENCES

1. Parr, I., Br. J. Cancer 26 (1972) 174.
2. Wiener, F., Fenyö, E.M., Klein, G., Harris, H., Nature New
    Biology 238 (1972) 155.
3. Schirrmacher, V., Shantz, G., Clauer, K., Komitowski, D.,
    Zimmermann, H.-P., Lohmann-Matthes, M.-L., (1978) Submitted.
4. Davey, G.C., Currie, G.A., Alexander, P., Br. J. Cancer 33
    (1976) 9.
5. Hamlin, I.M.E., Br. J. Cancer 24 (1969) 653.
6. Eccles, S.A., Alexander, P., Nature 250 (1974) 667.
7. Currie, G.A., Alexander, P., Br. J. Cancer 29 (1974) 72.
8. Alexander, P., In: Fundamental Aspects of Neoplasia. Eds.
    Gottlieb, A.A., Plescia, O.J., Bishop, D.H.L., Springer Verlag,
    N.Y. (1975)

ACKNOWLEDGEMENTS

The cooperation of Dr. Lohmann-Matthes and Dr. Schleich in the
test of in vitro invasiveness is gratefully acknowledged. We also

thank Mrs. Eva Bolzan from the EMBL Heidelberg for the electron-micrographs and Mrs. Karin Clauer for expert technical assistance. In particular we have to thank Prof. Peter Alexander for kindly sending us his tumor lines.

CHARACTERIZATION OF LYMPHOCYTES INVADING EXPERIMENTAL TUMORS

P.K. Lala, S. Garnis, L. Kaizer, S. Jacobs and V. Santer

Department of Anatomy, McGill University

Montreal, Canada

Over the last several years we have examined host cellular responses to tumor development at the systemic as well as local level in a number of host-tumor systems. Part of these studies was designed to characterize the mononuclear cells - lymphocytes in particular, that migrate into several tumors - Ehrlich ascites tumor grown intraperitoneally in CF_1 or CBA mice, and TA-3 (st) mammary tumor grown subcutaneously in A strain mice:

Post mitotic age: Lymphocytes accumulating within these tumors did not show any evidence of local proliferation as evaluated by 1 hour 3H thymidine (3HTdR) uptake; thus they must be emigrants from circulation. Post-mitotic age of these cells was studied by pre-labeling hosts with repeated 3HTdR injections prior to tumor trans-plantation (1,2). They were found to be newly formed cells selec-tively invading the tumor,in contrast to a random exchange of cells found between blood and normal tissue space, e.g. peritoneal cavity under physiological conditions. Tumor-invading monocytes were also found to be younger than those found in the normal circulation; They were found capable of a rapid transformation into macrophages.

Source of mononuclear cells: The source of the tumor-invading lymphocytes was further evaluated by comparing the extent of lympho-cyte accumulation within ascites tumors in mice subjected to different protocols of irradiation prior to tumor transplantation (3): Irradi-ation was either given to the whole body or to the limbs alone (containing about a half of the total bone marrow) or whole body minus the limbs (containing about a half of the total bone marrow, as well as other lymphoid organs inclusive of thymus). The patterns of resultant lymphocyte depletions in the tumors indicated bone

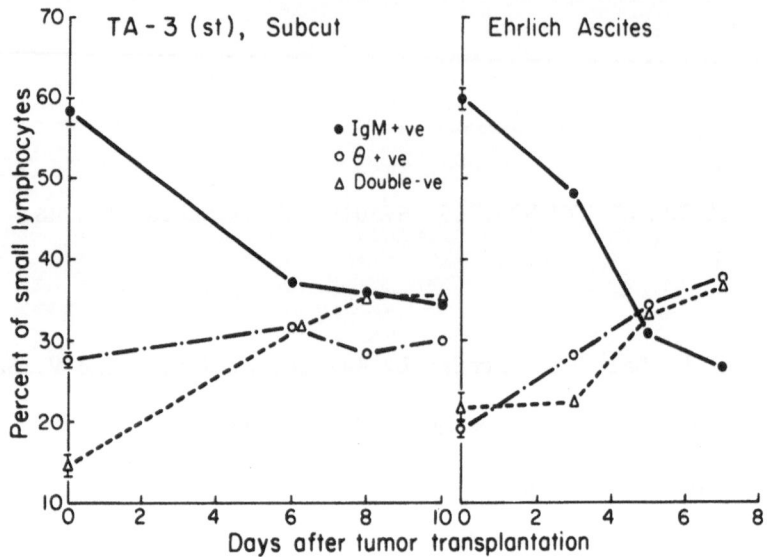

<u>FIG. 1</u>:   Incidence of small lymphocyte subsets within tumors.

marrow as the major source. A similar early influx of newly formed
marrow derived lymphocytes was also seen into the spleen (3,4).

   <u>Lymphocyte surface markers</u>:   Lymphocytes appearing at the
tumor site as well as in host lymphoid tissues (spleen and blood)
were further characterized at different stages of tumor development
on the basis of two well established surface markers – surface IgM
(S-IgM) for B cells and θ (Thy 1) antigen on T cells (5,6). S-IgM
bearing B lymphocytes were identified radioautographically from
their direct binding of radioiodinated anti-IgM. Exposure of
samples to anti θ serum prior to ^{125}I-anti IgM labeled both B and
T cells. Lymphocytes remaining unlabeled in the latter samples
were considered as "double negative", i.e. lacking in either
marker.

   Small lymphocytes accounted for a significant proportion of
host derived leukocytes accumulating in the TA-(st) solid tumor as
well as the Ehrlich ascites tumor. When surface markers were
examined on these cells (Fig.1), the incidence of IgM-bearing small
lymphocytes was found to decline with increasing tumor age. This
was unexpected because of our earlier findings of an increase in
the incidence of newly formed, marrow derived lymphocytes. However,

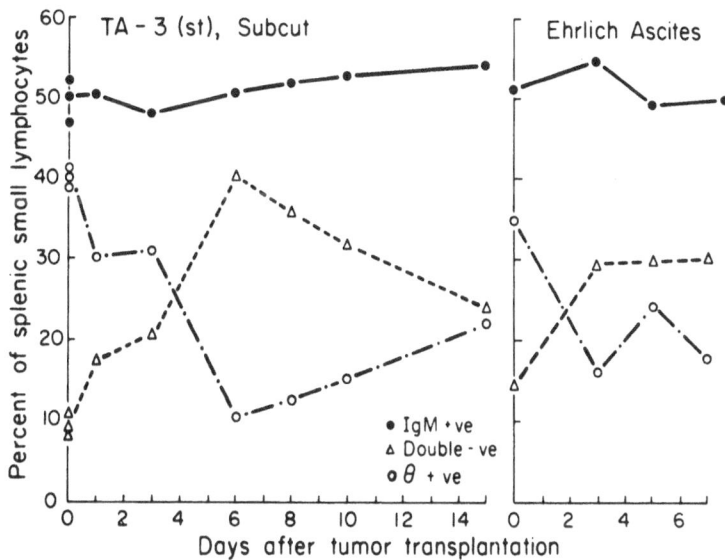

FIG. 2:   Incidence of small lymphocyte subsets within the spleen.

the proportion of double-negative small lymphocytes increased
substantially; this cell class was found to account for a majority
of the young marrow derived lymphoid cells. The proportion of θ +
ve cells was either unchanged (TA-3 (st) tumor) or increased
(Ehrlich ascites tumor). When the incidences were translated into
absolute numbers, all the three lymphocyte subsets were found to
increase at the tumor site – double negative cells, in particular.

When the incidences of various small lymphocyte subsets were
examined within the spleen (Fig.2), the IgM + ve population was
found to remain unchanged, the θ + ve population declined and the
double negative population increased in both tumor-host combinations.
Despite a rapid increase in the splenic size, absolute numbers of
splenic T cells remain level, but the other subsets, double negative
class in particular, increased. The latter population also increased
in incidence in the circulation. In summary, lymphocyte subsets in
peripheral organs did not reflect the local picture at the tumor
site, except for the double negative class. Since this cell class
became the predominant population at all the sites including the
tumor, we attempted to characterize them further.

Characteristics of splenic double negative small lymphocytes
in tumor-bearing hosts: Several lines of evidence suggested that
these were a subset of B cell lineage lacking in S-IgM:

a)   this cell class was found to be most abundant in the normal
bone marrow (5);

b)   this cell class could only reconcile the discrepancy between
the observed increase in the proportion of young marrow derived
lymphocytes at the tumor site and spleen, and the observed decline
(at the tumor site) or constancy (in the spleen) in the incidence
of S-IgM-bearing population;

c)   we found a rapid increase in the incidence of B lymphocyte
colony forming cells (BL-CFC) in the spleen (7), the time course
of which was very similar to that found for the double negative
lymphocytes.

For these reasons,we examined several other B cell markers, viz.,
C'3 receptors, Fc receptors and Ia antigens, on splenic double
negative cells in tumor bearing mice, as well as their ability to
produce B lymphocyte colonies in agar.

Radio-immunolabeling of B as well as T cells (as discussed
above) and S-RBC rosetting (8) techniques (for C'3 or Fc receptors)
were combined for the same cell population to examine directly the
presence of C'3 or Fc receptors on the double negative cells. Most
double negative cells, both in the normal CBA spleen or spleen of
tumor bearing mice, were found to be lacking in C'3 or Fc receptors.
This finding would fit with the idea that they represent the "null"
component of B cell lineage. However, other findings indicated that
they may belong to a specific subset. Splenic double negative cells
were purified by a rosette-exclusion technique or sorted by a
fluorescence activated cell sorter. They were then labeled for Ia
antigens by a sandwich technique using ^{125}I-labeled anti mouse IgG
or Protein A. Similar fractions were also grown in agar to examine
the incidence of BL-CFC. Results revealed a two-fold higher incidence of Ia^{+} cells as well as BL-CFC amongst the splenic double
negative cells from tumor bearing hosts compared to those present
in the normal spleen. They may thus belong to a special subset of
B cell lineage. An alternate possibility, which has not been
completely excluded, is that they may represent an Ig receptor
modulation in vivo due to an excess of circulating tumor antigens.
Surface marker studies on suspension cultures of double negative
cells have not resolved this issue. Incidence of IgM + ve cells
increases in such cultures after a day, which could either be due
to further maturation or resynthesis of S-IgM. Functional potentials
of this cell class (e.g. "NK" activity) are currently under study.

REFERENCES

1. Lala, P.K., Cell Tiss. Kinet. 7 (1974) 293.
2. Kaizer, L., Lala, P.K., Cell Tiss. Kinet. 10 (1977) 279.
3. Lala, P.K., Cancer Treatment Reports 60 (1976) 1781.
4. Lala, P.K., Terrin, M., Lind, C., Kaizer, L., Exp. Haematol. in press (1978).
5. Garnis, S., Lala, P.K., Immunol. 34 (1978) 539.
6. Lala, P.K., Kaizer, L., J. Nat. Cancer Inst., 59 (1977) 237.
7. Keeb, G., Lala, P.K., Europ. J. Cancer in press (1978).
8. Parish, C.R., Hayward, J.A., Proc. Royal Soc. London. B. 187 (1974) 65.

ACKNOWLEDGEMENTS

This study was supported by NCI Canada and U.S.P.H.S. grant CA-1117.

FUNCTIONAL ACTIVITY OF HUMAN TUMOR-INFILTRATING MACROPHAGES

B.M. Vose

Department of Immunology, Paterson Laboratories,
Christie Hospital and Holt Radium Institute
Manchester M20 9BX,   England

In the present investigation adherent cells have been isolated from disaggregated human tumours and tested for cytotoxic potential against autologous and allogeneic tumour cells and against antibody coated human erythrocytes (Holm 1972).

ISOLATION OF ADHERENT CELLS

Tumour material was obtained from patients with lung, breast and gastric carcinoma. Tumour was dissected free of fatty and connective tissue and necrotic areas and minced with scissors. Cell suspensions were prepared from lung and gastric tumours by pressing through a 60-mesh stainless steel grid into RPMI. Dead cells were removed by treatment of this suspension with 0.1 percent trypsin for 1 minute at 4°C in the presence of DNAse which prevented clumping. Breast tumours were disaggregated by treatment with 0.25 percent collagenase, 0.01 percent hyaluronidase and 0.01 percent DNAse for 3 hours at room temperature with stirring.

The cell suspensions were applied to discontinuous Ficoll-Triosil gradients as previously described (Vose et al 1977). Following centrifugation (900 g for 10 minutes) a fraction enriched for macrophages and viable tumour cells could be removed from the top of the gradient which corresponded to a 3:4 dilution in saline of the Ficoll-Triosil solution (density 1.077) used in lymphocyte separation. Cells were washed twice and aliquots (approximately 2.5×10^5) cells plated into the wells of Sterilin M29ARTL Microtest plates in RPMI containing 10 percent heat inactivated autologous plasma. Non-adherent cells were removed after 30 minutes incubation

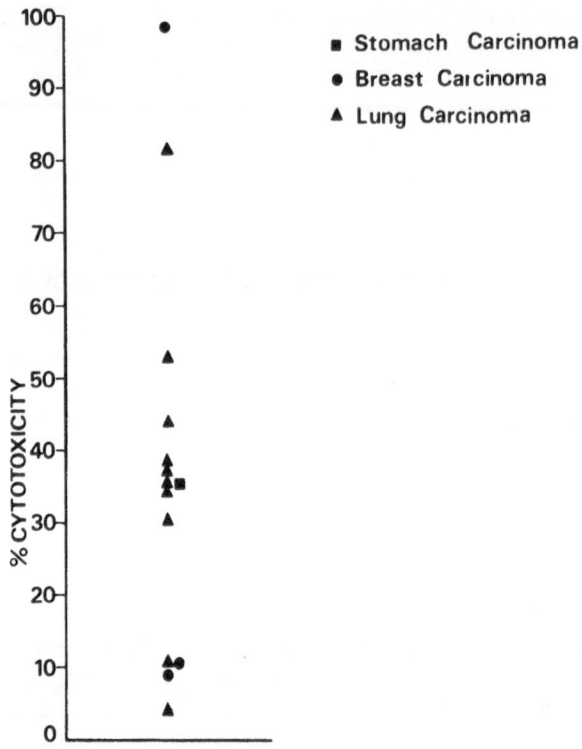

FIG. 1: Cytotoxicity of adherent cells from human tumours for anti-body coated human erythrocytes. Effector:target ratio 1:1. Values of greater than 10 percent were statistically significant.

at 37°C in a humidified atmosphere and further separated to produce tumour target cells (Vose et al 1977). Adherent cells were counted and used as effectors in cytotoxicity assays. Samples were also incubated with latex particles or neutral red or stained for morpho-logical examination.

RESULTS AND DISCUSSION

Cells have been isolated from disaggregated human tumours by adherence. These cells represented 0.2 - 8.5 percent of the cells plated. No differences in the proportion of adherent cells were noted between the different groups of patients with 2×10^3 3×10^4 cells adherent per well. The majority of these cells showed macro-phage characteristics, 64 - 88 percent showing phagocytosis of latex

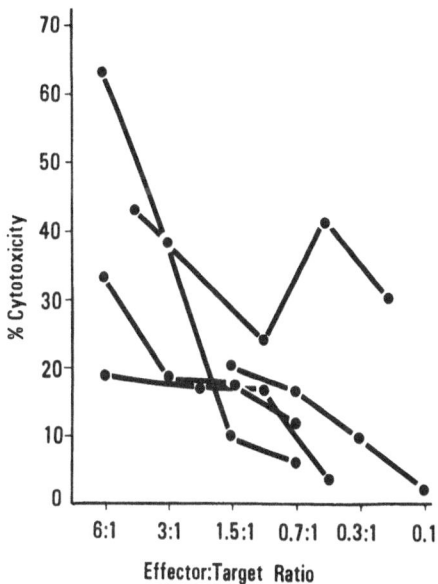

<u>FIG. 2</u>:   Dose relationship between cytotoxicity against autologous
tumour cells and the number of adherent cells. A constant number of
targets were plated to wells containing differing numbers of
effectors.

particles (1.1 μ diameter) in 2 hours and 77 - 94 percent pinocytosed
neutral red solution. The number of adherent lymphocytes and polymorphs in the preparations was less than 2 percent.

The monolayers of adherent cells were capable of inducing lysis
of antibody coated human erythrocytes in the assay described by Holm
(1972) (Fig.1). Dose relationships revealed that high cytotoxic
potential was demonstrable to ratios of 32 targets to 1 adherent
cell in experiments where numbers of ^{51}Cr labelled red cells were
kept constant and decreasing numbers of cells plated for the preparation of adherent cell monolayers. This marker has been extensively
studied in human blood preparations and appears to be a function of
monocyte/macrophages (Holm 1972; Poplack et al 1976). Polymorphonuclear cells have less lytic activity (MacDonald et al 1975; Moore
personal communication). The activity of the adherent cell monolayers
containing only low numbers of polymorphs in this assay would therefore

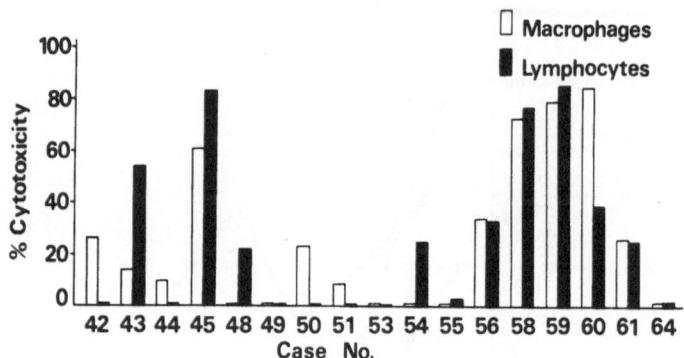

FIG. 3:   Cytotoxicity of peripheral blood lymphocytes and adherent cells from human tumours against autologous tumour cells. Lymphocyte: target ratio 50:1, macrophage:target ratio 1:1.

strongly support the isolation of monocyte macrophages from human tumours which are capable of effector function.

The monolayers also showed the capactiy to induce cell damage as detected in an 18 hour ^{51}Cr release assay against autologous tumour cells. Significantly increased ^{51}Cr release over background was detected in 16 of 24 cases studied. Again cytotoxicity showed a dose relationship with decreasing numbers of adherent cell effectors associated with decreasing cytotoxic potential (Fig.2). Cytotoxicity was also manifested in allogeneic plasma and foetal calf serum supplements. Similar lytic activities were detected against allogeneic targets. Significant reactivity was recorded in $5/10$ cases. Preliminary data suggested that cells derived from normal lung tissue was less susceptible to lysis. Effectors from tumour and normal lung induced increased ^{51}Cr release in lung tumour targets in $11/14$ combinations. With normal lung targets cytotoxicity was detected in $3/10$ tests. In two of these cases histological examination revealed degenerative changes associated with gross infection distal to the lesion.

In parallel studies using previously described methodology (Vose et al 1977) it was possible to detect lymphocyte-mediated cytotoxicity against the autologous tumour cells in a 4 hour ^{51}Cr release assay (Fig.3). Cytotoxicity was not found in the adherent cells in this shorter assay. The two cytotoxicities occured most frequently together. In 17 cases examined both lymphocytes and macrophages were cytotoxic together in 7 tests and negative together in 6. The difference between the two activities lay in the specificity of the lymphocyte mediated lysis. In an extended series in which these cases are included lymphocyte cytotoxicity against the autologous tumour was detected in 12 of 44 tests. Only 3 of 38 showed reactivity against allogeneic targets. This indicates that the parallel is not simply associated with target susceptibility. It may be considered that, as suggested by Evans and Alexander ('972) macrophages can be armed by humoral factors from specifically sensitized T lymphocytes and thereby become nonspecifically cytostatic or cytotoxic. The interaction between lymphocyte products and macrophages in the facilitation of cytotoxic effects is currently under investigation in this department.

REFERENCES

1.   Evans, R., Alexander, P. Immunology 23 (1972) 615.
2.   Holm, G. Int. Arch. Allergy 43 (1972) 671.
3.   MacDonald, H.R., Bonnard, G.D., Sondat, B., Zawodnik, S.A. Scand. J. Immunol. 4 (1975) 487.
4.   Poplack, D.G., Bonnard, G.D., Holimen, B.J., Blease, R.M. Blood 48 (1976) 809.
5.   Vose, B.M., Vánky, F., Klein, E. Int. J. Cancer 20 (1977) 512.

ACKNOWLEDGEMENTS

This study was supported by grants from the Medical Research Council and the Cancer Research Campaign.

APPROACHES TO EFFECTIVE TUMOR IMMUNOTHERAPY WITH CELLS AND THE ENZYME NEURAMINIDASE

H.H. Sedlacek, H.J. Bengelsdorff, A. Lemmer[*] and F.R. Seiler

Research Laboratories of Behringwerke AG,
3550 Marburg/Lahn, West Germany

[*]Clinic for Small Animals, 3550 Marburg-Heskem, W. Germany

INTRODUCTION

In a tumor therapy model with spontaneous mammary tumors in mongrel dogs (1) using Vibrio cholerae neuraminidase (VCN)-treated autologous tumor cells success has been shown to depend on the number of cells injected. Tumor enhancement (1×10^8 cells), long-lasting tumor regression (2×10^7 cells) or only a transient therapeutic effect (2×10^6 cells) could be demonstrated. Moreover, it has been shown that distinct amounts of active VCN remain attached to the cell surface of VCN-treated cells (2,3,4) and that VCN admixed to a variety of antigens either structurally containing or lacking sialic acid, dose dependently acts as an adjuvant (5), predominantly for the cellular immune response (6).

Thus, cell-membrane-bound VCN might be involved in the dose dependency of the tumor therapy experiments. Attempting to overcome the inherent risk of tumor enhancement by an inadequate tumor cell dose in tumor immunotherapy with VCN-treated cells, an immunization procedure was proposed by us, named chessboard vaccination (7). This chessboard vaccination consisted of intradermal injections of combinations of varying numbers of autologous tumor cells with various amounts of VCN in mammary tumor-bearing dogs. In this paper, the diagnostic and therapeutic results of this chessboard vaccination in spontaneous mammary tumors of dogs will be summarized. Moreover, data of a mouse model derived from that of Mackaness (8) will be shown in which the mechanism incited by chessboard-type vaccination was further investigated.

TAB. 1:   Number of dogs with increased DTH reaction induced by VCN within the chessboard vaccination with autologous tumor cells.

Tumor cells	0	0.65	6.5	65	VCN (mU)
10^5	-	-	2	2	
10^6	-	-	2	2	
10^7	-	1	3	1	
5 x 10^7	-	-	3	1	
10^8	-	1	1	-	

Chessboard Vaccination in Spontaneous Mammary Tumors in Dogs

Mongrel dogs of different races and ages bearing at least two spontaneous mammary tumors were selected. Exstirpation of one of the two tumors, isolation of single tumor cells and the histopathological examination were performed as described (1). Dogs were randomly distributed into two groups, treated differently.

As a positive control, dogs in group 1 were subcutaneously injected with a total of 2 x 10^7 autologous tumor cells, treated with mitomycin and Vibrio cholerae neuraminidase (M-VCN) exactly as described earlier (1). This treatment, given at the day of operation and at the day thereafter, has been shown in the past to be therapeutically effective. Dogs of group 2 underwent the chessboard vaccination: various numbers of autologous, mitomycin-treated tumor cells (10^5, 10^6, 10^7, 5 x 10^7 and 10^8 cells) were combined each with various amounts of purified (9) VCN (0; 0.65; 6.5; 65 mU VCN). Within about 1 hour after mixing and at the day of operation, the various combinations were separately and intradermally injected in the regio inguinalis of each dog. The skin reactions (possibly delayed-type hypersensitivity reactions (DTH)) at the various injection sites were observed 24 and 48 hours thereafter. Moreover, at certain time intervals the dogs were examined clinically and the diameters of the residual tumors were measured. Altogether, clinical data of 19 dogs (9 in group 1 and 10 in group 2) recorded over a period of about 150 days are summarized in Tables 1 and 2. In most dogs (8 of 10) the DTH reaction against the intradermal injection of autologous tumor cells could be slightly but significantly increased by the addition of VCN. Hereby low amounts of enzyme combined with a high number of tumor cells or high amounts of enzyme mixed with a low number of tumor cells induced a maximal response (Tab.1). Moreover, the chessboard vaccination proved to be at least as effective and possibly even more than the injection of 2 x 10^7 M-VCN tumor cells,

TAB. 2:   Therapeutical effect of chessboard vaccination on the
mammary tumor of dogs.

| Malignancy (by histology) | chessboard vaccination | | $2x10^7$ (M-VCN-treated | | |
	benign	malignant	benign	?	malignant
complete regression	4	4	1	1	-
complete regression with subsequent local recidives	-	1	-	-	1
partial regression	-	-	1	-	1
regression with subsequent progression	-	-	-	1	-
no change	-	1	-	1	-
progression	-	-	2	-	-
progression with subsequent local recidives	1	-	-	-	-

which again had a diminishing effect on the growth of the mammary
tumor (Tab.2) as compared with and in confirmation of results of
previous experiments (1),

Chessboard Vaccination with SRBC in Mice

Modifying the mouse model of Mackaness (8), mice (15 per group)
were injected intraveneously with either 10^3, 10^5 or 10^8 SRBC (0.1 ml
in phosphate-buffered saline, PBS) or as control with PBS at day O.
Chessboard vaccinations were performed on day 5. Various numbers of
SRBC (10^6, 10^7, 10^8) were combined with various amounts (0; 0.65;
6.5 mU VCN) of purified enzymatically active or heat-inactivated
(100°C, 15 min) VCN. The various mixtures were injected intradermally
in the back. On day 6, 5 mice of each group were killed by exsan-
guination, the skin was taken off and the diameters of the injection
site areas, visible by the red color of the located SRBC, were
estimated from the subcutis site. Moreover, the injection sites were
investigated histologically by conventional methods. The residual
mice were challenged on day 10 with 10^8 SRBC in the footpad and 24
hours later footpad swelling was recorded (8). The following results
were found: addition of enzymatically active VCN to SRBC within the
chessboard vaccination increased skin swelling, reduction of the red
colored injection site area, mononuclear cell infiltration and phagocytosis of SRBC predominantly in pre-immunized (Fig.1), less in non-

TAB. 3:   Effect of the chessboard vaccination with SRBC in mice on the cellular immune response after challenge into the footpad.

Pre-immunization i.v. (SRBC)	Chessboard (10^6, 10^7, 10^8 SRBC/ 0; 0.65; 6.5 mU VCN)	Footpad swelling after challenge with 2×10^8 SRBC (%)
–	VCN active	$19.0 + 4.0$
–	VCN (100°C/15 min)	$17.3 + 2.9$
10^3	VCN active	$36.1 + 4.1$
10^3	VCN (100°C/15 min)	$29.5 + 5.8$
10^5	VCN active	$40.9 + 5.5$
10^5	VCN (100°C/15 min)	$39.0 + 4.8$
10^8	VCN active	$27.1 + 4.0$
10^8	VCN (100°C/15 min)	$24.3 + 3.7$

immunized mice (Fig.2). The combination of 10^8 SRBC and 6.5 mU VCN proved to be maximally stimulating. However, between animals which underwent a chessboard vaccination with either enzymatically active or with heat-inactivated VCN on day 5 no difference in footpad swelling after challenge with SRBC on day 10 could be observed. Animals pre-immunized with 10^8 SRBC showed a lower footpad swelling after challenge on day 10 than those pre-immunized with 10^5 SRBC, similar as known from the original Mackaness Model in spite of chessboard vaccination on day 5. Thus, the chessboard vaccination does not seem to have any influence on footpad swelling after challenge at least in the time and dose schedule applied.

                                DISCUSSION

     It has been shown in mammary tumor-bearing dogs that skin reactions against autologous tumor cells (possibly DTH reactions) were increased at the intradermal injection sites when VCN had been added to the tumor cells. This effect of VCN depended on its amount and on the number of tumor cells, as revealed by the chessboard vaccination. In cases where high amounts of VCN with low cell numbers or where low amounts of VCN with high cell numbers had been combined, a maximal DTH response was found. Similarly, the cellular skin response against SRBC as revealed by the chessboard vaccination in mice was increased by addition of VCN. As pre-immunized mice exhibited a significantly higher response than non-immunized mice, the skin response within the chessboard vaccination seems to be correlated with the immunological state of the individuum tested and, therefore, may be regarded at least partly as a DTH reaction.

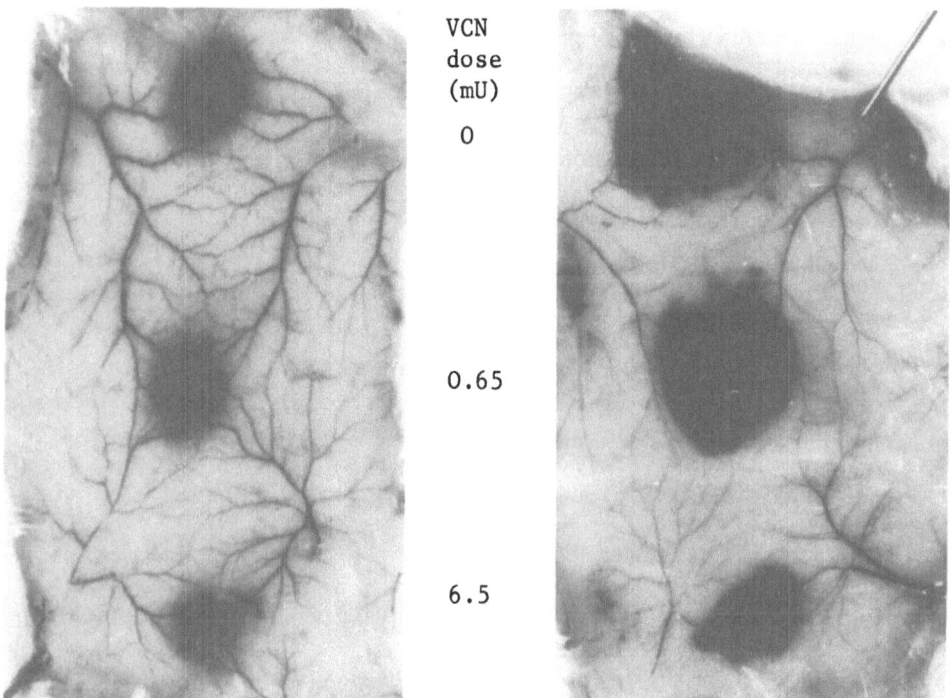

FIG. 1: (pre-immunized mouse)   FIG. 2: (untreated control)

DTH reaction after chessboard vaccination with 10^8 SRBC combined with 0; 0.65; 6.5 mU VCN in pre-immunized (10^8 SRBC i.v.) or untreated mice.

Thus, an increase of the skin response by VCN within a chessboard vaccination might point to a pre-immunized and immunocompetent situation. This assumption might even be of value in tumor systems. Indications for this are the results of the chessboard vaccination-like skin tests in dogs with low mammary tumor burden, presented above. An additional point of support might be the results of chessboard vaccinations with autologous tumor cells in 4 dogs with high tumor burdens (metastasizing melanoma and struma) and a suspected decreased specific immunological response where no DTH response increased by VCN and no therapeutic effect could be found (Sedlacek, Lemmer, Seiler - unpublished data).

The chessboard vaccination induced tumor regression in most of the mammary tumor-bearing dogs. However, no significant difference on the cellular immune response against a challenge of SRBC after chessboard vaccination could be found between mice immunized with enzymatically active and inactive VCN. Indeed, this result may be influenced by an inadequate time schedule and an overdosage of antigen. Thus, it has to be clarified 1) whether the chessboard vaccination induces an enhanced systemic cellular immune dependent of the antigen dose applied before or by the chessboard vaccination, 2) whether there is a relationship between an increased local DTH response within the chessboard and the subsequent specific immunological reactivity, and 3) whether enzymatically active VCN is an essential factor in the systemic or therapeutic effect of the chessboard vaccinations.

REFERENCES

1. Sedlacek, H.H., Seiler, F.R., Develop. biol. Standard 38 (1978) 399, Int. symp. on biolog. prepartions in the treatment of cancer, London, (1977) (S. Karger, Basel).
2. Sedlacek, H.H., Seiler, F.R., Behring Inst. Mitt. No. 55 (1974) 254.
3. Lüben, G., Sedlacek, H.H., Seiler, F.R., Behring Inst. Mitt. No. 59 (1976) 30.
4. Petitou, M., Rosenfeld, G., Sinay, P., Cancer Immunol. Immunotherapy 2 (1977) 135.
5. Knop, J., Sedlacek, H.H., Seiler, F.R., Immunology 34 (1978) 181.
6. Sedlacek, H.H., Seiler, F.R., Z. Immun. Forsch. 153,4 (1977) 353.
7. Seiler, F.R., Sedlacek, H.H.,(1978) Chessboard vaccination:A pertinent approach to immunotherapy of cancer with VCN and tumor cells? Proc. Symp. Immunotherapy of Malignant Diseases, Vienna, Nov. 1977, in press (Schattauer Verlag, Stuttgart).
8. Mackaness, G.B., Lagrange, P.H., Miller, T.E., Ishibashi, T., In: Activation of Macrophages, Ed. W.H. Wagner, H. Hahn, R. Evans, Excerpta Medica, Amsterdam, pp. 193-209 (1974).
9. Schick, H.J.,Zilg, H., Develop. biol. Standard. 38 (1978). Int. symp. on biological preparations in the treatment of cancer, London (1977) 81-85 (S. Karger, Basel).

SUMMING-UP

M. G. Hanna, Jr.

Frederick Cancer Research Center

P.O. Box B, Frederick, Md. 21701, U.S.A.

Over the last 10 years the field of tumor immunology and its technological transfer, immunotherapy, has gone from a state of optimistic liberalism to intraspective conservatism. This is probably the logical metamorphosis of a new field which has produced a large number of data generating experimental models, most of which have not yet been critically evaluated for their general relevance and usefulness.

It can now be accepted that tumor immunity is an autogenous or inducible host factor. This fact supports the early attention devoted to the role of T and B lymphocytes, both in vitro and in vivo, as tumoricidal effector cells. In spite of the fact that the majority of the original studies were performed with highly antigenic, experimentally induced tumors, which may or may not be associated in a relevant manner with spontaneous tumors, current investigations have characterized the "armamentarium" of the immune system, which is functional in the host-tumor relationship. Several of the presentations in this symposium further support the role of these various immunocompetent cells in tumor-directed, cell-mediated immunity, either with regard to cytotoxicity or immunodiagnosis and/ or prognosis. For instance, it is clear now that tumor antigens can cause T lymphocyte subpopulations to undergo sensitized proliferation, possibly through blastogenesis, to cytotoxic T lymphocytes, which are directly tumoricidal. These cells have been characterized in experimental models as well as spontaneous tumors of man. T lymphocyte subpopulations are known to produce several macrophage-inhibitory or macrophage-activating factors which can, along with tumor antigen, induce activated macrophages that are indiscriminantly cytotoxic to tumor target cells. Other known or suspected components of cell-mediated immunity are the "null" cells and the natural killer cells, both of which are less well characterized in terms of their cellular origin, but which have been demonstrated in vitro to be cytotoxic either specifically or nonspecifically to tumor target cells. Finally, tumor antigen-induced immunocompetent B lymphocytes working dependently through T lymphocyte subpopulations are known to produce antibody which can act directly on tumor target cells or act through K (killer) cells in antibody-dependent complement-mediated cytotoxicity. These effector mechanisms of the host-tumor interaction have been exhaustively studied and characterized by in vitro techniques.

It is now recognized, however, that the in vitro approach may only be of potential relevance in vivo. Important differences between immune-mediated tumor regression in vivo and tumor cell destruction in vitro involve the complexities of the former. Clearly, tumor regression in vivo is limited by the ability of effector cells to search and find the tumor, and then destroy it. In contrast, in an in vitro assay the need to search for the tumor cell is eliminated. The only measurable phenomenon involves the capacity of various effector cells at appropriate ratios to destroy relatively few tumor cells confined to an in vitro environment. Thus, although there is ample biological evidence in vitro for acquired immunity to specific tumor antigens of transformed cells, it may be of limited relevance since the immunity generally does not operate optimally and the tumor ultimately overwhelms the syngeneic host.

Acquired tumor immunity has also been demonstrated in a variety of transplantable experimental tumor systems and to a limited degree in spontaneous tumors. It is not unreasonable then to assume that immunotherapy for malignancy would evoke a quantitative alteration of a normal host protective mechanism. The limitations of immunotherapy as a function of tumor stage, both in experimental animal systems and in man, are well documented. Thus, in the untreated patient, the balance between host responses and tumor proliferation favors progressive tumor growth. Nevertheless, when malignancy consists of localized solid tumor with regional lymph node metastasis and probable subclinical micrometastatic disease in visceral organs, immunotherapy can be used as an adjunct treatment to the standard control of the primary tumor. Among the various strategies of immunotherapy for localized and/or disseminated minimal residual tumor, nonspecific immunopotentiation by microbial agents has received the greatest attention. These clinical procedures, however, have been carried out with limited guidance from experimental and animal models and thus far, for the most part, have been problematic and relatively unsuccessful. Improvement of immunotherapeutic procedures, with development of efficacious active specific immunotherapeutic protocols, requires more information on the complex interactions among tumor, host response, and therapy. Investigations such as those presented

in this session are contributing toward this goal. Considerably
more information is required, which will have to be gained from
experimental models that can be manipulated. If the experimental
models approximate the clinical reality, then insights can be gained
that will contribute to the treatment of cancer in humans.

IMMUNOPROPHYLAXIS AND
THERAPY OF INFECTIOUS DISEASES

CHAIRPERSON:

G.J.V. Nossal

INTRODUCTION

G.J.V. Nossal

The Walter and Eliza Hall Institute of Medical Research
Post Office, Royal Melbourne Hospital
Victoria 3050, Australia

I wish to take as a theme for my brief opening remarks the
provocative title of a recent paper by Dr. H. Mayer, Director of
the Bureau of Biologics of the U.S. Department of Health, Education
and Welfare. He asked: "Are vaccines an endangered species?"
Noting that vaccination had undoubtedly been the most powerful and
cost-effective tool in scientific medicine, he documented in this
paper the flight of major pharmaceutical manufacturers from the
vaccine field. Nine major firms geared up for poliomyelitis
vaccination originally; now there are 2 manufacturers on the North
American continent. Six started on the path towards measles vaccine,
there is now one manufacturer remaining. It would require only some
major production catastrophe within such a leading firm for vaccine
supply positions in the U.S. to become critical, not to speak of the
many countries that rely on imports of vaccines. Vaccine production
is caught in a two way squeeze: Increasing costs because of increasing
demands of the regulatory agencies as regards quality control and proof
of efficacy on the one hand; and decreasing price because of consumer
activism on the other. These have made vaccine production unprofitable
except for a few remaining big firms.

What has all of this to do with us, the immunological research
community? A great deal, I believe. I think it means that much of
the exploratory work for new vaccines will have to revert back to
academia, as will work for the improvement of existing vaccines. And
the challenges are still enormous. In the developed countries, we
remain without vaccines for hepatitis A, for any venereal disease,
for the gram-negative enterobacteria whose antibiotic resistance
plagues us in post-operative and many other situations, and for many
of the organisms that attack in old age or debility from chronic

disease. As regards the diseases of developing countries, immediate
challenge is posed by dengue haemorrhagic fever, where a quadrivalent
vaccine may be close; but no vaccine exists for any parasitic disease,
or for leprosy.

And what about the vaccines we already have? No one would deny
the urgent need for research to improve the current cholera or typhoid
vaccines, which remain at best partially effective and short-lasting.
Similarly influenza, pertussis and tuberculosis vaccines fall far
short of the ideal. Let me now pose the question: how seriously do
we all think about these problems? The answer must be: not enough.
The whole vast immunology research explosion, one of the epic phenomena in the recent history of science, has very nearly neglected its
ancestiral base in infectious diseases. At last count, there were
13,000 "card-carrying" immunologists in the world, adhering to the
International Union of Immunological Societies. It would be interesting to hear how many of these have ever seriously addressed a
communicable disease problem. Even for those who prefer not to think
about third world issues, it is time to re-examine this position, as
infectious diseases taken together compete with accidents for third
place in the list of causes of death, after heart and arterial
diseases and cancer.

The organizers of this conference expressed mild disappointment
about the small number of abstracts received for the Session on Immunoprophylaxis and Therapy of Infectious Diseases. All the more, we must
express our thanks to those speakers who did respond, and on whom I
shall now call.

THE PRODUCTION AND ROLE OF CYTOTOXIC T CELLS IN INFLUENZA VIRUS
INFECTION IN MICE: DO THE SAME RULES APPLY IN THE RESPONSE TO ANY
FOREIGN ANTIGEN?

K.L. Yap and G.L. Ada

Department of Microbiology, John Curtin School of Medical
Research, Australian National University, Canberra,
Australia

INTRODUCTION

One of the most remarkable developments in immunology in the
last decade has been the demonstration that the interaction between
the various T cell subsets and other cells in the immune system is
controlled by products of the genes in the major histocompatibility
complex. Helper (T_h), delayed type hypersensitivity (T_d) and
suppressor (T_s) T lymphocytes are controlled by genes in the I
region, whereas cytotoxic (T_c) T lymphocytes are controlled by genes
in the K and D region of the mouse H-2 gene complex. This distribution of control suggests that the K and D gene products are
important to those reactions where intimate contact between effector
and target cells is necessary as is the case in T_c reactions.
Furthermore, it is known that K and D glycoproteins are poorly
secreted from the cell. In contrast, the I region may be involved
in those responses where interaction between cells may occur via
secreted, soluble products, such as those described by Feldmann (1).
The two major phenomena where K and D gene products are of major
importance are T_c mediated lysis of either allogeneic cells or of
virus-infected target cells. It has been proposed (2) that the
latter phenomenon has been an important driving force during
evolution for the development of this class of lymphocyte as recognition and destruction of virus-infected cells must have been a very
early requirement for survival. What has become known as H-2
restriction of T cell-mediated lysis of virus-infected target cells
was discovered first by Doherty and Zinkernagel (3) in the LCM virus
murine system. It now seems likely that all classes of viruses where
viral antigens are expressed at the cell surface during the viral
replication cycle demonstrate this requirement of histocompatibility

between effector and target cell (4), though it is easier to demonstrate with some viruses than with others.

IS THE GENERATION OF SPECIFIC T_C AN
IMPORTANT RESPONSE DURING INFECTION BY VIRUS?

Neutralizing antibody is the most efficient method for preventing
infection by any virus, as it prevents the virus from infecting susceptible cells. Such antibody is likely to be present only in primed
hosts, however, and the question therefore arises – what are the
important factors which may contribute to the defence of a naive
host against a viral infection? These may include intracellular
killing by macrophages, the formation of interferon and specific
responses of T and B lymphocytes. Antibody formation during a viral
infection is important in many viral infections, notably those that
display viraemia; cell-mediated immune reactions have been clearly
implicated in only a few viral infections. The most extensively
studied system is ectromelia infection of mice and it was very clearly
shown that this is the primary mechanism involved in the process of
recovery from infection (5). This work was later followed by the
demonstration that the main effector T cells were T_c (6). Transfer
of specific cytotoxic T cells to infected mice reduced the titre of
virus in target organs (spleen, liver) within 24 hr. Such an
important role for the CMI response and particularly for T_c was
perhaps not unexpected with an agent which may pass directly from
cell to cell.

ARE SPECIFIC T_C AN IMPORTANT FORM OF RESPONSE
DURING INFECTION WITH INFLUENZA VIRUS?

Although the usual form of influenza viral infection in man is
mainly in the upper respiratory tract, influenzal pneumonia can
occur in man and the manifestations of this are considered to be
similar in many respects to this form of the disease in mice. Influenza virus infection is usually regarded as a disease in which the
humoral arm of the defence system is of paramount importance as it
has been well established (7,8,9,10) that specific antibody may play
a protective role in humans and in mice although this was not shown
to be so in ferrets (11). There has in fact been remarkably little
information available on the CMI response to infection by this virus.
Virion antigens were shown to induce CM reactions in humans (12) and
in animals (13,14), but it has not been shown that such reactivity
may be important in host protection. An investigation on the susceptibility of bursectomized chickens to influenza suggested that the
antibody response was more important than the cell-mediated immune
response (15). An investigation in mice (10) suggested that T_h had
an indirect role in protection; in these experiments, the cells were
obtained from spleens removed from mice more than a month after viral
challenge.

The findings with ectromelia and LCM resulted in several other viral systems being examined. Within a short time, several groups had demonstrated the presence in spleen, after intravenous injection or intranasal inoculation of infectious influenza virus, of cell-mediated cytotoxic activity which was mediated by T cells, was virus specific and required compatibility in the K or D region of the H-2 complex (16,17,18,19). Two questions could now be examined. 1) Would the availability of a system using a virus whose composition and structure was well known facilitate the determination of the nature of the antigenic pattern on the target (stimulator) cell recognized by the T cell? —— and perhaps the nature of the structure(s) on T cells which recognize these antigenic patterns. 2) Did these T_c have an important role in the recovery of the host from infection? If so, could conditions be determined which influenced their production? The second question will be examined here.

If the T_c were important in controlling a respiratory infection, they should be found at the site of the infection —— in the lungs. After a lethal dose of virus is given intranasally (i.n.), high levels of infectious virus are found in the lungs within 24 hr, and thereafter titres rise steadily until the mice die at 7-9 days. T_c can be first detected in the lung tissues and broncho-alveolar washings (BAW) at 3-4 days and thence the activity rises steeply. Their appearance occurs well before antibody can be detected in BAW using the standard H.I. test (20). A series of experiments gave results which suggested that if the virus level in the lungs did not get too high, the T_c might have a protective role. If this were so, transfer of specific immune cells should reduce lung virus levels and this proved to be so. Lung virus titres were reduced 1-2 $\log_{10}$ EID_{50} after transfer of primary immune spleen cells or 2-4 $\log_{10}$ EID_{50} after transfer of secondary immune cells, and in this case the recipient mice were protected from death. Protection from death occurred even if the cells were transferred as much as 3 days after infection. Fractionation experiments and susceptibility to the action of anti-Thy 1 sera and complement indicated that T cells were the cells responsible for the effect (21). Finally, the use of anti-Ly 1 or anti Ly 2,3 sera and complement and other experiments involving transfer of cells into hosts which differed in selected regions of H-2 showed clearly that T_c were almost, if not entirely, responsible for the reduction in lung virus levels (22). The results indicated that T_c formation is a defence mechanism of the host which, as in ectromelia infection, is provoked rapidly in response to influenza virus infection. This finding raised two further questions: 1) How important were T_c in recovery from influenza virus infection relative to other responses? What factors during the immune response control the generation and persistence of T_c during the infectious process?

THE RELATIVE IMPORTANCE OF T_c PRODUCTION
DURING AN INFLUENZA INFECTION

It is not easy to assess the importance of different mechanisms and responses during the course of an infectious process. The closest we have been able to come to an answer was to examine the course of the disease in congenitally athymic (nude) mice relative to their normal littermates. Graded doses of infectious virus were administered intranasally. At low doses both groups survived equally well and at high doses both groups were equally susceptible to a lethal infection. In the 2 $\log_{10}$ range, between 100% survival or death, the athymic mice were clearly more susceptible than their normal littermates. This was examined more closely by measuring infectious virus titres in the lungs during a period of 21 days after inoculation of a 50% lethal dose (for athymic mice) of virus. In both the normal mice and the surviving athymic mice, lung virus titres were similar when the peak was reached at about 3 days. Thereafter, virus levels in the normal mice fell steadily so that no infectious virus could be detected at day 17, and all mice survived. In contrast, the surviving athymic mice still had substantial levels of infectious virus at 18 days and demonstrated extensive pathological lesions in their lungs.

Transfer of immune T cells to the athymic mice produced a result similar to that shown by the normal mice, i.e., a more rapid clearance of virus (K.L. Yap, T. Braciale and G.L. Ada, submitted for publication). These results suggest: 1) that T_c play a really important role when the virus burden becomes a little higher than can be dealt with by "non-specific" mechanisms. If the virus titre is too high, the host is overwhelmed and possibly the T_c become infected and are destroyed; 2) that the role of the T_c is to aid recovery after the infection is well under way. It will be important to find out why the protective effect of the transferred T_c takes several days to be manifested.

FACTORS INFLUENCING THE PRODUCTION OF T_c

If the immune response to the infectious disease is to be manipulated, the mechanism involved in the stimulation of different cell responses must be understood much better. This certainly applies to the production of T_c. Two factors have already become apparent. One is the striking finding (23) that injection of equivalent doses of UV-irradiated (non-infectious) influenza virus does not result in T_c production, whereas the antibody response (to haemagglutinin) is essentially unchanged, suggesting that the replication process is necessary for viral antigens to be expressed adequately in the plasma membrane. The second observation, first reported by Effros and colleagues (17), is that the T_c response to a second injection of homologous virus is depressed. Under these conditions, previous work would show that there would be an enhanced secondary antibody response. We have confirmed and extended the finding of depression of T_c production which it has been suggested (17) may be due to antibody. These findings point to significant differences in the requirement for the T_c generation versus antibody production, both in a primary and in a secondary response.

THE SPECIFICITY OF THE T_c RESPONSE TO INFLUENZA VIRUS INFECTION

This question has been discussed elsewhere (24) and in this paper we wish to refer mainly to the recognition of viral antigen. A discussion of the association between viral antigen and K or D product is outside the scope of this article, except to say that a "minimal" model proposes that for a cell which supports viral replication, most cell surface associated viral antigen is not associated with K or D glycoprotein and that any complex which is recognized by T_c may not only involve a small portion of the total antigen present but that the association between a viral antigen and K or D product may be by non-covalent linkages.

The influenza virus has two external antigens — haemagglutinin and neuraminidase which differ antigenically in the different A type viruses. Beneath the lipid envelope of the virion are two proteins which occur in large amounts and are antigenically similar if not identical in all A strain viruses. These are the nucleoprotein and the matrix protein, the latter being adjacent to the lipid envelope. There is good evidence that the haemagglutinin on the surface of stimulator and target cells are recognized by T_c or their precursors. To date, the same cannot be said for neuraminidase. There was a surprise, however: T_c raised in mice against a given A type virus would lyse target cells infected with any other A type virus (17,18, 19). Evidence involving susceptibility to lysis by specific antibody and complement (25,26) and biosynthetic studies using an immune precipitation technique (27) clearly showed the expression of matrix protein on the surface of virus-infected cells. In some cases, it could be shown that almost as much matrix protein as haemagglutinin might be exposed (G.L. Ada and K.L. Yap, submitted for publication). That recognition of matrix protein is the explanation for the observed cross reactivity is supported by recent experiments which show that reduction in lung virus titres can occur following transfer of T_c which do not recognize either the haemagglutinin or neuraminidase of the challenge virus (K.L. Yap and G.L. Ada, submitted for publication). At present, the evidence indicates that T_c raised during an influenza infection may contain two subpopulations which recognize haemagglutinin and (at least) one common antigen — probably matrix protein.

It now seems not unreasonable to postulate that T_c will be formed in response to infection by most of those viruses whose form of replication in a cell involves the integration of viral coded antigens into the plasma membrane. There are certainly factors important in T_c generation about which we know little and the influenza virus model seems to be a very suitable system to be investigated for the elucidation of these mechanisms.

SOME REQUIREMENTS FOR A T_c RESPONSE TO BE GENERATED AGAINST A FOREIGN ANTIGEN

What determines whether there will be a T_c response to the expression of a foreign antigen on a cell surface? Can such a frank viral system be used as a model for studying systems such as a malignant cell? This aspect has been discussed previously (28), but here we would like to re-emphasise some of the features. The first most crucial point is: are unique antigens, the tumour-specific transplantation antigens, expressed on the surface of malignant cells? Unless this is so, one would assume the opportunities for any type of immune response, let alone a useful one, is very limited. From our current knowledge, in order for the malignant cell to act as a stimulator for T_c generation, the cell must also express K or D (or the host equivalent) antigen, and presumably in such a way that the appropriate association between molecules of the two antigens can associate (24).

The next most important requirement is another property of the cell displaying the antigen. This is the requirement for the cell to produce a second signal. The cell to be stimulated — the precursor of the T_c or the T_h — which is also involved in the process must not only recognize the foreign antigen, but also receive another "non-specific" signal in order for the process of stimulation to take place (29). A preparation which "duplicates" this activity — the costimulator — has been prepared and its use is described elsewhere in this meeting.

There are other factors which could interfere with this whole process — the generation of T_s and possible roles for specific antibody. Very little is known about these. But the influenza virus system may be a useful model to work on from the point of view of establishing principles in T_c generation and role.

REFERENCES

1.   Feldmann, M., Baltz, M., Erb, P., Howie, S., Kontiainen, S., Woody, J., Zwaifler, N.   Prog. Immunol. 3 (1977) 331.
2.   Blanden, R.V., Ada, G.L.   Scand. J. Immunol. 7 (1978) 181.
3.   Doherty, P.C., Zinkernage., R.M.   Nature 251 (1973) 547.
4.   Blanden, R.V.   Prog. Immunol. 3 (1977) 463.
5.   Blanden, R.V.   J. exp. Med. 133 (1971) 1074.

6. Kees, U., Blanden, R.V. J. exp. Med. 143 (1976) 450.
7. Fyzekaf de St Groth, S., Donnelley, M. Aust. J. exp. Biol. med. Sci. 28 (1950) 61.
8. Davenport, F.M. Am. Rev. resp. Dis. 83 (1961) 146.
9. Schulman, J.L., Khakpour, M., Kilbourne, E.D. J. Virology 2 (1968) 778.
10. Virelizier, J-L. J. Immunol. 115 (1975) 434.
11. Small, P.A., Waldman, R.H., Bruno, J.C., Gifford, G.E. Infection & Immunity 13 (1976) 417.
12. Beveridge, W.I.B., Burnet, F.M. Med. J. Aust. (i) (1944) 85.
13. Feinstone, S.M., Beachey, E.H., Rytel, M.W. J. Immunol. 103 (1969) 844.
14. Wetherbee, R.E. J. Immunol. 111 (1973) 157.
15. Portnoy, J., Bloom, K., Merigan, T.C. Cell. Immunol. 9 (1973) 251.
16. Yap, K.L., Ada, G.L. Immunol. 32 (1977) 151.
17. Effros, R.B., Doherty, P.C., Gerhard, W., Bennink, J. J. exp. Med. 145 (1977) 557.
18. Braciale, T.J. Cell. Immunol. 33 (1977a) 433.
19. Zweerink, H.J., Courtneidge, S.A., Skehel, J.J., Crumpton, M.J., Askonas, B.A. Nature 267 (1977) 354.
20. Yap, K.L., Ada, G.L. Scand. J. Immunol. 7 (1978a) 73.
21. Yap, K.L., Ada, G.L. Scand. J. Immunol. 7 (1978b).
22. Yap, K.L., Ada, G.L., McKenzie, I.F.C. Nature 273 (1978) 236.
23. Braciale, T.J., Yap, K.L. J. exp. Med. 147 (1978) 1236.
24. Braciale, T.J., Ada, G.L., Yap, K.L. Cont. Topics. Molec. Immunol. 7 (1978) in press.
25. Braciale, T.J. J. exp. Med. 146 (1977) 673.
26. Biddison, W.E., Doherty, P.C., Webster, K.G. J. exp. Med. 146 (1977) 690.
27. Ada, G.L., Yap, K.L. Immunochemistry 14 (1977) 643.
28. Ada, G.L., Yap, K.L. Blood Cells (1978) in press.
29. Lafferty, K.J., Woolnough, J. Immunol. Reviews 35 (1977) 231.

VIRUS SPIKE PROTEIN COMPLEXES AND VIROSOMES AS EFFECTIVE SUBUNIT

VACCINES

B. Morein, A. Helenius, K. Simons and V. Schirrmacher

European Molecular Biology Laboratory and Institute of
Immunology and Genetics, DKFZ,
6900 Heidelberg, W. Germany

INTRODUCTION

There is a trend regarding killed virus vaccine towards
purified subunit vaccines which contain only the viral surface
antigens (the membrane glycoproteins) to avoid nucleic acid and
toxic components in the virus preparations (1-4). However, subunit
vaccines available have generally proved less efficient than whole
virus vaccine in stimulating protective immunity. Little is,
however, known about the physical state of the glycoproteins in the
vaccine preparations used. It seems conceivable that the procedures
to isolate the proteins have been too harsh, and that the form in
which the proteins have been administered is not optimal (5).

To study these questions we have prepared subunit vaccines from
Semliki Forest virus (a Toga virus) the lethal strains of which
cause acute encephalomyelitis in mice (6,7). The viral glycoproteins
were isolated in nondenaturated form using mild nonionic detergents.
The proteins were then infected into mice either in a monomeric form,
an octameric form, or in a reconstituted phospholipid-bound form.
It was found that the protective immune response depended dramatically
on the physical state of the proteins, the two latter forms inducing
protection against a 10^3 fold higher challenge dose of virus than the
monomers.

Preparation of the vaccines

The molecular structure of Semliki Forest virus has been studied
in detail. The surface glycoproteins are integral membrane proteins
forming spike-like projections on the external surface of the virus

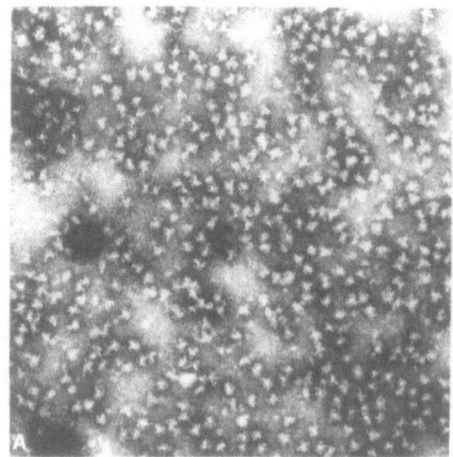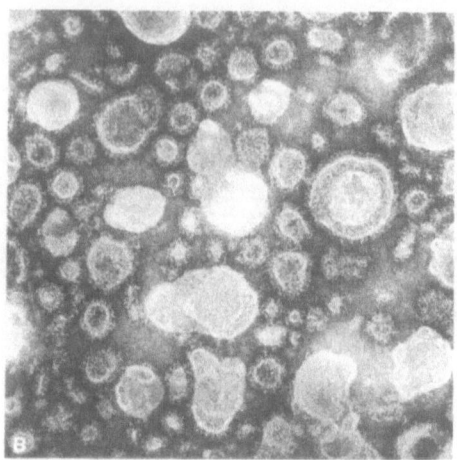

FIG. 1:   Electron micrographs of 29S complexes (A) and the
virosomes (B) used for vaccination. The preparations were
negatively strained.

particle. Each spike is a three chain structure containing three
glycopolypeptides E1 (no molecular weight 40 x 10^3), E2 (52 x 10^3)
and E3 (10 x 10^3) (8,9). The spikes span the lipid bilayer membrane
by hydrophobic carboxy terminal polypeptide segments in E1 and E2.
The spikes can be solubilized in lipid-free form using nonionic
detergents such as Triton X-100. (p-tert-octylphenolpolyoxyethylene
9-10). In Triton X-100 the spikes occur as monomers complexed to a
micelle of Triton X-100 (4.5S complexes) (10). When the detergent
is removed in absence of added lipid octameric spike aggregates
(29S complexes) (Fig.1A) are formed (11). When detergent is removed
in the presence of egglecithin reconstitution occurs and vesicles
(virosomes) are obtained which contain spike proteins inserted into
egglecithin bilayers in a way similar to the viral membrane (12,13),
(Fig.1B).

Virosomes and 29S complexes induce a high degree of protection

Groups of 10 mice were first vaccinated with 0.05-10µg of the
29S-complexes (a single immunization with one third S.C. and two
thirds i.p.). The mice were challenged 2 weeks later with 50LD$_{50}$
(10^4 pfu) virus intraperitoneally. It was found that 0.5µg induced
protective immunity in 50% of the mice and that all mice were
protected following vaccination with 10 µg. In subsequent
vaccinations 10µg spike protein was used irrespective of vaccine

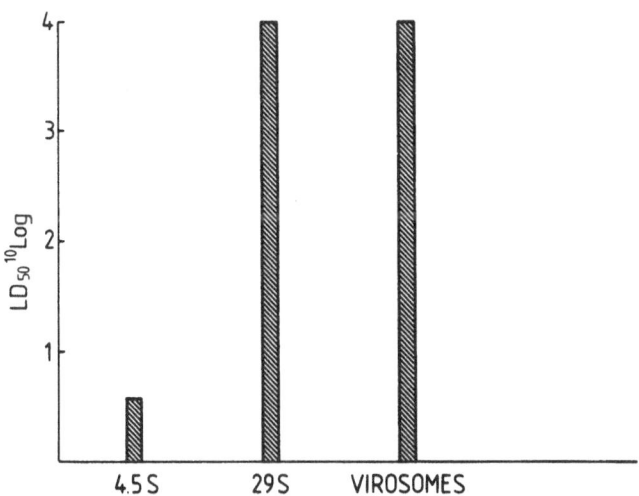

FIG. 2:   Vaccination against SFV encephalomyelitis in BALB/c mice:
the protective effect induced by different forms of purified spike
protein vaccine.

used.   Challenge was performed intraperitoneally with 50 to 10^7 pfu.

     As shown in Figure 2 most of mice vaccinated with 29S complexes
or virosomes survived a challenge dose of 10^7 pfu, the largest dose
tested.   Mice vaccinated with the monomer form (4.55 complexes)
resisted a challenge of only $10^{3.4}$.   These doses correspond to 10^4
and $10^{0.8}$ LD_{50} of non vaccinated mice respectively.   To verify the
small difference in resistance between mice vaccinated with 4.5S
protein and non vaccinated mice (Fig.2) the survivals after the first
challenge from these groups of mice were given a second challenge of
10^4 pfu of virulent virus.   Practically all of the non vaccinated
died regardless of the previous challenge dose, indicating that no
memory type of immunity was induced by the challenge virus itself,
a result which is in accord with those of Bradish & Allner (6).   The
mice vaccinated with monomer vaccine which survived a first challenge
dose higher than $1LD_{50}$ of non vaccinated mice, resisted the second
challenge but only 4 out of 17 mice which at the first challenge had
survived a challenge dose less than $1LD_{50}$ survived a second challenge.
The low protective effect afforded by the monomer form vaccine was
apparently enhanced at the first challenge.

     The dependence on T-cells for induction of protective immunity

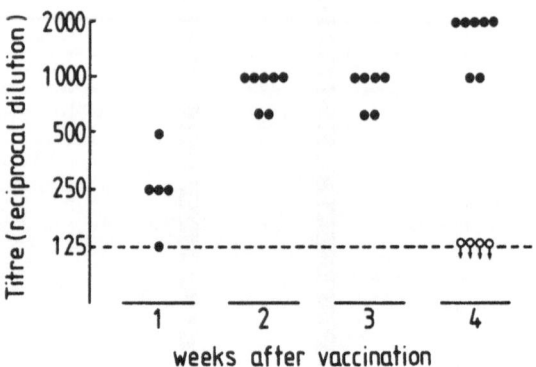

FIG. 3:   The antibody responses in serum of normal BALB/c (nu/nu) mice following vaccination with 10μg SFV spike protein in virosomes. The nude mice were challenged with 10^3 pfu virulent virus two weeks after vaccination and after further two weeks the sera from survivor were collected.

●   indicates titres from individual normal BALB/c mice

o   indicates titres from individual nude BALB/c mice. The arrow indicates that the titre was below dilution tested.

---   indicates threshold level of the test, i.e. the lowest dilution tested.

was studied by comparing the response of BALB/c mice with that of BALB/c nude (nu/nu) mice. The mice were vaccinated with virosomes. No difference in survival time or rate was found between non-vaccinated and vaccinated mice. The LD_{50} for non immunized nude mice was higher than that for normal BALB/c. In compensation for their deficient immune system the nude mice seem to have alternative mechanisms for resistance against Semliki Forest virus infection.

The total antibody response was measured in serum with radio-immunoassay. No antibodies were detected in vaccinated nude mice which were challenged after two weeks and tested after four weeks, whereas the antibody titres kept rising from the first to the fourth week after immunization of normal mice. Our results thus suggest that T-cells are required for protective immunity as well as for antibody formation against Semliki Forest virus as earlier shown for other viruses (14,15).

The high protective effect, resistance to more than 10^4 LD_{50}, induced by the 29S and virosome vaccines shows that highly effective subunit vaccines can be prepared when these proteins are assembled into multimer aggregates. Monomeric spike proteins give only a low degree of protection. Earlier studies have shown that solubilization of Toga viruses with different mild detergents leads to vaccines with low efficacy (7). From other enveloped viruses stable monomeric forms of spike proteins have been isolated, and they are poor immunogens. The Friend leukemia virus spike glycoprotein (gp 70) is in contrast to the Semliki Forest virus spike protein a typical peripheral membrane protein which does not need detergent for solubility. It is attached to the viral membrane through another membrane protein (see ref.16). This glycoprotein had to be injected with adjuvant in two doses of about 100µg per mouse to give partial protection against leukemia (16,17). A monomer preparation of the influenza virus hemaglutinin can be isolated by cutting off its hydrophobic tail by protease treatment (18). This was only weakly immunogenic in hamsters (19) and in man (20). Spike protein monomers water soluble as such or complexed to detergent appear not to be suitable as subunit vaccines.

REFERENCES

1.   Salk, J., Salk, D., Science 195 (1977) 834.
2.   Gross, P.A., Ennis, F.A., Gaerlan, P.F., Denson, L.J., Denning, C.R., Schiffmann, D., J. Infect. Dis. 136 (1977) 623.
3.   Marine, M.W., Stuart-Harris, C., J. Pediatr. 88 (1976) 26.
4.   Bachmayer, H., in Influenza (ed. Salby, P.), pp. 149-162 Academic Press, New York (1976).
5.   Chanock, R.M., Richman, D.D., Murphy, B.R., Spring, S.B., Schnitzer, T.J., Richardson, L.S., In Viral Immunology and Immunopathology (ed. A.L. Notkins) pp. 308-316 Academic Press, New York (1975).
6.   Bradish, C.J., Allner, B., Marber, H.B., J. Gen. Virol. 12, 141.
7.   Mussgay, M., Weiland, E., Intervirology 1 (1973) 529.
8.   Garoff, H., Simons, K., Renkonen, O., Virology 61 (1964) 493.
9.   Ziemiecki, A., Garoff, H., J. Mol. Biol. in press.
10. Simons, K., Helenius, A., Garoff, H., J. Mol. Biol. 80 (1973) 119.
11. Helenius, A., Von Bonsdorff, C.H., Biochem. Biophys. Acta 436 (1976) 895.
12. Almeida, J.D., Brand, C.M., Edwards, C.D., Heath, T.D., Lancet 2 (1975) 899.
13. Helenius, A., Fries, E., Kartenbeck, J., J. Cell Biol. 75 (1977) 866.

14. Vierelizier, J.L., Postlethwaite, R., Schild, G.C., Allison,
     A.C., J. Exp. Med. 140 (1974) 1559.
15. Bloom, B.R., Rager-Zisman, B., in Viral Immunology and Immuno-
     pathology (ed. A.L. Notkins) pp. 113-133 Academic Press, New
     York (1975)
16. Schäfer, W., Bolognesi, D.P., Contemp. Top. Immunobiol. 6 (1977)
     127.
17. Hunsmann, G., Moening, V., Schäfer, W., Virology 66 (1976) 327.
18. Brand, C.M., Skehel, J.J., Nature, New Biology 238 (1972) 145.
19. Jennings, R., Brand, C.M., McLaren, C., Shephard, L., Potter,
     C.W., Med. Microbiol. Immunol. 160 (1974) 295.
20. Tyrrell, D.A.J., J. Infect. Dis. 129 (1974) 766.

POSTTRANSFUSION HEPATITIS (PTH): FREQUENCY, SEROLOGICAL TYPE AND

POSSIBLE ROLE OF PRE-EXISTING ANTI-HB$_s$ IN PROTECTION

Harald Lehmann and Max Schlaak

Department of General Internal Medicine

University of Kiel, Schittenhelmstraße 12

2300 Kiel, West Germany

INTRODUCTION

Since 1971 we have performed a prospective study on posttrans-fusion hepatitis (1) (PTH) following major cardiac surgery with extracorporal circulation (ECC) and massive blood-transfusions.

This special situation serves as a model to study different aspects of hepatitis. In comparison to other studies of acute hepatitis, information about the preoperative immune status of our patients and data from the incubation period before clinically manifest hepatitis could be collected.

Although problems of protracted and chronic liver diseases are still a major hazard of PTH, we want to limit this presentation to the following questions:

1. What serological types of PTH are observed?

2. Does pre-existing anti-HB$_s$ protect against PTH?

PATIENTS AND METHODS

184 patients, 80 females and 104 males, undergoing major cardiac surgery were included in the study. The mean age was 45 years. The sera were collected and stored preoperatively and post-operatively on the 1st, 3rd, 7th, 14th and 28th days, and thereafter monthly for 6 months and in most cases longer. On the average 10

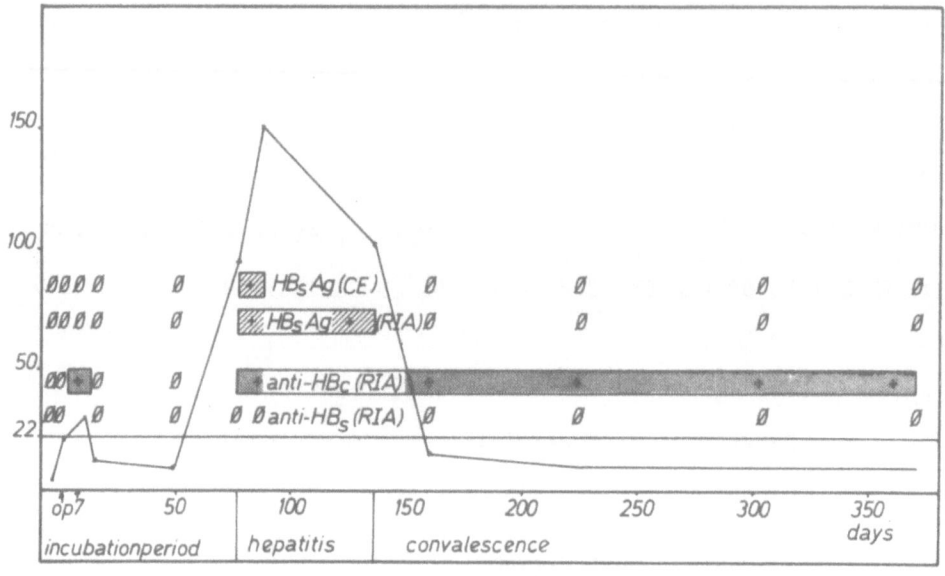

FIG. 1:   HB$_s$ -Ag positive posttransfusion hepatitis type B.   CE^s =
Counterimmune-electrophoresis.   RIA = Radioimmune assay.

blood units (500 ml each) per operation were transfused.

HB$_s$-Ag, anti HB$_s$ and anti HB$_c$ were tested by a standard solid
phase radioimmune assay (2).

Bilirubin levels and transaminase activities were investigated
by routine laboratory tests.   Statistical significances were
determined by χ^2-test without using the so-called Yates' correction.

RESULTS

Posttransfusion hepatitis occured in 68 patients, i.e. 37%.
The mean incubation period was 60-70 days.   One fatal outcome in the
acute phase was observed.

Three types of serological patterns predominated.   Fig.1 shows
the serological pattern of a case of HB$_s$-Ag positive PTH.   Anti-HB$_c$
was detected during the HB$_s$-Ag-aemia and has now persisted for more
than a year.   During the incubation period we were unable to identify

TAB. 1:   Frequency of different serological patterns of post-transfusion hepatitis during 1971-1975 and 1976-1977.

HEPATITIS 68 (37 %)	1971 - 1975 N = 54 (38 %)	1976 - 1977 N = 14 (31 %)
$HB_s AG$ POSITIVE	25	-
ANTI-HB_s POSITIVE	21	6
$HB_s AG$/ANTI-HB_s NEGATIVE	8	8

HB_s-Ag or anti-HB_s in the serum. In one postoperative serum specimen anti-HB_c was found temporarily; it was probably acquired from blood transfusion.

The second type of PTH demonstrated only an impressive drop of pre-existing anti-HB_s during the incubation period; some cases showed only a primary anti-HB_s response. We call this type "anti-HB_s-positive hepatitis B". Finally, some cases did not show this classic serological pattern. We call these cases "HB_s-Ag/anti-HB_s-negative PTH", probably being cases of a non-A non-B hepatitis.

Tab.1 shows the frequency of these different types during the course of our study.

Tab.2 demonstrates that anti-HB_s did not protect against PTH ($p < 0.05$).

DISCUSSION

The data clearly indicate that there has been an impressive change in the frequency of serological types of PTH since 1971. Up

TAB. 2:   Data demonstrating the missing protection of pre-existing
anti-HB$_s$ against PTH (p< 0.05) after massive blood transfusion in
cardiac surgery.

PREEXISTING	HEPATITIS N = 65	NO HEPATITIS N = 104	N 169
ANTI-HB$_s$ POSITIVE	11	10	21
ANTI-HB$_s$ NEGATIVE	54	94	148

to 1975 we observed only 8 (15%) HB$_s$-Ag- and anti-HB$_s$-negative cases
of PTH, which have now become the major type of PTH. This type of
PTH might be identical with non-A non-B hepatitis (3).

     The overall hepatitis morbidity decreased only slightly. But
the shift in the serological pattern of PTH from classical type B
to the non-A non-B type is obvious. As a matter of fact other
variants of hepatitis, e.g. cytomegaly (4) and mononucleosis, did
not play a significant role. This holds for hepatitis A in PTH as
well (5).

     There is considerable clinical interest in the question whether
PTH can be prevented by anti-HB$_s$. Looking at our data we must state
that pre-existing anti-HB$_s$ quite definitely does not prevent PTH.
On the contrary, we observe a trend towards higher hepatitis
morbidity in anti-HB$_s$ carriers. If a selection is performed
according to the pre-existing anti-HB$_c$, a similar trend is regarded
but without statistical significance on the 5% level.

                              SUMMARY

     During the past years a rather drastic shift occured in the
serological type of PTH without overt differences in the clinical
course of the disease between HB$_s$-Ag-positive, anti-HB$_s$-positive

and the non-A non-B hepatitis. The overall PTH morbidity after cardiac surgery with massive whole blood transfusions decreased to a minor degree.

Pre-existing anti-HB$_s$ did not protect against posttransfusion hepatitis.

REFERENCES

1. Lehmann, H., Schlaak, M., Ergebnisse einer fünfjährigen prospektiven Studie zur Hepatitis nach Massentransfusionen. Verh. dtsch. Ges. Inn. Med. (1976) 397.
2. Overbey, L.R., Miller, J.P., Smith, I.D., Decker, R.M., Ling, C.M., Radioimmunassay of hepatitis B virus-associated (Australia) antigen employing ^{125}J-antibody. Vox. Sang. 24 (1973) 102.
3. Prince, A.M., Brotman, B., Grady, G.F., Kuhns, W.J., Hazzi, C., Levine, R.W., Millian, S.J., Long-incubation post-transfusion hepatitis without serological evidence of exposure to hepatitis B virus. Lancet 2 (1974) 241.
4. Prince, A.M., Szmuness, W., Millian, S.J., David, D.S., A serologic study of cytomegalvirus infections associated with blood transfusions. New Engl. J. Med. 284 (1971) 1125.
5. Lehmann, H., Frösner, G.G., Maas, M., Schlaak, M., Hepatitis A-Antikörper und ihre Bedeutung für die posttransfusionelle Hepatitis. Verh. dtsch. Ges. Inn. Med. (1978) in press.

ACKNOWLEDGEMENTS

This study was sponsered by the Deutsche Forschungsgemeinschaft, Schwerpunktprogramm "Virushepatitis".

IMMUNOPATHOLOGICAL ALTERATIONS OF LYMPHATIC TISSUES IN MICE

INFECTED WITH LYMPHOCYTIC CHORIOMENINGITIS VIRUS

J. Löhler and F. Lehmann-Grube

Heinrich Pette-Instit für Experimentelle Virologie und
Immunologie an der Universität Hamburg
2 Hamburg 20, W. Germany

The LCM disease of the central nervous system (CNS) of the
mouse is a well studied example of a T-lymphocyte-mediated immunopathological host reaction against virally induced new antigens
(1). Less is known of organs other than the CNS. We have studied
the lymphoid system which may be heavily involved. Colony bred NMRI
mice infected with 10^4 infectious units (IU) of WE strain virus were
used as standard system. Virus was injected intraperitoneally in
order to circumvent the CNS disease with its 100% lethality after
intracerebral inoculation.

First pathological alterations could be detected on the 3rd
day after infection. In the spleen blast cells appeared in the
marginal zone and around the central artery of the white pulp. In
their vicinity small lymphocytes underwent necrosis. Similar alterations were observed in the marginal and internodular cortex, and in
the paracortical region of lymph nodes (Fig.1a,b). In contrast to
lymphocytes, which were destroyed early in the process, reticular
cells of the marginal zone of spleen and internodular and deep
cortex of lymph nodes showed initially proliferation, and histochemical staining for acid phosphatase and unspecific esterase
revealed marked activation of macrophages. Later, these cells too
were destroyed and destruction of all tissue elements progressed
and expanded until on days 6 and 7 the entire lymphatic tissue was
involved leading to nearly total depletion of lymphocytes and
fibrinoid necrosis of the reticulum (Fig.1d).

Thymic alterations, consisting of cortical lymphocytolysis,
proliferation of cells of the medulla, and proliferation of macrophages began later; on day 8 after infection there was marked thymic

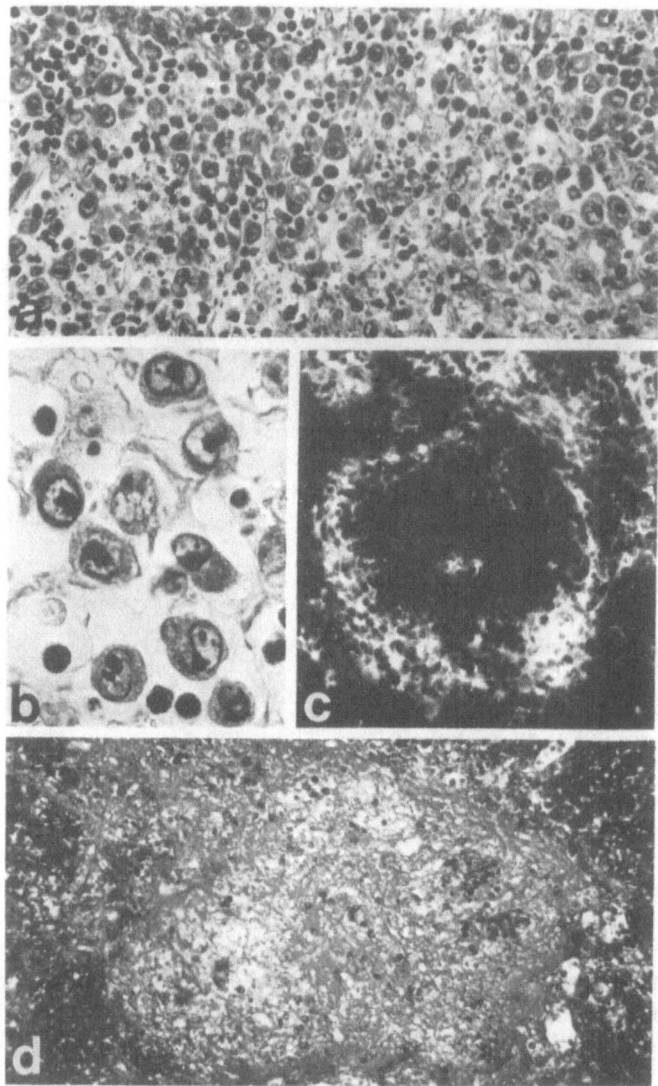

FIG. 1:   Histopathological and immunofluorescence findings in
lymphatic tissues of NMRI mice after intraperitoneal infection with
10^4 IU LCM virus, strain WE.   a) Paracortical region of lymph
node; day 4 p.i.   Proliferation of lymphoblasts and necrosis of
small lymphocytes. H. and E. x 380.   b) Paracortical region of
lymph node; day 5 p.i.   Lymphoblasts lying within the reticular
meshwork. Van Gieson stain. x 950.   c) White pulp of spleen;
day 4 p.i.   LCM virus antigen mainly in cells of the marginal
zone. Frozen section, indirect immunofluorescence. x 240.   d)
White pulp of spleen; day 6 p.i.   Fibrinoid necrosis. Dichrome
PAS reaction. x 100. (Reduced 40% for purposes of reproduction.).

TAB. 1:   Findings in different strains of mice infected by intraperitoneal inoculation with 10^4 IU LCM virus, strain WE.

Mice			Findings	
	H-2	Disease[a]	Histo-[b] pathology	Footpad-[c] response
NMRI col. bred.	?	++	+++	+++
A/J	a/a	++	++	++
C57BL/6J	b/b	−	++	++
DBA/2	d/d	−	++	++
BALB/c	d/d	−	+	+
CBA/J	h/h	−	+	+
AKR	h/h	++	+++	+++
SWR	q/q	+	+++	+++
SJL/J	s/s	+	++	+++
STU	?	−	++	++

[a] Severe signs of disease leading frequently to death: ++; light
disease leading rarely to death: +; no apparent disease: −.

[b] Severe: +++; moderate: ++; low: +.

[c] High: +++; intermediate: ++; low: +.

involution.   Inflammatory changes were also seen in liver, lungs
and intestinal mucosa.

Virus multiplied in lymphoid organs.   In the spleen the peak
of 10^9 IU per g was attained on the 3rd day.   In the thymus infectivity increased slower, reaching maximal concentration around the
7th day after infection, which corresponded with the onset of
pathological alterations in this organ.

Immunofluorescence methods exhibited virus-specific antigen in
macrophages, reticular cells and lymphoblasts.   In the spleen
immunofluorescence was most prominent in the marginal zone of the
white pulp (Fig.1c) from where it spread towards inner parts of the
white pulp and towards the red pulp.   In lymph nodes virus-specific
immunoflurescence first appeared in macrophages and reticular cells
of the marginal sinus and internodular cortex and later expanded to
medulla and deep cortex.   Immunofluorescence was maximal 2 days
later than infectivity.   It rapidly diminished from day 6 after
infection onwards at a time, when fibrinoid necrosis of the lymphatic
tissue became apparent.   As detected by immunofluorescence, small

unstimulated lymphocytes, either in frozen sections or in fractionated spleen cell suspensions, were never found to contain viral antigens.

Since the pattern of lymphocytolysis in these animals was reminiscent of the effects of experimental stress or cortisone treatment adrenalectomized and cortisone-substituted mice were infected. The outcome was increased destruction of lymphocytes as well as increased lethality and we may conclude that the histopathological alterations of lymphatic tissues do not result from acute stress. In contrast, cyclophosphamide treatment prevented the occurrence of histopathological lesions and reduced lethality, although virus replication was not affected. Furthermore, when spleen cells from hyperimmune syngeneic donors were injected into LCM virus-infected and cyclophosphamide-protected mice, the recipients died and developed typical lesions in the lymphoid organs. To evaluate the possible pathogenetic role of activated macrophages, mice were inoculated with silica or carrageenan before infection. This treatment had no beneficial effect.

Not all mice respond to infection with LCM virus in the same fashion as NMRI mice, and there is a considerable variation between strains regarding the expression of disease signs and pathological lesions (Tab.1). The question arose whether differences between mouse strains resulted from differences in their ability to respond immunologically to the LCM virus. As an independent parameter of cell-mediated immunity the footpad reaction after innoculation of 10^4 IU of the virus into the planta of the foot was measured. Ten mouse strains were thus compared and a correlation was found to exist between the extent of pathological alterations and the degree of footpad swelling. Virus multiplication was essentially identical in these mice (data not shown). It should be noted that linkage to the major histocompatibility locus was not disclosed by our data.

We conclude that the severe lesions in the lymphoid system of LCM virus-infected mice are just as immunopathological in nature as the CNS disease following intracerebral inoculation of the virus. It may appear paradoxical that an immunological response, in which the lymphoid organs play a central role, should lead to preferential destruction of just these organs.

REFERENCES

1. Cole, G.A., Nathanson, N., Lymphocytic choriomeningitis: Pathogenesis, Prog. Med. Virol. 18 (1975) 94.

LIGHT AND ELECTRON MICROSCOPIC CHARACTERISTICS OF SINUS REACTIONS AND CELLULAR TRAFFIC IN THE HILAR LYMPH NODE COMPLEX (HLNC) IN RABBITS UNDERGOING A PULMONARY CELL-MEDIATED IMMUNE REACTION

Q.N. Myrvik, P. Racz and Klara Tenner-Racz

Department of Microbiology and Immunology, Bowman Gray
School of Medicine of Wake Forest University
Winston-Salem, N.C., 27103, USA

INTRODUCTION

In rabbits undergoing BCG-induced pulmonary granulomatous reactions we observed (1) a hyperplasia of bronchial associated lymphoid tissue (BALT), enlargement of the HLNC and histologic evidence of increased lymph flow and cellular traffic from the lung toward the HLNC.

The present investigation describes 3 important forms of the sinus reactions that occur in the HLNC during a pulmonary CMI reaction:

1.   In the submarginal sinuses and, especially in the medullary sinuses, clusters of macrophages were frequently seen. The aggregation of macrophages was called the "Sinus Macrophage Clumping Reaction" (SMCR).

2.   Sinus lymphocytosis (plugging of the paracortical sinuses with small lymphocytes).

3.   Immature sinus histiocytosis which has been described only in human beings.

In addition, the reaction of the sinus endothelial (SE) cells were also studied to distinguish between the different forms of macrophages and the activated SE cells.

MATERIALS AND METHODS

White New Zealand outbred rabbits of either sex were sensitized
subcutaneously (s.c.) with 200 μg heat-killed BCG suspended in 0.2
ml mineral oil (2). Three weeks later the animals were skin tested
with PPD to detect tuberculin positivity. The rabbits that were
skin test positive (24 hr) were challenged intratracheally (i.t.)
2 days later with 3 mg of heat-killed BCG suspended in phosphate-
buffered saline (pH 7.4). Groups of animals were sacrificed at 9,
16 and 24 hr, 2 days, 1, 2 and 3 weeks after the challenge dose.
Control groups consisted of 10 non-treated animals. These rabbits
were sacrificed at time points corresponding to those in the
experimental group. Sample pieces from lung and HLNC were fixed
and processed for light and electron microscopy (1).

RESULTS AND DISCUSSION

In normal non-treated animals we found that the inner wall of
the subcapsular sinus, the paracortical sinus as well as the
medullary sinus were lined by a discontinuous endothelium. This
endothelium exhibited a mosaic-like structure having a limited
number of macrophages or lymphocytes in the gaps between the SE
cells.

Following the i.t. challenge of sensitized animals, the number
of gaps increased. In addition, the parenchymal side of the sinus
linings as well as the endothelium surrounding the fibrous trabeculae
displayed dramatic changes. Some of the SE cells underwent severe
degeneration and death. The desquamated SE cells were replaced
mainly by macrophages. At later time intervals, SE cells showed
signs of activation in certain areas of the sinus system. This
phenomenon was observed especially in those portions of the sinuses
where intense cellular reactions took place in the lumen.

In the lymph node sinuses of control animals, 2 types of free
macrophages were predominant: 1) Immature macrophages; 2) Large
free macrophages (sparse numbers), similar to the type 1 macrophages
described by Lennert et al. (3).

During the early intervals (24 hr) after the challenge of
sensitized animals there was a marked increase in the number of
large free macrophages suggesting that the resident (fixed) macrophages had detached from the SE cells that ensheath the trabeculae.
Large numbers of macrophages arrived also through the afferent
lymphatics. At 16 hr after challenge, loosely formed aggregations
of macrophages were observed both in the subcapsular (Fig.1a) and
medullary sinuses (SMCR). The clumps regularly contained large
numbers of macrophages and several lymphocytes. At 48 hr

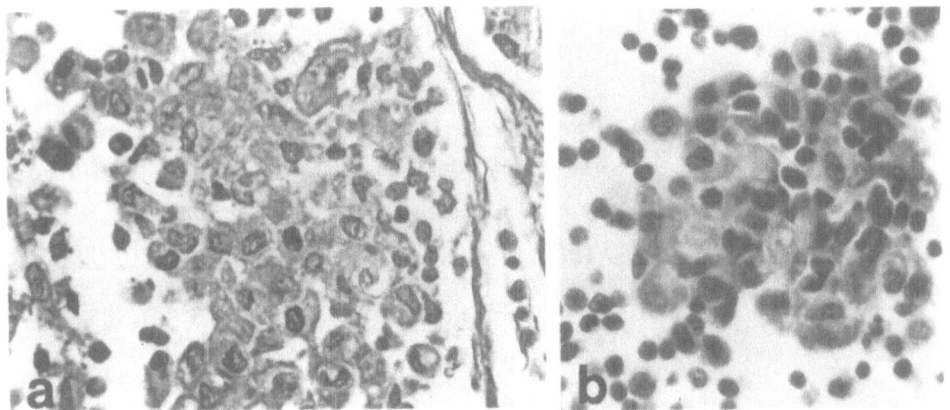

FIG. 1a: Initial stage of SMCR.   Silver impr.

FIG. 1b: SMCR (H and E).

the clumps appeared to be more compactly organized (Fig. 1b).
Similar clusters were seen in the lymphatics around the BALT (Fig.1c)
and in the alveoli of the lung. The cell aggregates in the lymph
node sinuses were free or loosely attached around the trabeculae.
Frequently, the cell clumps blocked different parts of the sinus
system.

To the best of our knowledge, there are no published experimental data describing macrophage-lymphocyte aggregation in the
sinuses of the draining nodes during a CMI reaction. However, there
are several reports concerning antigen-induced aggregation of macrophages in vitro (see references in 4). In our laboratory it was
demonstrated that the CMI reaction elicited in the rabbit lung
generated a macrophage agglutinating factor (MAgF) (2) which has
been identified as a hyaluronic acid-protein complex (5). The
lymph obtained from the HLNC 2 days after i.t. challenge agglutinated
normal alveolar macrophages. In addition, hyaluronidase rapidly
dispersed the cell clumps. These findings indicate that HA probably
plays a major role in the early phase of the SMCR.

At 1 to 2 weeks after challenge, the initial clumps developed
into epithelioid granulomas (Fig.1e). The changes in the morphology
of the macrophages participating in the SMCR were similar to those
observed by Adams (6) who studied BCG-induced epithelioid granulomas
in the fat pad of guinea pigs. During the first 2 weeks, in our
experiment, the macrophages underwent a maturation process and showed
the morphologic characteristics of immature and mature macrophages,
immature epithelioid cells and finally, mature epithelioid

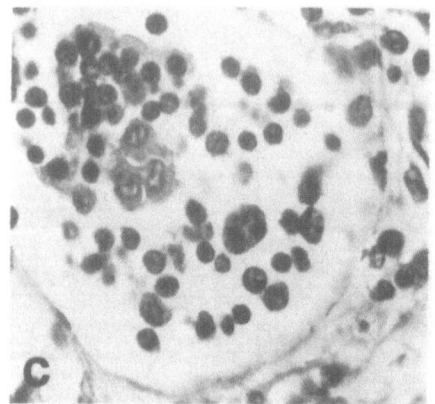 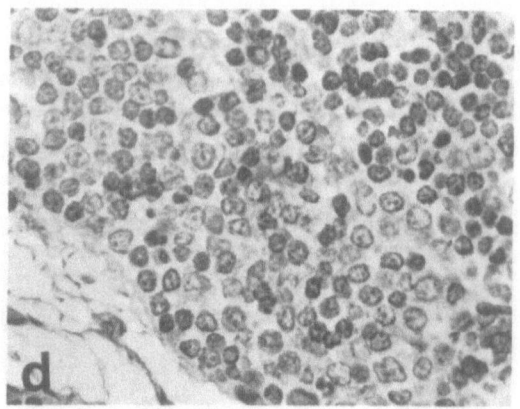

FIG. 1c: Macrophage aggregate in a lymphatic around the BALT.(H & E).

FIG. 1d: Immature sinus histiocytosis. Giemsa's stain.

cells. A similar maturation was observed in the granulomas of the
lung of the same animal.   The hypertrohpy and hyperplasia of the
Golgi apparatus and that of rough endoplasmic reticulum, the
presence of large numbers of coated vesicles and dense bodies in
the epithelioid cells support the idea that the mature epithelioid
cells have secretory activity.

Characteristic interdigitations among the epithelioid cells
were frequently observed (Fig.1f). The contacts between epithelioid
cells and activated lymphocytes participating in the SMCR were also
intimate. Moderate electron dense material was frequently seen
between macrophages, and macrophages and lymphocytes.

Our results indicate that the aggregation of immunologically
activated macrophages and lymphocytes in the cavities or the lumens
of tubular structures represents the initial stage of epithelioid
granuloma formation. Accordingly, the SMCR illustrates the basic
mechanism by which granulomata can originate in the course of a CMI
reaction.

At 1 to 2 weeks following the i.t. challenge, we noted regularly
a sinus lymphocytosis reaction. At the same time hyperplasia of the
follicles and parenchyma was noted. These findings indicate that
increased emptying of cells from the parenchyma into the subfollicular
and paracortical sinuses can produce a jam between the paracortical
and medullary sinuses. Our results suggest that the sinus lymphocytosis or "plugging" is only a transient reaction which does not
represent, necessarily, an immunologic event.

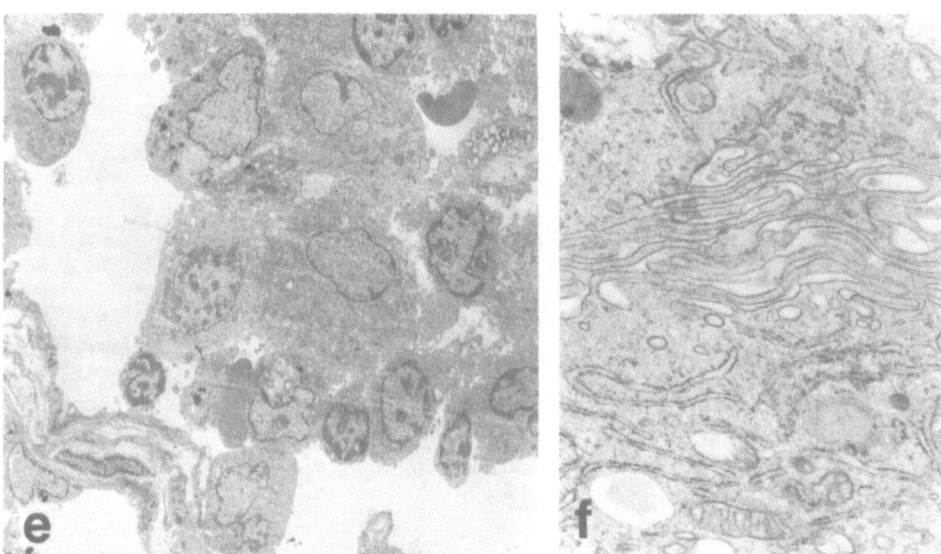

FIG. 1e: Late stage of SMCR. 1 week after the challenge.
Electron micrograph.

FIG. 1f: Interdigitations between two epithelioid cells. (High
power view from Fig.1e).

At 2 days (in about 20% of the animals) an immature sinus
histiocytosis was observed in the subcapsular sinuses (Fig.1d).
This unique response showed all of the characteristic features of
immature sinus histiocytosis described in human beings (7).

This response consisted of characteristic cells, concommittant
capsulitis, lack of argentophil fibers among the cells, focal
appearance in the subcapsular sinuses, and the presence of PMN in
limited numbers. This condition retained the same morphology during
the entire course of the experiment.

REFERENCES

1.   Racz, P., Tenner-Racz, K., Myrvik, Q.N., Fainter, L.K., J.
     Reticuloendothel. Soc. 22 (1977) 59.
2.   Galindo, R., Myrvik, Q.N., Love, S.H., J. Reticuloendothel.
     Soc. 18 (1975) 295.
3.   Lennert, K., Niedorf, H.R., Blumcke, S., Virchows Arch. Abt.
     B. Zellpath. 10 (1972) 14.
4.   Preston, P.M., D'Arcy Hart, P., Brown, T.N., Immunology 32
     (1977) 33.

5.   Love, S.H., Shannon, B.T., Myrvik, Q.N., Lynn, W.S., J. Retic-
      uloendothel. Soc. 22 (1977) 44a.
6.   Adams, D.O., Amer. J. Path. 76 (1974) 17.
7.   Lennert, K., Frankf. Z. Pathol. 69 (1958) 103.

PERIPHERAL BLOOD LYMPHOCYTE SUBPOPULATIONS IN MULTIPLE MYELOMA

I. Schedel, P. Beck, D. Peest, K.-D. Schneider, M.
Fricke, G. Eckert, H. Deicher

Division of Clinical Immunology and Blood Transfusion
Department of Medicine, Medical School, Hannover,
West Germany

INTRODUCTION

Human myeloma is regarded as a monoclonal malignancy of B-type
secretory lymphoid cells and has been classified as plasmocytic
immunocytoma by Lennert et al. (1). Plasma cells carrying the
morphological appearance of tumor cells can be identified in the
bone marrow of these patients (2,5,6). Myeloma cells disseminate
to multiple skeletal sites and may spread to other organs, but
malignant plasma cells are only rarely demonstrable in peripheral
blood as judged by light microscopy (3). The idiotypic determinant
(I.D.) of the myeloma protein, which is also carried by the surface-
immunoglobulin (SmIg) of the myeloma cell clone, represents an
individual and tumor-specific antigenic determinant (2,5). Previous
investigations using FITC-labelled heterologous anti-idiotypic
antisera (AIAS) have shown that a varying percentage of peripheral
blood lymphocytes (PBL) bear the I.D. of the patient's myeloma
protein, proving that they must also belong to the individual tumor
cell clone (2,4,5). The percentage of PBL detected by AIAS closely
parallels the clinical course of multiple myeloma (2,7).

The present study was performed in order to characterize the
population of lymphoid cells in the peripheral blood carrying the
idiotypic determinant in patients with multiple myeloma (MM) and
Waldenström's macroglobulinemia, using PBL preparations obtained by
a cell separation technique.

TAB. 1: Chromatography of PBL of healthy adults using Sepharose 6MB coated with heterologous anti-Ig-serum (% of total).

cell surface determinant	input ($\pm$ SD)	passed unretarded cells ($\pm$ SD)	eluted cells ($\pm$ SD)	P
SmIg	14.4 ($\pm$ 9.4)	10.9 ($\pm$ 9.8)	79.2 ($\pm$ 6.7)	i/p <0.0025 i/e <0.0005
E - rosetting	65.9 ($\pm$ 6.5)	73.6 ($\pm$ 5.9)	19.9 ($\pm$ 8.9)	i/p <0.01 i/e <0.0005
EA$_{human}$-rosetting	18.7 ($\pm$ 10.3)	15.3 ($\pm$ 5.8)	13.6 ($\pm$ 17.6)	i/p <0.15 i/e <0.15
EA$_{ox}$-rosetting	16.9 ($\pm$ 7.9)	11.7 ($\pm$ 5.5)	40.0 ($\pm$ 16.3)	i/p <0.01 i/e <0.005
EAC - rosetting	16.8 ($\pm$ 7.2)	10.3 ($\pm$ 5.6)	56.2 ($\pm$ 18.3)	i/p <0.0025 i/e <0.0005

9 tests

TAB. 2: Chromatography of PBL of multiple myeloma patients using Sepharose 6MB coated with heterologous anti-idiotypic-serum (% of total).

cell surface determinant	input ($\pm$ SD)	passed unretarded cells ($\pm$ SD)	eluted cells ($\pm$ SD)	P
SmIg	11.0 ($\pm$ 3,8)	16.0 ($\pm$ 9,2)	49.2 ($\pm$ 11,2)	i/p < 0.15 i/e < 0.0005
idiotypic determinant	18.6 ($\pm$ 11,7)	31.4 ($\pm$ 12,3)	56.6 ($\pm$ 16,5)	i/p < 0.05 i/e < 0.0025
E-rosetting	73.0 ($\pm$ 9,8)	75.9 ($\pm$ 9,6)	80.3 ($\pm$ 14,6)	i/e < 0.25
EA$_{human}$-rosetting	22.8 ($\pm$ 7,3)	20.0 ($\pm$ 5,4)	18.3 ($\pm$ 17,4)	i/e < 0.35
EA$_{ox}$-rosetting	24.4 ($\pm$ 5,8)	24.6 ($\pm$ 9,3)	46.7 ($\pm$ 3,5)	i/e < 0.0005
EAC-rosetting	20.8 ($\pm$ 8,5)	18.3 ($\pm$ 14,5)	28.3 ($\pm$ 24,0)	i/e < 0.3

5 tests

MATERIALS AND METHODS

Preparation of Anti-Idiotypic-Antisera (AIAS)

Antisera against the variable region of the myeloma protein were raised in rabbits by repeated immunisation with 1 mg of purified myeloma proteins isolated from the patients' sera by amonium sulphate precipitation and subsequent gel filtration on Sephadex G-200- and Sephadex DEAE-A 50 (Pharmacia, Uppsala). Antisera were adsorbed with purified polyclonal immunoglobulin preparations coupled to activated Sepharose 4 CnBr, and with PBL prepared by Ficoll-density centrifugation from healty individuals. Idiotypic specificity was assessed by Ouchterlony and solid-phase Elisa-techniques (6).

Preparation of Peripheral Blood Lymphoid Cells

Lymphoid cells from 10 healthy adults, from 3 patients with IgG-myeloma, and from 2 patients with Waldenström's macroglobulinemia were collected by means of a continuous flow blood cell separator (AMINCO). Cell preparations containing $3 - 6 \times 10^9$ leucocytes were defibrinated, iron-phagocytosing cells were eliminated with lymphocyte separating reagent, and were further purified by Ficoll-gradient centrifugation.

Cell-Separation by Column Chromatography

Activated Sepharose 6 MB (Pharmacia/Uppsala/Sweden) was coated with goat anti-human-Ig or with rabbit AIAS (ca. 0.8 mg specific antibody protein were given to 1 g of Sepharose 6 MB) (6). 2×10^8 PBL lymphocytes, suspended in 20 ml M 199 medium containing 0.5 g of Albumin/100 ml, were used for column chromatography at a flow rate of 0.5 ml/min. Unbound cells were removed by washing with 150 ml medium (flow rate 5 ml/min/4°C). Subsequently the cells were separated from the Sepharose mechanically by repeated batch washing. Cell surface marker determinations (E-, EA-, EAC-rosettes) and direct immuno-fluorescence techniques using FITC-labelled specific goat-anti-human-Ig (Hyland, München) or FITC-labelled rabbit AIAS were applied for further characterization of PBL subpopulations.

RESULTS

As shown in Table 1, lymphoid cells bearing SmIg as well as complement receptor positive lymphoid cells and cells showing Fc-receptors, were enriched by column chromatography using heterologous anti-Ig sera. A five fold concentration of SmIg-positive lymphocytes was thus achieved as compared to the "input" cell suspension. In contrast, the percentage of sheep red blood cell (SRBC)-receptor

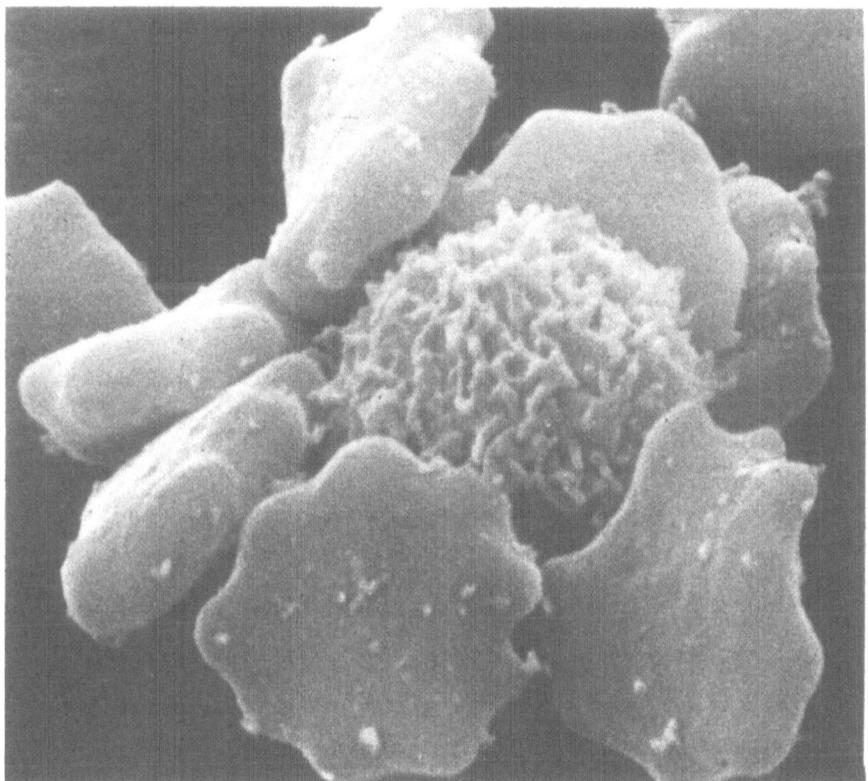

FIG. 1:   PBL in MM-patients carrying the corresponding idiotypic
determinants as seen by rosette formation with goat-anti-rabbit-Ig-
coated SRBC after incubation with AIAS. The cell surface is
characterized by the existence of microvilli and plicae (scanning-
electronmicroscopy).

bearing cells was diminished in the eluted cell suspension. When
AIAS was used instead to coat the adsorbing columns, lymphoid cells
carrying the corresponding idiotypic determinant of the individual
serum myeloma protein were enriched approximately four fold (Tab.2).
However, the cell suspensions eluted from the AIAS-coated columns
were heterogeneous with respect to surface markers usually applied
for differentiating lymphocyte populations: 80% of the eluted cells
displayed SRBC receptors, ca. 30% carried C3 receptors, and close to
50% showed some type of Fc-receptor. The observed overlap of
percentage values for different cell surface determinants in the
eluted cell fraction indicated that a portion of cells must carry
more than one receptor. Recent experiments have shown the existence
of lymphoid cells among myeloma PBL which - as judged by their

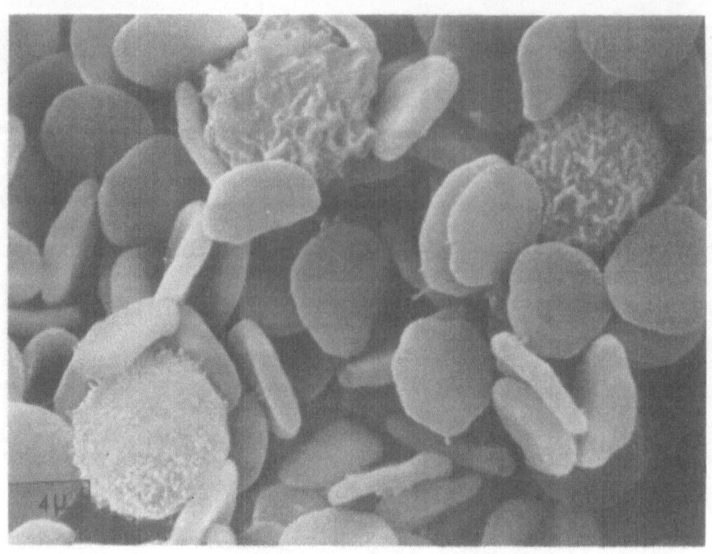

FIG. 2:   PBL in MM-patients displaying the same surface characteristics as the cell shown in Fig.1, giving spontaneous rosette-
formation with uncoated SRBC.   At the lift a typical T-cell with a
predominantly smooth surface showing also rosette-formation.

morphological appearance – carry the idiotypic marker as well as a
receptor for SRBC (Figs.1,2).

     In control experiments, no significant enrichment of SmIg-
bearing cells from healthy individuals was seen using individually
specific AIAS-coated columns.

                              DISCUSSION

     Columns coated with heterologous anti-(polyclonal-) Ig are
capable of enriching SmIg bearing cells from PBL of healthy adults.
Cells eluted from these columns display EAC- and also EA-rosetting
in a high percentage, whereas the percentage of E-rosetting cells
representing T-lymphocytes, is decreased.   Thus normal B-PBL defined
by conventional surface markers, are successfully enriched by this
technique.

     The marked heterogeneity of lymphoid cells eluted from the AIAS-
coated columns with respect to surface markers usually applied for
differentiating normal lymphocyte populations was a surprising finding,
since in analogy to the results with normal PBL, one had expected an
enrichment of B-type lymphocytes by this technique.   Preud' Homme et

al. (4) have reported similar results in one case without separating their PBL. The overlap of surface determinant percentages indicated that a considerable fraction of I.D.-positive cells must also carry other markers, in particular an SRBC-receptor, usually regarded as a typical marker for T-lymphocytes under normal conditions. It must be concluded that non-specific surface markers such as SRBC - or other receptors, in contrast to specific tumor markers, may only have limited value in characterizing lymphoid tumor clone cells. This conclusion is further strengthened by the finding that I.D.-positive and SRBC-rosetting lymphoid cells appear to be closely related, if not identical, as judged by their morphological appearance. Although these findings may be unique for M.M. and macroglobulinemia, and must not necessarily come true for other monoclonal B-cell lymphomas, they provide evidence that the use of idiotypic markers may allow a better recognition of the total tumor cell compartment, which may consist of cells with quite different morphological appearance and unusual distribution of non-tumor-specific cell surface markers.

SUMMARY

Antisera raised against idiotypic determinants of myeloma proteins and macroglobulins have been used to differentiate peripheral blood lymphocyte populations from individual patients. I.D.-positive lymphocytes not resembling plasma cells have been regularly found in peripheral blood in these diseases. This lymphocyte population is heterogeneous with respect to non-tumor-specific surface markers, such as SRBC-, Fc- and C-receptors. Tumor specific idiotypic determinants will thus allow a more correct recognition of the total tumor cell compartment in these diseases.

REFERENCES

1. Stein, H., Kaiserling, E., Lennert, K. Paper presented at the 10th Int. Congr. Int. Acad. Path., Hamburg, Abstract Book 105 (1974) 50.
2. Holm, G., Mellstedt, H., Petterson, D., Biberfeld, P. Transplant. Rev. 34 (1977) 139.
3. Kyle, R.A. Proc. Staff. Meet. Mayo Clin. 50 (1975) 29.
4. Preud' Homme, J.-L., Klein, M., Labaume, S., Seligmann, M. Eur. J. Immunol. 7 (1977) 840.
5. Schedel, I., Schöner, W., Ziegler, R., Kalden, J.R., Deicher, H. In: Immunological diagnosis of leukemias and lymphomas, Haematology and Blood Transfusion 20 (1977) 329.
6. Schedel, I., Peest, D., Schneider, K.-D., Stünkel, K., Eckert, G., Deicher, H. (in preparation).
7. Warner, T.F. C.S., Krueger, R.G. Lancet June 3 (1978) 1174.

GENERAL SUMMARY

G.J.V. Nossal

The Walter and Eliza Hall Institute of Medical Research
Post Office, Royal Melbourne Hospital
Victoria 3050, Australia

How well have we fulfilled the main trends set for the conference?

On structure-function relationships, I would say we have done reasonably well. This conference remains virtually the only forum in which the intricate and beautiful micro-architecture of the lymphoid system is discussed at all to any degree of sophistication, and we must draw some encouragement from the useful hints that have come from papers such as those of Smithyman, Klaus, Humphrey and Lennart.

On in vivo relevance of in vitro models, we have done less well. We do pay lip-service to this area, but in the main I think we are all still more interested in polishing our reductionist models than we are in performing the difficult continuous oscillations between a variety of in vitro models and a variety of highly complex real life situations. The task is difficult; we must struggle a bit harder.

On the clinical relevance of animal experimentation I think we are doing badly. It remains a sobering fact that most of the noteable advances in clinical medicine have not arisen from the labor of the basic scientists - in most cases we end up simply explaining how something that works really does work. Intelligent immunomanipulation based on scientific models boasts only one major triumph, namely the development of anti-D serum for the prevention of haemolytic disease of the newborn. One might reasonably assume that the explosive growth in our knowledge of allergy will soon impact on drug manufacture. But for the other main areas of concern to us, namely cancer, organ transplantation, autoimmunity and infectious diseases, the key life-saving

events came from disciplines other than the new immunology. The best
that we can hope is that the very dynamic interplay which now exists
will reverse this trend.

What of our most striking advances? First, I should mention Dr.
H. Warren and the demystification of immune signalling in the case of
the T cell. Dr. Warren is just a little way down the track of
resolving this problem, as supernatants from Concanavalin A-treated
spleen cells represent a veritable museum of factors - but she has
given us a conceptual framework on which to build.

Noteworthy progress was also made by Dr. Gerry Klaus and Dr.
John Tew. Dr. Ada and I discovered 15 years ago the remarkable
antigen-trapping function of certain dendritic cells in lymphoid
follicles; simultaneously and independently, so did R.G. White. We
also showed that, in contrast to macrophages, these dendritic cells
held antigen on their surface for very long periods. What Klaus and
Tew have done is to reveal the major functional role of these
dendritic cells in generating B memory cells, in the formation of
anti-idiotypic antibody and in long-term antibody synthesis and
memory.

Another great achievement of the Conference has been to bring
the immunoparasitologists into our midst. Their contributions were
of great importance both theoretically and practically.

I was very struck by the work of Dr. Smithyman in preparing pure
germinal centres. If these can be maintained in organ culture or
suspended cell tissue culture, much might be learned about the B cell
subsets generated in germinal centres.

What are the great problems of the future? We still have to
resolve the great anatomic-physiologic problem of collaborative and
suppressive intercellular interactions in the lymphoid system. There
has been great progress in our visions of T cells always recognizing
antigen X in the context of some "self"-MHC gene product, the "self-
ness" being learnt by the cells during their sojourn in the thymus.
We are making progress in integrating this new work with older problems such as the great polymorphism of the MHC; the nature of immune
response genes; the special immunogenicity of allogeneic lymphoid
cells; the MHC gene influence on certain diseases; and the presence
of MHC gene products in cell interaction factors. But in all this
work, one dimension is missing. Where are the T cell - B cell interactions going on? How does the architecture of the lymphoid system
promote cellular interactions?

Next, I should welcome further progress in our structural understanding of lymphokines and monokines. This is slow and patient work,
given the low molarities at which these factors work, but it is very

important. It should aid drug development considerably. The relationship, if any, between the molecules the immunologist works with
and the colony-stimulating factors so well known to the students of
haemopoietic differentiation will be of considerable interest. Some
of the latter are now pure and being sequenced.

Finally, we must continue to give attention to what germinal
centres really do. This is intimately tied into questions of B cell
subsets, which we must seek to define with a wider variety of
techniques including the use of monoclonal antibodies made by hybridomas. These could be very useful in the tissue localization of B
cell subsets. How do germinal centres come into Shortman's idea
about pre-progenitor and direct progenitor B cells? Do germinal
centres act as sites of post-antigenic mutation, as noted by Cunningham and Pilarski? Are germinal centres involved in the affinity
broadening noted during the second week of life in the mouse of
Siskind? Are they the chief sites of affinity maturation in prolonged
immune responses? Could the role of germinal centres be further
illuminated by studies on the ontogeny or phylogeny of the dendritic
antigen-capturing network that seems to precede germinal centre
formation? These problems are no less urgent now than when this
series of conferences was initiated, and must give us heart to
continue.